Concussions in Athletics

Semyon M. Slobounov
Wayne J. Sebastianelli
Editors

Alexa E. Walter
Assistant Editor

Concussions in Athletics

From Brain to Behavior

Second Edition

Springer

Editors
Semyon M. Slobounov
Kinesiology and Neurosurgery
Pennsylvania State University
University Park, PA
USA

Wayne J. Sebastianelli
Department of Orthopedics
Pennsylvania State University
State College, PA
USA

Assistant Editor
Alexa E. Walter
Department of Kinesiology
Pennsylvania State University
University Park, PA
USA

ISBN 978-3-030-75566-9   ISBN 978-3-030-75564-5 (eBook)
https://doi.org/10.1007/978-3-030-75564-5

© Springer Nature Switzerland AG 2014, 2021
This work is subject to copyright. All rights are reserved by the Publisher, whether the whole or part of the material is concerned, specifically the rights of translation, reprinting, reuse of illustrations, recitation, broadcasting, reproduction on microfilms or in any other physical way, and transmission or information storage and retrieval, electronic adaptation, computer software, or by similar or dissimilar methodology now known or hereafter developed.
The use of general descriptive names, registered names, trademarks, service marks, etc. in this publication does not imply, even in the absence of a specific statement, that such names are exempt from the relevant protective laws and regulations and therefore free for general use.
The publisher, the authors, and the editors are safe to assume that the advice and information in this book are believed to be true and accurate at the date of publication. Neither the publisher nor the authors or the editors give a warranty, expressed or implied, with respect to the material contained herein or for any errors or omissions that may have been made. The publisher remains neutral with regard to jurisdictional claims in published maps and institutional affiliations.

This Springer imprint is published by the registered company Springer Nature Switzerland AG
The registered company address is: Gewerbestrasse 11, 6330 Cham, Switzerland

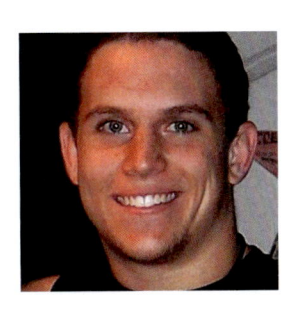

Injuries in athletics remain in the spotlight for many reasons. Healthy, young, vibrant athletes expect to participate forever in the activities they so love. This book focuses on a specific injury that continues to be nebulous but endemic to sport. Mild traumatic brain injury, or concussion, occurs with high frequency and in every sport. The understanding of the pathophysiology of concussion continues to develop; however, our ability to diagnosis, treat, and prevent such injury is far from complete. Tragically, we occasionally lose an athlete to injury or illness. This book is dedicated to Derek Sheely: a bright, talented young man who gave his life to the sport he loved as a result

of a concussion. May we continue, as providers and researchers dedicated to athlete and patient welfare, in our quest to eliminate such heartache.

Wayne J. Sebastianelli, MD
Semyon M. Slobounov, PhD
Alexa E. Walter, PhD

Foreword

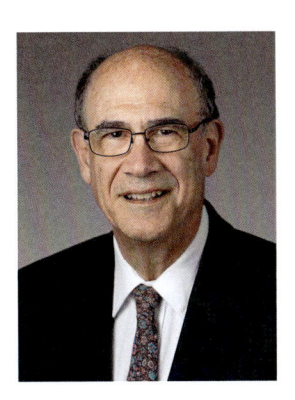

In my neurology clinic, I saw a 16-year-old cheerleader who had suffered five concussions. She dropped from an A student to a C student who needs special help. Another patient, a 12-year-old former cheerleader, after two concussions has had to drop back to the first-grade level in school.

Concussion in sport is a big deal. It is a common problem with consequences. There is the short-term issue of a period of time where the athlete cannot continue to play. But then there are longer-term issues of post-concussive symptoms including increased sensitivity for subsequent concussions (second impact syndrome). And even though there is no obvious damage to the brain on routine neuroimaging, there may well be brain damage leading to reduction in cognitive abilities or even, in severe cases, post-traumatic encephalopathy. It is also a big deal for another reason: it is a problem occurring in children and young adults, and concussion can change their lives forever. Of course, concussion can also occur with auto accidents and with war injuries, as well as in everyday life, and similar issues emerge; thus, studies of athletes can well be generalized to other situations.

With an acute injury, it is important to recognize that a concussion has occurred and determine its severity. There can be a variety of symptoms including difficulty in thinking, concentrating, or remembering; headache; nausea; dizziness; and imbalance. Clinical assessment can include drowsiness, disorientation, slow reaction time, memory loss, difficulty with balance and coordination, and emotional lability. In post-concussion syndrome, all of these symptoms and signs can persist for variable periods of time.

There are almost 3 million sports-related concussions annually in the USA. It is interesting to consider in what sports they occur. An informative paper by Marar et al. (*Am J Sports Med* 2012) looked in detail at the epidemiology of concussions in high school athletes. They reported on 1936 concussions in 7,778,064 athletic exposures. Boys' football leads to the largest number of concussions with more exposures and with the highest rate overall. After that, in numbers of concussions comes girls' soccer, boys' wrestling, girls' basketball, and boys' soccer.

Thus, we are dealing with a common problem. But we certainly do not understand it well enough. What is happening in the acute and chronic states? Why does sensitivity increase for subsequent concussions? There are clinical issues all along the recovery trajectory. What is the best way to recognize and grade the severity of concussion? When is it relatively safe to return to the sport? Is clinical assessment enough? Can laboratory testing help? Are there ways to prevent concussion? How should it be treated? All these topics and more are dealt with in the second edition of this book edited by Drs. Slobounov and Sebastianelli. They have enormous experience themselves at Penn State and have put together a distinguished group of authors to speak to the important issues in this field.

The second edition of this textbook is welcome since the science and knowledge in this field is advancing rapidly, and it is important to present updated topics. Moreover, there are new chapters dealing with the role of the playing surface, the role of biomarkers, and the advances in relevant basic science. In recent years, there have been major advances in neuroimaging and blood biomarker domains that have provided information about the nature of concussion but also helped with diagnosis. It is clear that the effects of concussion may last a very long time, but what does this mean for prognosis or for clinical decision making? Advice from the experts who wrote the chapters in this book is needed to begin to address these many questions. Many thanks to Drs. Slobounov and Sebastianelli for putting this all together.

This book should be of value to anyone dealing with persons with concussion—and that is almost everyone.

Mark Hallett
Chief, Human Motor Control Section
Distinguished NIH Investigator
Medical Neurology Branch
National Institute of Neurological Disorders and Stroke
National Institutes of Health
Bethesda, MD, USA

Athletics Foreword

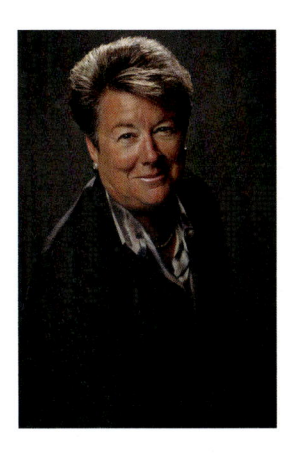

The role of coaches and athletic administration in the management of sports-related concussion has changed drastically over the years. It used to be completely acceptable for a player to "get their bell rung" and continue competing in practice or game scenarios. In fact, this type of competitiveness was heavily encouraged. As our knowledge and understanding of sports-related concussion has developed over the years, this mentality has also been forced to change. It is no longer acceptable from a coaching perspective to instill this type of attitude in players: the consequences can be too drastic. Historically, there has been pushback when coaches or players have publicly spoken out about safety concerns, new practice techniques, or rule changes. But thankfully, due to an increasing public awareness and a willingness to create change from within, this pushback has been significantly diminished.

The involvement of coaches and athletic administration in the management and prevention of sports-related concussion is crucial. Athletes participating in sports do it because they love it and have a passion for it: their long-term health should not have to be compromised because of it. Unfortunately, injury is unavoidable at times, but through knowledge and a willingness to embrace basic science, coaches have the ability to protect their players.

Here at Penn State, we pride ourselves on integrating sport, clinical, and research personnel – creating a team of individuals that in some way, big or small, have contributed to a successful program. Success can be measured in many ways – athletic, academic, or health – and we are grateful to all who have contributed and helped make Penn State a leading institution on sports-related concussion.

As researchers trying to solve a clinical problem affecting athletes, a strong partnership with coaching and athletic administration is fundamental; without this, timely access to injured athletes would not be possible. We collectively strive for success with safety.

Sandy Barbour
Vice President for Intercollegiate Athletics
Pennsylvania State University
University Park, PA, USA

Introduction

Concussion in Athletics: Current Understanding from Basic Brain Science to Clinical Research

Introduction

Participation in and enjoyment of sport has been a large part of culture in the United States. It is estimated that 45 million children participate in youth sports [1], 8 million continue sport at the high school level, and approximately 480,000 continue at the college level [2]. Involvement in sport has proven to provide numerous physical, mental, and social benefits ranging from reduced body fat and increased bone health, to decreased symptoms of depression and anxiety, to better social skills and self-esteem [3, 4]. However, despite the numerous benefits of sport, over the past few decades there has been growing concern surrounding the overall brain health and well-being of participating athletes.

Sports-related concussion (SRC) has gained significant attention within the clinical and basic brain research communities. With some researchers reporting 1.6–3.8 million concussions occurring in sports [5], "mild concussions" account for 80% of all reported traumatic brain injuries [6]. The annual rate of diagnosed concussions over the past 10 years in high school sports demonstrated an annual increase of 16.5% [7]. Despite advances in coaching knowledge and strategies, policy changes, and improved understanding of the mechanisms of SRC, the annual rate of this type of traumatic injury continues to grow [8]. With such high rates of sports-related brain injury occurring during adolescence and young adulthood, an emphasis has to be placed on fully understanding the short- and long-term consequences of this complex and puzzling neurological disorder [8]. This textbook, contributed to by world-renowned experts in the field, aims to provide a multi-modal approach including topics of clinical relevance, motor control, biomechanics, modeling, neuroimaging, genetics, and blood biomarkers to better understand the nature and signs of the most puzzling sports-related injury.

Clinical Research of Sports-Related Concussion

Each year, thousands of first responders, athletic trainers, coaches, and medical professionals face a critical question: What is the time frame for safe return-to-sports participation after SRC? A concussed athlete must be completely *asymptomatic* at rest, with cognitive and exercise-induced exertion, and with activities of daily living prior to the initiation of a stepwise "Return-to-Play" protocol. Current clinical efforts are examining the role of rest, exercise and activity, physical and vestibular therapy, and psychological interventions in their effectiveness in the treatment of athletes recovering from SRC. However, it remains that our definition of *recovery* is largely based on clinical features, symptom self-reports, and restoration to baseline normative executive function. Therefore, our current clinical best practice still lacks the inclusion of serially measured physiological biomarkers of recovery from SRC.

An athlete is defined as *asymptomatic* once they have returned to baseline levels on self-reported symptom scales and clinical examinations. While the current clinical standard of neuropsychological testing, postural control measures, physical signs, and behavior and symptoms checklists have been reported to be sensitive, there is no indication that resolution of these overt indices corresponds to recovery of the complex pathophysiology induced by SRC. Overall, there is current consensus in the literature that *clinical symptom resolution may not be equivalent to physiological injury resolution.*

Allied health professionals treating concussed people have been using the same approach to treatment for nearly two decades. Initially, focused on classification systems, clinicians would choose a system based on their general preference. With 41 different classification systems [9] and a return-to-play protocol based on a clinical construct [10], practitioners have been held to management and return-to-play standards that were based less on well-researched physiologic data and more on clinical intuition and consensus statements from leaders in the field of neuropsychology [11]. Even with increased awareness of concussion and an increased presence of trained allied health professionals such as athletic trainers monitoring high schools and college sports, concussion is still commonly misunderstood by some clinicians and can be oversimplified in terms of its diagnosis and recovery [12, 13]. Athletes typically present clinically with a variety of physical and cognitive symptoms which can be reasonably detected with a thorough clinical evaluation both on the field and in the clinic or athletic training room [14].

Previous controversy surrounding the effects of SRC centered around the idea of *structural* versus *functional* recovery. It was stated in consensus statements [11, 14–16] that "concussion may result in neuropathologic changes, but the clinical symptoms largely reflect a functional disturbance rather than a structural injury." This clinical sentiment is repeated and reexamined in clinical research in which neuropsychologists and other clinical concussion researchers continue to promote the idea of cognitive functional recovery being representative of clinical recovery [16]. Objectively, this basic statement represents a construct flaw in their hypothesis: all of the supporting data are mainly based on the restoration of cognitive functioning measured by neuropsychological testing and not on the healing of the brain microstructure.

However, this sentiment has become less accepted in recent years as numerous animal and human studies on the physiology of concussion have demonstrated lasting physiological changes post injury. These studies have demonstrated a complex series of neurometabolic cascades, neurovascular compromise, and neurophysiologic impairment [17–20] stemming from the mechanical forces of sports-related concussion. The mechanical stretch of axons produces injury to the cytoarchitecture of the axon [21, 22] and surface architecture of the axon [23], which significantly impairs normal neurologic function [24] and leaves the neuron vulnerable to more significant repeated insult [23]. These forces are also capable of inducing short-term and lasting vascular changes [25–27].

Unfortunately, these findings are largely overlooked and underappreciated in the clinical management of sports-related concussion due to the burden of obtaining the data. Inclusion and implementation of these findings, upon validation, should be considered in the clinical management of concussion.

Furthermore, given the increase in awareness of the fact that symptom resolution does not mean physiological resolution, the fields of genetics and blood-based biomarkers have gained great traction in SRC. Much work has been done in the past decade to better identify the genetic and metabolic underpinnings of SRC and in ways that are more clinically feasible than, for example, a research MRI.

More recently, there has been a shift in public concern from SRC solely to the accumulation of impacts to the head in contact and collision sports. An inherent part of many sports involves forces being applied to the head repetitively throughout practice and game settings. These repetitive impacts have been called subconcussion, subconcussive impacts, receptive head impacts, and repetitive head acceleration events (HAEs), among others.

Part of the concern surrounding HAEs is their potential link to neurodegenerative diseases including Alzheimer's, chronic traumatic encephalopathy (CTE), and amyotrophic lateral sclerosis (ALS) [28, 29]. CTE, a neurodegenerative disease marked by tau accumulation, has recently been diagnosed in many former contact sport players, at many levels of experience ranging from high school to professional athletes [30]. The marked degeneration present, in combination with the clinical symptoms reported, has increased concern regarding the safety of contact sports. Unfortunately, at this time, CTE can only be diagnosed upon autopsy, so many questions continue to remain surrounding its link to contact sports.

We understand that at present, many modalities, such as advanced imaging studies, are often not easily accessible, and their full implication is not yet established. Continuing research should indicate what will be cost effective in better protecting athletes and determining safe return-to-play after brain injuries. However, it becomes clear that the proposed solution for existing controversies in sport concussion research needs to result in a combination of multiple modalities that will be able to concurrently record performance (functional) variables as well as structural/functional brain imaging (fMRI, DTI, MRS, EEG) variables. Clinicians and coaching staff should be interested not only in the restoration of successful functional performance (memory, attention, balance, executive functions) but also the structural (neural) network responsible for maximum performance outcomes. Numerous multimodal findings and modeling biomechanical studies obtained in many research laboratories are indicative of the types of results to which clinicians should be attentive. These studies seek to find a behavioral and structural resolution after SRC. Is there ever ultimate restoration of normal structural components and functional integrity, or permanent "brain damage and/or reorganization"? With combined modality longitudinal studies, we can come closer to answering this critical question. In brief below we describe some of the major findings found in this textbook. This is by no means a comprehensive description, instead highlighting key points and discoveries over the past decade.

EEG Research

High-temporal resolution EEG signal is highly suitable for examining neurophysiological correlates of fast sensori-motor and cognitive functions [31–33], susceptable to concussive impacts. Not suprisingly, electroencephalography (EEG) was the first monitoring assessment tool to demonstrate the alteration of brain functions in subjects suffering from traumatic brain injury (TBI) [32–36]. Presence of pathophysiology in their definition of concussion has finally been accepted in the clinical literature. Thus, it seems appropriate to utilize a physiological measure such as EEG in the clinical setting of concussion.

Historically, EEG was first demonstrated in humans by Hans Berger in 1924. Since then, considerable empirical evidence has been accumulated indicating both (a) the clinical value of EEG in terms of the accuracy of assessement of mTBI, and (b) the conceptual significance of EEG in enabling the examination of neural substrates underlying neurological, behavioral, and neuropsychological alterations in SRC [34, 37–40].

There is a line of recent research indicating the efficacy of EEG-based ERP (event-related potentials) in detecting subtle and pervasive alterations of cognition-related waveforms in athletes suffering from SRC, including multiple concussions [41, 42]. It appeared that the athletes with a history of previous concussions exhibited significantly attenuated amplitude of posterior contralateral negativity (SPCN) compared to normal volunteers in absence of working memory abnormalities [42]. Similarly, Broglio et al. reported significant decrement in the N2 and P3b amplitude of the stimulus-locked ERP in athletes with a history of concussion on average of 3.4 years post injury [43]. Most importantly, no significant alterations were observed based on commonly used clinical and neuropsychological tests. *These EEG findings strongly support the notion that SRC can no longer be considered a transient injury.*

Overall, serially implemented EEG studies, in conjunction with clinical assessements over the course of SRC, clearly document residual cerebral dysfunction. Specifically, alteration of EEG alpha power dynamics in conjunction with balance data in the acute phase of injury, with respect to baseline measures, may predict the rate of recovery from a single concussive blow. As such, EEG measures (if properly executed in conjunction with other behavioral variables) are excellent tools to assess the status and prognosis of patients with concussion. Details regarding the nature of EEG signal, signal processing in both time and frequency domains, and EEG concussion research can be found in the relevant chapters (Chaps. 4 and 19) within this textbook.

Advanced Neuroimaging Research

Functional MRI (fMRI) One of the more recent and popular advancements in neuroimaging, fMRI, has become a widely used research tool in probing the complexities of the brain [44]. Functional MRI uses the principle of Blood Oxygen Level-Dependent (BOLD) contrast as an index of neuronal activity [45]. The BOLD signal in fMRI is sensitive to blood-based properties, specifically the local magnetic susceptibility produced by deoxyhemoglobin which causes a reduction in signal. The assumption in BOLD fMRI is that an increase in neuronal activity within a brain region results in an increase in local blood flow, leading to reduced concentrations of deoxyhemoglobin in nearby vessels [46]. Therefore, the higher concentrations of oxyhemoglobin associated with neuronal activity results in higher signal intensities due to a reduction in local field inhomogeneities and signal dephasing caused by deoxyhemoglobin. For a more detailed review of MR physics or fMRI methodological and conceptual pitfalls, see Horowitz [47] and Hillary et al. [48] respectively.

Most recent brain imaging research, particularly evoked fMRI, revealed alteration of the BOLD signal in concussed individuals while performing various neurocognitive tasks. For example, a seminal study using the N-back task suggested a complex relationship between cognitive load and functional activation at one-month post concussive injury, with hyperactivation observed within the dorsolateral prefrontal cortex (DLPFC) and lateral parietal cortex during moderate load, whereas hypoactivation was observed during low and high load compared to healthy controls [49]. More recently, a longitudinal study of student athletes indicated that hyperactivation of the inferior parietal lobe in concussed subjects when compared to the control group persisted 2 months post injury, despite there being no differences in neurobehavioral performance [50]. Overall, these studies provide support for changes in neuronal activity of brain regions implicated in working memory following SRC. However, there is still debate in the literature regarding the values of fMRI data in a clinical assessment of concussion, at least as this pertains to athletics (see Chap. 11 for details).

Resting State Functional MRI (rs-fMRI) There has been a recent trend in studies using MRI BOLD signal to examine neuronal health following SRC, specifically to incorporate baseline or "resting state" measurement of the BOLD signal. Conceptually, the human brain has two contradictory properties: (1) "segregation," which means localization of specific functions and (2) "integration," which means combining all the information and functions at a global level within the conceptual framework of a "global integrated network" [51, 52]. Consistent with this conceptual framework, Biswal et al. were the first to document the spontaneous fluctuations within the motor system and high potential for functional connectivity in resting state fMRI (rs-fMRI) using intrinsic activity correlations [53]. Since this discovery of coherent spontaneous fluctuations, many studies have shown that several brain regions engaged during various cognitive tasks also form coherent large-scale brain networks that can be identified using rs-fMRI [54].

As noted in Chap. 11 of this book, rs-fMRI has several advantages over more traditional evoked studies. Foremost, using a relatively simple task (i.e., passively maintaining fixation), it is possible to probe the neuronal integrity of the multiple sensory, motor, and cognitive networks that exist in the human brain. This can occur without concerns about practice effects or decreased novelty associated with multiple administrations of a task, potentially confounding the results. Moreover, rs-fMRI eliminates the complex requirements for presenting sensory stimuli and monitoring motor responses (e.g., interfacing with a computer, projecting stimuli, special non-ferrous motor response devices), rendering it more feasible for performing clinical scans.

Default Mode Network (DMN) The existence of a "default mode network" in the brain during the resting state was reported by Greicius et al. [55]. Both functional and structural connectivity between brain regions were examined to detect whether there are orderly sets of regions that have particularly high local connections (forming families of clusters) as well as a limited number of regions that serve as relay stations or hubs [56]. It was suggested that the neural network of the brain has a small-world structure, namely, high-cluster coefficients and low average path length allowing optimization of information processing [57].

As one of the resting state networks (RSN) of the brain, the DMN includes the precuneus/posterior cingulate cortex (PCC), medial prefrontal cortex (MPFC), and medial, lateral, and inferior parietal cortices [58]. Although the DMN is active during rest, it is not actively involved in attention or goal-oriented tasks [59]. Despite the fact that the DMN is deactivated during specific tasks, the presence of the DMN during rs-fMRI has been reported and validated in several studies [59–61].

At present, there are a growing number of reports focusing on alteration of DMN in SRC. Mayer et al. [62] investigated the resting state DMN of sub-acute SRC and showed that these subjects displayed decreased BOLD connectivity within the DMN and hyper-connectivity between the right prefrontal and posterior parietal cortices involved in the fronto-parietal task-related network (TRN). However, inhomogeneities such as (a) differential diagnosis of SRC including the presence or absence of loss of consciousness (LOC); (b) time since injury; and (c) subject's detailed medical history that includes information on past head injuries influence fMRI data. In our own study, we examined DMN in SRC athletes using resting state fMRI with specific focus on recruiting a homogeneous subject population and controlling for the number of previous concussions [63]. We have also reported that there were disruptions in the connections that make up the DMN in concussed subjects [64]. More recent imaging studies using dynamic complementary functional analysis of resting state MRI showed potential benefits to further examining abnormalities in brain network communication in response to SRC [65] (see further details on this MRI issue in the imaging chapters).

Diffusion Tensor Imaging (DTI) Diffusion tensor imaging (DTI) is an advanced imaging technique that exploits the molecular diffusion or Brownian motion of water due to thermal energy. Due to this random diffusion, the displacement and motion of molecules can be used to gain information on microscopic tissue structures and characteristics that are beyond the basic resolution of MRI [66]. Brownian motion is random, and this free diffusion is described as being isotropic, yet the direction and mobility of water molecules can be restricted by certain tissue characteristics and structures that result in anisotropy [67]. In the white matter of the brain this diffusion anisotropy becomes ever apparent as myelinated axonal fibers organized into bundles and tracts allow for quicker diffusion along axonal fibers as compared to diffusion oriented perpendicular to the fiber [68]. As the name implies, a tensor model is fitted in order to obtain certain indices, λ_1, λ_2, and λ_3, that allow for a quantitative description of this anisotropic diffusion, where λ_1 is the axial diffusivity, and λ_2 and λ_3 are combined to form the radial diffusivity [63]. Another important scalar measure reported in the literature is the fractional anisotropy (FA). The FA value is between 0 and 1, with 0 representing free diffusion in all directions and 1 representing diffusion confined to only one direction. More precisely, the FA value is the ratio of the direction of maximal diffusion to the diffusion that is perpendicular to that main direction [69]. Further metrics include apparent diffusion coefficient (ADC), which tries to correct image contrasts due to relaxation effects or diffusion, and mean diffusivity (MD), which is an averaged value of diffusion.

A voxel-based analysis of DTI of high school athletes by Bazarian and colleagues performed DTI within a 3-month interval pre and post season [70]. Despite the small sample size, one athlete received a concussion during the season and had the largest number of affected voxels in the white matter as compared to the individual's exposure to repetitive impacts. Another investigation examined ten concussed collegiate athletes and scanned them with DTI at least 1 month post injury [71]. A voxel-based analysis was implemented and revealed significant increases in MD only in the left hemisphere. A recent systematic review on DTI findings in adult civilian, military, and sports-related concussion revealed (a) widespread but inconsistent differences in white matter diffusion metrics (primarily FA, MD and RD, and AD) following concussion and (b) significant overlap in white matter abnormalities reported in concussed subjects with those commonly affected by socio-economic status or the presence of major depressive disorder and attention-deficit hyperactivity disorder (ADHD) [72].

In addition, as noted in Chap. 8, trauma-induced edematous reactions in the brain compress parenchyma, which in turn may influence water diffusion potentially detected by DTI. Using the FA metric, alterations in the FA outside of baseline levels may indicate neuroinflammation and secondary membrane dysfunction creating fluid shifts. Since brain trauma may induce dynamic changes over time, differences in FA over acute, subacute, and chronic time frames post injury may differ as well. Thus, in SRC low FA may reflect white matter degeneration while increased FA beyond normative baseline may indicate neuroinflammation. Overall, DTI may offer valuable structural and molecular information and insight into the brain as it becomes more commonplace in neuroimaging studies of SRC (see Chap. 9 for an in-depth look at DTI). It should be noted, however, that more research needs to be done to optimize its effectiveness and clinical utility.

Magnetic Resonance Spectroscopy (MRS) Magnetic resonance spectroscopy (MRS), also known as proton magnetic resonance spectroscopy (H-MRS), is a useful tool that allows for identification and quantification of cellular metabolites connected to nervous cell energetics in vivo [73]. As with many MRI applications, there are a number of different parameters and pulse sequences that can be used in order to acquire MRS data, all of which have their advantages and disadvantages and can make comparisons between studies difficult.

The metabolites in the brain that are most often studied are N-acetylaspartate (NAA), choline (Cho), and creatine-phosphocreatine (Cr) [74–76]. NAA is used as an indicator of neuronal and axonal integrity as decreased levels are seen after injury and associated with neuronal loss, metabolic dysfunction, or myelin repair [77].

Another common MRS finding after head trauma is increases in Cho levels [78, 79], which are a marker of cell membrane turnover [78]. The Cr peak, which is a combination of the two creatine-containing compounds creatine and creatine phosphate, is an accepted indicator of cell energy metabolism [80, 81]. Despite the information MRS can yield on the metabolic response of the brain to injury, there are still limited numbers of studies that utilize it to evaluate metabolic alterations induced by SRC (see Chap. 10 for more detail).

It is worth noting that the original studies from different laboratories reported connections between the alteration of NAA homeostasis and changes in amino acids linked to post-brain injury excitotoxic phenomena, and possibly to transitory increases in the number of dysfunctional mitochondria [82]. A previous MRS study of "asymptomatic" collegiate athletes recovering from SRC reported a reduction in NAA/Cr and NAA/Cho in the genu and splenium of the corpus callosum [83]. The general findings from more recent MRS studies suggest that brain cells might be defined as biochemically, metabolically, and genetically vulnerable after concussive injury. Thus, a *window of vulnerability* after SRC might last much longer than symptoms clearance. Overall, there is growing empirical evidence from MRS, in isolation and in combination with other advanced MRI studies (e.g., fMRI, DTI, etc.), that metabolic and ultrastructural SRC-mediated brain-compromised architecture persists far beyond clinical and neuropsychological clearance.

Biomarkers and Genetic Basis of SRC Research

The use of blood-based biomarkers as diagnostic and prognostic tools for risk stratification of SRC has increased exponentially but is still limited in its clinical utility.

As biomarker levels can vary over time post injury, they present a potentially useful tool for identifying individuals by severity of injury, monitoring responses to treatment, or predicting functional outcomes. Commonly studied proteomic biomarkers for mild TBI and SRC are markers of the central nervous system functioning including astroglia (GFAP, S100β) and neuronal cells, with specific areas of the neuron such as the cell body (UCH-L1) and axon (Tau, Neurofilament). Furthermore, transcriptomic biomarkers, called microRNAs, have also been gaining traction as promising biomarkers of injury as they are relatively abundant in biofluids (cerebrospinal fluid, serum, urine), and are relatively stable at variable pH conditions, and resistant to repeated freeze thaw and enzymatic degradation. Due to these properties, miRNA may have advantages over protein-based markers.

GFAP and UCH-L1 have been well studied, and even FDA-approved for specific use with CT scans. GFAP was detectable in serum within an hour of concussion and remained elevated for several days after and consistently identified concussion over 7 days. GFAP also detected with good accuracy traumatic intracranial lesions on head computed tomography (CT), and neurosurgical intervention over a week [84]. In contrast, UCH-L1 rose rapidly within 30 minutes of injury, peaked at 8 hours after injury, and decreased steadily over 48 hours with small peaks and troughs over 7 days – making UCH-L1 a very early marker of concussion [84].

In early 2018, GFAP and UCH-L1 were FDA-approved for clinical use in adult patients with mild to moderate TBI to help determine the need for CT scan within 12 hours of injury [85]. The approval was based on the ability to find lesions on a CT scan, but they were not approved to diagnose a concussion.

Other promising biomarkers include S100β, neuron-specific enolase, tau, neurofilament, amyloid beta, and brain-derived neurotrophic factor (see Chap. 13 for more details). Some correlate with number of hits to the head (soccer), acceleration/deceleration forces (jumps, collisions, and falls), post-concussive symptoms, trauma to the body versus the head, and dynamics of injury [86].

The role of genetics in susceptibility to SRC and recovery trajectory after injury has grown exponentially in the past decade. Previous research mainly focused on the role of Apolipoprotein E (*APOE*), specifically ε4; however, there were mixed findings on the involvement of APOE in risk of obtaining an SRC. There has been more evidence that the APOE ε4 allele plays a role in recovery from injury as studies have demonstrated that those with the ε4 allele have greater impairments in neurocognitive standardized scores [87, 88] and higher symptom severity [89, 90].

Further work has been done on other single nucleotide polymorphisms (SNPs) including Brain Derived Neurotrophic Factor (*BDNF*), dopamine receptors (DRD), catechol-O-methyl transferase (*COMT*), interleukins (*IL*), tau, *KIAA0319*, *SLC17A7*, and *CACNA1A* (see Chap. 14 for more details). The use of individuals' genetics for health purposes has been a growing area of research, and it can be assumed that there is a link between concussion and genetics. However, at this time, the findings are still fairly limited and, overall, there is limited evidence of a genotype predicting previous concussion history. In future, more comprehensive work is needed to fully understand some of the genetic underpinnings of SRC.

Concluding Statement

The main goal of this textbook is to provide empirical evidence from clinical research, advanced neuroimaging, biomarkers, and genetic studies that resist the conventional wisdom that *typically quick and spontaneous* recovery following an SRC is rapid and complete, with no residual deficits. There is growing evidence that *atypical evolution* of concussive injury may be more prevalent due to the fact that clinical, behavioral, neurocognitive, emotional, and underlying neural and other biological alterations persist months or even years post injury. Specifically, the findings of recent brain imaging and biomarkers studies (see details in the following chapters) challenge the conventional wisdom based solely upon clinical and neurocognitive assessment of concussion.

Overall, this summation of the chapters highlights research being done employing various techniques, ranging from clinically focused to more physiologically based approaches, to study the athletes involved in sports. The continued overlap between basic science and clinical science is needed for the field to move forward, and these chapters highlight possible paths. While this updated version of this volume demonstrates the great strides made in the past decade, more work is needed to continue our understanding of the complex factors relating to these injuries. Since these injuries are indeed a complex pathophysiological process affecting the brain, proper tools have to be validated and implemented. When the physiology of the brain after different levels of injury is better defined, we will have a better understanding of the true definition of injury, its diagnosis, risk, and the threshold of energy causing injury. This, in turn, will lead to improved understanding of the resultant cognitive, imaging, and biomarker changes. With increased knowledge of the complex physiology of the brain after exposure to SRC, or repetitive HAEs, both scientific and clinical questions will be easier to answer. Thus, overall, we will be better able to protect the neurologic health and well-being of athletes involved in sports.

References

1. The Aspen Institute Project Play. Kids sports facts: participation rates [Internet]. [cited 2020 Jan 20]. Available from: https://www.aspenprojectplay.org/kids-sports-participation-rates.
2. smeyers@ncaa.org. Estimated probability of competing in college athletics [Internet]. NCAA.org – the official site of the NCAA. 2015. [cited 2020 Jan 20]. Available from: http://www.ncaa.org/about/resources/research/estimated-probability-competing-college-athletics.
3. health.gov. Advisory report – 2008 physical activity guidelines [Internet]. [cited 2020 Jan 20]. Available from: https://health.gov/paguidelines/2008/report/.
4. Eime RM, Young JA, Harvey JT, Charity MJ, Payne WR. A systematic review of the psychological and social benefits of participation in sport for children and adolescents: informing development of a conceptual model of health through sport. Int J Behav Nutr Phys Act. 2013;10:98.

5. Langlois JA, Rutland-Brown W, Wald MM. The epidemiology and impact of traumatic brain injury: a brief overview. J Head Trauma Rehabil. 2006;21:375–8.
6. Ruff RM. Mild traumatic brain injury and neural recovery: rethinking the debate. NeuroRehabilitation. 2011;28:167–80.
7. Lincoln AE, Caswell SV, Almquist JL, Dunn RE, Norris JB, Hinton RY. Trends in concussion incidence in high school sports: a prospective 11-year study. Am J Sports Med. SAGE Publications Inc STM. 2011;39:958–63.
8. Cantu RC, Aubry M, Dvorak J, Graf-Baumann T, Johnston K, Kelly J, et al. Overview of concussion consensus statements since 2000. Neurosurg Focus. 2006;21:E3.
9. Anderson T, Heitger M, Macleod AD. Concussion and mild head injury. Pract Neurol. BMJ Publishing Group Ltd. 2006;6:342–57.
10. Guidelines for assessment and management of sport-related concussion. Canadian Academy of Sport Medicine Concussion Committee. Clin J Sport Med. 2000;10:209–11.
11. Aubry M, Cantu R, Dvorak J, Graf-Baumann T, Johnston K, Kelly J, et al. Summary and agreement statement of the First International Conference on Concussion in Sport, Vienna 2001. Recommendations for the improvement of safety and health of athletes who may suffer concussive injuries. Br J Sports Med. 2002;36:6–10.
12. Chrisman SP, Schiff MA, Rivara FP. Physician concussion knowledge and the effect of mailing the CDC's "Heads Up" toolkit. Clin Pediatr (Phila). 2011;50:1031–9.
13. McCrea M, Prichep L, Powell MR, Chabot R, Barr WB. Acute effects and recovery after sport-related concussion: a neurocognitive and quantitative brain electrical activity study. J Head Trauma Rehabil. 2010;25:283–92.
14. McCrory P, Meeuwisse W, Johnston K, Dvorak J, Aubry M, Molloy M, et al. Consensus statement on concussion in sport: the 3rd International Conference on Concussion in Sport held in Zurich, November 2008. J Athl Train. 2009;44:434–48.
15. McCrory P, Meeuwisse WH, Aubry M, Cantu RC, Dvořák J, Echemendia RJ, et al. Consensus statement on concussion in sport--the 4th International Conference on Concussion in Sport held in Zurich, November 2012. PM R. 2013;5:255–79.
16. Moser RS, Iverson GL, Echemendia RJ, Lovell MR, Schatz P, Webbe FM, et al. Neuropsychological evaluation in the diagnosis and management of sports-related concussion. Arch Clin Neuropsychol. 2007;22:909–16.
17. Giza CC, Hovda DA. The neurometabolic cascade of concussion. J Athl Train. 2001;36:228–35.
18. Barkhoudarian G, Hovda DA, Giza CC. The molecular pathophysiology of concussive brain injury. Clin Sports Med. 2011;30:33–48, vii–iii.
19. Kan EM, Ling E-A, Lu J. Microenvironment changes in mild traumatic brain injury. Brain Res Bull. 2012;87:359–72.
20. Goetz P, Blamire A, Rajagopalan B, Cadoux-Hudson T, Young D, Styles P. Increase in apparent diffusion coefficient in normal appearing white matter

following human traumatic brain injury correlates with injury severity. J Neurotrauma. 2004;21:645–54.
21. Browne KD, Chen X-H, Meaney DF, Smith DH. Mild traumatic brain injury and diffuse axonal injury in swine. J Neurotrauma. 2011;28:1747–55.
22. Yuen TJ, Browne KD, Iwata A, Smith DH. Sodium channelopathy induced by mild axonal trauma worsens outcome after a repeat injury. J Neurosci Res. 2009;87:3620–5.
23. Flamm ES, Ommaya AK, Coe J, Krueger TP, Faas FH. Cardiovascular effects of experimental head injury in the monkey. Surg Forum. 1966;17:414–6.
24. Grundl PD, Biagas KV, Kochanek PM, Schiding JK, Barmada MA, Nemoto EM. Early cerebrovascular response to head injury in immature and mature rats. J Neurotrauma. 1994;11:135–48.
25. Lewine JD, Davis JT, Bigler ED, Thoma R, Hill D, Funke M, et al. Objective documentation of traumatic brain injury subsequent to mild head trauma: multimodal brain imaging with MEG, SPECT, and MRI. J Head Trauma Rehabil. 2007;22:141–55.
26. Chason JL, Hardy WG, Webster JE, Gurdjian ES. Alterations in cell structure of the brain associated with experimental concussion. J Neurosurg. 1958;15:135–9.
27. Nevin NC. Neuropathological changes in the white matter following head injury. J Neuropathol Exp Neurol. 1967;26:77–84.
28. McKee AC, Cantu RC, Nowinski CJ, Hedley-Whyte ET, Gavett BE, Budson AE, et al. Chronic traumatic encephalopathy in athletes: progressive tauopathy after repetitive head injury. J Neuropathol Exp Neurol. 2009;68:709–35.
29. Omalu BI, DeKosky ST, Minster RL, Kamboh MI, Hamilton RL, Wecht CH. Chronic traumatic encephalopathy in a National Football League player. Neurosurgery. 2005;57:128–34; discussion 128–134.
30. Mez J, Daneshvar DH, Kiernan PT, Abdolmohammadi B, Alvarez VE, Huber BR, et al. Clinicopathological evaluation of chronic traumatic encephalopathy in players of American football. JAMA. 2017;318:360–70.
31. Glaser M, Sjaardema H. The value of the electroencephalograph in craniocerebral injuries. West J Surg. 1940;48:6989–96.
32. Jasper H, Kershman J, Elvidge A. Electroencephalographic study in clinical cases of injury of the head. Arch Neurol Psychiatr. 1940;44:328–50.
33. Williams D. The electro-encephalogram in acute head injuries*. J Neurol Psychiatry. 1941;4:107–30.
34. Arciniegas DB. Clinical electrophysiologic assessments and mild traumatic brain injury: state-of-the-science and implications for clinical practice. Int J Psychophysiol. 2011;82:41–52.
35. Geets W, Louette N. Early EEG in 300 cerebral concussions. Rev Electroencephalogr Neurophysiol Clin. 1985;14:333–8.
36. McClelland RJ, Fenton GW, Rutherford W. The postconcussional syndrome revisited. J R Soc Med. 1994;87:508–10.

37. Tebano MT, Cameroni M, Gallozzi G, Loizzo A, Palazzino G, Pezzini G, et al. EEG spectral analysis after minor head injury in man. Electroencephalogr Clin Neurophysiol. 1988;70:185–9.
38. Montgomery EA, Fenton GW, McClelland RJ, MacFlynn G, Rutherford WH. The psychobiology of minor head injury. Psychol Med. 1991;21:375–84.
39. Pratap-Chand R, Sinniah M, Salem FA. Cognitive evoked potential (P300): a metric for cerebral concussion. Acta Neurol Scand. 1988;78:185–9.
40. Watson MR, Fenton GW, McClelland RJ, Lumsden J, Headley M, Rutherford WH. The post-concussional state: neurophysiological aspects. Br J Psychiatry. 1995;167:514–21.
41. Duff J. The usefulness of quantitative EEG (QEEG) and neurotherapy in the assessment and treatment of post-concussion syndrome. Clin EEG Neurosci. 2004;35:198–209.
42. Gosselin N, Thériault M, Leclerc S, Montplaisir J, Lassonde M. Neurophysiological anomalies in symptomatic and asymptomatic concussed athletes. Neurosurgery. 2006;58:1151–61. discussion 1151-1161
43. Broglio SP, Pontifex MB, O'Connor P, Hillman CH. The persistent effects of concussion on neuroelectric indices of attention. J Neurotrauma. 2009;26:1463–70.
44. Logothetis NK. What we can do and what we cannot do with fMRI. Nature. 2008;453:869–78.
45. Ogawa S, Lee TM, Kay AR, Tank DW. Brain magnetic resonance imaging with contrast dependent on blood oxygenation. Proc Natl Acad Sci U S A. 1990;87:9868–72.
46. Ogawa S, Menon RS, Tank DW, Kim SG, Merkle H, Ellermann JM, et al. Functional brain mapping by blood oxygenation level-dependent contrast magnetic resonance imaging. A comparison of signal characteristics with a biophysical model. Biophys J. 1993;64:803–12.
47. Horowitz AL. MRI physics for radiologists – a visual approach [Internet]. 3rd ed. New York: Springer; 1995. [cited 2020 Dec 23]. Available from: https://www.springer.com/gp/book/9780387943725.
48. Hillary FG, Steffener J, Biswal BB, Lange G, DeLuca J, Ashburner J. Functional magnetic resonance imaging technology and traumatic brain injury rehabilitation: guidelines for methodological and conceptual pitfalls. J Head Trauma Rehabil. 2002;17:411–30.
49. McAllister TW, Sparling MB, Flashman LA, Guerin SJ, Mamourian AC, Saykin AJ. Differential working memory load effects after mild traumatic brain injury. NeuroImage. 2001;14:1004–12.
50. Dettwiler A, Murugavel M, Putukian M, Cubon V, Furtado J, Osherson D. Persistent differences in patterns of brain activation after sports-related concussion: a longitudinal functional magnetic resonance imaging study. J Neurotrauma. 2014;31:180–8.

51. Varela F, Lachaux JP, Rodriguez E, Martinerie J. The brainweb: phase synchronization and large-scale integration. Nat Rev Neurosci. 2001;2:229–39.
52. Reijneveld JC, Ponten SC, Berendse HW, Stam CJ. The application of graph theoretical analysis to complex networks in the brain. Clin Neurophysiol. 2007;118:2317–31.
53. Biswal B, Yetkin FZ, Haughton VM, Hyde JS. Functional connectivity in the motor cortex of resting human brain using echo-planar MRI. Magn Reson Med. 1995;34:537–41.
54. Smith SM, Fox PT, Miller KL, Glahn DC, Fox PM, Mackay CE, et al. Correspondence of the brain's functional architecture during activation and rest. Proc Natl Acad Sci U S A. 2009;106:13040–5.
55. Greicius MD, Krasnow B, Reiss AL, Menon V. Functional connectivity in the resting brain: a network analysis of the default mode hypothesis. Proc Natl Acad Sci U S A. 2003;100:253–8.
56. Sporns O, Honey CJ, Kötter R. Identification and classification of hubs in brain networks. PLoS One. 2007;2:e1049.
57. Broyd SJ, Demanuele C, Debener S, Helps SK, James CJ, Sonuga-Barke EJS. Default-mode brain dysfunction in mental disorders: a systematic review. Neurosci Biobehav Rev. 2009;33:279–96.
58. Raichle ME, MacLeod AM, Snyder AZ, Powers WJ, Gusnard DA, Shulman GL. A default mode of brain function. Proc Natl Acad Sci U S A. 2001;98:676–82.
59. Beckmann CF, DeLuca M, Devlin JT, Smith SM. Investigations into resting-state connectivity using independent component analysis. Philos Trans R Soc Lond Ser B Biol Sci. 2005;360:1001–13.
60. Damoiseaux JS, Rombouts SARB, Barkhof F, Scheltens P, Stam CJ, Smith SM, et al. Consistent resting-state networks across healthy subjects. Proc Natl Acad Sci U S A. 2006;103:13848–53.
61. De Luca M, Beckmann CF, De Stefano N, Matthews PM, Smith SM. fMRI resting state networks define distinct modes of long-distance interactions in the human brain. NeuroImage. 2006;29:1359–67.
62. Mayer AR, Mannell MV, Ling J, Gasparovic C, Yeo RA. Functional connectivity in mild traumatic brain injury. Hum Brain Mapp. 2011;32:1825–35.
63. Wilde EA, Merkley TL, Bigler ED, Max JE, Schmidt AT, Ayoub KW, et al. Longitudinal changes in cortical thickness in children after traumatic brain injury and their relation to behavioral regulation and emotional control. Int J Dev Neurosci. 2012;30:267–76.
64. Stulemeijer M, Vos PE, van der Werf S, van Dijk G, Rijpkema M, Fernández G. How mild traumatic brain injury may affect declarative memory performance in the post-acute stage. J Neurotrauma. 2010;27:1585–95.
65. Churchill NW, Hutchison MG, Graham SJ, Schweizer TA. Scale-free functional brain dynamics during recovery from sport-related concussion. Hum Brain Mapp. 2020;41:2567–82.
66. Le Bihan D, Mangin JF, Poupon C, Clark CA, Pappata S, Molko N, et al. Diffusion tensor imaging: concepts and applications. J Magn Reson Imaging. 2001;13:534–46.

67. Snook L, Paulson L-A, Roy D, Phillips L, Beaulieu C. Diffusion tensor imaging of neurodevelopment in children and young adults. NeuroImage. 2005;26:1164–73.
68. Sharp DJ, Ham TE. Investigating white matter injury after mild traumatic brain injury. Curr Opin Neurol. 2011;24:558–63.
69. Shah S, Yallampalli R, Merkley TL, McCauley SR, Bigler ED, Macleod M, et al. Diffusion tensor imaging and volumetric analysis of the ventral striatum in adults with traumatic brain injury. Brain Inj. 2012;26:201–10.
70. Bazarian JJ, Zhu T, Blyth B, Borrino A, Zhong J. Subject-specific changes in brain white matter on diffusion tensor imaging after sports-related concussion. Magn Reson Imaging. 2012;30:171–80.
71. Cubon VA, Putukian M, Boyer C, Dettwiler A. A diffusion tensor imaging study on the white matter skeleton in individuals with sports-related concussion. J Neurotrauma. 2011;28:189–201.
72. Asken BM, DeKosky ST, Clugston JR, Jaffee MS, Bauer RM. Diffusion tensor imaging (DTI) findings in adult civilian, military, and sport-related mild traumatic brain injury (mTBI): a systematic critical review. Brain Imaging Behav. 2018;12:585–612.
73. Shekdar K, Wang D-J. Role of magnetic resonance spectroscopy in evaluation of congenital/developmental brain abnormalities. Semin Ultrasound CT MR. 2011;32:510–38.
74. Cecil KM, Hills EC, Sandel ME, Smith DH, McIntosh TK, Mannon LJ, et al. Proton magnetic resonance spectroscopy for detection of axonal injury in the splenium of the corpus callosum of brain-injured patients. J Neurosurg. 1998;88:795–801.
75. Belanger HG, Vanderploeg RD, Curtiss G, Warden DL. Recent neuroimaging techniques in mild traumatic brain injury. J Neuropsychiatry Clin Neurosci. 2007;19:5–20.
76. Govind V, Gold S, Kaliannan K, Saigal G, Falcone S, Arheart KL, et al. Whole-brain proton MR spectroscopic imaging of mild-to-moderate traumatic brain injury and correlation with neuropsychological deficits. J Neurotrauma. 2010;27:483–96.
77. Gasparovic C, Yeo R, Mannell M, Ling J, Elgie R, Phillips J, et al. Neurometabolite concentrations in gray and white matter in mild traumatic brain injury: an 1H-magnetic resonance spectroscopy study. J Neurotrauma. 2009;26:1635–43.
78. Ross BD, Ernst T, Kreis R, Haseler LJ, Bayer S, Danielsen E, et al. 1H MRS in acute traumatic brain injury. J Magn Reson Imaging. 1998;8:829–40.
79. Signoretti S, Di Pietro V, Vagnozzi R, Lazzarino G, Amorini AM, Belli A, et al. Transient alterations of creatine, creatine phosphate, N-acetylaspartate and high-energy phosphates after mild traumatic brain injury in the rat. Mol Cell Biochem. 2010;333:269–77.
80. Vagnozzi R, Signoretti S, Cristofori L, Alessandrini F, Floris R, Isgrò E, et al. Assessment of metabolic brain damage and recovery following mild traumatic brain injury: a multicentre, proton magnetic resonance spectroscopic study in concussed patients. Brain. 2010;133:3232–42.

81. Walz NC, Cecil KM, Wade SL, Michaud LJ. Late proton magnetic resonance spectroscopy following traumatic brain injury during early childhood: relationship with neurobehavioral outcomes. J Neurotrauma. 2008;25:94–103.
82. Di Pietro V, Amorini AM, Tavazzi B, Vagnozzi R, Logan A, Lazzarino G, et al. The molecular mechanisms affecting N-acetylaspartate homeostasis following experimental graded traumatic brain injury. Mol Med. 2014;20:147–57.
83. Johnson B, Zhang K, Gay M, Neuberger T, Horovitz S, Hallett M, et al. Metabolic alterations in corpus callosum may compromise brain functional connectivity in MTBI patients: an 1H-MRS study. Neurosci Lett. 2012;509:5–8.
84. Papa L, Brophy GM, Welch RD, Lewis LM, Braga CF, Tan CN, et al. Time course and diagnostic accuracy of glial and neuronal blood biomarkers GFAP and UCH-L1 in a large cohort of trauma patients with and without mild traumatic brain injury. JAMA Neurol. 2016;73:551–60.
85. US Food & Drug Administration. FDA authorizes marketing of first blood test to aid in the evaluation of concussion in adults. 2018.
86. Papa L, Ramia MM, Edwards D, Johnson BD, Slobounov SM. Systematic review of clinical studies examining biomarkers of brain injury in athletes after sports-related concussion. J Neurotrauma. 2015;32:661–73.
87. Cochrane GD, Sundman MH, Hall EE, Kostek MC, Patel K, Barnes KP, et al. Genetics influence neurocognitive performance at baseline but not concussion history in collegiate student-athletes. Clin J Sport Med. 2018;28(2):125–9.
88. Merritt VC, Rabinowitz AR, Arnett PA. The influence of the apolipoprotein E (APOE) gene on subacute post-concussion neurocognitive performance in college athletes. Arch Clin Neuropsychol. 2018;33:36–46.
89. Merritt VC, Ukueberuwa DM, Arnett PA. Relationship between the apolipoprotein E gene and headache following sports-related concussion. J Clin Exp Neuropsychol. 2016;38:941–9.
90. Merritt VC, Arnett PA. Apolipoprotein E (APOE) ε4 allele is associated with increased symptom reporting following sports concussion. J Int Neuropsychol Soc. 2016;22:89–94.

Semyon M. Slobounov
Wayne J. Sebastianelli
Alexa E. Walter

Contents

Part I Evaluation of Concussion

1 **Consequences of Ignorance and Arrogance for Mismanagement of Sports-Related Concussions: Short- and Long-Term Complications** 3
Robert C. Cantu and Madeline Uretsky

2 **Neuropsychological Testing in Sports Concussion Management: Test of an Evidence-Based Model When Baseline Is Unavailable** 19
Peter Arnett, Jessica Meyer, Victoria Merritt, Erin Guty, Kaitlin Riegler, and Garrett Thomas

3 **Feasibility of Virtual Reality for Assessment of Neurocognitive, Executive, and Motor Functions in Concussion**................... 37
Semyon M. Slobounov, Wayne J. Sebastianelli, Karl M. Newell, and Alexa E. Walter

4 **Feasibility of Electroencephalography for Direct Assessment of Concussion**.. 55
William J. Ray, Elizabeth Teel, Michael Gay, Semyon M. Slobounov, Robert Fornini, and Owen Griffith

Part II Biomechanics and Motor Control Mechanisms of Concussion

5 **Biomechanical Studies of Impact and Helmet Protection**........... 81
Andrew S. Mcintosh

6 **Acute and Lingering Impairments in Post-Concussion Postural Control** 95
Thomas A. Buckley, Kelsey N. Bryk, Katherine J. Hunzinger, and Alexander L. Enrique

7 **The Role of the Playing Surface in Mitigating the Deleterious Effects of Head Impacts in Field Sports**............ 119
Breana Cappuccilli, Nicolas Leiva-Molano, Thomas M. Talavage, and Eric A. Nauman

Part III Physiology of Concussion and Subconcussive Injuries

8 **Neuropathology of Mild Traumatic Brain Injury: Relationship to Structural Neuroimaging Findings** 147
Erin D. Bigler

9 **Advanced Neuroimaging of Mild Traumatic Brain Injury** 173
Zhifeng Kou and E. Mark Haacke

10 **Analytical Monitoring of Brain Metabolism: Not a Research Tool for Elite Academy but an Essential Issue for Return to Play Following Concussion** 193
Stefano Signoretti, Francesco Saverio Pastore, Barbara Tavazzi, Giuseppe Lazzarino, and Roberto Vagnozzi

11 **Functional Magnetic Resonance Imaging in Sport-Related Concussions** 221
Veronik Sicard, Danielle C. Hergert, and Andrew R. Mayer

12 **Sports-Related Subconcussive Head Trauma** 249
Brian D. Johnson

13 **Biomarkers for Concussion** 271
Linda Papa

14 **Genetics in Concussion** 285
Alexa E. Walter

Part IV Sport-Related Concussion in Pediatric Populations

15 **Predicting Postconcussive Symptoms After Mild Traumatic Brain Injury in Children and Adolescents: 2020 Update** 299
Keith Owen Yeates

16 **Long-Term Effects of Pediatric Mild Traumatic Brain Injury** 317
Rimma Danov

17 **Multimodal Approaches to Preventing Asymptomatic Repetitive Head Injury in Adolescent Athletes** 333
Thomas M. Talavage, Eric A. Nauman, and Taylor A. Lee

Part V Clinical Management and Rehabilitation of Concussions

18 **Management of Collegiate Sport-Related Concussions** 359
Allyssa K. Memmini, Vinodh Balendran, Steven E. Pachman, and Steven P. Broglio

19	**The Role of the Quantitative EEG (QEEG) in the Assessment and Treatment of the Brain Injured Individual**................... 377 Kirtley E. Thornton	
20	**Treatment of Sports-Related Concussion**....................... 389 Michael Gay	
21	**Narrowing the Knowledge Gap Between Basic Neuroscience Research and Management of Concussive Injury**................ 415 Jeffrey Wisinski, James R. Wilkes, and Peter H. Seidenberg	

Index... 435

Contributors

Peter Arnett, PhD Department of Psychology, Penn State University, University Park, PA, USA

Vinodh Balendran, BS Michigan Concussion Center, University of Michigan, Ann Arbor, MI, USA

Erin D. Bigler, PhD Department of Psychology and Neuroscience Center, Brigham Young University, Provo, UT, USA

Departments of Psychiatry and Neurology, University of Utah, Salt Lake City, UT, USA

Steven P. Broglio, PhD Michigan Concussion Center, University of Michigan, Ann Arbor, MI, USA

Kelsey N. Bryk, PhD Interdisciplinary Program in Biomechanics and Movement Science, Department of Kinesiology and Applied Physiology, University of Delaware, Newark, DE, USA

Thomas A. Buckley, EdD Interdisciplinary Program in Biomechanics and Movement Science, Department of Kinesiology and Applied Physiology, University of Delaware, Newark, DE, USA

Robert C. Cantu, MD Department of Neurosurgery, Emerson Hospital, Concord, MA, USA

Concussion Legacy Foundation, Boston, MA, USA

Boston University Alzheimer's Disease Research and Chronic Traumatic Encephalopathy Centers, Boston University School of Medicine, Boston, MA, USA

Departments of Neurology and Neurosurgery, Boston University School of Medicine, Boston, MA, USA

Breana Cappuccilli, MSc. Mechanical Engineering School of Mechanical Engineering, Purdue University, West Lafayette, IN, USA

Rimma Danov, PhD Private Neuropsychology Clinic, Brooklyn, NY, USA

Alexander L. Enrique, MS Interdisciplinary Program in Biomechanics and Movement Science, Department of Kinesiology and Applied Physiology, University of Delaware, Newark, DE, USA

Robert Fornini, BS Center for Sports Concussion Research and Services, Department of Kinesiology, Pennsylvania State University, University Park, PA, USA

Michael Gay, PhD, ATC Center for Sports Concussion Research and Services, Department of Kinesiology, Pennsylvania State University, University Park, PA, USA

Department of Intercollegiate Athletics, Penn State Center for Sports Concussion Research and Services, Penn State University, University Park, PA, USA

Owen Griffith, BS Center for Sports Concussion Research and Services, Department of Kinesiology, Pennsylvania State University, University Park, PA, USA

Erin Guty, MS Department of Psychology, Penn State University, University Park, PA, USA

E. Mark Haacke, PhD Department of Radiology, Wayne State University School of Medicine, Detroit, MI, USA

Danielle C. Hergert, PhD The Mind Research Network/Lovelace Biomedical and Environmental Research Institute, Albuquerque, NM, USA

Katherine J. Hunzinger, MS Interdisciplinary Program in Biomechanics and Movement Science, Department of Kinesiology and Applied Physiology, University of Delaware, Newark, DE, USA

Brian D. Johnson, PhD, MS, RT (MR)(N) Philips Healthcare, Gainesville, FL, USA

Department of Radiology, University of Texas Southwestern Medical Center, Dallas, TX, USA

Zhifeng Kou, PhD Departments of Biomedical Engineering and Radiology, Wayne State University School of Medicine, Detroit, MI, USA

Giuseppe Lazzarino, PhD Department of Biomedical and Biotechnological Sciences, Division of Medical Biochemistry, University of Catania, Catania, Italy

Taylor A. Lee, MS School of Mechanical Engineering, Purdue University, West Lafayette, IN, USA

Nicolas Leiva-Molano, MSc. Biomedical Engineering Weldon School of Biomedical Engineering, Purdue University, West Lafayette, IN, USA

Andrew R. Mayer, PhD The Mind Research Network/Lovelace Biomedical and Environmental Research Institute, Albuquerque, NM, USA

Department of Psychiatry and Behavioral Sciences, University of New Mexico, Albuquerque, NM, USA

Department of Neurology, University of New Mexico, Albuquerque, NM, USA

Department of Psychology, University of New Mexico, Albuquerque, NM, USA

Andrew S. Mcintosh, BAppSci (PT), MBiomedE, PhD McIntosh Consultancy and Research, Sydney, NSW, Australia

The Australian Centre for Research into Injury in Sport and its Prevention (ACRISP), School of Engineering, Edith Cowan University, Joondalup, WA, Australia

Allyssa K. Memmini, MS Michigan Concussion Center, University of Michigan, Ann Arbor, MI, USA

Victoria Merritt, PhD Department of Psychology, Penn State University, University Park, PA, USA

Jessica Meyer, PhD Department of Psychology, Penn State University, University Park, PA, USA

Eric A. Nauman, PhD School of Mechanical Engineering, Purdue University, West Lafayette, IN, USA

Weldon School of Biomedical Engineering, Purdue University, West Lafayette, IN, USA

Department of Basic Medical Sciences, Purdue University, West Lafayette, IN, USA

Karl M. Newell, PhD Department of Kinesiology, Pennsylvania State University, University Park, PA, USA

Steven E. Pachman, Esq. Montgomery McCracken Walker & Rhoads LLP, Philadelphia, PA, USA

Linda Papa, MD.CM, MSc Department of Emergency Medicine, Orlando Regional Medical Center, Orlando, FL, USA

University of Central Florida College of Medicine, Orlando, FL, USA

University of Florida College of Medicine, Gainesville, FL, USA

Florida State University College of Medicine, Tallahassee, FL, USA

Department of Neurology and Neurosurgery, McGill University, Montreal, QC, Canada

Francesco Saverio Pastore, MD, PhD Institute of Neurosurgery, Department of System's Medicine, University of Rome Tor Vergata, Rome, Italy

William J. Ray, PhD Center for Sports Concussion Research and Services, Department of Kinesiology, Pennsylvania State University, University Park, PA, USA

Kaitlin Riegler, MS Department of Psychology, Penn State University, University Park, PA, USA

Wayne J. Sebastianelli, MD Pennsylvania State University, University Park, PA, USA

Departments of Orthopaedics and Sports Medicine, Penn State Hershey, Bone and Joint Institute, State College, PA, USA

Peter H. Seidenberg, MD, MA Department of Family Medicine, Louisiana State University Health School of Medicine, Shreveport, LA, USA

Veronik Sicard, PhD The Mind Research Network/Lovelace Biomedical and Environmental Research Institute, Albuquerque, NM, USA

Stefano Signoretti, MD, PhD Division of Emergency-Urgency, UOC of Neurosurgery, S. Eugenio Hospital, Rome, Italy

Semyon M. Slobounov, PhD Center for Sports Concussion Research and Services, Department of Kinesiology and Neurosurgery, Pennsylvania State University, University Park, PA, USA

Thomas M. Talavage, PhD Department of Biomedical Engineering, University of Cincinnati, Cincinnati, OH, USA

Barbara Tavazzi, PhD Department of Basic Biotechnological Sciences, Intensive and Perioperative Clinics, Section of Biochemistry, Catholic University of Rome, Rome, Italy

Fondazione Policlinico Universitario Agostino Gemelli IRCCS, Rome, Italy

Elizabeth Teel, PhD Center for Sports Concussion Research and Services, Department of Kinesiology, Pennsylvania State University, University Park, PA, USA

Garrett Thomas, MS Department of Psychology, Penn State University, University Park, PA, USA

Kirtley E. Thornton, PhD The Neuroscience Center, Charlotte, NC, USA

Madeline Uretsky, BS Boston University Alzheimer's Disease Research and Chronic Traumatic Encephalopathy Centers, Boston University School of Medicine, Boston, MA, USA

Department of Neurology, Boston University School of Medicine, Boston, MA, USA

Roberto Vagnozzi, MD, PhD Institute of Neurosurgery, Department of System's Medicine, University of Rome Tor Vergata, Rome, Italy

Alexa E. Walter, PhD Department of Kinesiology, Pennsylvania State University, University Park, PA, USA

James R. Wilkes, PhD, MEd, ATC Department of Kinesiology, Penn State University, University Park, PA, USA

Jeffrey Wisinski, DO Penn State Health Orthopaedics and Sports Medicine, Penn State Health Family and Community Medicine, University Park, PA, USA

Keith Owen Yeates, PhD Department of Psychology, University of Calgary, Calgary, AB, Canada

Alberta Children's Hospital Research Institute, University of Calgary, Calgary, AB, Canada

Hotchkiss Brain Institute, University of Calgary, Calgary, AB, Canada

About the Editors

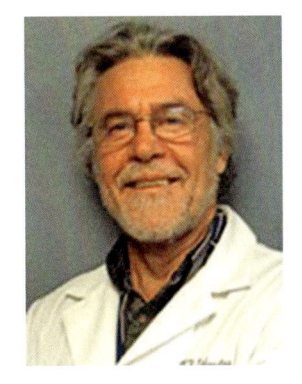

Semyon M. Slobounov is the director of the Virtual Reality/Traumatic Brain Injury research laboratory at Pennsylvania State University. He is a professor in the Department of Kinesiology, College of Health and Human Development, and an adjunct professor of Neurosurgery with Penn State Milton S. Hershey Medical Center. In addition to research, his primary responsibilities include teaching undergraduate and graduate courses in the areas of psychology of injury, neuropsychology, and psychophysiology. He received his first PhD from the University of Leningrad, Department of Medical Psychology, USSR, in 1978 and his second PhD from the University of Illinois at Urbana-Champaign, Department of Kinesiology, in 1994. Slobounov has an extensive coaching background and clinical experience working with numerous injured athletes for more than 30 years. His research focuses on the neural basis of human movements with special emphasis on rehabilitation medicine, neuroimaging, and neurophysiology, especially in regard to concussive injuries. He has published more than 120 papers in refereed journals including *Experimental Brain Research*, *Clinical Neurophysiology*, *Psychophysiology*, the *Journal of Neurotrauma, Neuroscience Letters*, and *Neuroimage*. He is the author/co-editor of three published books by Springer: *Foundations of Sport-Related Injuries*, *Injury in Athletics: Causes and Consequences*, and *Concussion in Athletics: From Brain to Behavior*. His research had been previously funded by the NIH, DOD, NCAA, and NFL Medical Charity grants.

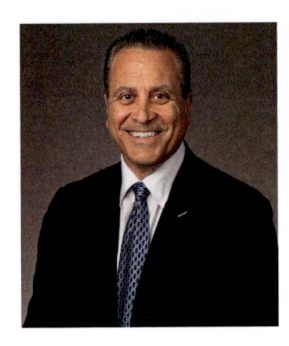

Wayne J. Sebastianelli is Associate Chief Medical Officer for Penn State Health, Centre County Region; Associate Dean for Clinical Affairs at the University Park Regional Campus; Kalenak Professor in Orthopaedics; Medical Director at Penn State Sports Medicine; and Director of Athletic Medicine at Penn State University. He is also the Chief of Staff at Mount Nittany Medical Center and Mount Nittany Surgical Center. He received his BA (1979) in Biology and Anthropology, Magna Cum Laude, and MD with honors (1983) from the University of Rochester. He completed his orthopaedic surgery residency in 1988 and his sports medicine fellowship at Hershey Medical Center in 1989. He became board certified in 1991 in Orthopaedic Surgery. Sebastianelli received his Subspecialty Certificate in Sports Medicine in 2007, the very first year it was created, the culmination of a rigorous evaluation and testing procedure recognizing excellence in his specialty.

Sebastianelli's research and teaching interests are in orthopaedic and sports medicine. His clinical interests are in knee, shoulder, ankle, hand, and ligament Surgery. Sebastianelli has served as a principal and co-investigator for several NIH grants including Investigation of Athletes at Risk for Traumatic Brain Injuries. Sebastianelli has co-authored several books, including *Foundations of Sports-Related Brain Injuries and Concussion in Athletics: From Brain to Behavior*. He has also published more than 85 articles in multiple peer-reviewed journals.

Sebastianelli is a member of multiple societies including the American Academy of Orthopaedic Surgeons, American Orthopaedic Association, American Medical Association, and American Orthopaedic Society for Sports Medicine. Sebastianelli is a manuscript reviewer for the *Journal of Orthopaedics and Sports Physical Therapy* and the *American Journal of Sports Medicine*. He is a long-time oral examiner for the American Board of Orthopaedic Surgery and serves on the Board of Directors for the American Board of Orthopaedic Surgery. Most recently, he was elected to the position of Second President-Elect on the Executive Committee of the American Orthopaedic Association.

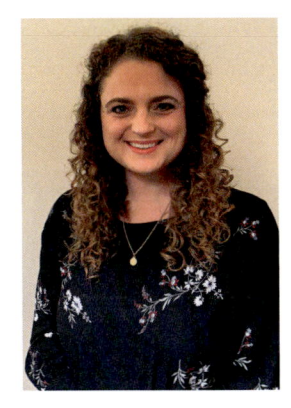

Alexa E. Walter is currently a postdoctoral fellow in the Department of Neurology, Center for Brain Injury and Repair, at the University of Pennsylvania Perelman School of Medicine. She graduated from Penn State University with a BS in Biology: Neuroscience (2015) and a PhD in Kinesiology (2020). At Penn State, she was involved in research and teaching, focusing on undergraduate courses related to psychology and neuroscience. Her research aimed to examine the susceptibility and resiliency to sports-related concussion and exposure to repetitive head impacts. Jointly, her work employed various techniques, ranging from clinically focused to more physiologically based approaches, to study the athletes involved in contact sports with the goal to begin to identify and distinguish factors that may differentiate individuals in regard to their susceptibility or resiliency to injury. Walter has published peer-reviewed articles in top-tier academic journals, contributed to textbooks, and presented at national and international conferences.

Part I

Evaluation of Concussion

Consequences of Ignorance and Arrogance for Mismanagement of Sports-Related Concussions: Short- and Long-Term Complications

Robert C. Cantu and Madeline Uretsky

Short-Term Risks of Concussion Mismanagement

It is fun to think about how history may have changed if we knew centuries ago what we now know. A number of drivers were praising, as we would too, Dale Earnhardt Jr. for bringing forward his concussion symptoms after the Talladega crash. He did this because he was aware himself, that he had had a concussion a few weeks before in Kansas, and had concerns about his health. Drivers that were commenting were saying that this just would not have happened 10 years ago and that is probably true. NASCAR drivers driving cars are similar to fighter pilots on wheels. Their reaction times and their vision need to be 100%. We are very glad to see that he brought concussion issues to doctors even though it cost his team a great deal of money.

R. C. Cantu (✉)
Department of Neurosurgery, Emerson Hospital, Concord, MA, USA

Concussion Legacy Foundation, Boston, MA, USA

Boston University Alzheimer's Disease Research and Chronic Traumatic Encephalopathy Centers, Boston University School of Medicine, Boston, MA, USA

Departments of Neurology and Neurosurgery, Boston University School of Medicine, Boston, MA, USA
e-mail: rcantu@emersonhosp.org

M. Uretsky
Boston University Alzheimer's Disease Research and Chronic Traumatic Encephalopathy Centers, Boston University School of Medicine, Boston, MA, USA

Department of Neurology, Boston University School of Medicine, Boston, MA, USA
e-mail: muretsky@bu.edu

So, What Are the Short-Term Risks of Mismanaging a Concussion?

The most common result of not imposing physical and cognitive rest after a concussion is greatly exacerbating concussion symptoms, and causing something that would have recovered in a matter of days to weeks into something that may now go on for months to years, and become post-concussive syndrome (PCS). Also, a much less common, but potentially fatal risk is *second impact syndrome* (SIS), which Bob Harbaugh and Dick Saunders first described in a *JAMA* article in 1984 [1]. It is interesting to us to see how our own practice has greatly changed in recent years, because of the awareness of concussions and PCS. We are actually inundated with post-concussive syndrome patients, most of whom have months of symptoms before we ever see them.

Approximately 8 years ago, one of my colleagues and I (R.C.C.), along with one of his graduate students, wrote a paper looking at a retrospective analysis of 215 consecutive post-concussion patients. Those that had post-concussive syndrome had a disproportionate amount of a history of multiple prior concussions, as opposed to this being their first injury [2]. Many of them took a double hit, which means your first hit may be to the head, and then you fall to the turf and slam your head a second time.

Double hits do seem to be associated with symptoms that last longer than a single hit and may actually involve rotational forces, which are in one direction, and then rebound in the other opposite direction. Some suggest we should be thinking of those rotational forces as being summated or added. We will leave that up to further research that the biomechanists are doing, but it is a very interesting theory and it does correlate with what we see [3, 4]. The most common occurrence with PCS is athletes who are playing while still symptomatic. We wrote a paper a few years ago, not about post-concussive syndrome, but catastrophic injuries. It was found that 38% of individuals were playing while still symptomatic from a previous head injury that was sustained that season [5]. We are finding the same thing with post-concussive syndrome.

Two young children cracking heads is unacceptable, and what we are realizing today, and what we are measuring today, are primarily linear forces. For several years, we have associated concussion risk being much higher with linear forces of 80–100 g. We have also seen from the work of Dr. Kevin Guskiewicz and others that just because you have 100 g impact, it is not necessarily associated with a concussion [6]. Conversely, concussions can occur with *g* forces that are well under 100 g. We now realize that it is not just those higher hits that are important. Today, we realize concussion occurrence is multifactorial and there is no known threshold of force required to produce symptoms. We also recognize that the tools measuring linear and rotational accelerations have significant accuracy challenges that contribute to the problem.

Various laboratory and clinical studies over the last 10 years have demonstrated that the subconcussive hits, those hits that do not result in overt clinical symptoms, count as well. Helmet accelerometer data for youth, high school, and college-level football players have shown the tremendous variability in the number of hits and repetitive trauma young people are taking over a single season. At the college level [7], while the mean is not terribly high, the extremes that the individuals are taking can be very high. Certainly at the high school level, over 1000 hits a season is not uncommon [8]. While every hit does not result in a symptomatic concussion, the accumulation of hits to the head over a single season, both in football and in soccer, has shown to result in changes in functional connectivity, decreased cognitive performance, white matter, and cerebrospinal fluid markers, demonstrating that seemingly routine and minor hits can have a profound impact [9]. We believe this emerging evidence should give us all cause for concern but of course needs to be replicated by other investigators. We have studies that show structural changes in individuals' brains that have headed more than 1300 times in a given soccer season as well [10].

It is not just metabolic magnetic resonance spectroscopy (MRS) studies that have shown changes, but diffusion tensor imaging (DTI) studies have also shown changes similarly when comparing baseline cognitive assessments prior to and after an athletic season. The integrity of fiber tracts tends to decrease over the course of the season [10, 11]. Presumably, this is due to subconcussive blows. Some of the studies have also used computer-based neuropsychological testing and found deterioration in the test scores over the course of the season when compared with baseline. By using neuropsychological, fiber tract, and metabolic data, there is a suggestion that it may be these subconcussive blows that are producing deleterious effects on brains. It is an accumulation of these data that led me, the senior author (R.C.C.), to write a book 8 years ago, and certainly the more controversial parts of the book are focusing on children in sports. I suggest taking tackle football away from youngsters *until the age of 14*, no body checking in ice hockey until the age of 14 (which has since led to the age moving from 11 to 13), and no heading in soccer until the age of 14 (which has since led to US Soccer banning headers under age 11 and limit heading for ages 11–13).

Further changes suggested were regarding helmets and officiating. It does not make sense that you have a very good batting helmet for baseball players, but then the helmet falls off of the players' heads as they round the bases. This subjects them to epidural hematomas due to skull fractures from a thrown ball, when it would be so simple to put a chin strap that holds the helmet on the head.

Also, in sports that do not have helmets right now, but the mechanism of injury is a focal blow, meaning a stick or ball to the head or face, like women's field hockey and lacrosse, we believe there should be helmets, rather than simply face shields. Additionally, we feel very strongly and passionately that we are giving our officials a pass they do not deserve. They should either start calling sports appropriately or they should be replaced.

With regard to neck strength, force equals mass times acceleration (g), or force divided by mass equals acceleration. Acceleration is what the brain is experiencing during a hit. If we look at it a different way, with change of velocity over time, you have a decreased opportunity for change in velocity with a well-developed neck. Dom Comstock and I (R.C.C.), as well as a few others, have been working for a number of years on a study, testing neck strength with regard to concussion incidence. The data have correlated that the strongest necks have the lowest number of concussions, and the weakest necks have the highest number of concussions. Others have found the same theory that neck strength reduces your risk of concussion [12, 13]. For example, the woodpecker has a large, strong neck, and it moves only in a linear straightforward manner—a woodpecker does not experience concussions. We strongly believe that any athlete who is involved with a contact or collision sport should strengthen their neck muscles as well as their other core muscles as much as they can. Youngsters and females do not have nearly the testosterone compared to adult males, and are not going to bulk up their neck muscles, so they are not going to look any different, but they can strengthen them.

We do not know the exact combination of linear and rotational forces necessary to reach threshold for a concussion, but we do know that there are curves which suggest that the risk of sustaining a concussion certainly increases as the linear forces go up. Many of us feel that the rotational forces are more important than the linear, and that is really what should be researched further. This is especially true in sports where the head is swiveled on the neck from a hit like a helmeted football, ice hockey, or lacrosse player. The reason that we believe that we do not yet have concussion thresholds despite a lot of good research is that we are not dealing with just biomechanical issues when we think about concussion. It is a complex situation. Yes, linear accelerations need to be known, and rotational accelerations would be ideally known as well. But duration of impact, location of impact, and tissue strain issues are all very relevant and in need of study.

However, there are also biological and social factors at play. There are rarely situations where the biological issues are matched up with the biomechanical situations to truly allow you to look at the whole picture when you talk about concussions. Some of these risk factors include history (how many concussions has somebody had, how severe were they, and what is the proximity in time of them), neck strength, age, gender (girls are more prone), hydration/volume (some science suggests that a dehydrated brain moves more inside the skull and is at greater risk of injury than a well-hydrated brain) [14, 15], as well as underreporting.

Concussions: Structural Versus Functional Brain Disorder

Expert neuropathologist and colleague Dr. Ann McKee has found diffuse axonal swelling and axonal damage in some individuals that have died by suicide shortly after a concussion. Concussion in part involves a neural metabolic cascade, a metabolic issue, but also in part, at least in some concussions, there is a *structural issue*. We believe that as we learn more through neuroimaging studies, like the use of DTI [16], we are going to be able to see those structural changes in concussion that we cannot currently see with routine clinical MRIs or CT scans.

Subjects' Reports Versus Pure Evaluation

It is common knowledge that concussions are prevalent without loss of consciousness more than 90% of the time, and that presents a problem. For those of us that have been on the sideline, and I (R.C.C.) was for a lot of years, it is not a great feeling knowing that we are probably missing multiple concussions for every one of which we are aware. Theoretically by asking after the season, when there is no longer a feeling of possibly letting down their coaches or teammates, the athlete will be more likely to give honest answers. The incidence of concussion reported by individuals from these post-event studies is six to seven times what is known on the sideline. Some years ago, we were a part of a Canadian study in which Paul Echlin was the lead author. This study looked at the incidence of concussion in junior "A" ice hockey that was reported from people on the bench, as opposed to physician observers in the stands. The physician observers in the stands had the responsibility of looking at people on the ice. When somebody got up slowly and seemed to have a problem but stayed in, they would go down between periods and examine them to determine if they had a concussion [17]. A seven times greater incidence of concussion was found from the physician observers, as compared with medical personnel on the bench [17].

The National Football League knows this is true as well; they instituted a policy in 2012 for the use of independent, certified athletic trainers to act as spotters in stadium booths at every game to spot potential injuries that are missed on the field, including concussions. Looking at the same television feeds that the public sees when we watch the game on television, the same feeds are now fed to the medical personnel on the sideline to be used as part of the concussion assessment. When this was deemed insufficient, the 2017–2018 NFL season introduced the placement of an unaffiliated neurotrauma consultant (UNC) in the league's command center for all games, and later on-site UNCs. There have been multiple examples of individuals who were sent off the field, and a body part was examined that was not the head, when it was a concussion that they had sustained. Former Cleveland Browns quarterback Colt McCoy is the most notable of them.

I am very pleased that Dr. Chris Nowinski, co-founder of the Concussion Legacy Foundation (formerly the Sports Legacy Institute), and I (R.C.C.) held a meeting, dedicated to documenting the number of impacts occurring as well as potentially identifying what the threshold number should be for cumulative hits. We know that the numbers that youngsters are receiving are appreciable, with published data showing that roughly 60–70% of those hits in the past have occurred during practice [18].

Coaching Preventive Strategies

If you change the way that practice occurs, you can dramatically reduce the number of hits individuals are taking to the head. The *winningest* college coach in this country is John Gagliardi from St. John University outside of Minneapolis St. Paul. He has over 800 victories, and during the season over the last 50 years he has never allowed tackling, only games are full contact. During practice the skill drills are all done with people thud tackling, wrapping arms around but not bringing players to the ground. Similarly, Dartmouth College football uses tackling dummies and even a tackling robot in practices so that they are not hitting each other. The NFL certainly gets that message too, because in the collective bargaining agreement during the 18-week long NFL season, players can only hit 14 times, less than once a week! Things are changing, and what we are doing is taking the head trauma out of practice.

We protect little league pitcher's arms with good intentions, without question, when we limit the number of pitches they can throw. However, medial collateral ulnar ligaments can be replaced and the arms can come back from high school to pitch in the big leagues. There are many examples of that including some big league players that are on their third Tommy John surgery operation, and still pitching in the big leagues. For a correctable condition, we have pitch counts for youngsters. We think there should be hit counts to the head because obviously the brain cannot be replaced. We can modify how practices occur, and to their credit, Pop Warner football has reduced drastically the amount of hitting that they allow in practice.

Second Impact Syndrome

SIS [19, 20] is simply an individual that has sustained an initial brain injury, who while still symptomatic sustains another brain injury that may be incredibly mild. What usually happens is that within minutes, there is a loss of autoregulation, which leads to massive blood flow inside the head and increasing intracranial brain pressure. It is the capillary beds in our brain that have the ability to be dilated and hold extra blood, as do the arterials. In *SIS* this autoregulation, which keeps a constant flow of blood to our brain, is disrupted. In a normal situation, if your blood pressure goes up, you find a constriction occurring in the arterial bed to keep a constant amount of blood flowing to the capillaries, and then to the tissue that needs it. On the other hand, the blood pressure returns to normal and the arterials go back to their normal size keeping the same amount of blood flow. When blood pressure goes down, we have dilation in that arterial bed to keep the same amount of blood in your capillaries.

With *SIS*, the autoregulation is lost, and with blood pressures that are normal or even above normal because of adrenaline flowing from either pain or exertion, you find dilation in the arterial bed [19]. When that happens with normal or heightened blood pressure, you have a massive accumulation of blood in the capillaries of the brain. The brain inside the skull houses spinal fluid, brain, and blood. If you quickly increase the amount of blood that is inside the blood vessels, you will increase intracranial pressure and cause brain herniation. Essentially, that is what we are seeing happen. *SIS* is usually bilateral and symmetrical, but it can occur unilaterally, and it can occur with a small sliver of subdural hematoma [19]. The subdural is not causing much mass effect; however, it is this vascular engorgement of the brain that is causing detrimental outcomes. This is not vasogenic edema, because there is gray and white matter differentiation. It is a drastic increase in the volume of the brain due to blood in the arteriolar-capillary bed.

Long-Term Risks of Mismanaging Multiple Concussions

Historical Perspective

One of the long-term risks is prolonging your post-concussion syndrome if a concussion is mismanaged, and the other is the issue of chronic traumatic encephalopathy (CTE). CTE is a distinct, progressive, neurodegenerative disease characterized by a pathognomonic lesion of *hyperphosphorylated tau protein* accumulated around blood vessels at the depths of cortical sulci believed to develop due to, at least in part, to repetitive head impacts (RHI) [21, 22].

Do you know who first described CTE? I (R.C.C.) asked this question recently at a conference, and immediately a hand went up and said Bennett Omalu. He did describe the first cases of CTE in National Football League players [23, 24], but not the distinct pathology or the associated clinical syndrome itself. In 1928, forensic pathologist Dr. Harrison Martland described "punch drunk," the clinical syndrome of boxers, which is akin to the clinical features of traumatic encephalopathy syndrome (TES) seen today in CTE [25], but without using those words. In a book that was a tribute to Clovis Vincent that came out in 1949, a number of individuals were solicited to write chapters, and in the book, there was one chapter written in English. In that volume, the CTE of boxers was written by Macdonald Critchley (1949); therefore, it was the first time that the neurological syndrome of boxers was described as "chronic traumatic encephalopathy." Pathologically, the first description was by Corsellis in 1973, who connected neuropathological findings to a retrospective pattern of behaviors seen in a sample of 15 retired boxers. Since Martland first described the disease in 1928, until Dr. Omalu's report in 2005, there were fewer than 50 confirmed cases of CTE in the literature; there are now nearly 400 published cases. However, there are only three confirmed cases of women with CTE—one with a history of domestic violence described in 1990 by Dr. Roberts, one in 1991 by Dr. Hof with a history of autistic head-banging behaviors, and one in 2021 of a 29-year-old with a history of domestic violence.

Boston University School of Medicine Chronic Traumatic Encephalopathy Center

At Boston University School of Medicine, we started with four directors at the Center for the Study of Traumatic Encephalopathy in 2008 (now the BU CTE Center), a part of the BU Alzheimer's Disease Research Center, which was established in 1996 [26]. Original directors included Chris Nowinski, concussion advocate and former professional wrestler, neuropathologist Dr. Ann McKee, famous for her work in neurodegenerative disease, Dr. Bob Stern, neuropsychologist and clinical research director, and myself (R.C.C.). The Center was established to focus on the study of repetitive head impacts, including the clinical and pathological features associated with contact sport play and military service. Partnerships with the Boston VA Healthcare System, as well as the Concussion Legacy Foundation (formerly Sports Legacy Institute), enhanced collaboration and formation of the VA-BU-CLF Brain Bank, now the largest tissue repository in the world dedicated to the study of CTE. We established an online brain donation registry in 2015 to de-mystify and normalize the process of brain donation; this registry now has over 6,000 people enrolled. We are hoping to register and study brains of asymptomatic individuals that live normal lives, and yet play contact sports. The brain donation registry has greatly accelerated brain donation post-mortem. In the early stages of the Center, we were examining just a handful of cases a year. We have since received over 100 donations in each of the last 3 years. At this time, the VA-BU-CLF Brain Bank houses over 1,000 brains of former athletes and military veterans, the vast majority of whom were symptomatic. Donors range in age from 13 to 99, from youth through professional and Olympic levels of play and 98% are men. Additionally, as a neurodegenerative disease brain bank, it is quite striking that 35% of our donors are under the age of 50. While the majority of donations are from former football players (about 70%), we are increasingly receiving a wider variety of athletes, including several lacrosse, soccer, and rugby players, as well as motocross and BMXers, and amateur wrestlers. Most of these people were symptomatic and were predicted to have CTE by their emotional, behavioral, and cognitive symptoms reported by family members upon donation.

The VA-BU-CLF Brain Bank currently lacks a repository of brains of individuals that were not symptomatic, but they will likely come from that registry. Dr. Stern as P.I., along with Dr. Nowinski, Dr. McKee, myself (R.C.C.), and a crew of graduate students, are doing a longitudinal clinical research study on over a hundred NFL players compared to a group of individuals with no recognized brain trauma over the course of their lives. Structural issues using a variety of MRI modalities, magnetic spectroscopy, DTI, volume averaging MRI, and biomarkers are being used to see whether or not we can have a profile that correlates highly enough to make a diagnosis of CTE in living people. Dr. Stern is also one of the P.I.s on the NIH-funded DIAGNOSE CTE Research Project, a larger, multisite study examining college and NFL players and age-matched controls. Currently, CTE can only be diagnosed with certainty after death. You can actually have a very high clinical suspicion if the right clinical profile is there, as demonstrated by the high rate of CTE in our brain bank, but you cannot be 100% certain until a neuropathological examination is performed.

Dr. McKee's first case was John Grimsley in 2008, a former NFL player who had advanced CTE. The medial temporal lobe was just riddled with this staining identifying *hyperphosphorylated tau protein*. Other notable NFL players examined by Dr. McKee, and that were later publicized, were Dave Duerson, Cookie Gilchrist, Bubba Smith, John Mackey, Ken Stabler, Aaron Hernandez, and three members of the 1972 Miami Dolphins, Bill Stanfill, Earl Morrall, and Bob Kuechenberg. An important study from 2012 by Lehman et al. examined causes of mortality in former NFL players [27]. They looked at death certificates of a number of NFL players who played over a 10-year period, and they all had to play 5 years or more to be included in the study. When looking at the death certificates of these individuals, they found that the incidence of Alzheimer's disease and amyotrophic lateral sclerosis (omitting Parkinson's disease) was four times higher than what would have been predicted by the national average. These brains were not studied, only the death certificates were examined. These death certificates are filled out by a doctor, which is never a happy task—and often a task that subsequently ends up being done as quickly as possible. This leads the information to not necessarily be as thorough as one would hope, particularly when Alzheimer's disease can look like CTE.

We do not know from our work in Boston what the incidence of CTE is, and what the prevalence of it is in any population. We know it occurs, and we know that it occurs in a very high percentage of those brains that we examine, but we also know that those brains are in a skewed sample. However, just because a sample is skewed toward symptomatic, high-level exposed individuals does not mean that the work is invalid. In fact, there have been a number of extremely valuable studies over the last few years using VA-BU-CLF Brain Bank data.

We published our first case series of autopsy-confirmed CTE in 2009, where we reviewed 48 cases of boxers, football players, wrestlers, and others with repetitive head impacts [21]. Subsequent papers over the last 10 years have examined the pathology in depth, as well as the various risk factors that we think are involved. Many of these studies examining risk factors, both antemortem in clinical studies, and post-mortem using donated brain tissue, have been led by additional BU colleagues Dr. Jesse Mez, Dr. Michael Alosco, Dr. Jon Cherry, Dr. Lee Goldstein, Dr. Dan Daneshvar, and Dr. Thor Stein. CTE in the context of motor neuron disease [28], epidemiological considerations with concussion [29], subconcussive head trauma [30], military blast exposure [31], clinical presentation [32], research criteria for traumatic encephalopathy syndrome [25], age of first exposure to football and later-life impairments [33–35], corpus callosum and white matter microstructural changes [36, 37], beta-amyloid deposition [38], inflammation [39, 40], MRI, MRS, and PET imaging markers [41–45], cerebrospinal fluid markers [46, 47], Lewy bodies [48], cerebral amyloid angiopathy [49], genetics [46, 50], and duration of play [8, 51, 52] have all been described. Dr. McKee has also led the international effort to characterize the neuropathology of the disease through a series of consensus conferences that have brought together the world's leading experts in tauopathies.

Doctor, Do I Have CTE?

CTE in most people is a progressive neurodegenerative disease believed to be caused by repetitive trauma to the brain which includes subconcussive blows. This is NOT a prolonged post-concussive syndrome, nor is it solely the cumulative effects of concussions. Symptoms characteristically, although not always, begin years to decades after the individual has stopped sustaining brain trauma. One sport with a fairly high incidence of CTE is boxing. It is fairly common that individuals in their 30s have already started to lose some foot speed, developed slurred speech, etc. We need to know about the risk factors for CTE, and we need to know how we can differentiate them from other neurodegenerative diseases, psychiatric conditions, and post-concussive syndrome before being able to diagnose the disease in living people. The Center receives countless calls and emails every week from families and individuals concerned they have CTE. We always suggest seeing a neurologist, neuropsychologist, or other professional experienced in treating brain trauma to treat the symptoms, which may or may not be associated with CTE. There is no treatment for CTE, but there are ways to manage symptoms and everyday life with neurological and psychiatric conditions [53]. Building a strong network of support from family and friends, eating healthy foods to properly fuel the brain, getting enough sleep, exercising appropriately, and finding meaningful hobbies and activities are just some of the ways in which individuals and families can cope with symptoms. Unfortunately, many cases of CTE have been reported due to those individuals dying by suicide. Suicide is associated with head trauma, including concussion. In terms of increased incidence, it is also associated with CTE; however, we do not yet fully understand all of the factors involved, as suicide in itself is a complex issue. It is certain that we do not know the prevalence or incidence of the disease, but we certainly know that we do not want to see any more of our heroes having their brains examined because of suicide.

In Summary: 10 Myths About Concussion

Myth Number One: You Have to Be Hit in the Head to Have a Concussion

We think that most people now know this is not true. Just from whiplash you can have a concussion, from a blow to your back that snaps your head back or a blow to your chest which snaps it forward, or from a fall on your butt where the forces go up the spine. Of course, when we look at our blast victims, at least in our models, it is not the pressure wave that is producing the concussion. It is the blast winds that are associated with it that are causing the head to shake violently and oscillate 10–14 times. This event can give somebody a lifetime of concussions from one blast.

Myth Number Two: You Have to Be Rendered Unconscious to Sustain a Concussion

More than 90% of athletic concussions do not involve loss of consciousness.

Myth Number Three: Helmets Prevent Concussions

It is possible this could be true, if it were big enough, paired with enough energy attenuating materials maybe, but it is not practical. This would also be putting the neck at risk, so it is not going to happen. We are, however, getting better helmets all the time, and I (R.C.C.) personally am a strong advocate of going in that direction and not going in the direction of less protection. It is amazing how topics such as this have made their way into the media, because they are things that society in general needs to think about and know.

Myth Number Four: Mouth Guards Prevent Concussions

No, it is not only mouth guards that claim to prevent concussions, but headbands and a plethora of unproven products too. While we encourage research in concussion prevention, we are against claims that cannot be substantiated.

Myth Number Five: You Can Always See a Concussion

You can always see if somebody is unconscious or if they cannot stand up, but you are not going to see most concussions. Most concussions are subtle, and it takes time, especially with mild concussions, to sort out whether somebody has had one or not.

Myth Number Six: Your Next Concussion Will Be Worse Than Your Last

Wrong. A professional ice hockey player I (R.C.C.) cared for had his first concussion that consisted of four and a half months of symptoms, causing him to lose a season. With his second concussion, he experienced 2 weeks of symptoms, lost a month of playing, and was back playing the rest of that season. With his third concussion, he had 4 days of symptoms and was back in 2 weeks. That was an exception, and it is not usually what we see, but it demonstrates that every concussion is unique. You cannot predict what the next one is going to be, unless somebody is on a trajectory that they are more easily concussed and each concussion is lasting longer.

Myth Number Seven: Three Concussions and You Are Out

This myth really frustrates us because it is essentially saying in a very naive way that all concussions are created equally, when they are not. Concussions are not created equally, and each one needs to be handled on an individual basis. We strongly believe that you need to record in verbiage how long the symptoms lasted with each concussion. This way in the future, others working on managing an individual's concussion can have an idea about how severe their previous concussions were. If symptoms lasted months, that is not the same injury as symptoms that lasted hours or only a day. It is ultimately a combination of factors, and a larger discussion between a patient, provider, and the family in deciding to retire from contact sports.

Myth Number Eight: Signs and Symptoms Occur Immediately

Incorrect. Some individuals have very little in the way of symptoms immediately, and some are not aware that they have had a concussion immediately. How much of that is related to adrenaline and rationalization we are not sure, but it is a reality that many people worsen hours after the incident. Some may not have symptoms really worsen until later that night or the next morning.

Myth Number Nine: Boys Suffer More Concussions Than Girls

The number of girls are now almost equal to boys in most sports, in part due to Title IX legislation in the 1970s. In ice hockey, basketball, and soccer, in fact, girls have almost twice as many recognized concussions as boys. We stress "recognized" and keep repeating it because we do not really know that they have twice as many concussions; but twice as many are recorded. It is possible that this is due to the fact that they are more honest in reporting their symptoms, or due to their weak necks. It could also be both, but only time and research will tell.

Myth Number Ten: Concussions Determine Risk of CTE

This has not shown to be true in the work we have done at the VA-BU-CLF Brain Bank. Our work suggests that individuals that take the greatest amount of brain trauma are most likely to wind up with CTE, not the people that suffered spectacular concussions. We have found the best measure of repetitive head impacts, or concussion and subconcussive blows combined, to be the length of one's playing career. If you play in a sport that takes a higher amount of brain trauma, like boxing or football, you are going to have a greater chance for CTE than if you play a sport like basketball which has less head trauma. If you play football, the linemen are going to take a lot more hits to the head than the wide receivers or the quarterbacks, although the wide receivers and the quarterbacks may take a more spectacular hit. In a sport like ice hockey, you are going to take hits equal to or greater than a football player occasionally, but not as frequently. As we accumulate more and more cases going forward at the Brain Bank, we expect to see a similar trend—that boxing seems to have the greatest incidence and football is second. Sports like ice hockey, rugby, lacrosse, and soccer, although they certainly have cases of CTE, now appear to have a lower risk for CTE, but various risk factors other than contact sport participation are still being studied.

Acknowledgments We gratefully acknowledge all of the collaborative efforts that have made this work possible, including the faculty and staff at the Boston University School of Medicine Chronic Traumatic Encephalopathy Center, the Dr. Robert C. Cantu Concussion Center at Emerson Hospital, the Concussion Legacy Foundation, and all of the patients, brain donors, and donor families.

References

1. Saunders RL, Harbaugh RE. The second impact in catastrophic contact-sports head trauma. JAMA. 1984;252(4):538–9.
2. Cantu RC, Guskiewicz K, Register-Mihalik JK. A retrospective clinical analysis of moderate to severe athletic concussions. PM R. 2010;2(12):1088–93.
3. Tagge CA, Fisher AM, Minaeva OV, Gaudreau-Balderrama A, Moncaster JA, Zhang X-L, et al. Concussion, microvascular injury, and early tauopathy in young athletes after impact head injury and an impact concussion mouse model. Brain. 2018;141(2):422–58.
4. Mihalik JP, Guskiewicz KM, Marshall SW, Blackburn JT, Cantu RC, Greenwald RM. Head impact biomechanics in youth hockey: comparisons across playing position, event types, and impact locations. Ann Biomed Eng. 2012;40(1):141–9.
5. Boden BP, Tacchetti RL, Cantu RC, Knowles SB, Mueller FO. Catastrophic head injuries in high school and college football players. Am J Sports Med. 2007;35(7):1075–81.
6. Guskiewicz KM, Mihalik JP, Shankar V, Marshall SW, Crowell DH, Oliaro SM, et al. Measurement of head impacts in collegiate football players: relationship between head impact biomechanics and acute clinical outcome after concussion. Neurosurgery. 2007;61(6):1244–52.
7. Rowson S, Duma SM, Greenwald RM, Beckwith JG, Chu JJ, Guskiewicz KM, et al. Can helmet design reduce the risk of concussion in football? J Neurosurg. 2014;120(4):919–22.
8. Montenigro PH, Alosco ML, Martin BM, Daneshvar DH, Mez J, Chaisson CE, et al. Cumulative head impact exposure predicts later-life depression, apathy, executive dysfunction, and cognitive impairment in former high school and college football players. J Neurotrauma. 2017;34(2):328–40.
9. Cantu RC. Role of diffusion tensor imaging MRI in detecting brain injury in asymptomatic contact athletes. World Neurosurg. 2013;80(6):792–3.
10. Lipton ML, Kim N, Zimmerman ME, Kim M, Stewart WF, Branch CA, et al. Soccer heading is associated with white matter microstructural and cognitive abnormalities. Radiology. 2013;268(3):850–7.
11. Shenton ME, Hamoda HM, Schneiderman JS, Bouix S, Pasternak O, Rathi Y, et al. A review of magnetic resonance imaging and diffusion tensor imaging findings in mild traumatic brain injury. Brain Imaging Behav. 2012;6(2):137–92.
12. Collins CL, Fletcher EN, Fields SK, Kluchurosky L, Rohrkemper MK, Comstock RD, et al. Neck strength: a protective factor reducing risk for concussion in high school sports. J Prim Prev. 2014;35(5):309–19.
13. Schmidt JD, Guskiewicz KM, Blackburn JT, Mihalik JP, Siegmund GP, Marshall SW. The influence of cervical muscle characteristics on head impact biomechanics in football. Am J Sports Med. 2014;42(9):2056–66.
14. Lariviere K, Bureau S, Marshall C, Holahan MR. Interaction between age, sex, and mental health status as precipitating factors for symptom presentation in concussed individuals. J Sports Med Hindawi Publ Corp. 2019;2019:9207903.
15. Patel AV, Mihalik JP, Notebaert AJ, Guskiewicz KM, Prentice WE. Neuropsychological performance, postural stability, and symptoms after dehydration. J Athl Train. 2007;42(1):66–75.

16. Bigler ED, Maxwell WL. Neuropathology of mild traumatic brain injury: relationship to neuroimaging findings. Brain Imaging Behav. 2012;6(2):108–36.
17. Echlin PS, Tator CH, Cusimano MD, Cantu RC, Taunton JE, Upshur REG, et al. A prospective study of physician-observed concussions during junior ice hockey: implications for incidence rates. Neurosurg Focus. 2010;29(5):E4.
18. Campolettano ET, Rowson S, Duma SM. Drill-specific head impact exposure in youth football practice. J Neurosurg Pediatr. 2016;18(5):536–41.
19. Cantu RC, Gean AD. Second-impact syndrome and a small subdural hematoma: an uncommon catastrophic result of repetitive head injury with a characteristic imaging appearance. J Neurotrauma. 2010;27(9):1557–64.
20. Cantu RC. Dysautoregulation/second-impact syndrome with recurrent athletic head injury. World Neurosurg. 2016;95:601–2.
21. McKee AC, Cantu RC, Nowinski CJ, Hedley-Whyte ET, Gavett BE, Budson AE, et al. Chronic traumatic encephalopathy in athletes: progressive tauopathy following repetitive head injury. J Neuropathol Exp Neurol. 2009;68(7):709–35.
22. McKee AC, Cairns NJ, Dickson DW, Folkerth RD, Keene CD, Litvan I, et al. The first NINDS/NIBIB consensus meeting to define neuropathological criteria for the diagnosis of chronic traumatic encephalopathy. Acta Neuropathol (Berl). 2016;131(1):75–86.
23. Omalu BI, DeKosky ST, Minster RL, Kamboh MI, Hamilton RL, Wecht CH. Chronic traumatic encephalopathy in a National Football League player. Neurosurgery. 2005;57(1):128–34.
24. Omalu BI, DeKosky ST, Hamilton RL, Minster RL, Kamboh MI, Shakir AM, et al. Chronic traumatic encephalopathy in a National Football League player: part II. Neurosurgery. 2006;59(5):1086–92.
25. Montenigro PH, Baugh CM, Daneshvar DH, Mez J, Budson AE, Au R, et al. Clinical subtypes of chronic traumatic encephalopathy: literature review and proposed research diagnostic criteria for traumatic encephalopathy syndrome. Alzheimers Res Ther. 2014;6(5):68.
26. Baugh CM, Stamm JM, Riley DO, Gavett BE, Shenton ME, Lin A, et al. Chronic traumatic encephalopathy: neurodegeneration following repetitive concussive and subconcussive brain trauma. Brain Imaging Behav. 2012;6(2):244–54.
27. Le MN, Kim W, Lee S, McKee AC, Hall GF. Multiple mechanisms of extracellular tau spreading in a non-transgenic tauopathy model. Am J Neurodegener Dis. 2012;1(3):316–33.
28. McKee AC, Gavett BE, Stern RA, Nowinski CJ, Cantu RC, Kowall NW, et al. TDP-43 proteinopathy and motor neuron disease in chronic traumatic encephalopathy. J Neuropathol Exp Neurol. 2010;69(9):918–29.
29. Daneshvar DH, Nowinski CJ, McKee AC, Cantu RC. The epidemiology of sport-related concussion. Clin Sports Med. 2011;30(1):1–17.
30. Gavett BE, Stern RA, McKee AC. Chronic traumatic encephalopathy: a potential late effect of sport-related concussive and subconcussive head trauma. Clin Sports Med. 2011;30(1):179–88.
31. Goldstein LE, Fisher AM, Tagge CA, Zhang X-L, Velisek L, Sullivan JA, et al. Chronic traumatic encephalopathy in blast-exposed military veterans and a blast neurotrauma mouse model. Sci Transl Med. 2012;4(134):134ra60.
32. Stern RA, Daneshvar DH, Baugh CM, Seichepine DR, Montenigro PH, Riley DO, et al. Clinical presentation of chronic traumatic encephalopathy. Neurology. 2013;81(13):1122–9.
33. Stamm JM, Bourlas AP, Baugh CM, Fritts NG, Daneshvar DH, Martin BM, et al. Age of first exposure to football and later-life cognitive impairment in former NFL players. Neurology. 2015;84(11):1114–20.
34. Alosco ML, Mez J, Tripodis Y, Kiernan PT, Abdolmohammadi B, Murphy L, et al. Age of first exposure to tackle football and chronic traumatic encephalopathy. Ann Neurol. 2018;83(5):886–901.
35. Alosco ML, Kasimis AB, Stamm JM, Chua AS, Baugh CM, Daneshvar DH, et al. Age of first exposure to American football and long-term neuropsychiatric and cognitive outcomes. Transl Psychiatry. 2017;7(9):e1236.

36. Stamm JM, Koerte IK, Muehlmann M, Pasternak O, Bourlas AP, Baugh CM, et al. Age at first exposure to football is associated with altered corpus callosum white matter microstructure in former professional football players. J Neurotrauma. 2015;32(22):1768–76.
37. Alosco ML, Stein TD, Tripodis Y, Chua AS, Kowall NW, Huber BR, et al. Association of white matter rarefaction, arteriolosclerosis, and tau with dementia in chronic traumatic encephalopathy. JAMA Neurol. 2019;
38. Stein TD, Montenigro PH, Alvarez VE, Xia W, Crary JF, Tripodis Y, et al. Beta-amyloid deposition in chronic traumatic encephalopathy. Acta Neuropathol (Berl). 2015;130(1):21–34.
39. Cherry JD, Stein TD, Tripodis Y, Alvarez VE, Huber BR, Au R, et al. CCL11 is increased in the CNS in chronic traumatic encephalopathy but not in Alzheimer's disease. PLoS One. 2017;12(9):e0185541.
40. Cherry JD, Tripodis Y, Alvarez VE, Huber B, Kiernan PT, Daneshvar DH, et al. Microglial neuroinflammation contributes to tau accumulation in chronic traumatic encephalopathy. Acta Neuropathol Commun. 2016;4(1):112.
41. Koerte IK, Hufschmidt J, Muehlmann M, Tripodis Y, Stamm JM, Pasternak O, et al. Cavum septi pellucidi in symptomatic former professional football players. J Neurotrauma. 2016;33(4):346–53.
42. Alosco ML, Tripodis Y, Koerte IK, Jackson JD, Chua AS, Mariani M, et al. Interactive effects of racial identity and repetitive head impacts on cognitive function, structural MRI-derived volumetric measures, and cerebrospinal fluid tau and Aβ. Front Hum Neurosci. 2019;13:440.
43. Alosco ML, Koerte IK, Tripodis Y, Mariani M, Chua AS, Jarnagin J, et al. White matter signal abnormalities in former National Football League players. Alzheimers Dement Amst Neth. 2018;10:56–65.
44. Schultz V, Stern RA, Tripodis Y, Stamm J, Wrobel P, Lepage C, et al. Age at first exposure to repetitive head impacts is associated with smaller thalamic volumes in former professional American football players. J Neurotrauma. 2017;35(2):278–85.
45. Stern RA, Adler CH, Chen K, Navitsky M, Luo J, Dodick DW, et al. Tau positron-emission tomography in former National Football League Players. N Engl J Med. 2019;380(18):1716–25.
46. Alosco ML, Tripodis Y, Fritts NG, Heslegrave A, Baugh CM, Conneely S, et al. Cerebrospinal fluid tau, Aβ, and sTREM2 in former National Football League players: modeling the relationship between repetitive head impacts, microglial activation, and neurodegeneration. Alzheimers Dement J Alzheimers Assoc. 2018;23
47. Alosco ML, Tripodis Y, Jarnagin J, Baugh CM, Martin B, Chaisson CE, et al. Repetitive head impact exposure and later-life plasma total tau in former National Football League players. Alzheimers Dement Amst Neth. 2017;7:33–40.
48. Adams JW, Alvarez VE, Mez J, Huber BR, Tripodis Y, Xia W, et al. Lewy body pathology and chronic traumatic encephalopathy associated with contact sports. J Neuropathol Exp Neurol. 2018;77(9):757–68.
49. Standring OJ, Friedberg J, Tripodis Y, Chua AS, Cherry JD, Alvarez VE, et al. Contact sport participation and chronic traumatic encephalopathy are associated with altered severity and distribution of cerebral amyloid angiopathy. Acta Neuropathol (Berl). 2019;138(3):401–13.
50. Cherry JD, Mez J, Crary JF, Tripodis Y, Alvarez VE, Mahar I, et al. Variation in TMEM106B in chronic traumatic encephalopathy. Acta Neuropathol Commun. 2018;6(1):115.
51. Mez J, Daneshvar DH, Abdolmohammadi B, Chua AS, Alosco ML, Kiernan PT, et al. Duration of American football play and chronic traumatic encephalopathy. Ann Neurol. 2020;87(1):116–31.
52. Mez J, Daneshvar DH, Kiernan PT, Abdolmohammadi B, Alvarez VE, Huber BR, et al. Clinicopathological evaluation of chronic traumatic encephalopathy in players of American football. JAMA. 2017;318(4):360–70.
53. Cantu R, Budson A. Management of chronic traumatic encephalopathy. Expert Rev Neurother. 2019;19(10):1015–23.

Neuropsychological Testing in Sports Concussion Management: Test of an Evidence-Based Model When Baseline Is Unavailable

Peter Arnett, Jessica Meyer, Victoria Merritt, Erin Guty, Kaitlin Riegler, and Garrett Thomas

Introduction

Barth and colleagues' [1] seminal study using baseline neuropsychological testing as a model for sports concussion management set a standard that continues to be influential today. Many school-based sports medicine programs have adopted variations of their approach, and a range of recommendations have been made for the use of neuropsychological testing within that framework. Although the literature is variable regarding how best to use neuropsychological testing, most investigators recommend the use of pre-injury baseline neuropsychological testing as the best practice for sports concussion management [1–7]. Still, baseline data are not always available, and there is recognition that guidelines are needed for interpretation in such cases. In their "Consensus Statement on Concussion in Sport" article, McCrory and colleagues [6] suggested that an important area for future research was determining "best-practice" neuropsychological testing in cases where baseline data are not available. Also, in a position paper published under the aegis of the National Academy of Neuropsychology (NAN), Moser et al. [3] noted that neurocognitive tests can play a meaningful role in concussion management even in the absence of baseline testing. Nonetheless, neither article provides guidelines for how neuropsychological tests should be used when no baseline testing has been conducted. The most recent consensus statement published by McCrory and colleagues [8] indicated that baseline or preseason neuropsychological testing should not be mandatory, but also stating that it could be helpful in some situations. The consensus panel also indicated that conducting neuropsychological testing post concussion would be optimal.

The central goal of this chapter is to provide a test of the evidence-based model for using neuropsychological testing in the management of sports-related concussion when no baseline is available that we laid out in our chapter in the first edition

---

P. Arnett (✉) · J. Meyer · V. Merritt · E. Guty · K. Riegler · G. Thomas
Department of Psychology, Penn State University, University Park, PA, USA
e-mail: paa6@psu.edu

© Springer Nature Switzerland AG 2021
S. M. Slobounov, W. J. Sebastianelli (eds.), *Concussions in Athletics*,
https://doi.org/10.1007/978-3-030-75564-5_2

of this book. We first summarize and evaluate existing approaches, focusing on the merits and limitations of baseline testing, the timing of testing post concussion, and the additional value of neuropsychological tests in a sports concussion context. We then lay out the framework of our model and provide a test of it using five cognitive outcome variables not included in the algorithm itself by comparing "Recovered" and "Not Recovered" groups based upon the algorithm. It is not our intent to suggest that the model presented in this chapter should replace the baseline model. Furthermore, a discussion of the case for or against the use of neurocognitive testing in a sports concussion framework goes well beyond the scope of this chapter and has been discussed at length by other investigators [9, 10]. However, we do touch upon the merits and limitations of such tests, as well as the pros and cons of conducting baseline testing.

Summary of Literature Recommendations for the Use of Neuropsychological Testing in Sports Concussion

Use of Baseline Testing

Although the literature is variable regarding how best to use neuropsychological testing, many investigators recommend the use of pre-injury baseline neuropsychological testing as best practice for sports concussion management [1–7]. As Guskiewicz et al. [2] and Echemendia and colleagues [11] have articulated, the use of baseline testing for comparison with post-injury scores helps to control for idiosyncratic interindividual differences at baseline (e.g., ADHD, possible cumulative cognitive impact of prior concussions, cultural/linguistic differences, learning disorders, age, education, and proneness to psychiatric issues). Controlling for such extraneous factors by using baseline testing should make neuropsychological tests more sensitive to the impact of concussions on specific individuals.

Still, the baseline paradigm for sports concussion is not without limitations. It has been criticized because there is no empirical evidence that the use of baseline testing improves diagnostic accuracy [9, 12], reduces risk of further injury [10], or predicts decline better than would be expected by chance alone [11].

Another significant limitation of the baseline model is that, for the types of intervals often used in sports concussion testing, the test-retest reliability is not known for many typically used neuropsychological tests [10, 13–15]. Furthermore, the time between baseline and post-injury intervals can be years apart, whereas test-retest reliabilities are typically assessed over about 4–8 week intervals. Finally, commonly used neurocognitive tests in sports concussion often have less than optimal test-retest reliabilities for clinical decision-making [13, 15].

Consideration of test-retest reliability coefficients is critical because they are central to calculating the reliable change indices (RCIs) that are typically used to determine clinically significant change. If these reliability coefficients are low, then confidence intervals will be large and greater declines will be required post concussion for change to be detected. Tests with low test-retest reliability coefficients, then, will be less sensitive to changes post concussion than those with higher values.

In practical terms, baseline testing is logistically complex and expensive. Also, practice effects are commonly seen with neuropsychological tests, something that can reduce sensitivity post concussion [16]. Overall, despite its utility in controlling for interindividual differences, the baseline model does have limitations. Given these considerations, using neuropsychological tests in the sports concussion framework when no baseline has been conducted should be considered.

Timing of Post-concussion Testing

There is no clear consensus on the timing of post-concussion neurocognitive testing. In Guskiewicz et al.'s [2] National Athletic Trainers' Association (NATA) Position Statement, the authors suggest that neurocognitive testing should ideally be conducted in the acute injury period to help determine the severity of the concussion, and then again when the athlete is symptom-free to help with return-to-play decisions. However, they do not provide any clear indication of when during the acute injury period that testing might ideally occur.

In the ImPACT Technical Manual [17] on the "Best Practices" page from the ImPACT website, the authors recommend post-concussion ImPACT testing 24–72 hours post concussion to assess whether declines have occurred from baseline and to help with concussion management in general. They also recommend testing after this acute period once the athlete is symptom free both at rest and with cognitive exertion.

The most recent consensus conference [8] recommended that neurocognitive testing be conducted when clinically indicated and when athletes are symptom free by their own self-report; however, these authors provided the caveat that some cases (especially children and adolescents) may warrant neurocognitive testing prior to symptom resolution. They reasoned that such testing could help with school and home management. A position statement published by the American Medical Society for Sports Medicine [18] was agnostic on this issue, asserting that the evidence was unclear regarding the optimal timing of post-concussion neuropsychological testing. In sum, the available literature indicates that there is no clear consensus on the timing of neuropsychological testing post concussion.

The "Value-Added" of Neuropsychological Tests in a Sports Concussion Framework

Some investigators have argued that there is no "value added" to neuropsychological testing in the management of sports concussion, and that return-to-play decisions should strictly be based upon athletes' self-reported symptoms [9, 10]. However, research on this topic has revealed two important findings that counter such a recommendation: (1) A significant percentage of concussed athletes who report full symptom resolution still show objective neurocognitive deficits—either declines from baseline [19] or when no baseline is available, worse neurocognitive performance than control participants [20]; and (2) neurocognitive tests can identify concussed athletes in the acute post-concussion period (within 2 days post concussion) who deny any symptoms but show objective declines from baseline [7].

Although the additional value of neurocognitive tests to the concussion management process is controversial, beyond such considerations there are problems with relying exclusively on self-report of cognitive functioning in guiding return-to-play decisions. First, athletes have a high motivation to minimize symptoms following concussion because of their desire to return to play (RTP), a process articulated in Echemendia and Cantu's [21] "Dynamic Model for Return-to-Play Decision Making." Second, there is extensive literature demonstrating that self-reports of cognitive functioning are only weakly correlated with actual performance on objective cognitive tests, even in individuals who are motivated and who have not experienced any injury to the brain [22].

Harmon and colleagues [18] argue that there are at least three circumstances where post-concussion neurocognitive testing may be warranted: (1) In situations where athletes are presumed to be at high-risk because of prior concussion; (2) with athletes who are likely to minimize or deny symptoms so that they can RTP; and (3) to identify athletes with persistent deficits. Thus, these authors appear to recommend post-concussion neurocognitive testing under limited circumstances. One problem with only administering neurocognitive tests to athletes who are likely to minimize or deny symptoms is that such individuals can only be definitively identified if neurocognitive testing is conducted. Otherwise, how does one know? A limitation of only administering tests to identify athletes with persistent deficits is that, again, how does one know if athletes have "persistent deficits" if they are not actually tested? As indicated above, self-report of symptoms is suspect for a variety of well-established reasons, so relying on an athlete's self-report of symptoms is not going to be useful in identifying persistent deficits.

A Proposed Evidence-Based Model for Neurocognitive Concussion Management When No Baseline Is Available

Following Ellemberg and colleagues' [14] observation that the absence of scientifically validated algorithms for neuropsychological test interpretation has resulted in clinicians and researchers using idiosyncratic decision rules, as well as McCrory et al.'s [8] recommendation for "Best-Practice" guidelines, we articulate a model for the use of neuropsychological tests in a sports concussion framework when no baseline is available. We then provide an empirical test of this model.

Figure 2.1 illustrates our algorithm. Before going into the details of this, we outline the tests in the battery on which the algorithm is based, which includes both computerized and paper-and-pencil tests. We then describe the evidence basis for each step of the algorithm. Note that there are separate decision rules for males and females. This is due to findings of sex differences

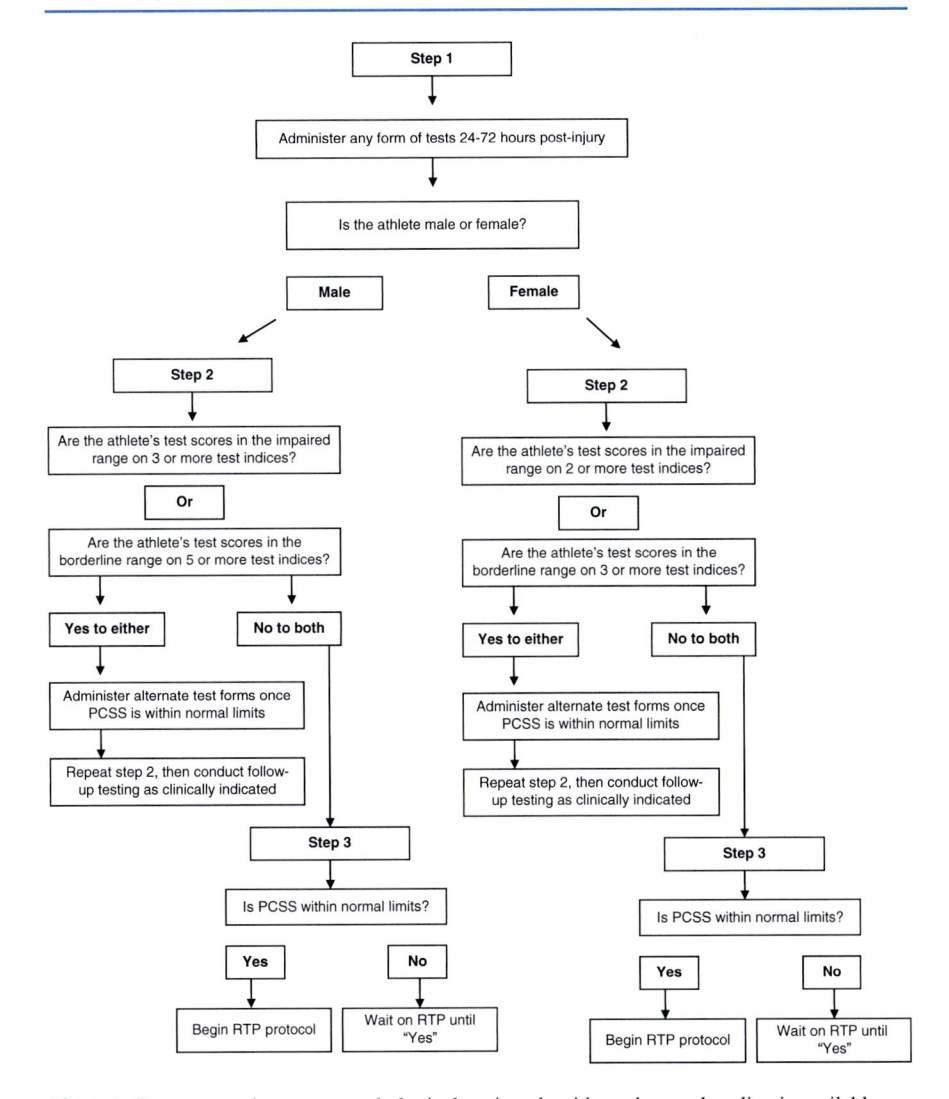

Fig. 2.1 Post-concussion neuropsychological testing algorithm when no baseline is available

in base rates of impairment using this same battery in Division I collegiate athletes [23].

Measures

The battery we use as the basis for our model includes both computerized and paper-and-pencil measures. Although the use of paper-and-pencil measures can be logistically more complex and expensive than using computerized tests alone because they require face-to-face administration, including such tests is likely to increase the sensitivity of the battery. Also, if neuropsychological tests are only used post concussion, then the cost of administration is considerably lower.

Computerized tests Computerized tests include the ImPACT [24] and the Vigil Continuous Performance Test (CPT) [25]. The following summary indices from the ImPACT are included: Verbal Memory Composite, Visual Memory Composite, Visuomotor Speed Composite, and Reaction Time Composite. Although more recent versions of the ImPACT are available, we based our algorithm on the 2.0 version because of the availability of data for our evidence-based model. This version appears to be highly correlated with more recent (including online) versions of the ImPACT. Average Delay (a reaction time index) is used for the Vigil.

Paper-and-pencil tests These measures include: the Hopkins Verbal Learning Test-Revised (HVLT-R) [26] (total correct immediate and delayed recall), the Brief Visuospatial Memory Test-Revised (BVMT-R) [27] (total correct immediate and delayed recall), the Symbol-Digit Modalities Test (SDMT) [28] (total correct within 90 seconds), a modified Digit Span Test [29] (total correct forward and backward sequences), the PSU Cancellation Task [30] (total correct within 90 seconds), Comprehensive Trail Making Test Trails 2 and 4 or 3 and 5 (CTMT) [31] (completion times for both parts), and the Stroop Color-Word Test (SCWT) [32] (time to completion for both Color-Naming and Color-Word conditions). Thus, across computerized and paper-and-pencil measures, there are 17 test indices.

When multiple assessments are completed, we suggest that alternate forms be used at each repeated administration of the test battery. The ImPACT has such alternate forms built into the program; alternate forms are available for all of the above paper-and-pencil tests with the exception of the modified Digit Span Test and Stroop Color-Word Test.

Self-report To measure post-concussion symptoms, we use the Post-Concussion Symptom Scale (PCSS). This measure includes a list of 22 common post-concussion symptoms. Examinees rate the extent to which they are currently experiencing each symptom on a scale from 0 to 6, with 0 indicating the absence of the symptom, and 6 indicating severe symptoms.

Algorithm of Decision Rules

As Fig. 2.1 shows, each step of the algorithm after the initial neuropsychological testing involves a question, and then an action depending on the answer to the question.

Step 1 The action at Step 1 is to administer the test battery at 24–72 hours post injury. The evidence basis for this stems from animal models showing that many elements of the neurochemical cascade in the brain following concussion peak at about 48 hours post injury, and the decrease in glucose metabolism that occurs at about 48 hours post injury, are correlated with cognitive dysfunction in adult rats [33–35]. Also, neurocognitive research in humans has shown that the greatest cognitive impact post concussion typically occurs within 24–72 hours post injury [1, 16, 36, 37], though there is considerable individual variability [37]. As such, testing athletes during this time interval should provide a likely estimate of the full impact of the concussion on the brain as manifested by neurocognitive test results. Also, if the athlete is free of neurocognitive impairment at this early stage (relative to base rates), then no further neurocognitive testing would necessarily need to be conducted post concussion, and the return-to-play (RTP) decision could be made based on other factors (e.g., self-reported symptoms, vestibular signs, etc.). If the athlete does show signs of neurocognitive impairment at this point, then the objective neurocognitive data could be used to assist in getting temporary academic accommodations while symptomatic (e.g., deferral of exams and other assignments, testing in a room free from distraction, extra time on exams, etc.). A more detailed rationale for testing at this early time point post concussion, and possibly before self-reported symptom resolution, is provided below in the section entitled, "Why Recommend Testing During the Acute Concussion Phase?"

Step 2 The algorithm has different Step 2s for males and females because the study on which these specific decision rules are based revealed slightly different base rates for males and females. In this study, we examined baseline performance in 495 collegiate athletes on the same test battery outlined in this article [23], and impairment on a test was defined as performing 2 SDs or more below the mean of other athletes; borderline impairment was defined as 1.5 SDs or more below the mean. These criteria were used since currently there is no agreed upon definition of abnormally poor test performance on neuropsychological tests following concussion, and also to allow for some flexibility in decision-making.

In this study, less than 10% of males had five or more borderline scores, and less than 10% of females had three or more borderline scores. Additionally, less than 10% of males had three or more impaired scores, and less than 10% of females had two or more impaired scores. We used these base rates as a foundation for the decision rules in our model. In light of such data, male athletes who are tested post concussion who show impairment on 3 or more tests and female athletes who show impairment on 2 or more tests evidence highly unusual performance that is likely to reflect the impact of their concussion (see Fig. 2.1). Similarly, male athletes who are tested post concussion who show borderline scores on 5 or more tests and female athletes who show borderline scores on 3 or more tests display highly unusual performance that is likely to reflect the impact of their concussion. The application of these data in decision rules is shown at Step 2 in Fig. 2.1. Ideally, concussion programs adopting this algorithm would be advised to use base rate of impairment data collected from athletes participating in their specific programs. In this way, the data used are likely to be most valid for that group of athletes for a particular neurocognitive test battery. If such base rates differ from what we report, relevant values could simply replace what we report from our athletes in the algorithm. If base rates of impairment are not available, it should be noted that other studies using test batteries of comparable length have reported similar base rates of impairment using a similar number of test indices in healthy older adults [38, 39], as well as children and adolescents [40].

If male or female athletes receive a "yes" response at Step 2, for either the impaired or borderline criterion, then the action is to "Administer Alternate Test Forms Once PCSS is Within Normal Limits." The evidence basis for this stems from findings showing that even when athletes report that they are symptom free, many still show evidence for objective cognitive impairment [19]. Additionally, relying on self-report of cognitive functioning when determining when athletes can RTP may be inaccurate given the consistently replicated low correlation found between objective neurocognitive test performance and self-reported neurocognitive functioning [22]. Thus, any athlete should have to perform within normal limits neurocognitively prior to returning to play, and such decisions should not be based on self-reported cognitive functioning alone. Following this recommendation after a "yes" response, the algorithm indicates, "Repeat Step 2, Then Conduct Follow-Up Testing as Clinically Indicated."

Step 3 If either male or female athletes have a "no" response at Step 2, then the algorithm moves to Step 3 to consider the following question: "Is PCSS Within Normal Limits?" The determination of "within normal limits" is made using normative data from our sample of collegiate athletes at baseline on the PCSS. Scores falling within the broad average range (i.e., standard score of 80 or above) are considered "within normal limits." If the answer to this question is "yes," then the recommendation is to begin the Return-to-play (RTP) protocol. If the answer is "no," then the recommendation is to wait on starting the RTP until the PCSS is within normal limits.

One complicating issue involves cases where athletes have a "yes" response at Step 2 (meeting the below base rate impaired or borderline criterion), yet report being within normal limits in terms of their symptom report. Given that the recommendation following such an outcome is to "Administer Alternate Test Forms Once PCSS Is Within Normal Limits," how does one proceed? There are no clear evidence-based guidelines for how to proceed here in terms of the precise timing of the next post-concussion testing point. A broad guideline would be to recommend testing the athlete again between 5 and 10 days post concussion, given that many studies show that most collegiate athletes show full cognitive recovery by that point [1, 16, 30, 36, 41–43]. With that said, other research shows that some collegiate athletes do not recover within that window and take longer than 2 weeks for their neurocognitive functioning to normalize [43, 44]. Thus, more research will clearly be needed to refine this broad guideline. Studies that examine the duration for normalization of brain functioning in athletes who report being normal in terms of symptom report but show impairments neurocognitively would be ideal. Given the current state of the literature, the most prudent approach would be to rely more on individualistic clinical concussion management strategies employed by skilled clinicians to determine temporal sequencing of testing in these cases [45]. Factors such as the urgency with which a return-to-play decision needs to be made (e.g., if a crucial game is imminent vs. the athlete's sport not being "in season"), as well as other individualistic factors (e.g., prior concussion history, the presence of clinically significant depression) would need to be considered. Thus, the model allows for considerable flexibility at this stage due, in part, to the absence of clear research evidence to guide decision-making, but also due to idiosyncratic factors that are nearly always going to be at play in the clinical management of concussion.

Why Recommend Testing During the Acute Concussion Phase?

One potentially controversial recommendation in our algorithm is to routinely test athletes in the acute stage more systematically post concussion. Many athletes are likely to still be experiencing some symptoms at the 24–72 hour post-concussion point, and some investigators and clinicians have asserted that such testing should be avoided on a number of grounds. First, given that athletes are still symptomatic, some posit that such testing cannot contribute anything to the RTP decision, because clinicians are typically not going to put athletes back to play who are still experiencing self-reported symptoms. Second, it has been suggested that such testing could exacerbate the athlete's symptoms, and there is some evidence to support this concern [46]. These are reasonable concerns; however, we assert that the value of such acute testing outweighs the potential minor risk of a temporary increase in symptoms. The caveat to this, of course, involves cases where symptoms are so severe that testing could be harmful in exacerbating already severe symptoms, or where the nature of such symptoms would likely substantially interfere with test performance (e.g., severe dizziness, nausea, or headache, among others). This is where individualistic concussion management again becomes important [45].

One benefit of such testing in the early acute phase is to help document the severity of the concussion. Athletes who show more impairments at this acute stage could be managed more conservatively once RTP procedures have begun than those who were back to their likely premorbid cognitive level, or nearly back to such a level. Another benefit, as noted earlier, is that early objective documentation of deficits could result in athletes quickly being able to secure needed academic accommodations during their recovery period. A third benefit of acute testing is that it may show that the athlete is in fact back to baseline neurocognitively, even at this early stage. If this is the case, then more rapid RTP could potentially occur. Although an athlete's medical well-being must always be the most important consideration of sports medicine professionals, athletes performing at a high level of sport (e.g., Division I college, the basis of our algorithm) could suffer significant harm in terms of their status on the team and ability to compete in important games and maintain their scholarships, as well as their mental health, if they are held out of play for an unnecessarily long period of time.

A final benefit of conducting systematic testing during this acute period post concussion and at other systematic time points is that the neurocognitive results following any future concussion could be compared with the results from the previous concussion to assess whether the range and severity of cognitive impairments increases. If an athlete is tested at different points following different concussions, then such systematic comparisons would not be possible. Athletes who suffer multiple concussions and show an increased range and severity of cognitive impairments with each successive concussion can then be treated more conservatively.

Limitations

Our algorithm represents an initial attempt to develop systematic guidelines for decision-making post concussion in cases where baseline data are not available. Although we provide systematic decision rules, there is much room for individualistic concussion management, and we spell out a number of examples where such factors come in to play. The neuropsychological test battery we recommend is relatively lengthy and logistically complex; however, applying it in cases where baseline testing has not been conducted significantly reduces such complexity. Also, the algorithm can be adapted to different (possibly shorter) test batteries and different athlete groups when base rates of impairment data can be derived from such groups.

Testing the Model

In this section, we provide a preliminary test of our model in a group of concussed collegiate athletes. We aimed to test the validity of the model by comparing algorithm-determined "Recovered/Not Recovered" groups of concussed collegiate athletes along a number of dimensions. Our primary hypothesis concerned examining post-injury cognitive tests between these groups that we conceptualized as other indicators of recovery beyond the number of cognitive impairments used for the algorithm.

Primary Hypothesis Compared with the Not Recovered group, the Recovered group will show significantly better performance on indices from five cognitive test indices not included in the algorithm itself when tested post concussion: Immediate and Delayed Recall on the Story subtest from the Rivermead Behavioral Memory Test (RBMT); Immediate and Delayed Recall from the Affective Word List (AWL); and the Controlled Oral Word Association Test (COWAT).

Method

Participants

The sample was derived from athletes who were referred to us for evaluation between 2002 and 2019 at our Division I university. All participants were referred by either an athletic trainer or team physician for concussion testing after sustaining a sports-related concussion (SRC).

Recovered Versus Not Recovered Participants Using Base Rate of Impairment at Baseline Algorithm

In terms of dichotomizing groups using this algorithm, participants were included in the "Not Recovered" group if they met criteria for either the "borderline" or "impaired" algorithm (see Fig. 2.1). Participants were included in the "Recovered" group if they fell below the threshold for both the "borderline" and "impaired" algorithm. As shown in Table 2.1, this resulted in a total of 96 (80%) "Recovered" athletes and 24 (20%) "Not Recovered" athletes.

Measures

Post-Concussion Cognitive Outcome Variables Not Included in the Algorithm

The RBMT—Story Memory involves examinees having to recall two different stories read to them. They are asked to recall these immediately and then after about a 30-minute delay. The Affective Word List (AWL) [47] has a similar format as a traditional list-learning task. The examinee is read three trials of a list of 16 words, 8 positively valenced and 8 negatively valenced, and is then asked to recall as many of the words as possible. After a 20- to 25-min delay, examinees are again asked to recall as many of the words as they can remember. The AWL was developed to measure affective bias, specifically to assess the proportion of positive versus negative words recalled as a way of detecting depressive tendencies through a performance-based task. However, we have also found that it can be used as a traditional list-learning task, and it has been shown to have good convergent and discriminant validity as a memory test [48]. The COWAT is a speeded measure of verbal fluency that requires examinees to generate as many words as they can that begin with a particular letter of the alphabet. Total words generated across three letter trials was used as the dependent variable for the COWAT.

Results

Preliminary Analyses: Recovered Versus Not Recovered Participants Using Combined Algorithm

As shown in Table 2.1, the groups did not differ significantly in age or days since concussion. However, the groups did differ in terms of sex distribution. Specifically, a much higher proportion of females comprised the Not Recovered group (45.8%) compared with the Recovered (20.3%) group, X^2 (N = 120) = 11.37, p = 0.001. Given these differences, we conducted some post-hoc analyses (see below) to try and understand these differences further.

The groups were also compared on the number of borderline and impaired scores. Not surprisingly, given the selection criteria for the groups, the Not Recovered group had significantly more borderline scores (mean = 6.58 (3.41),

Table 2.1 Participant demographic and impairment variables for recovered versus not recovered groups using combined algorithm criteria

	Recovered ($n = 96$)		Not recovered ($n = 24$)			
Continuous variables	M	SD	M	SD	t-value	p
Age (years)	18.96	1.27	18.83	1.27	−0.43	0.67
Days since concussion	20.56	51.38	26.79	45.22	0.54	0.59
Impaired scores[1]	0.44	0.65	4.58	2.98	6.78[3]	<0.001
Borderline scores[2]	0.88	1.00	6.58	3.41	8.11[3]	<0.001
Categorical variables	N	%	N	%	X^2	p
Sex					11.37	=0.001
Male	82	85.4	13	54.2		
Female	14	14.6	11	45.8		
Ethnicity						
Caucasian	109	77.9	17	53.1		
African American	22	15.7	11	34.4		
Asian American	4	2.9	0	0.0		
Biracial/multiracial	3	2.1	4	12.5		
Other	2	1.4	0	0.0		
Sport						
Baseball	3	3.1	0	0.0		
Cheerleading	1	1.0	0	0.0		
Football	25	26.0	9	37.5		
Golf	2	2.1	0	0.0		
Men's basketball	17	17.7	0	0.0		
Men's ice hockey	6	6.3	1	4.2		
Men's lacrosse	16	16.7	1	4.2		
Men's soccer	2	2.1	1	4.2		
Rugby	12	12.5	0	0.0		
Softball	1	1.0	1	4.2		
Swimming/diving	1	1.0	0	0.0		
Women's basketball	1	1.0	4	16.7		
Women's ice hockey	0	0.0	2	8.3		
Women's lacrosse	2	2.1	2	8.3		
Women's soccer	1	1.0	2	8.3		
Wrestling	6	6.3	0	0.0		
Other	0	0.0	1	4.2		

Note: M = Mean, SD = Standard deviation. [1] Number of impaired scores reflects the number of scores out of the 17 indices from the algorithm that are 2 SD or more below the mean of 100 (i.e., at or below a standard score of 70). [2] Number of borderline impaired scores reflects the number of scores out of the 17 indices from the algorithm that are 1.5 SD or more below the mean of 100 (i.e., at or below a standard score of 78). [3] Degrees of freedom for this t-score = 1, 24, because of significant Levene's Test for Equality of Variances for this variable

median = 6.50) compared with the Recovered group (mean = 0.88 (1.00), median = 1.00), t (1, 24)[1] = 8.11, $p < 001$. The Not Recovered group also had significantly more impaired scores (mean = 4.58 (2.98), median = 4.00) compared with the Recovered group (mean = 0.44 (0.65), median = 0.00), $t(1, 24)^1 = 6.78, p < 001$.

---

[1] The dfs are lower here because of an adjustment in the degrees of freedom due to the fact that Levene's test for Equality of Variances between the groups was significant.

Hypothesis Testing Analyses on Recovered Versus Not Recovered Participants Using Combined Algorithm

Primary Hypothesis: A Multivariate ANOVA (MANOVA) was conducted comparing the Recovered and Not Recovered groups on all five cognitive indices. The Multivariate F was significant, indicating that the groups were different on the five factors overall, $F(5, 114) = 4.69$, $p = 0.001$, $\eta_p^2 = 0.17$. Univariate tests showed that the groups were significantly different on the RBMT—Immediate Recall ($F(1, 118) = 4.89$, $p < 0.05$, $\eta_p^2 = 0.04$), RBMT—Delayed Recall ($F(1, 118) = 10.75$, $p = 0.001$, $\eta_p^2 = 0.08$), and AWL—Immediate Recall ($F(1, 118) = 12.98$, $p < 0.001$, $\eta_p^2 = 0.10$). There was a statistical trend for AWL—Delayed Recall ($F(1, 118) = 3.49$, $p < 0.10$, $\eta_p^2 = 0.03$), and the effect for the COWAT was not significant ($F(1, 118) < 1.0$, ns). Consistent with predictions, all effects were in the direction of the Not Recovered group having lower scores than the Recovered group (See Table 2.2).

Post Hoc Analyses

Unexpectedly, females comprised more than twice the percentage of the Not Recovered compared with the Recovered group. Using our base rate algorithm, fewer tests need to fall in the impaired or borderline range in females compared with males for selection in the Not Recovered group. Given this, we wanted to explore whether the males in our Not Recovered group had more impaired tests than the females. Although the males had more impairments (5.5 vs. 3.5) and more borderline impairments (7.6 vs. 5.4), the differences between groups were not significant, $t(1, 22) = 1.62$, ns, and $t[1, 20] = 1.67$, ns, respectively. Still, these mean differences were relatively large.

Table 2.2 Mean performance on key outcome variables for recovered versus not recovered groups using combined borderline and impaired criteria

Measure	Recovered		Not recovered		F-test	p	η_p^2
	M	SD	M	SD			
Cognitive Indices[1]							
Multivariate F (df = 5, 114)					4.69	<0.001	0.17
Univariate F (1, 170)							
RBMT—Immediate Recall	101.62	14.39	94.11	16.75	4.89	<0.05	0.04
RBMT—Delayed Recall	100.93	14.61	89.93	15.05	10.75	=0.001	0.08
AWL—Immediate Recall	26.20	5.62	21.54	5.83	12.98	<0.001	0.10
AWL—Delayed Recall	7.14	3.79	5.58	2.95	3.49	=0.06	0.03
COWAT	16.34	7.36	15.00	3.22	0.76	ns	0.01

Note: M = Mean, SD = Standard deviation. Cognitive indices include the RBMT—Story subtest Immediate and Delayed Recall, AWL—Immediate and Delayed Recall, and the COWAT. *RBMT* Rivermead Behavioral Memory Test, *AWL* Affective Word List, *COWAT* Controlled Oral Word Association Test. RBMT indices are in standard scores; AWL and COWAT indices are raw scores. η_p^2 effect size magnitudes: small = 0.01 to 0.05; medium = 0.06 to 0.13; large = 0.14 and above

Next, we explored whether females in the Not Recovered group had worse scores on the key cognitive outcome indices compared with males, such that the disproportionate number of females in this group might be driving the group difference with the Recovered group. A MANOVA was conducted with sex as the grouping variable and the five cognitive outcome indices as the dependent variables. The multivariate F was significant, F [5, 16] = 2.95, $p < 0.05$, $\eta_p^2 = 0.45$, with all of the univariate F values being significant (p at least <0.05) for all of the individual tests. Remarkably, all of the effects were in the direction of females performing better than males in the Not Recovered group.

We also examined whether the female athletes were different from males in terms of the number of days post concussion when they were tested, and the groups did not significantly differ, t [1, 20] = −0.28, ns. Finally, we examined whether there were motivational/effort differences between males and females in the Not Recovered group. Using the ImPACT Impulse Control Composite (ICC), as well as an Examiner Rating (scale of 1–7, with higher scores reflecting higher motivation), the groups were again not different, t [1, 20] = −0.53, ns, and t [1, 20] = −0.28, ns, respectively.

Discussion of Model Test

Our test of the model showed partial support. We found that the "Not Recovered" group performed significantly worse than the "Recovered" group on three of the five outcome variables: the RBMT Immediate and Delayed Recall, and the AWL Immediate Recall. One interesting finding from the study was that there were a highly disproportionate number of females in the Not Recovered group, over double the percentage found in the Recovered group. With follow up analyses, we found that females performed significantly better than males on all of the cognitive outcome variables. As such, it appears that the worse performance of the Not Recovered compared with the Recovered group was largely driven by poorer performance of *males* in the Not Recovered group. These differences may be due to the fact that, using our base rate algorithm, fewer tests need to fall in the impaired or borderline range in females compared with males for selection in the Not Recovered group. Although there were no significant differences in number of impairments between males and females in the Not Recovered group, the mean differences were fairly large. It seems likely that, given that more cognitive impairments are necessary for males to reach criteria for being "Not Recovered," their overall greater cognitive difficulties were manifested in our cognitive outcome variables, even though the latter were not part of the algorithm.

We conducted other follow-up tests and found that males did not differ from females in the Not Recovered group on two motivational indices (ICC from the ImPACT, and an Examiner Rating of observed effort on testing), so such factors could not explain the sex differences observed on the cognitive outcome variables.

Future Directions

Future work should include additional studies to validate the algorithm in other samples independent of our lab group. Ideally to extend what we have presented as a preliminary test in this chapter, groups of collegiate athletes with and without concussions could be tested at the same time intervals as suggested by our model. Examining base rates of impairment on the test battery in individuals with ADHD and/or learning disorders would also be a valuable focus for future work.

Our recommendations are tentative, given the limited evidence available for some aspects of the proposed algorithm. For example, several factors still need to be empirically established, including the ideal timing of post-concussion testing during the acute injury period, and the ideal temporal sequence of testing once athletes are normative symptomologically, but still impaired neurocognitively. However, we hope that our algorithm provides a template for improving neurocognitive concussion management in collegiate athletes.

Acknowledgments There are no conflicts of interest involved with this manuscript, and no sources of financial support.

References

1. Barth JT, Alves WM, Ryan TV, Macciocchi SN, Rimel RW, Jane JA, et al. Mild head injury in sports: neuropsychological sequelae and recovery of function. In: Levin HS, Eisenberg HM, Benton AL, editors. Mild head injury. New York: Oxford University Press; 1989. p. 257–75.
2. Guskiewicz KM, Bruce SL, Cantu RC, Ferrara MS, Kelly JP, McCrea M, et al. Recommendations on management of sport-related concussion: summary of the National Athletic Trainers' association position statement. Neurosurgery. 2004;55:891–5.
3. Moser RS, Iverson GL, Echemendia RJ, Lovell MR, Schatz P, Webbe FM, et al. NAN position paper: neuropsychological evaluation in the diagnosis and management of sports-related concussion. Arch Clin Neuropsychol. 2007;22:909–16.
4. Aubry M, Cantu R, Dvorak J, Graf-Baumann T, Johnston K, Kelly J, et al. Summary and agreement statement of the first International Conference on Concussion in Sport, Vienna 2001. Br J Sports Med. 2002;36:3–7.
5. McCrory P, Johnston K, Meeuwisse W, Aubry M, Cantu R, Dvorak J, et al. Summary and agreement statement of the 2nd International Conference on Concussion in Sport, Prague 2004. Br J Sports Med. 2005;39:196–204.
6. McCrory P, Meeuwisse W, Johnston K, Dvorak J, Aubry M, Molloy M, et al. Consensus Statement on Concussion in Sport – the 3rd International Conference on Concussion in Sport held in Zurich, November 2008. Br J Sports Med. 2009;43(Suppl 1):i76–90.
7. Van Kampen DA, Lovell MR, Pardini JE, Collins MW, Fu FH. The "value added" of neurocognitive testing after sports-related concussion. Am J Sports Med. 2006;30:1630–5.
8. McCrory P, Meeuwisse W, Dvořák J, Aubry M, Bailes J, Broglio S, et al. Consensus statement on concussion in sport—the 5th international conference on concussion in sport held in Berlin, October 2016. Br J Sports Med. 2017;51:838–47.
9. Randolph C, McCrea M, Barr WB. Is neuropsychological testing useful in the management of sport-related concussion? J Athl Train. 2005;40:139–54.
10. Randolph C. Baseline neuropsychological testing in managing sport-related concussion: does it modify risk? Curr Sports Med Rep. 2011;10(1):21–6.

11. Echemendia RJ, Bruce JM, Bailey CM, Sanders JF, Arnett PA, Vargas G. The utility of post-concussion neuropsychological data in identifying cognitive change following sports-related MTBI in the absence of baseline data. Clin Neuropsychol. 2012;26:1077–91.
12. Randolph C, Kirkwood MW. What are the real risks of sport-related concussion, and are they modifiable? J Int Neuropsychol Soc. 2009;15:1–9.
13. Broglio SP, Ferrara MS, Macciocchi SN, Baumgartner TA, Elliott R. Test–retest reliability of computerized concussion assessment programs. J Athl Train. 2007;42:509–14.
14. Ellemberg D, Henry LC, Macciocchi SN, Guskiewicz KM, Broglio SP. Advances in sport concussion assessment: from behavioral to brain imaging measures. J Neurotrauma. 2009;26:2365–82.
15. Mayers LB, Redick TS. Clinical utility of ImPACT assessment for postconcussion return-to-play counseling: psychometric issues. J Clin Exp Neuropsychol. 2012;34:235–42.
16. Rosenbaum AM, Arnett PA, Bailey CM, Echemendia RJ. Neuropsychological assessment of sports-related concussion: measuring clinically significant change. In: SSWS, editor. Foundations of sport-related brain injuries. Norwell, MA: Springer; 2006. p. 137–71.
17. Lovell M. ImPACT version 2.0 clinical user's manual. Pittsburgh, PA: ImPACT Applications Inc.; 2002.
18. Harmon KG, Drezner JA, Gammons M, Guskiewicz KM, Halstead M, Herring SA, et al. American Medical Society for Sports Medicine position statement: concussion in sport. Br J Sports Med. 2013;47:15–26.
19. Broglio SP, Macciocchi SN, Ferrara MS. Neurocognitive performance of concussed athletes when symptom free. J Athl Train. 2007;42:504–8.
20. Fazio VC, Lovell MR, Pardini JE, Collins MW. The relation between post concussion symptoms and neurocognitive performance in concussed athletes. NeuroRehabilitation. 2007;22:207–16.
21. Echemendia RJ, Cantu RC. Return to play following brain injury. In: Lovell MR, Echemendia RJ, Barth JT, Collins MW, editors. Traumatic brain injury in sports: an international neuropsychological perspective. Lisse, the Netherlands: Swets & Zeitlinger B.V.; 2004.
22. Lezak MD, Howieson DB, Loring DW. Neuropsychological assessment. 4th ed. New York: Oxford University Press; 2004.
23. Barwick FH, Rabinowitz AR, Arnett PA. Base rates of impaired neuropsychological test performance among healthy collegiate athletes. in revision.
24. Lovell M, Collins M, Podell K, Powell J, Maroon J. ImPACT: immediate post-concussion assessment and cognitive testing. Pittsburgh, PA: NeuroHealth Systems, LLC; 2000.
25. Cegalis JA, Cegalis S. The vigil/W continuous performance test (manual). New York: ForThought; 1994.
26. Benedict RHB, Schretlen D, Groninger L, Brandt J. Hopkins verbal learning Testñrevised: normative data and analysis of inter-form and test-retest reliability. Clin Neuropsychol. 1998;12(1):43–55.
27. Benedict RHB. Brief visuospatial memory test – revised: professional manual. Psychological Assessment Resources: Odessa, FL; 1997.
28. Smith A. Symbol digit modalities test (SDMT) manual (revised). Western Psychological Services: Los Angeles; 1982.
29. Wechsler D. Wechsler adult intelligence scale-III (WAIS-III). New York: Psychological Corporation; 1997.
30. Echemendia RJ, Putukian M, Mackin RS, Julian L, Shoss N. Neuropsychological test performance prior to and following sports-related mild traumatic brain injury. Clin J Sport Med. 2001;11:23–31.
31. Reynolds CR. Comprehensive trail making test (CTMT). Pro-Ed: Austin, TX; 2002.
32. Trenerry MR, Crosson B, DeBoe J, Leber WR. Stroop neuropsychological screening test. Psychological Assessment Resources: Odessa, FL; 1989.
33. Barkhoudarian G, Hovda DA, Giza CC. The molecular pathophysiology of concussive brain injury. Clin Sports Med. 2011;30:33–48.

34. Giza CC, DiFiori JP. Pathophysiology of sports-related concussion. Sports Health. 2011;3:46–51.
35. Giza CC, Hovda DA. The neurometabolic cascade of concussion. J Athl Train. 2001;36:228–35.
36. Belanger HG, Vanderploeg RD. The neuropsychological impact of sports-related concussion: a meta-analysis. J Int Neuropsychol Soc. 2005;11:345–57.
37. Wilde EA, McCauley SR, Barnes A, Wu TC, Chu Z, Hunter JV, et al. Serial measurement of memory and diffusion tensor imaging changes within the first week following uncomplicated mild traumatic brain injury. Brain Imaging Behav. 2012;6:319–28.
38. Brooks BL, Iverson GL, White T. Substantial risk of 'accidental MCI' in healthy older adults: base rates of low memory scores in neuropsychological assessment. J Int Neuropsychol Soc. 2007;13:490–500.
39. Palmer BW, Boone KB, Lesser IM, Wohl MA. Base rates of "impaired" neuropsychological test performance among healthy older adults. Arch Clin Neuropsychol. 1998;13:503–11.
40. Brooks BL, Sherman EMS, Iverson GL. Healthy children get low scores too: prevalence of low scores on the NEPSY-II in preschoolers, children, and adolescents. Arch Clin Neuropsychol. 2010;25:182–90.
41. Covassin T, Schatz P, Swanik CB. Sex differences in neuropsychological function and post-concussion symptoms of concussed collegiate athletes. Neurosurgery. 2007;61:345–51.
42. Covassin T, Elbin R, Harris W, Parker T, Kontos A. The role of age and sex in symptoms, neurocognitive performance, and postural stability in athletes after concussion. Am J Sports Med. 2012;40:1303–12.
43. Echemendia RJ, Iverson GL, McCrea M, Broshek DK, Gioia GA, Sautter SW, et al. Role of neuropsychologists in the evaluation and management of sport-related concussion: an inter-organization position statement. Arch Clin Neuropsychol. 2012;27:119–22.
44. McClincy MP, Lovell MR, Pardini J, Collins MW, Spore MK. Recovery from sports concussion in high school and collegiate athletes. Brain Inj. 2006;20:33–9.
45. Lovell M. The management of sports –related concussion: current status and future trends. Clin J Sport Med. 2009;28:95–111.
46. Meyer JE, Arnett PA. Changes in symptoms in concussed and non-concussed athletes following neuropsychological assessment. Dev Neuropsychol. 2015;40(1):24–8.
47. Ramanathan DN, Rabinowitz AR, Barwick FH, Arnett PA. Validity of affect measurements in evaluating symptom reporting in athletes. J Int Neuropsychol Soc. 2012;18:101–7.
48. Meyer J, Arnett PA. Validation of the affective word list as a measure of verbal learning and memory. J Clin Exper Neuropsychol. 2015;37:316–24.

Feasibility of Virtual Reality for Assessment of Neurocognitive, Executive, and Motor Functions in Concussion

Semyon M. Slobounov, Wayne J. Sebastianelli, Karl M. Newell, and Alexa E. Walter

Introduction

Mild traumatic brain injury (mTBI), the most common variant of what is known as concussion, has an annual reported incidence of 1.4 million cases in the United States alone [1, 2] and accounts for 80% of all traumatic brain injuries (TBIs) [3, 4]. There are a number of immediate physical, cognitive, and emotional symptoms that arise from mTBI that include headache, dizziness, unsteady posture and gait, nausea, slurred speech, poor concentration, and short-term memory loss. For most sport-related concussions (80–90%) the recovery is rapid, with spontaneous symptoms resolution within 10 days post injury, thus referred to as *uncomplicated mTBI* [5, 6]. Yet when more challenging testing protocols are implemented [7], as many as 15–38% of individuals suffering from mTBI have clinical symptoms that persist and may be detected for months or even years post injury [8–10]. Prolonged clinical symptoms resolution exceeding 1 month post injury associated with positive standard neuroimaging findings is referred to as *complicated mTBI* [11]. The definitional problems often are reflected in the lack of consistency and consensus among clinical practitioners and researchers dealing with mild TBI.

S. M. Slobounov (✉)
Center for Sports Concussion Research and Services, Department of Kinesiology and Neurosurgery, Pennsylvania State University, University Park, PA, USA
e-mail: sms18@psu.edu

W. J. Sebastianelli
Pennsylvania State University, University Park, PA, USA

Departments of Orthopaedics and Sports Medicine, Penn State Hershey, Bone and Joint Institute, State College, PA, USA
e-mail: wsebastianelli@hmc.psu.edu

K. M. Newell · A. E. Walter
Department of Kinesiology, Pennsylvania State University, University Park, PA, USA
e-mail: aow5128@psu.edu

There is consensus among clinical practitioners dealing with sports-related concussions (mTBI) that motor (predominantly whole body posture and balance), executive functions (i.e., decision making and reaction time (RT)), and neurocognitive functioning are the most prominent deficits that concussed athletes experience at least within the acute phase of injury [8, 12, 13]. The Zurich (2009) and Berlin (2016) Consensus Statement recommended that working memory, attention/vigilance, visual learning and memory, reasoning/problem solving, and speed of information processing are the most important neurocognitive functions that need to be accurately assessed to define the degree of brain damage induced by a concussive blow [5, 14]. While current clinical management is based on neuropsychological testing, balance assessment, and symptom evaluation, this can be largely subjective [15]. Furthermore, ecologically valid, sports-concussion-specific, and reliable assessment tools for detection of these neurocognitive functions have yet to be defined.

Several previous studies have identified a negative effect of mTBI on postural stability [15–17]. The use of postural stability testing for the management of sport-related concussion is gradually becoming more common among sport medicine clinicians. A growing body of controlled studies has demonstrated postural stability deficits, as measured by the Balance Error Scoring System (BESS), on post-injury day 1 [12, 18–24]. In the case of an *uncomplicated mTBI*, the recovery of balance occurred between day 1 and day 3 post injury for most of the brain-injured subjects [23]. It appeared that the initial 2 days after an mTBI are the most problematic for subjects standing on the foam surfaces, which was attributed to a sensory interaction problem using visual, vestibular, and somatosensory systems [19, 24]. However, more recent studies by Cavanaugh et al. [25–27] have shown that advanced methods from nonlinear dynamics (i.e., approximate entropy, ApEn) may detect changes in postural control in athletes with *normal* postural stability measures based upon conventional balance testing, longer than 3–4 days after *uncomplicated* concussions. Our own recent study has also shown alteration of virtual-time-to-contact (VTC) measures in the absence of traditional measures of postural instability in concussed individuals [28]. Overall, there is an agreement that when more challenging testing modalities are introduced, balance deficiency in concussed athletes may be observed far beyond 7–10 days post injury even after clinical symptoms resolution [10, 21, 28–37]. Specifically, application of nonlinear methods [25–27] and virtual reality tools [10, 21, 28–37] for assessment of postural data may reveal abnormal balance in the subacute phase of brain injury evolution even in *uncomplicated mTBI*.

Regardless of overall advances, both technological and conceptual, there is still no *gold standard* for accurate assessment of concussion in athletics. There are a few factors that exacerbate the problems with accurate assessment of mTBI. First, conventional neuropsychological (NP) tests are not designed to perform repeated measurements [38], and thus suffer from the so-called *practice effect*. Practice effects are particularly troublesome for post-injury cognitive impairment tracking since they can confound interpretation [39]. Moreover, computerized conventional neuropsychological tests that have validity for single assessments does not make them any more valid than the original paper and pencil versions for repeated testing, particularly at high frequency intervals. It provides administration, standardization, and data management advantages, but the tests are fundamentally the same as when given manually. Therefore, it is not surprising that the results of follow-up tests in the acute phase of injury often appear to be better than those obtained from the initial baseline test.

Second, it should be noted that NP deficits persist in a significant minority (38%) of concussed athletes even after they self-report that they are symptom free [8]. Overall, currently used NP modalities, including computerized assessment of neurocognitive performance, cannot detect long-term cognitive decrement in majority of concussed individuals [8].

Third, most of the NP tests are lengthy and often boring which may induce mental and even physical fatigue. Several recent papers indicate that even normal volunteers may experience both self-reported and EEG-evidenced fatigue while taking NP tests [40]. This confounding factor may be exacerbated by the lack of control for subjects' efforts during administering NP tests (Iverson, personal communication 2010) that makes the interpretation of data at least questionable.

Finally, there is a growing concern regarding the lack of *ecological validity* and *transferability* of data obtained in a clinical setting to real-life situations. For example, a concussed subject may be *asymptomatic* based on traditional memory testing but cannot recall the coaches' instructions and immediate play actions required by coaches. 3D environments are more realistic, can provide feedback more comparable to athletic situations, for example, and require more brain resources than a 2D environment [41]. Furthermore, behaviors, like visual search or decision-making, in 2D situations can differ from behaviors in 3D situations [42, 43]. VR has the potential to overcome some of the aforementioned challenges and ultimately be used as a complementary tool for accurate assessment of the degree of damage induced by concussive blows. In fact, the Zurich Consensus Statement on concussion in sport [14] identified VR among the key areas of future research and possible clinical application.

VR is an interactive, computer-generated 3D environment that simulates the real world and provokes a sensation of immersion in the individual. In fact, VR has recently emerged as a promising method in various domains of therapy, including brain damage rehabilitation, offering the potential to achieve significant successes in assessment, treatment, and improved outcome. Continuing advances in VR technologies along with cost reductions have stimulated both research and development of VR systems aimed at psychological, physical/behavioral, and emotional assessment/rehabilitation of brain-injured individuals. A growing number of diverse occupations that currently use the immersive and interactive properties of VR include athletes, drivers, parachutists, fire fighters, soldiers, divers, and surgeons. However, with respect to implication for clinical practice, it is still yet to be determined whether VR is vulnerable to practice and fatigue effects, similar to the modalities currently used in clinical practice. The overall objective of this chapter is to address these critical questions in two separate experiments.

Virtual Reality Applications, Methods, and Procedures

VR Visual Spatial Memory Test

The assessment of memory functions (i.e., spatial memory and its underlying distinct processes such as encoding, retention, and retrieval) was implemented via presentation of 3D simulation of a *virtual corridor*. TBI patients commonly experience memory problems, specifically in assessing their spatial location with respect to some external objects in the surrounding environment. For example, if the patient left the hospital room, he/she would have difficulty in finding his/her way back to the room, not remembering whether to turn *left* or *right*, move *forward* and/or *backward* in the hospital corridors.

The subjects (a) were shown the navigation route to encode (E) and then (b) requested to navigate purposefully with the goal of reaching specific target room location (active navigation, AN) using a high-resolution joystick (www.magconcept.com). The subjects *moved* around using their right thumb to freely navigate in forward, backward, and side-to-side directions. The virtual corridor (see Fig. 3.1, including the floor plan of the *virtual corridor*) was generated by a VTC Open GL developing kit (HeadRehab, LLC, USA— http://www.headrehab.com/) which provides a realistic VR environment and sense of presence (see also [44] for details). A total of three trials were allowed to successfully complete this test.

VR Recognition "A" Test

This test aimed to measure a subject's visual recognition performance in remembering and recognizing objects found within a virtual environment. This module can be used in conjunction with the recognition B test (see below). The subject's task is to passively navigate through the virtual corridor. Along his/her way, there are seven objects that should be memorized. Both types and color of these objects are

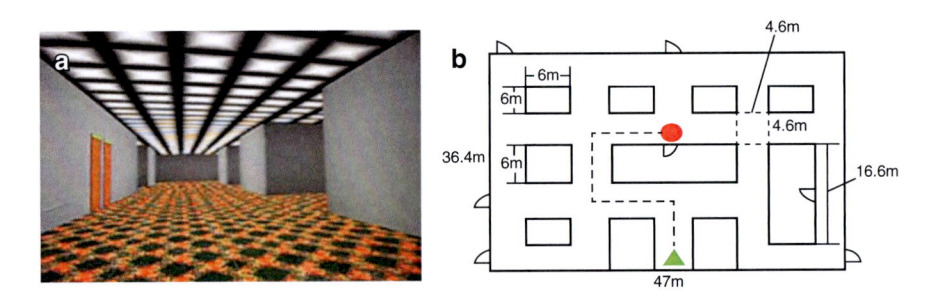

Fig. 3.1 (**a**) View of the virtual corridor used for navigation tasks under study, and (**b**) floor plan, and a sample of the route for one of the runs. The subjects were instructed to reproduce (e.g., retrieval) the previously shown routes (e.g., encoding) via navigating through virtual corridor by the joystick and to find the target location. It should be noted that starting position was the same for all runs

important to remember. Then, the subject is presented with a display panel of 14 different objects and given 120 s to select *only* the same seven objects previously seen in the virtual corridor. The number of correct/incorrect responses and time to perform the test are computed and converted into the scoring format from 10 to 0 (Fig. 3.2).

VR Recognition "B" Test

The subject is shown seven different objects slowly rotating for 60 s to memorize before passive navigation through the virtual corridor. Both the type and color of the objects are important memorizing properties. The subject is then passively navigated through the virtual corridor. If the subject recognizes an object from the seven objects previously shown in the display panel, he/she must press the trigger/button on the interactive device to select the recognized object. The total number of correct/incorrect responses is computed and converted into the scoring format from 10 to 0.

VR Assessment of Sustained Attention

Sohlberg and Matter in 1989 [45] proposed a clinical model of attention processes that outlined hierarchically organized levels of attention. Our personal experience in dealing with TBI patients on a daily basis is clearly in support of this clinical model of attention. Specifically, TBI patients, especially in acute stage of injury, most often are unable to sustain attention even for a short period of time. Their distractibility level increases significantly, affecting both everyday life and academic/learning activities. The rate of recovery of this cognition function is influenced by numerous factors, such as the initial impact, degree of structural damage, and/or initial functional deficits, although not well documented in clinical research.

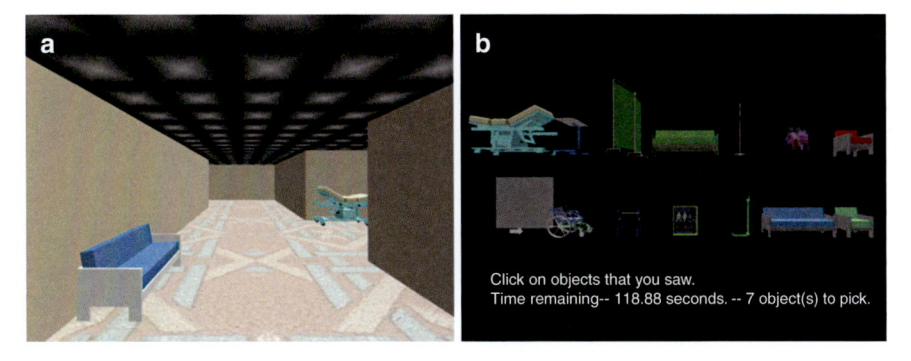

Fig. 3.2 (**a**) Different objects (total $n = 7$) are displayed to memorize while passively navigating via virtual corridor; (**b**) fourteen objects are displayed to recognize that were shown while navigating via virtual corridor

The attention deficit in TBI, specifically deficits in visual selective and sustained attention, is a prominent aspect of cognitive dysfunction after TBI. TBI patients frequently complain of distractibility and difficulty attending to more than one thing at a time. We designed the VR prototype of Everyday Attention [46] within the context of a *dual-task* paradigm to assess attention deficits in mild TBI. Our design of the VR attention module, *Virtual Elevator* (VE), was implemented by HeadRehab, LLC and is currently utilized in our laboratory for baseline and follow-up testing of concussed athletes (Fig. 3.3).

The VR advanced prototype of the Test of Everyday Attention (TEA) using the Virtual Elevator was implemented as the following:

- Sustained attention is being tested similar to the "Elevator Counting" test (1). The subjects are situated in the Virtual Elevator (VE) moving up (from floor 1 to floor 12) and down (from floor 12 to floor 1). There are visual separations that a subject should count in order to identify the floor indicator upon arrival (stop). There are numerous random trials that last for 10 min. The number of correct and incorrect counts assessed is used as an input to the comprehensive report.
- Elevator floor counting with distractions. Similar to (Λ) while additional sources of noise (external visual stimuli, i.e., adjacent buildings, windows, trees, and people coming in and out) are being added.
- Dual-task version of VE is also elaborated to test the properties of "Divided Attention."

These data were used as an input for normalized reports of success rate ranges from 10 to 0 for each subject under study. It should be noted, we were able to detect attention deficits in concussed individuals in subacute phase of injury, although diagnosed as *asymptomatic* based upon conventional neurocognitive assessment

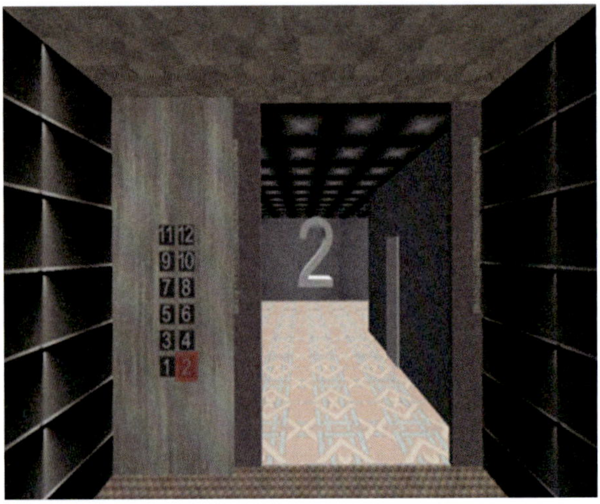

Fig. 3.3 The image of the Virtual Elevator module as perceived by the subject

tools, such as STROOP, SDMT, WMS-R Digit Span, Ruff 2 s and 7 s Selective Attention Test, and PASAT [47]. Current research is in progress to evaluate both convergent and discriminant validity of VR sustained attention module in the context of concussion evaluation that will be published elsewhere.

VR Assessment of Balance

Balance abnormalities specifically evident during visual-kinesthetic tasks are the most common symptoms in TBI patients suffering from sport-related concussions [19]. It should be noted that balance symptom resolution varies among mTBI patients and may last up to more than 1 year post injury [10]. Our previous research has shown the presence of balance abnormalities and visual-kinesthetic disintegration, induced by VR visual field motion up to 30 days post injury [30, 32, 48]. We have designed the VR moving room paradigm to examine postural stability via introducing the visual perturbation balance tasks [30]. The VR moving room appears to be an advanced tool allowing the detection of residual postural abnormalities as evidenced by impaired visual-kinesthetic integration [10].

The VR system that was used in this study includes: (a) VisMini portable stereo 3D projection system; (b) Draper Inc. 6 × 8 portable Cinefold surface screen; and (c) AMTI force plate for assessment of postural responses to visual field motion.

The field sequential stereo images were separated into right and left eye images using liquid crystal shutter glasses. An additional sensor was located on the subject's head to interact with the visual field motion. The visual field motion consists of a realistic looking moving room (see Fig. 3.4).

Preprogrammed manipulations of the VR moving room included the following: (1) viewing stationary VR room; (2) VR room forward–backward oscillatory translation within 18 cm displacement at 0.2 Hz; (3) VR room *Roll* around heading y-axis between 10 and 30° at 0.2 Hz; (4) VR room *Pitch* around interaural x-axis between 10 and 30° at 0.2 Hz; (5) VR room *Yaw* around vertical z-axis between 10 and 30° at 0.2 Hz; and (6) VR room translation along x-axis within 18 cm displacement at 0.2 Hz. The subjects were instructed: (a) to acquire the Romberg stance and stand as still as possible on the force platform while viewing the computer-generated *moving room* visual scenes for 30 s trial duration (VR—balance 1 test); and (b) to produce whole body oscillations in synchrony with the motion of the VR room along x, y, and z axes (VR—balance 2 test).

Normalized Assessment of Postural Stability

The area of the center of pressure (COP) was calculated from AMTI force platform data sampled at 100 Hz. A specially developed MATLAB program was used to estimate the subject response data obtained from the force platform similar to

Fig. 3.4 AMTI force platform and 6° of freedoms ultrasound IS-900 micromotion tracking technology from "InterSense, Inc." was used to control the head and body kinematics and postural responses to visual manipulations of VR scenes

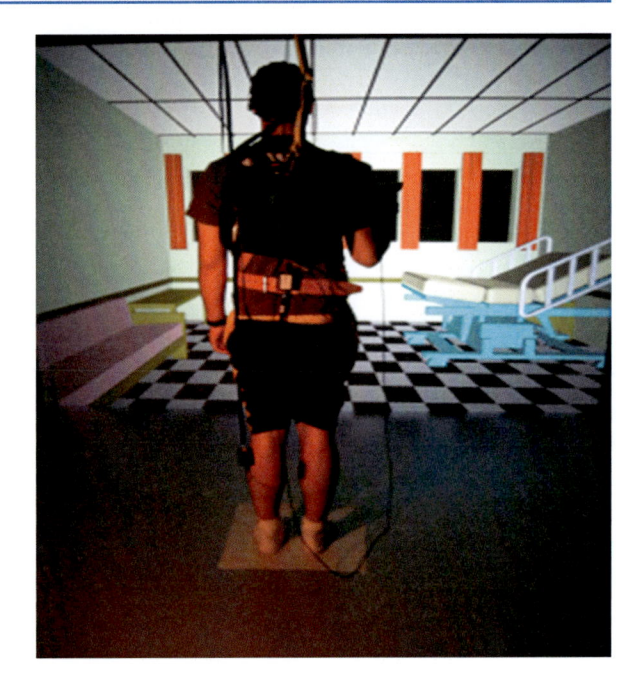

Slobounov et al. [36]. The COP area calculated from the data obtained for each individual subject (with respect to 450 records from normal age-matched volunteers) was used as an input for normalized reports of success rate (stable vs. unstable posture) ranges from 10 to 0 (loss of balance during the test).

Coherence values between quantities of moving room and subject responses were assessed using a specially developed MATLAB code. The auto-spectra for each signal were calculated by using Welsh's averaged periodogram method. Coherence was calculated based on the cross-spectra fxy and auto-spectra fxx, fyy with the spectra estimated from segments of data and the coherence Rxy estimated from the combined spectra:

$$Rxy(\lambda)|2 = |fxy(\lambda)|2 / (fxx(\lambda) fyy(\lambda)); \tag{3.1}$$

The significance of coherence was also calculated. That is the confidence limit for zero coherence at the α %, and L is the number of disjoint segments: sig $(\alpha) = 1 - (1 - \alpha)1/(L - 1)$. In addition, continuous wavelet transform (CWT) was performed to track the dynamics of coupling between subject body motion and visual scenes oscillation over the entire trial duration (30 s). The CWT is able to resolve both time and scale (frequency) events better than the short Fourier transform (STFT). In mathematics and signal processing, the CWT of a function f is defined by (1):

$$\gamma(\tau,s) = \int_{-\infty}^{+\infty} f(t) \frac{1}{\sqrt{|s|}} \overline{\psi\left(\frac{t-\tau}{s}\right)} \, dt; \qquad (3.2)$$

where τ represents translation, s represents scale which is related to frequency, and ψ is the mother wavelet. $\overline{z}$ is the complex conjugate of z. The mother wavelet is a complex Morlet wavelet, as it has both good time and frequency accuracy. The degree of coherence was converted to normalized score ranged from 10 (max dynamic balance) to 0 similar to Slobounov et al. [36, 48].

VR Assessment of Executive Function (Reaction Time)

Early and most recent research indicates that reaction time (RT), especially complex reaction time, significantly and reliably increased in mild TBI patients at least in acute phase of injury [13, 49–51]. Specifically, these finding have been replicated and confirmed in a number of studies [8, 44, 52]. Overall, it is widely accepted now that RT measures may serve as an index of the subject's integrity of executive functions, therefore may be used in clinical assessment of concussion [8, 13, 52] (Fig. 3.5).

We have designed a VR module of reaction time allowing the assessment of whole-body response to unpredictable manipulation of optic flow. The subject was requested to oscillate forward and backward to follow the anterior–posterior (A–P) translation of the moving room at 0.2 Hz for 30 s trial duration.

Unpredictable change of moving room from A–P to medial–lateral (M–L) directions was randomized requiring the subject to respond via whole body motion and

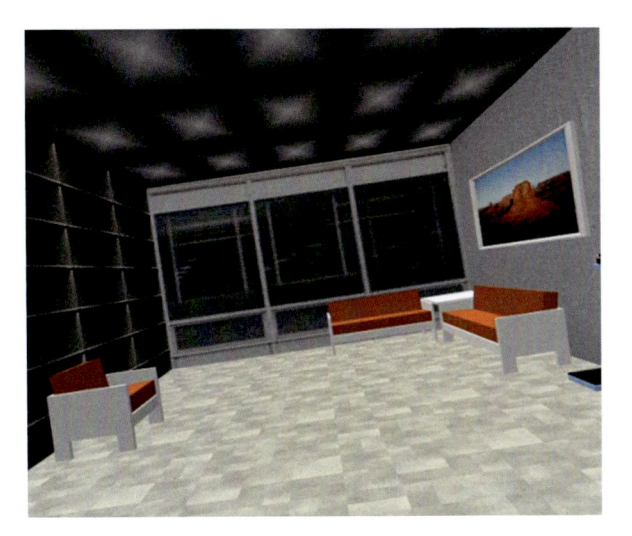

Fig. 3.5 Virtual room rolling to the left requiring subject to change direction of sway from AP to the left (ML) as fast as possible

follow the motion of the moving room. The measured reaction time (ranged from 250 to 750 plus ms) and errors of anticipation (wrong direction of response) were calculated, interpolated, and converted into scoring system from 10 (best score, less than 250 ms compared to 450 samples from normal student-athletes volunteers) to 0 (more than 800 ms) and included in comprehensive reports. Current research is in progress to evaluate both convergent and discriminant validity of VR reaction time module with respect to RTclin and RTcomp derived from CogState-Sport [13] in the context of concussion evaluation that will be published elsewhere.

Assessment of Sense of Presence and Practice Effect

In a study for sense of presence, 15 athletically active and neurologically normal undergraduate students recruited from the Pennsylvania State University. Average age was 21.4 years (SD = 1.3) and average estimated IQ, based upon Wechsler Test of Adult Reading (WTAR; The Psychological Corporation, 2001) test scores, was 108.9 (SD = 6.4). The sample was 70% male and 30% female. The reported racial/ethnic composition was 70% Caucasian American, 10% African American, 10% Asian American, and 10% mixed. All participants had become involved in sports between ages 4 and 8 and had maintained their involvement, at either the recreational or collegiate level, as students at the university. We ensured that participants were neurologically normal through a telephone screening questionnaire. All participants reported that they had slept 7–8 h the night before testing. Half of the subjects were tested between 10:00 am and noon, and the other half was tested between noon and 2:00 pm. Subjects were requested to avoid taking any beverages containing caffeine at least 3 h prior to testing.

Subjects were visiting our lab every other day for a total of three visits and performed sequence of (a) VR spatial memory navigation; (b) VR sustained attention; and (c) VR recognition, A and B; (d) VR balance tests; and (e) reaction time (RT). The order of testing modalities was randomized and necessary time between modalities was provided if needed to control for subjects' fatigue. The total time of testing was within 45 min.

All subject reports indicated that navigation via immersive VR environment induced a strong sense of presence. The scores for sense of presence for the spatial memory task were 6.8 ± 2.4, for the sustained attention task were 7.4 ± 1.7, and for the balance task were 9.2 ± 1.4. All subjects under study reported significant amounts of mental effort during the encoding phase of spatial memory task (8 ± 2) and during the retrieval phase (6 ± 2), that is consistent with our previous research [34, 53].

A representative example of VR data obtained for three consequent testing sessions of one subject is shown in Fig. 3.6. The overall VR results obtained from all 15 subjects on three testing sessions are shown in Fig. 3.7. The ANOVA revealed neither main effect of testing day ($p > 0.05$) nor effect of VR testing modality ($p > 0.05$). In other words, no effect of practice was observed for either VR resting modalities.

SCORES	0.00	1.00	2.00	3.00	4.00	5.00	6.00	7.00	8.00	9.00	10.00
COMPREHENSIVE										9.10	
ATTENTION										9.11	
SPATIAL 1										9.23	
RECOGNITION A										9.09	
RECOGNITION B									8.91		
BALANCE										9.07	
REACTION TIME										9.20	

a Testing session 1

SCORES	0.00	1.00	2.00	3.00	4.00	5.00	6.00	7.00	8.00	9.00	10.00
COMPREHENSIVE									8.97		
ATTENTION										9.09	
SPATIAL 1										9.12	
RECOGNITION A									8.73		
RECOGNITION B									8.89		
BALANCE									8.97		
REACTION TIME									8.99		

b Testing session 2

SCORES	0.00	1.00	2.00	3.00	4.00	5.00	6.00	7.00	8.00	9.00	10.00
COMPREHENSIVE										9.05	
ATTENTION										9.16	
SPATIAL 1									8.93		
RECOGNITION A										9.08	
RECOGNITION B									8.96		
BALANCE										9.01	
REACTION TIME										9.15	

c Testing session 3

Fig. 3.6 Representative example from one subject on VR performance scores, including comprehensive, and those obtained from different testing modalities. Both visually and statistically, there are no significant differences in performance scores across testing sessions (session 1 (**a**), session 2 (**b**), and session 3 (**c**))

Assessment of Fatigue Induced by Full Contact Football Practices

Fifteen Penn State football players participated in this study. The subjects were males whose mean age was 20 ± 1.6 years. At the time of this study, none of the subjects were injured and all were cleared for full contact sport participation by the team physician. Complete medical history of all players under study was available only to one of the authors (Dr. Sebastianelli) and the other members of the research team were blind regarding the history of prior concussions until the completion of all results analysis.

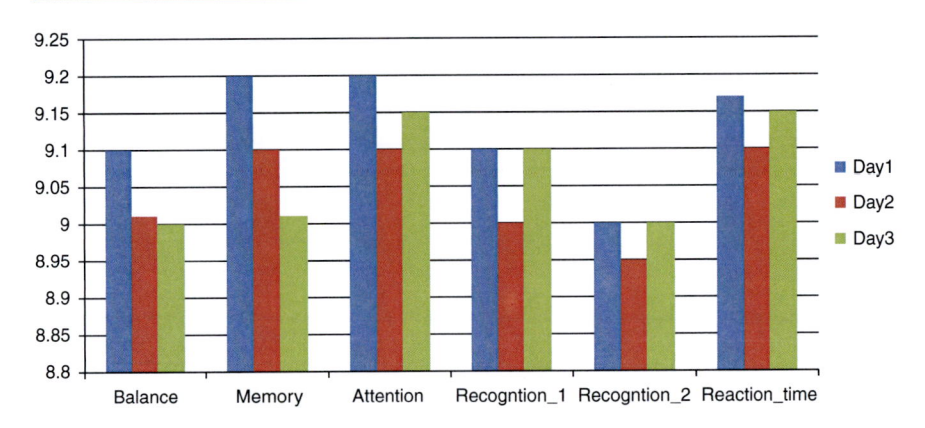

Fig. 3.7 Summary results of VR testing from all subjects under study ($n = 15$) as a function of testing day ($n = 3$). Both visually and statistically, no significant differences were observed within the testing modality and between tests indicating the lack of practice effect

Table 3.1 Subjects' performance on VR tests before and after full contact football practices inducing fatigue and the number of blows received

Players	Memory pre/post/post	Balance pre/post/post	RT pre/post/post	Impacts pr1/pr2
F001	8.3/8.7/8.4	8.6/9.1/8.8	9.4/9.1/8.3	46/38
F002	9.4/9.4/9.4	9.2/9.1/8.6	8.5/7.9/7.7	41/34
F003	7.5/7.9/8.1	9.3/9.0/9.1	8.6/8.9/8.0	37/42
F004	9.7/8.8/8.5	8.4/8.4/7.9	8.4/7.1/89	34/43
F005	6.9/8.3/8.1	7.4/7.9/6.8	8.5/7.2/8.3	36/38
F006	9.5/8.6/9.1	8.8/9.3/9.0	9.4/7.9/7.8	38/41
F007	8.1/8.6/5.4	9.3/7.8/5.6	7.7/5.5/4.2	37/43
F008	9.5/8.6/9.1	8.7/8.9/8.3	9.3/8.4/8.1	46/32
F009	8.4/8.9/9.3	8.3/8.1/7.6	7.9/8.1/8.3	41/39
F010	8.6/8.5/8/3	7.5/7.9/8.2	8.2/7.8/7.6	26/35
F011	8.6/8.5/5.3	7.8/5.6/5.1	9.2/8.8/4.9	29/35
F012	9.4/9.7/9.5	7.4/7.7/7.8	8.2/8.7/8.6	31/37
F013	7.4/6.7/5.2	8.6/8.1/6.1	9.5/6.7/4.2	34/31
F014	8.6/9.2/8.7	9.3/9.6/9/2	9.3/9.4/8.1	37/29
F015	9.3/9.6/9.0	7.8/8.5/8.1	8.4/7.8/8.4	35/41

The blow types included head-to-head, head-to-torso, blow to the back, blow to the torso, blow to the face, landing on the head, etc.

VR assessment of spatial memory, balance, and executive functions (RT) was conducted prior to and within 30 min post-full contact practices. The number of blows during the practice was measured via reconstruction of impacts captured on video [54]. In addition, our research assistants registered the frequency and various types of impact experienced by the *targeted players* using a specially developed observation chart. The similar pre-post-full contact practice VR assessment was conducted 1 week later at the peak of preseason training load.

The results from effect of fatigue on VR assessment of memory, balance, and executive functions are summarized in Table 3.1. The subjects' fatigue was assessed via verbal responses that ranged from 0 (no fatigue) to 10 (extreme exhaustion). All subjects under study had reported fatigue scored 7 ± 2.4 after full contact practice.

As can be seen from Table 3.1, the fatigue did not influence the VR data for either of the testing dates obtained from 12 of the football players ($p > 0.05$). However, there was a negative effect of fatigue on three of the subjects, and upon further investigation it was found that of all of the 15 subjects tested they were the only ones to have a history of previously diagnosed concussions. It is important to note that players received approximately equal number of blows during both practices. The effect of multiple blows, in conjunction with fatigue, on performance measurement needs further investigation.

Validation of Virtual Reality Modalities

The individual virtual reality modules (balance, reaction time, attention, spatial navigation) and the compositive, or comprehensive, score were examined for their sensitivity and specificity in comparing concussed and non-concussed subjects.

Balance A study by Teel and Slobounov [55] examined 60 normal controls and 21 concussed participants using standard balance assessments (force plate) and the VR balance module. Concussed participants were tested 7–10 days post injury to avoid any symptom provocation and to examine more subtle deficits after injury. Findings revealed that center of pressure (COP) with eyes open and eyes closed was significantly ($p < 0.01$) and negatively correlated with VR balance measures of yaw, pitch, roll, and total score. However, for both COP positions, the stationary balance scores were not significant. When examining group, there were significant and negative correlations (range: $r = -0.246$ to -0.641) with all VR balance outcome measures. The roll condition (around heading y-axis between 10 and 30° at 0.2 Hz) was the strongest correlation to group. Between groups, there were significant differences with the concussed group performing significantly worse on all VR balance measures compared to the control group.

To validate this module, another study was done by Teel and colleagues [56] on 94 normal controls and 27 concussed participants. The concussed participants were also tested between 7 and 10 days post injury. An ROC curve was run to establish cutoff scores and identify the sensitivity and specificity of the balance module. The AUC was 0.862 (95% CI: 0.767–0.958) and a cutoff score of 8.25 was identified to maximize sensitivity (85.7%) and specificity (87.8%). Additionally, the likelihood ratio was 18.28 and the odds ratio was 0.24.

The following modules were validated on the same group of participants [57]; 128 control participants (with no history of concussion) and 24 concussed participants (tested between 7 and 10 days post injury) were used. Group differences were examined, and the control group had significantly better performance ($p < 0.001$) on spatial navigation, reaction time, and comprehensive scores. There was no significant difference between group on the attention module ($p = 0.81$).

Reaction Time The whole-body reaction time module revealed a cutoff score of 6.75 to maximize sensitivity (95.2%) and specificity (89.1%). AUC was 0.952 (95% CI: 0.915, 0.985) and the likelihood ratio was 32.3.

Attention The attention module revealed a cutoff score of 9.50 to maximize sensitivity (54.2%) and specificity (30.5%). AUC was 0.593 (95% CI: 0.459, 0.728) and the likelihood ratio was 0.062.

Spatial Navigation The spatial navigation module revealed a cutoff score of 7.50 to maximize sensitivity (95.8%) and specificity (91.4%). AUC was 0.962 (95% CI: 0.934, 0.990) and the likelihood ratio was 57.2.

Comprehensive Score The combination of all modules (balance, attention, reaction time, spatial navigation) into a comprehensive score revealed a cutoff score of 7.55 to maximize sensitivity (95.8%) and specificity (96.1%). AUC was 0.989 (95% CI: 0.976, 1.000) and the likelihood ratio was 88.8.

The sensitivity and specificity of the comprehensive score are comparable to previously reported values of sensitivity (81.95–96.6%) and specificity (69.7–97.3%) in traditional neuropsychological testing [7, 58].

Overall Application of Virtual Reality as a Research and Clinical Tool

There is a considerable debate in the literature regarding the best practices in treatment of athletes suffering from concussion. Up to date, there is still no "gold standard" and the absence of definite biomarkers for an accurate diagnosis or prognostication of sports-related concussions continues [59]. The lack of consent among clinical practitioners is also exacerbated even more by the fact that the majority of subjects with *uncomplicated mTBI* appeared to be *asymptomatic* based on anatomical MRI, CT, and/or conventional clinical and neuropsychological (NP) assessments shortly after the injury [60]. Therefore, the search for more accurate complementary concussion assessment tools is ongoing.

This tool was developed on previous empirical findings; for example, there are no differences in planned agility between expert and novice athletes, although a reactive agility test was able to discriminate skill between levels due to the inclusion of the sport-specific visual stimuli [61]. Indeed, human vision is 3D. Therefore, depth perception is critical for successful performance in various sports environments [62]. Most recent research has attempted to improve visual stimuli realism for examining visual-perceptual skill via 2D/3D video projections of real-life opponents to elicit reactive movement [63]. In our own research, we observed differential patterns of brain activation (fMRI BOLD) while performing the spatial navigation memory task in 2D versus 3D virtual environment. Collectively, 3D realistic sports-specific virtual reality scenarios may enhance sensitivity of testing modalities used in a clinical setting. It is our ongoing line of research to examine the efficacy of 3D realistic sports-specific scenarios for assessment of performance indices in normal volunteers and student-athletes suffering the concussion.

VR modules aimed to assess balance, neurocognitive, and executive functions appeared to be resilient to a practice effect and, thus, may be implemented in repeated fashion to track evolution of a measured function, for example, as result of recovery from brain injury. Clearly, every single existing NP (and/or other) tool currently used in a clinical practice may have a possible practice effect. Therefore, it should not be overused while evaluating the concussed individuals during follow-up testing. The reported findings regarding virtual reality testing modalities' resilience to practice effect may indicate the feasibility of VR modules for multiple uses in a clinical practice.

The VR modules implemented in this study appeared to be resilient to a fatigue effect, for example, that may significantly confound evaluation of neurocognitive, balance, and executive functions as a sporting event is in progress. Clearly, comprehensive neuropsychological and behavioral evaluation of concussed individuals requires time and effort that may induce both physical and mental fatigue due to taking the tests [40]. Thus, dissociating fatigue symptoms due to concussion from those due to taking the tests is an important clinical issue. Moreover, it is also important to dissociate the athletes' performance level of neurocognitive, balance, and executive functions at different times during practices and/or games as a function of fatigue and/or concussion, if occurred. The resilience of VR modules to fatigue effect, but possible sensitivity to prior history of concussion, as reported in this study, may be considered as a valuable asset for sideline assessment of athletes in a clinical setting.

Furthermore, VR has been shown to have high sensitivity and specificity in identifying between control and concussed participants and has comparable normative values reported in traditional neuropsychological batteries used in clinical concussion management [64]. Additionally, it has shown utility in detecting residual cognitive abnormalities in concussed individuals who are considered asymptomatic and pass traditional clinical assessments. The inclusion of multiple modalities adds to the clinical utility of VR when using it in assessment of a concussed individual and may help provide more information on deficits post injury.

Acknowledgements This study was supported by NIH R01 grant: "Identification of Athletes at Risk for Traumatic Brain Injury." The authors would like to thank George Salvaterra, Katie Finelli, and Gregory Miskinis for their contribution to subjects' recruitment and data collection for this study.

References

1. Bazarian JJ, McClung J, Cheng YT, Flesher W, Schneider SM. Emergency department management of mild traumatic brain injury in the USA. Emerg Med J. 2005;22:473–7.
2. Langlois JA, Rutland-Brown W, Wald MM. The epidemiology and impact of traumatic brain injury: a brief overview. J Head Trauma Rehabil. 2006;21:375–8.

3. Risdall JE, Menon DK. Traumatic brain injury. Philos Trans R Soc Lond Ser B Biol Sci. 2011;366:241–50.
4. Ruff RM. Mild traumatic brain injury and neural recovery: rethinking the debate. NeuroRehabilitation. 2011;28:167–80.
5. McCrory P, Meeuwisse WH, Aubry M, Cantu RC, Dvořák J, Echemendia RJ, et al. Consensus Statement on Concussion in Sport: The 4th International Conference on Concussion in Sport, Zurich, November 2012. J Athlet Train (Allen Press). 2013;48:554–75.
6. Makdissi M, Darby D, Maruff P, Ugoni A, Brukner P, McCrory PR. Natural history of concussion in sport: markers of severity and implications for management. Am J Sports Med. 2010;38:464–71.
7. Iverson GL, Brooks BL, Collins MW, Lovell MR. Tracking neuropsychological recovery following concussion in sport. Brain Inj. 2006;20:245–52.
8. Broglio SP, Ferrara MS, Macciocchi SN, Baumgartner TA, Elliott R. Test-retest reliability of computerized concussion assessment programs. J Athl Train. 2007;42:509–14.
9. Sedney CL, Orphanos J, Bailes JE. When to consider retiring an athlete after sports-related concussion. Clin Sports Med. 2011;30:189–200. xi
10. Slobounov S, Sebastianelli W, Hallett M. Residual brain dysfunction observed one year post-mild traumatic brain injury: combined EEG and balance study. Clin Neurophysiol. 2012;123:1755–61.
11. Shenton M, Hamoda H, Schneiderman J, Bouix S, Pasternak O, Rathi Y, et al. A review of magnetic resonance imaging and diffusion tensor imaging findings in mild traumatic brain injury. Brain Imaging Behav. 2012;6:137–92.
12. Guskiewicz KM, McCrea M, Marshall SW, Cantu RC, Randolph C, Barr W, et al. Cumulative effects associated with recurrent concussion in collegiate football players: the NCAA Concussion Study. JAMA. 2003;290:2549–55.
13. Eckner JT, Kutcher JS, Richardson JK. Between-seasons test-retest reliability of clinically measured reaction time in National Collegiate Athletic Association Division I Athletes. J Athl Train. 2011;46:409–14.
14. McCrory P, Meeuwisse W, Johnston K, Dvorak J, Aubry M, Molloy M, et al. Consensus statement on concussion in sport: the 3rd International Conference on Concussion in Sport Held in Zurich, November 2008. J Athl Train. 2009;44:434–48.
15. Ingersoll CD, Armstrong CW. The effects of closed-head injury on postural sway. Med Sci Sports Exerc. 1992;24:739–43.
16. Lishman WA. Physiogenesis and psychogenesis in the "post-concussional syndrome". Br J Psychiatry. 1988;153:460–9.
17. Wöber C, Oder W, Kollegger H, Prayer L, Baumgartner C, Wöber-Bingöl C, et al. Posturographic measurement of body sway in survivors of severe closed head injury. Arch Phys Med Rehabil. 1993;74:1151–6.
18. Guskiewicz KM, Riemann BL, Perrin DH, Nashner LM. Alternative approaches to the assessment of mild head injury in athletes. Med Sci Sports Exerc. 1997;29:S213–21.
19. Guskiewicz KM. Postural stability assessment following concussion: one piece of the puzzle. Clin J Sport Med. 2001;11:182–9.
20. Guskiewicz KM, Ross SE, Marshall SW. Postural stability and neuropsychological deficits after concussion in collegiate athletes. J Athl Train. 2001;36:263–73.
21. Guskiewicz KM, Mihalik JP. The biomechanics and pathomechanics of sport-related concussion. In: Slobounov S, Sebastianelli W, editors. Foundations of sport-related brain injuries; 2006. p. 65–83.
22. Riemann BL, Guskiewicz KM. Effects of mild head injury on postural stability as measured through clinical balance testing. J Athl Train. 2000;35:19–25.
23. Peterson CL, Ferrara MS, Mrazik M, Piland S, Elliott R. Evaluation of neuropsychological domain scores and postural stability following cerebral concussion in sports. Clin J Sport Med. 2003;13:230–7.

24. Valovich TC, Perrin DH, Gansneder BM. Repeat administration elicits a practice effect with the balance error scoring system but not with the standardized assessment of concussion in high school athletes. J Athl Train. 2003;38:51–6.
25. Cavanaugh JT, Guskiewicz KM, Stergiou N. A nonlinear dynamic approach for evaluating postural control: new directions for the management of sport-related cerebral concussion. Sports Med. 2005;35:935–50.
26. Cavanaugh JT, Guskiewicz KM, Giuliani C, Marshall S, Mercer V, Stergiou N. Detecting altered postural control after cerebral concussion in athletes with normal postural stability. Br J Sports Med. 2005;39:805–11.
27. Cavanaugh JT, Guskiewicz KM, Giuliani C, Marshall S, Mercer VS, Stergiou N. Recovery of postural control after cerebral concussion: new insights using approximate entropy. J Athl Train. 2006;41:305–13.
28. Slobounov S, Cao C, Sebastianelli W, Slobounov E, Newell K. Residual deficits from concussion as revealed by virtual time-to-contact measures of postural stability. Clin Neurophysiol. 2008;119:281–9.
29. Slobounov S, Sebastianelli W, Simon R. Neurophysiological and behavioral concomitants of mild brain injury in collegiate athletes. Clin Neurophysiol. 2002;113:185–93.
30. Slobounov S, Slobounov E, Newell K. Application of virtual reality graphics in assessment of concussion. Cyberpsychol Behav. 2006;9:188–91.
31. Slobounov S, Sebastianelli W, Moss R. Alteration of posture-related cortical potentials in mild traumatic brain injury. Neurosci Lett. 2005;383:251–5.
32. Slobounov S, Slobounov E, Sebastianelli W, Cao C, Newell K. Differential rate of recovery in athletes after first and second concussion episodes. Neurosurgery. 2007;61:338–44; discussion 344.
33. Slobounov S, Cao C, Sebastianelli W. Differential effect of first versus second concussive episodes on wavelet information quality of EEG. Clin Neurophysiol. 2009;120:862–7.
34. Slobounov SM, Zhang K, Pennell D, Ray W, Johnson B, Sebastianelli W. Functional abnormalities in normally appearing athletes following mild traumatic brain injury: a functional MRI study. Exp Brain Res. 2010;202:341–54.
35. Slobounov SM, Gay M, Zhang K, Johnson B, Pennell D, Sebastianelli W, et al. Alteration of brain functional network at rest and in response to YMCA physical stress test in concussed athletes: RsFMRI study. NeuroImage. 2011;55:1716–27.
36. Slobounov S, Sebastianelli W, Newell KM. Incorporating virtual reality graphics with brain imaging for assessment of sport-related concussions. Ann Int Conf IEEE Eng Med Biol Soc. 2011;2011:1383–6.
37. Slobounov S, Gay M, Johnson B, Zhang K. Concussion in athletics: ongoing clinical and brain imaging research controversies. Brain Imaging Behav. 2012;6:224–43.
38. Bartels C, Wegrzyn M, Wiedl A, Ackermann V, Ehrenreich H. Practice effects in healthy adults: a longitudinal study on frequent repetitive cognitive testing. BMC Neurosci. 2010;11:118.
39. Schmidt JD, Register-Mihalik JK, Mihalik JP, Kerr ZY, Guskiewicz KM. Identifying impairments after concussion: normative data versus individualized baselines. Med Sci Sports Exerc. 2012;44:1621–8.
40. Barwick F, Arnett P, Slobounov S. EEG correlates of fatigue during administration of a neuropsychological test battery. Clin Neurophysiol. 2012;123:278–84.
41. Slobounov SM, Ray W, Johnson B, Slobounov E, Newell KM. Modulation of cortical activity in 2D versus 3D virtual reality environments: an EEG study. Int J Psychophysiol. 2015;95:254–60.
42. Cochrane JL, Lloyd DG, Besier TF, Elliott BC, Doyle TLA, Ackland TR. Training affects knee kinematics and kinetics in cutting maneuvers in sport. Med Sci Sports Exerc. 2010;42:1535–44.
43. Vaeyens R, Lenoir M, Williams AM, Mazyn L, Philippaerts RM. The effects of task constraints on visual search behavior and decision-making skill in youth soccer players. J Sport Exerc Psychol. 2007;29:147–69.
44. Schatz P. Long-term test-retest reliability of baseline cognitive assessments using ImPACT. Am J Sports Med. 2010;38:47–53.

45. Sohlberg MM, Mateer CA. Training use of compensatory memory books: a three stage behavioral approach. J Clin Exp Neuropsychol. 1989;11:871–91.
46. Bate AJ, Mathias JL, Crawford JR. Performance on the Test of Everyday Attention and standard tests of attention following severe traumatic brain injury. Clin Neuropsychol. 2001;15:405–22.
47. Gloyer K, Aukerman D, Sebastianelli W, Slobounov S. Application of virtual reality for assessment of concussion in sports. Salt Lake City, UT; 2011.
48. Slobounov S, Tutwiler R, Sebastianelli W, Slobounov E. Alteration of postural responses to visual field motion in mild traumatic brain injury. Neurosurgery. 2006;59:134–9; discussion 134–139.
49. MacFlynn G, Montgomery EA, Fenton GW, Rutherford W. Measurement of reaction time following minor head injury. J Neurol Neurosurg Psychiatry. 1984;47:1326–31.
50. Stuss DT, Stethem LL, Hugenholtz H, Picton T, Pivik J, Richard MT. Reaction time after head injury: fatigue, divided and focused attention, and consistency of performance. J Neurol Neurosurg Psychiatry. 1989;52:742–8.
51. Warden DL, Bleiberg J, Cameron KL, Ecklund J, Walter J, Sparling MB, et al. Persistent prolongation of simple reaction time in sports concussion. Neurology. 2001;57:524–6.
52. Iverson GL, Lovell MR, Collins MW. Validity of ImPACT for measuring processing speed following sports-related concussion. J Clin Exp Neuropsychol. 2005;27:683–9.
53. Jaiswal N, Ray W, Slobounov S. Encoding of visual-spatial information in working memory requires more cerebral efforts than retrieval: evidence from EEG and virtual reality study. Brain Res. 2010;1347:80–9.
54. Pellman EJ, Viano DC, Tucker AM, Casson IR, Waeckerle JF. Concussion in professional football: reconstruction of game impacts and injuries. Neurosurgery. 2003;53:799–814.
55. Teel EF, Slobounov SM. Validation of a virtual reality balance module for use in clinical concussion assessment and management. Clin J Sport Med. 2015;25:144–8.
56. Teel EF, Gay MR, Arnett PA, Slobounov SM. Differential sensitivity between a virtual reality balance module and clinically used concussion balance modalities. Clin J Sport Med. 2016;26:162–6.
57. Teel E, Gay M, Johnson B, Slobounov S. Determining sensitivity/specificity of virtual reality-based neuropsychological tool for detecting residual abnormalities following sport-related concussion. Neuropsychology. 2016;30:474–83.
58. Louey AG, Cromer JA, Schembri AJ, Darby DG, Maruff P, Makdissi M, et al. Detecting cognitive impairment after concussion: sensitivity of change from baseline and normative data methods using the CogSport/Axon cognitive test battery. Arch Clin Neuropsychol. 2014;29:432–41.
59. Bigler ED, Bazarian JJ. Diffusion tensor imaging: a biomarker for mild traumatic brain injury? Neurology. 2010;74:626–7.
60. Bigler ED, Maxwell WL. Neuropathology of mild traumatic brain injury: relationship to neuroimaging findings. Brain Imaging Behav. 2012;6:108–36.
61. Farrow D, Young W, Bruce L. The development of a test of reactive agility for netball: a new methodology. J Sci Med Sport. 2005;8:52–60.
62. Vickers JN. Perception, cognition, and decision training: the quiet eye in action; 2007.
63. Lee MJC, Tidman SJ, Lay BS, Bourke PD, Lloyd DG, Alderson JA. Visual search differs but not reaction time when intercepting a 3D versus 2D videoed opponent. J Mot Behav. 2013;45:107–15.
64. Broglio SP, Macciocchi SN, Ferrara MS. Sensitivity of the concussion assessment battery. Neurosurgery. 2007;60:1050–7; discussion 1057–1058.

Feasibility of Electroencephalography for Direct Assessment of Concussion

William J. Ray, Elizabeth Teel, Michael Gay, Semyon M. Slobounov, Robert Fornini, and Owen Griffith

Introduction

Recently, much research has focused on the role of concussion in athletics, particularly contact sports. An international conference on Concussion in Sport published a consensus statement that includes a summary of the most recently agreed-upon causes, diagnostic tools, symptoms, guidelines for return to sport and daily life, and prevention of sports-related concussion. The updated definition of sports-related concussion is:

> a traumatic brain injury induced by biomechanical forces, which may be caused either by a direct blow to the head, face, neck or elsewhere on the body with an impulsive force transmitted to the head, typically results in the rapid onset of short-lived impairment of neurological function that resolves spontaneously or evolve over a number of minutes to hours, and may result in neuropathological changes, but the acute clinical signs and symptoms largely reflect a functional disturbance rather than a structural injury and, as such, no abnormality is seen on standard structural neuroimaging studies [1].

With the growing public concern regarding these injuries, the National Football League has supported studies of the long-term effects of concussion in professional athletes and many universities have established centers for the study of concussion on their athletes. Additionally, many individual states within the United States have established laws related to concussion assessment and management in child-age athletics, as well as return to play and academic guidelines. In particular, high school athletes are at risk for repeat concussion since surveys suggest that this group believes that there is not a problem playing sports after injury. Furthermore, studies on high school athletes revealed common reasons for concussion not being reported including thinking the injury is serious enough to warrant medical attention, social and intrinsic motivation not to be withheld from competition, and lack of awareness of probable concussion [2–5]. The reasons for not self-reporting may also vary based on the stage, as motivation to stay in competition changes across age groups and level. In collegiate athletes for example, factors such as future professional career, scholarship, acceptance of peers, support from coaching staff, and personal identity as an athlete may all impact symptom reporting [6, 7]. Returning to play before the concussion has been fully resolved can increase the likelihood of long-term injures due to a higher risk of secondary injury during recovery. Athletes who suffer repeat concussion typically do so within the first 7–10 days after the initial injury [8]. Since adolescence is a time in which an individual's brain is still developing and goes through a series of cortical reorganizations, brain insults at this time can put the adolescent at greater risk for more serious injury or even death. For college and professional athletes, different internal, team, or societal pressures may cause players to ignore information concerning the effects of concussion. Overall, this can lead to a lack of candor when athletes describe their symptoms. Since, at this time, diagnosis is often based on the individual's self-reporting of their symptoms to a doctor, it is critical to utilize measures that can evaluate the effects of concussion beyond the traditional signs and symptoms, in a more objective way.

When the injury occurs, acceleration/deceleration forces are applied to the head and can often produce diffuse microstructural injury. Due to the diffuse nature of these injuries, standard structural imaging, such as MRI and CT, may not be able to identify all abnormalities [9]. Evidence collected from several animal studies implies that mTBI and SRC induce temporary variance in neuronal energy metabolism, excitatory neurotransmitter release, and cerebral blood flow [10, 11], establishing a functional injury, rather than solely a structural injury. With this evidence, numerous organizations have published position statements concluding that neuroimaging findings are generally normal in sports-related concussion individuals and imaging studies add little to the field of clinical concussion management [12–16]. Currently, authorities recommend that neuroimaging be used for patients in the acute phase of head injury, when there is suspicion of severe intracranial pathological conditions like subdural hematoma, epidural hematoma, or intraparenchymal hemorrhage (IPH), or in patients with extended disruption in consciousness, focal neurological deficits, or aggravated symptoms [12–18].

In summary, rather than the gross structural damage or lesions found in penetrating head injury or severe traumatic brain injuries, concussive episodes can be characterized by cognitive dysfunction, specifically in information processing and working memory [9].

Need for Physiologic Measurement in Clinical Concussion Diagnosis/Management

Athletic participation is unique in its requirement of the able-bodied participant. Physicians and allied health professionals making recommendations for athletes returning to sport from concussion must ultimately be comfortable with the concept of potential repeated injury. In other words, although unclear whether this is entirely possible, it is the clinician's goal to ensure that an athlete recovering from concussion and returning to full athletic participation be as resilient to head trauma as compared to an athlete with no previous head injury. Ultimately, clinicians must be assured that the athlete's risk of short-term or long-term effects from their concussive episode has been minimized as best as possible.

With these important clinical considerations in mind, management of sports-related concussion must evolve beyond the limitations in the currently accepted definition of concussion with *functional* recovery from concussion being representative of clinical healing. Considering the number of mTBI-linked short-term and long-term physical and mental health issues [19–22], clinicians and researchers alike must take important steps to ensure proper management of the recovering athlete. Intense scrutiny of residual physiological and functional deficits, as well as measuring and monitoring the athlete's rate of pathophysiological recovery from concussive injuries must become a primary focus. By increasing collective efforts, we can hope to reduce short- and long-term health issues. Yet, despite this need, clinical management of the mild head-injured athlete has evolved relatively slowly.

One of the reasons that clinical management of concussion has remained largely unchanged is due partly to a disproportionate focus on functional cognitive testing. Neuropsychological testing remains the mainstay in determining the clinical recovery for the concussed athlete. As neuropsychological testing is limited to cognitive functional performance, it has seemingly maximized its clinical utility at present. Therefore, clinical researchers need to push the constructs of other applicable and relevant diagnostic tools to provide athletes recovering from sports-related concussion with better assessment and management tools. These tools must be able to distinguish residual functional *and* structural (physiological) recovery from mTBI. As both diffuse functional and structural injury are present in mTBI [23, 24], clinicians and researchers must develop and research both functional and structural diagnostic tools when treating the athlete recovering from concussion.

Several organizations include the presence of pathophysiology in their definitions of concussion. Thus, it seems appropriate to utilize a physiological measure to denote the presence of concussion. Due to the diffuse nature of the injury and the consequential cognitive dysfunction, electroencephalograms or EEGs, which are able to systematically evaluate the underlying neural process that contributes to functional networks, are a sensitive and appropriate tool to evaluate the effects of concussive episodes.

EEG was first demonstrated in humans by Hans Berger in 1924 and published 5 years later [25]. Since the neurons of the brain and their connections are constantly active, EEG can be measured in an individual both during conscious and unconscious states as seen in sleep and brain trauma. As such, EEG was the first brain assessment tool that was able to establish an alteration in brain function in a traumatic brain injury population [26, 27] and has continued to be useful in the brain injury field.

Early EEG research including 300 patients clearly demonstrated the slowing of major frequency bands and focal abnormalities within 48 hours post injury [28]. A study by McClelland et al. has shown that EEG recordings performed during the immediate post-concussion period demonstrated a large amount of "diffusely distributed slow-wave potentials," which were markedly reduced when recordings were performed 6 weeks after injury [29]. Additionally, Tebano et al. showed a shift in the mean frequency in the alpha (8–10 Hz) band toward lower power and an overall decrease of beta (14–18 Hz) power in patients suffering from mTBI [30]. The reduction of theta power [31] accompanying a transient increase of alpha-theta ratios [32, 33] was identified as residual symptoms in concussion patients.

At the beginning of the twenty-first century, Gaetz and Bernstein [19] cited electrophysiological techniques as the most commonly used method to evaluate brain functioning, noting the relatively low cost, noninvasive nature of the test, and the long, well-documented history dating back to the 1930s. Leon-Carrion et al. [34] echo the benefits defined by Gaetz and Bernstein and also speak to the uncomplicated procedure, high test-retest reliability, and characteristic stability of EEGs as additional features that contribute to its appropriateness as a diagnostic testing tool.

The Nature of EEG

EEG reflects the electrical activity of the brain at the level of the synapse [35]. It is the product of changing excitatory and inhibitory currents. More specifically, graded postsynaptic potentials of the cell body and dendrites of vertically orientated pyramidal cells in cortical layers three to five give rise to the EEG recorded on the scalp. The ability to record the relatively small voltage at the scalp from these actions results from the fact that pyramidal cells tend to share a similar orientation and polarity and may be synchronously activated. Action potentials contribute very little to the EEG. However, since changes at the synapse do influence the production of action potentials, there is an association of EEG with spike trains [36]. The summation of these electrophysiological measures is precisely what makes EEGs better suited for the study of concussion compared to several other types of brain imaging techniques.

Historically, the system of locating electrodes in EEG is referred to as the International 10–20 system [37]. The name 10–20 refers to the fact that electrodes in this system are placed at sites 10% and 20% from four anatomical landmarks. One landmark is the front of the nasion (the bridge of the nose). In the rear of the head, the inion (the bump at the back of the head just above the neck) is used. The left and right landmarks are the preauricular points (depressions in front of the ears above the cheekbone). In this system, the letters refer to areas of the brain; 0 = occipital, P = parietal, C = central, F = frontal, and T = temporal. Numerical subscripts indicate laterality (odd numbers left, even right) and degree of displacement from the midline (subscripted z). Thus, C3 describes an electrode over the central region of the brain on the left side whereas Cz would refer to an electrode placed at the top of the scalp above the central area. With the development of dense array systems, the historical 10–20 system has been greatly expanded (see Fig. 4.1 for an example cap).

To record the EEG, electrical signals of only a few microvolts must be detected on the scalp. A signal can be found by amplifying the differential between two electrodes, at least one of which is placed on the scalp. Since the signal must be amplified almost one million times, care must be taken that the resulting signal is indeed actual EEG and not artifact. Where the electrodes are placed and how many are used depend on the purpose of the recording. Almost all EEG procedures currently use a variety of EEG caps with up to 256 electrodes built into the cap, although it is always possible to record EEG from only two electrodes. Those recording caps that use 128 to 256 electrodes are generally referred to as dense array EEG recordings and are used in most research settings. However, research in clinical situations, such as the hospital emergency room, has shown that as few as 5 electrodes can be used for the screening of mild traumatic brain injuries [38]. That study demonstrated that EEG showed a 94.7% accuracy rate when compared with computed tomography for detecting mild traumatic brain injuries, highlighting the potential of using even simple EEG montages for detecting concussions in a sports setting.

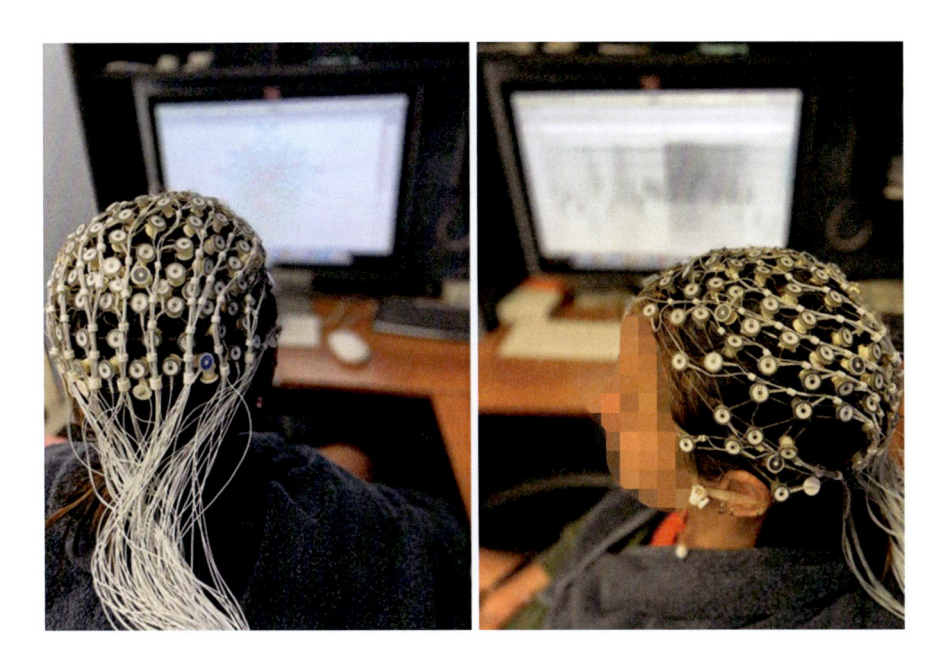

Fig. 4.1 128-electrode cap applied during routine EEG recording

EEG Frequency Bands

One important parameter of EEG is the determination of frequency. Although there are some minor discrepancies in the literature in terms of the beginning and ending of the specific frequency band, a general template is presented in Table 4.1. Frequency bands are generally determined through signal processing techniques such as Fourier analysis and wavelet analysis.

Alpha activity can be seen in about three-fourths of all individuals when they are awake and relaxed. Asking these individuals to further relax and close their eyes will result in recurring periods of several seconds in which the EEG consists of relatively large, rhythmic waves of about 8–12 Hz. This is the *alpha rhythm*, the presence of which has been related to relaxation and the lack of active cognitive processes. If someone who displays alpha activity is asked to perform cognitive activity such as solving an arithmetic problem in their head, alpha activity will no longer be present in the EEG. This is referred to as alpha blocking. Typically, cognitive activity causes the alpha rhythm to be replaced by high frequency, low amplitude EEG activity referred to as beta activity. Since the discovery of the alpha rhythm, a variety of studies have focused on its relationship to psychological processes and broad developments of the cognitive and affective neurosciences amplified this interest [see [39, 40] for reviews].

High-frequency activity occurs when one is alert. Traditionally, lower voltage variations ranging from about 18 to 30 Hz have been referred to as beta and higher frequency, lower voltage variations ranging from about 30 to 70 Hz or higher are referred to as gamma. Initial work suggests that gamma activity is related to the brain's ability to integrate a variety of stimuli into a coherent whole. For example, Tallon-Baudry and colleagues [41] showed individual pictures of a hidden Dalmatian dog that was difficult to see because of the black and white background. After training individuals to see the dog, differences in the gamma band suggested meaningful and non-meaningful stimuli produced differential responses.

Additional patterns of spontaneous EEG activity include delta activity (0.5–4 Hz), theta activity (4–8 Hz), and lambda and Kcomplex waves and sleep spindles, which are not defined solely in terms of frequency. Theta activity refers to EEG activity in the 4–8 Hz range. Grey Walter [42], who introduced the term theta rhythm, suggested that theta was seen at the cessation of a pleasurable activity. More recent

Table 4.1 Frequency ranges for each given bandwidth

Bandwidth name	Frequency	Brain function correlation
Delta	0.5–4 Hz	Deep sleep, memory consolidation, infant resting state
Theta	4–8 Hz	Beginning phases of sleep, working memory, information uptake and processing
Alpha	8–13 Hz	Relaxation/meditation, mind-body integration
Beta1	13–24 Hz	Active thinking, problem solving, decision making
Beta2	24–32 Hz	
Gamma	32–60 Hz	Heightened perception and processing

research associated theta with such processes as hypnagogic imagery, REM (rapid eye movement) sleep, problem solving, attention, and hypnosis, and source analysis of midline theta suggests that the anterior cingulate is involved in its generation [42]. In an early review of theta activity, Schacter [43] suggested that there are actually two different types of theta activity: (1) theta activity associated with low levels of alertness as would be seen as one falls asleep and (2) theta activity associated with attention and active and efficient processing of cognitive and perceptual tasks. This is consistent with the suggestion of Vogel et al. [44] that there two types of behavioral inhibition, one associated with a gross inactivation of an entire excitatory process resulting in less active behavioral states and one associated with selective inactivity as seen in over-learned processes.

Delta activity is low frequency (0.5–4 Hz) and has been traditionally associated with sleep in healthy humans as well as pathological conditions including cerebral infarct, contusion, local infection, tumor, epileptic foci, and subdural hematoma. The idea is that these types of disorders influence the neural tissue that in turn creates abnormal neural activity in the delta range by cutting off these tissues from major input sources. Although these observations were first seen with intracranial electrodes, more recent work has found similar results using MEG and EEG techniques. Additionally, EEG delta activity is the predominant frequency of human infants during the first 2 years of life.

EEG and Concussion

While conventional EEGs are not part of the current clinical "gold-standard" assessment battery, a number of studies show EEG differences in those individuals suffering from concussion compared to healthy controls [see [45] for an overview]. Of the differences observed on conventional EEGs, the most common abnormalities seen are generalized or focal slowing as well as weakened posterior alpha in mTBI patients [28, 46, 47]. These deficits were found in the immediate post-injury period (within a few hours of a concussive episode); however, similar findings have been reported even when there is a longer period between injury occurrence and evaluation.

These common abnormalities seen on conventional EEG recordings usually resolve within the first few months post injury [48], similar to the resolution of functional and symptomatic deficits in concussive recovery. However, up to 10% of individuals diagnosed with mTBI still show atypical electrophysiological readings in the late post-injury period [48, 49]. This small but significant portion of individuals who show electrophysiological abnormalities in the late post-injury period parallels those individuals who have atypical resolution of concussive symptoms and functioning.

Traditionally, in clinical settings, conventional EEGs were interpreted by the visual inspection of raw EEG signals. However, studies show that visual inspection of EEG lacks the sensitivity to detect changes following concussion. With the advancement of computerized signal processing techniques, there is a growing body of literature that suggests more complex EEG paradigms may be used to assess changes in functional status after concussive injuries [9]. Compared to visually inspected EEGs, computerized EEG analyses are advantageous because they can detect subtle differences in signal patterns and shifts not visible to the naked eye [23]. Due to these benefits, Cannon et al. [50] indicated the usefulness of EEG as an assessment tool for brain injury is due to its "direct signature of neural activity" and "ideal temporal resolution."

Several different types of variables can be isolated using quantitative EEG methods. Spectral analysis, relative amplitude, and power in particular frequency bandwidth, coherence, and phase are the most common types of analyses performed in EEGs. In terms of mTBI, frequency and coherence analyses of particular cortical areas can offer important information [9, 23, 51]. By examining the pattern of activity between the cortical areas, it is also possible to delineate brain networks, see how they are involved in different types of tasks, and determine how they differ under certain conditions such as the presence of a concussion.

Coherence analysis describes how the EEG signal at each of two electrodes is related to one another. In other words, coherence reflects the manner in which two signals "co-vary" at a particular frequency and represents the correlation of signal phase stability between two different electrodes. Coherence measurements within the same frequency band offer an estimate of the temporal relationships between adjacent neural systems. Like correlation, coherence is a measure between 0 and 1, where 1 represents a perfect phase correlation between two groups and 0 represents no correlation. Thus, in performing the coherence analysis, one can also obtain a measure of phase or synchrony (see Fig. 4.2 for an example of various EEG outputs).

The particular interest in EEG coherence is due to the biological nature of concussive injury. The brain structures involved in neural connectivity, such as the reticular system activation and thalamocortical tracts, are the structures most likely to be affected by concussion. Considering the probability that these areas are altered following concussion, frequency and coherence analyses are likely to be the most sensitive electrophysiological measures to indicate deficits due to concussive injury.

According to Arciniegas [23], frequency measures can vary with the number of neurons (smaller number, smaller amplitude/power), the integrity of the thalamocortical circuits in which the neurons contribute (injury to the circuit causes slower frequencies), and the influence of activation from the reticular system (increases in reticular system activity cause higher frequencies, while decreases in reticular system activity cause lower frequencies). Coherence, which by definition correlates the frequency measures between two different electrodes, may indicate the level of communication between different areas of the brain and signify neural network connectivity and dynamics [23]. Reduced coherence values can be attributed to damage in myelinated fibers and/or gray matter. If lowered coherence values are seen in concussion patients, it is still unknown which of these factors, or if a combination of all of them, produces these results.

Each concussive episode is individualized and may produce different changes in the brain. In turn, one might expect that the respective EEG measures would be different in each concussion patient. While the electrophysiological deficits found for

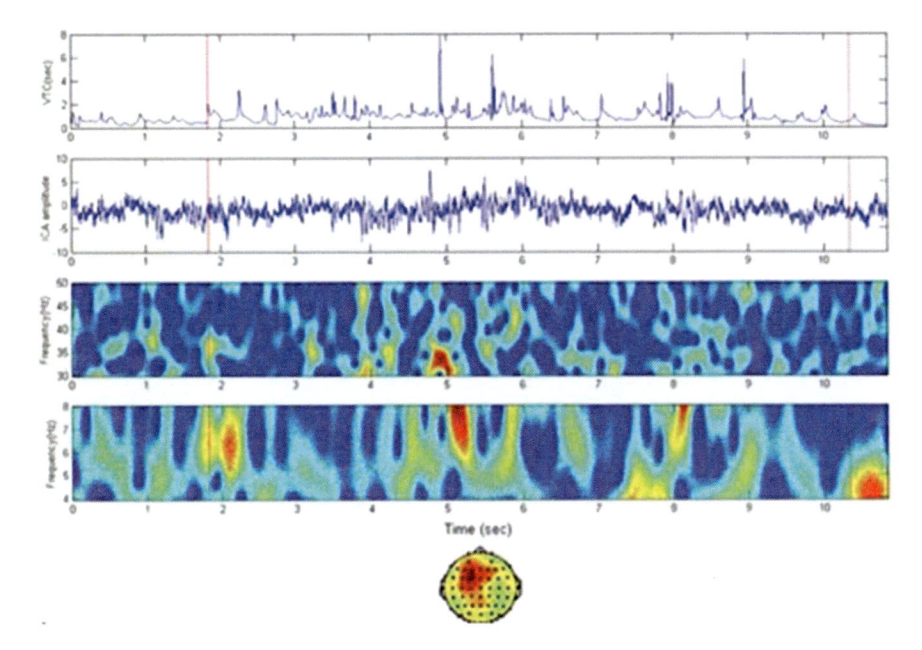

Fig. 4.2 An example of various EEG outputs: (top panel) wave frequency; (middle panel) example of ICA analysis; (bottom two panels) frequency domain color map where warm colors, that is, red, indicate higher activity. (Used with permission from Slobounov et al. [108])

each concussive episode remain unique, several consistent EEG patterns have been identified. According to a review by Arciniegas [23], the most common EEG findings in concussion include: (1) a decrease in mean alpha frequency [30, 33, 52–55], increase in theta activity [29, 31, 56, 57], or increased alpha-theta ratio [32, 33, 52, 55, 58], lessened alpha and beta power between anterior and posterior regions, weakened alpha power (posterior region), and increased coherence between frontal and temporal regions [59–61].

Along with these findings, a review by Nuwer et al. [47] listed other common EEG findings after concussive episodes. These findings concluded that changes in EEG measures resolved along the same timeline as symptoms, with gradual changes mainly occurring over weeks to months. They also found that left temporal slowing may correspond to lingering cognitive symptoms. Importantly, in all the studies evaluated by Nuwer, coherence was not correlated to outcome or diffuse axonal injury. Due to how quickly EEG patterns can change in an mTBI population [23], it is critically important that research involving individuals being tested after a concussive injury are evaluated at as similar time points as possible.

Evidence provided by Thornton [62] and Thatcher [63] indicates that the EEG patterns seen in a concussed athlete do not change over time and, therefore, should be present at the initial time of injury. While this is useful in describing EEG as a possible tool in diagnosing and evaluating concussed individuals, it also indicates that concussive episodes, even "mild" or "typical" episodes, cause long-lasting alterations in brain electrophysiology. Work by Barr et al. [64] showed that despite improvement or normal levels of cognitive functioning, brain patterns remain altered in mTBI patients. This further suggests that the brain may not completely heal from concussive episodes; instead, the individual learns to compensate for the deficit in order to achieve normal performance. The idea of compensation instead of recovery has been examined in a study by Thornton [65] and discussed in a book chapter [51].

A study by Theriault and colleagues revealed the cumulative effects of concussions in athletes by EEG abnormalities on visual working memory. They found that athletes with a history of three or more concussions exhibited significantly reduced sustained posterior contralateral negativity (SPCN) amplitude, relative to both athletes without concussion and those with only one or two prior concussions [66]. Sustained posterior contralateral activity has been shown to indicate the processing of visual stimulus, specifically in relation to a changing visual environment [67]. Additionally, SPCN amplitude was found to significantly correlate with the number of previous concussions, indicating visual working memory storage is further depleted with successive concussions [66].

Two prominent studies have examined the reproducibility of EEG absolute measures. First, a study by Corsi-Cabera et al. [68] tested nine subjects 11 times over a 1-month period. When looking at absolute amplitude, the median correlation coefficient over the 11 sessions was 0.94 while alpha and beta bands showed greater variability than any of the other bands. Pollock et al. [69] evaluated test-retest reliability in each bandwidth over a 20-week period on 46 normal controls. Absolute amplitude in theta, alpha, and beta1 had correlation coefficients that exceeded 0.60 while beta2 and delta correlation coefficients were found to be lower, with delta showing the poorest correlation. The authors also found that absolute amplitude has higher correlation coefficients than relative power and is, therefore, recommended for use in future studies. The high levels of correlation found in these studies, combined with the varying intervals between testing sessions (a common feature in concussion testing), imply that absolute amplitude is an appropriate measure for research purposes.

Although related to amplitude, several studies have separately analyzed the reproducibility of power (see Figs. 4.3 and 4.4 for an example of a power map). Salinksy et al. [70] tested absolute and relative power and found correlation coefficients of 0.84. Tests were run between 12 and 16 weeks apart on 25 normal controls. Cannon et al. [50] examined test-retest EEG power reliability by examining 19 normative controls over a 30-day testing period. Each participant was recorded for a 4-minute interval under an eyes open and eyes closed condition. Intraclass correlation coefficients for absolute power were 0.90 for eyes closed data and 0.77 for eyes open data. The results of these studies closely mimic those found when evaluating amplitude, with power having sufficiently high levels of reliability over both short (days) and long (months) testing periods.

Mathematically distinct from amplitude and power, researchers have spent time considering the reproducibility of coherence values. Studies by Harmony et al. [71] and Nikulin and Brismar [72] evaluated the reproducibility of coherence during rest

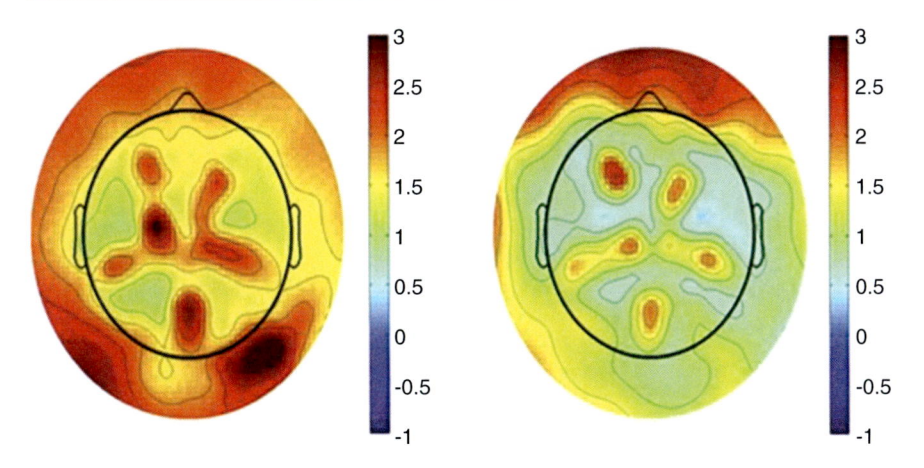

4 Feasibility of Electroencephalography for Direct Assessment of Concussion 65

Fig. 4.3 Power images for the beta frequency band during the eyes closed seated baseline EEG condition for the control (left) and concussed (right) groups. (Used with permission from Teel et al. [109])

a Theta Power (4-7 Hz) Evolution from pre-test to post-test on Stroop Interference Condition

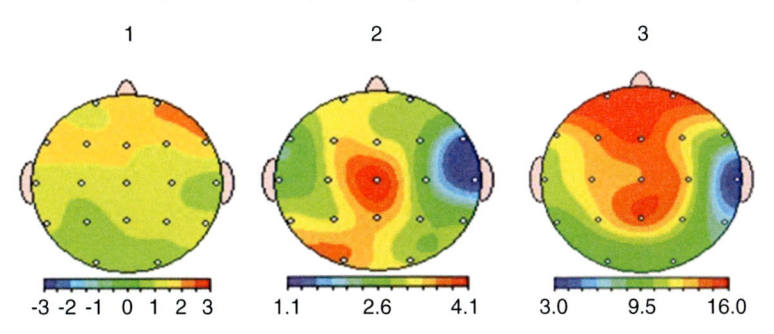

b Alpha Power (8-12 Hz) Evolution from pre-test to post-test on Stroop Interference Condition

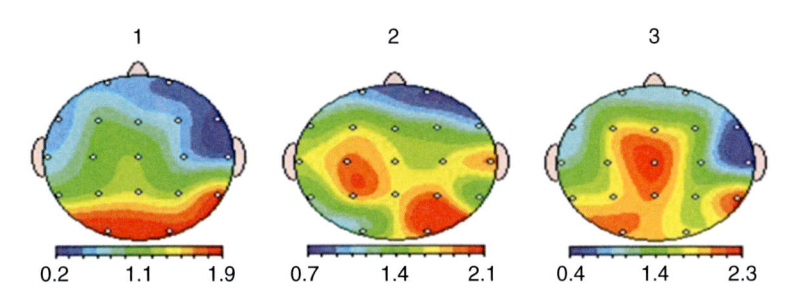

Fig. 4.4 An example EEG power map. (**a**) shows theta power map and (**b**) shows alpha power map. (Used with permission from Barwick et al. [110])

and cognitive tasks in individuals. Both studies found good correlations within a given task or under resting-state conditions, but Harmony et al. reported much lower correlation values between sessions, even within the same subject during the same condition.

While these early tests show low levels of reproducibility, even within testing sessions, more recent research has provided vastly different results. The Cannon et al. [50] study mentioned earlier also examined coherence over a 30-day testing period. For eyes closed coherence measures, intraclass correlation coefficients (ICCs) for delta, theta, alpha, and beta bandwidths were all greater than 0.90. For the eyes open condition, coherence in all bandwidths had ICCs above 0.85. This indicates "good" to "very good" reproducibility for all EEG variables examined and deems coherence as a reliable enough measure to use in both a research and clinical setting.

In all of the studies presented, roughly half of the variance seen in all EEG variables was reproducible within the given subject. These measures have all been determined to have a sufficient level of reproducibility to use in future research. However, it should be noted that these results do not necessarily indicate that EEG can currently be considered a reliable diagnostic tool and differentiate between concussed and healthy individuals.

Although there are many benefits to using EEGs in concussion research and a wealth of knowledge has been gained, the use of EEGs in this type of research is not without its criticisms and limitations. Nuwer et al. [47] questioned the use of EEG in concussion research, citing the lack of clear EEG features that are specifically unique to mTBI patients, especially late after injury. While there is merit to a lack of unique abnormalities, several studies [73, 74] have found deficits in concussed participants up to 3 years post injury. Additionally, another study found that relative to former athletes with no history of sports concussion, former athletes who sustained their last sports concussion more than 30 years ago reveal cognitive and motor system alterations that closely resemble those found in previous electrophysiological studies on asymptomatic concussed athletes tested at 3 years post concussion [75]. This implies that there may be lifetime effects of sports-related concussion that are measurable using EEG.

Most EEG and concussion research focuses on lower frequency bands, but several studies by Thornton [51, 62, 65, 74] demonstrated that extending the frequency to include gamma bands provides important additional information, particularly between correlating EEG variables and the participant's cognitive deficits. Additionally, most research and consequently normative databases provide information solely about eyes closed conditions. This severely limits the type of cognitive testing that can be simultaneously completed, restricting neuropsychological testing to auditory-based tests. While auditory-based cognitive research has provided valuable EEG patterns, such as those outlined in Thornton and Carmody [51], several cognitive domains cannot be adequately assessed via auditory tasks. As mentioned above, the link between EEG patterns and cognitive domains, such as visual memory and attention, remains weakly established, with further research ongoing.

Additionally, further consideration when validating EEG as a tool for "on field" concussion assessment should be given to the standardization of EEG baseline testing protocol, particularly with respect to the effects of exercise on baseline levels. Portable EEG devices can in theory be used "on field" as an objective measure of change in cortical activity directly after a head injury [76], but exercise, in addition to changes in cognitive function measures, also increase cortical activity measured by EEG. Although a limited amount of evidence shows that EEG spectrum differs before and after acute bouts of exercise, it has been identified in connection with changes in alpha and beta range [77–79].

In summary, reviews by Arciniegas [23] and Nuwer et al. [47] have cited numerous studies that have proven EEG is a useful tool for identifying and managing concussive injuries. While EEGs are one of the least expensive and easiest to use neuroimaging tools, the expertise needed to administer and evaluate EEG results, as well as the lack of research between EEG and concussion, has kept EEG evaluations from becoming part of the current clinical gold standard. The most comprehensive EEG study using a database of 608 mTBI subjects that were followed up to 8 years post injury revealed a number of findings. These include the following: (a) increased coherence in frontal-temporal regions; (b) decreased power differences between anterior and posterior cortical regions; and (c) reduced alpha power in the posterior cortical region, which was attributed to mechanical head injury [61]. A study by Thornton [71] has shown a similar data trend in addition to demonstrating the attenuation of EEG within the high-frequency gamma cluster (32–64 Hz) in mTBI patients. Overall, resting EEG has demonstrated alterations in power dynamics across electrical spectra [23], increased short-distance coherences [80], and decreases in connectivity across long-distance connections [80]. These consistent findings in resting EEG and mTBI research point to the sensitivity and validity of using EEG in the assessment and management of concussion. Resting-state electroencephalography (rs-EEG) may also be the most affordable, accessible, and sensitive method of assessing severity of brain injury and rate of recovery after a concussion [81]. However, it should be noted that one controversial report concluded that no clear EEG features are unique to mTBI, especially late after injury [47].

Current Work from Our Lab

In our previous work, a significant reduction of the cortical potentials amplitude and concomitant alteration of gamma activity (40 Hz) was observed in MTBI subjects performing force production tasks 3 years post injury [73]. More recently, we showed a significant reduction of EEG power within theta and delta frequency bands during standing postures in subjects with single and multiple concussions up to 3 years post injury [74] and reduced amplitude of cortical potentials (MRCP) up to 30 days post injury [82].

We applied advanced *EEG-wavelet entropy* measures to detect brain functional deficits in concussion subjects. These EEG measures were significantly reduced after the first and more significantly after the second concussion far beyond 7 days post injury. Most importantly, the rate of recovery of EEG entropy measures was significantly slower after second concussion compared to the first concussion [26]. Recently, we reported the alteration of EEG signals in concussion subjects detected by a novel measure of nonstationarity, named Shannon entropy of the peak frequency shifting [83]. These findings are complementary to our previously published concussion report indicating the presence of residual deficits in concussion subjects detected by multi-channel EEG signals classifier using support vector machine [84]. We also conducted an EEG resting-state study and reported the alteration of cortical functional connectivity in concussion subjects revealed by graph theory, ICA, and LORETA analyses. Overall, a clear departure from a *small world-like network* was observed in concussion subjects [80].

The presence of a residual disturbance of the neuronal network is involved in the execution of postural movement in concussion subjects incorporating EEG and VR-induced measures [85]. As shown in Fig. 4.5, there was a significant increase of *theta* power during the progression of a balance task. Specifically, this *theta* increase was obvious initially at central areas with further diffusion to frontal electrode sites bilaterally. Interestingly, no significant *theta* power was present in concussed subjects at either phase of postural task progression. Most recently, we reported that 85% of concussion subjects who showed significant alteration of alpha power in acute phase of injury did not return to pre-injury status up to 12 months [26].

Another recent EEG-related study in our lab examined the practical use of the supplement Enzogenol, an extract of the *Pinus radiata* tree with antioxidant, anti-inflammatory, and possible neuro-protective properties, as a combatant of the chronic effects of sports concussion (6 months–3 years). Post-concussion symptom scale, virtual reality, and neurocognitive testing were administered to subjects with history of concussion both prior to and after being provided either Enzogenol or a placebo daily for 3 months. EEG recording was administered during testing, examining differences in brain activity within groups.

EEG results showed mental fatigue during testing in subjects through alpha, beta, and theta frequencies, which reflect arousal levels of the brain. Increases in mental fatigue, a noted symptom of the acute and chronic phase of concussion, was further induced by the strenuousness of the virtual reality and neuropsychological

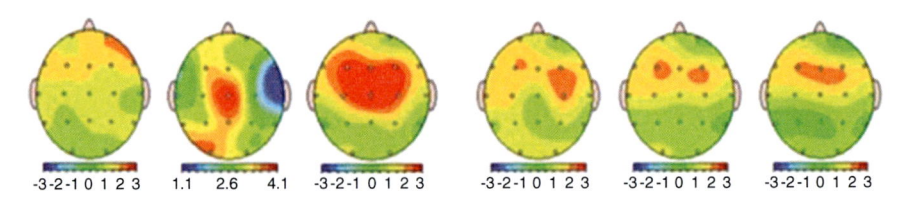

Fig. 4.5 Example 2D plots grand-average of theta power as the postural task progressed at 10, 15, and 27 seconds in before and after mTBI time points. EEG data included during the VR "roll" condition. Note a significant enhancement of theta power over frontal-central electrode sites as trial progressed during baseline, but not in concussed subjects. (Used with permission from: Slobounov et al. [111])

testing. Most notably, the EEG results during testing showed modulation and attenuation of FMT power, and parietal theta. The increase in FMT, more evident in the Enzogenol group, implied increases in brain resource allocation during focus and task completion, and with reference to previous findings could indicate that untreated subjects are less able to allocate brain resources during prolonged neuropsychological testing. With regard to the shift of theta bands to posterior regions; this has been connected to mental fatigue [86] and decreased efficiency of cognitive tasks [87]. The Enzogenol group did show less posterior theta which is certainly a promising indication of potential supplemental benefits on neurocognitive function in the chronic phase of concussion, but the most glaring conclusion of this study with regard to EEG, is its usefulness and sensitivity in measuring small changes in brain activity in concussion subjects [88].

Compensatory Approach During Concussion Assessment Batteries

Several studies have found electrophysiological deficits in asymptomatic concussed participants [26, 89, 90]. In these studies, concussed participants displayed normal levels of cognitive functioning, yet continue to show physiological dysfunction on EEG measures. The authors cite an unknown compensatory mechanism as an explanation for the findings. As part of our research, we sought to investigate this compensatory mechanism in more detail. In order to assess this, we chose to record EEG signals while participants were completing clinical concussion assessment measures. Subjects took the Immediate Post-Concussion Assessment and Cognitive Testing (ImPACT) neuropsychological assessment as well as completed VR balance and spatial navigation modules. They also participated in EEG resting-state evaluations in order to highlight the differences between clinical cognitive and balance performance and neuroelectric measures.

In a sample of 13 normal volunteers and 7 concussed participants, no differences were found between groups on ImPACT and VR composite outcome scores. When looking at outcomes, the only group difference was worse stationary balance in the concussed group. However, several significant group differences were found when looking at the EEG variables. For EEG resting-state and ImPACT conditions, the concussed group had significantly lower power in the theta and beta bandwidths. Additionally, the concussed group had significantly lower alpha power during the ImPACT conditions and significantly lower delta power in the VR conditions. Conversely, the concussed group displayed significantly higher levels of coherence during EEG resting-state and ImPACT evaluations, but lower levels of coherence during VR balance and spatial navigation testing.

Overall, for EEG resting state and ImPACT, results indicated that concussed participants could not establish enough local effort (seen via lower power), so they recruited additional long-distance network connections (seen via the increased coherence). By recruiting additional networks, the concussed participants were able to successfully compensate for their neuroelectric deficits and produce normal clinical results. This research indicates a disconnect between cognitive and neuroelectric resolution. Future research projects aim at determining whether cognitive functions resolve before physiological function or if current clinical concussion assessments are not sensitive enough to detect the residual effects of concussion.

"Return to Play" and EEG Concussion Research

One specific aspect of concussion injury that is still lacking in research is the area of return to work or play. In 2004, the World Health Organization (WHO) task force found no studies that demonstrate acceptable evidence to suggest when a person or athlete may safely return to work or the athletic field. A decade later, the International Collaboration on Mild Traumatic Brain Injury Prognosis (ICoMP) formed to update the original WHO Task Force publications, stating that although return to play guidelines are widely used, there are no studies of acceptable standard that assess their impact on fitness to play or prevention of additional injury [91]. They also stated that there is some evidence suggesting that the majority of athletes were assessed for return to play within the same game or within a few days post injury [91]. Despite the growing concern over return to play after sport concussion, research quality continues to be poor, establishing little to no methodological advances since the WHO Task Force review in 2004.

Additionally, return to play decision-making tools, like the Zurich Consensus guidelines, are based on expert opinion and clinical judgment, rather than scientific evidence [16]. As it has demonstrated its ability to identify physiological differences in the recovery from TBI, EEG should be considered as a feasible diagnostic tool for recommendations given to athletes returning to activity and sport.

EEG has been used to study concussion or mTBI throughout many phases of recovery from acute, sub-acute to chronic or long term. One clinical-stage EEG has not been used is within the "Return to Play" stepwise progression back into athletic participation. The "Return to Play" protocol is the internationally accepted method for the safe return to activity of an athlete recovering from concussion [16]. This formalized "Return to Play" protocol has been in place since the original 2001 Concussion in Sport Group (CISG) Consensus Statement and with continued updates is widely accepted as the "Gold Standard" for returning athletes to competition but without evidence to support either the progression sequence or the time spent in each stage [18].

Under this procedure, "Return to Play" after a concussion follows a stepwise progression of increasing efforts and risk as outlined in Table 4.2. An initial period of 24–48 hours of both relative physical rest and cognitive rest is recommended before beginning the RTS progression [1]. Once asymptomatic and cleared by a supervising physician, the athlete may progress to a light aerobic exercise such as walking or stationary cycling. This light aerobic challenge is limited by restricting an athlete to <70% of their calculated maximum heart rate.

With this activity progression, each stage of increasing efforts should be separated by 24 hours with health professionals monitoring the athlete and their

Table 4.2 Graduated "return to play" protocol

Stage/aim	Activity	Objective
1. Symptom-limited activity	Daily activities that do not provoke symptoms	Gradual reintroduction of work/school activities
2. Light aerobic exercise	Walking or stationary cycling at slow to medium pace. No resistance training	Increase heart rate
3. Sports-specific exercise	Running or skating drills. No head impact activities	Add movement
4. Non-contact training drills	Harder training drills, for example, passing drills. May start progressive resistance training	Exercise, coordination, and increased thinking
5. Full contact practice	Following medical clearance, participate in normal training activities	Restore confidence and assess functional skills by coaching staff
6. Return to play	Normal game play	

symptom status. If any of the athlete's post-concussion symptoms should manifest before, during, or after a stage within the protocol, the athlete is instructed to drop back to the previous asymptomatic stage and try to progress again after a further 24-hour period of rest.

In our lab, we investigated the use of EEG as a supplementary tool in the clinical assessment of concussion during the "Return to Play" phase of recovery. Specifically, we looked at the differential effect of exercise (modified YMCA Bike protocol) on the quantitative EEG measures of spectral absolute power and coherence in normal volunteers vs. concussion subjects. There were several major findings from this study. Of particular clinical significance was that all concussed subjects had met the clinical criteria for asymptomatic at rest [92] for a period of at least 24 hours prior to exercise testing. These athletes had also been cleared by a sports medicine physician for the initiation of the "Return to Play" protocol as outlined above.

When completing the modified YMCA bike protocol, there were no group differences in dynamic measures of heart rate at any time and both groups demonstrated no differences in symptom presentation after completion. However, some differences were evident when reviewing the physiological data from the EEG evaluation. Both groups demonstrated no regional power differences at rest and at 24-hour follow-up. In addition, both groups demonstrated no significant differences in mean or regional coherence values at rest or at 24-hour follow-up. Historically within the literature, abnormal attenuation of alpha power and an increase in focal slow wave distribution is short lasting and typically returns to normal within the sub-acute phase of experimental concussion [93–95]. Further, in a recent quantitative EEG examination by McCrea et al. no resting-state differences in athletes recovering from concussion at days 8 and 45 post injury were found when compared to age-matched controls [96]. Within the neural imaging research, resting-state fMRI findings of concussion cohorts at rest do not vary significantly from normal volunteers [97]. This is an important finding as researchers look to develop the clinical significance of EEG as a diagnostic tool for concussion. Resting-state EEG measurement remains largely normal as reported throughout the literature.

There were group differences however with the modified YMCA Bike protocol causing an increase in Alpha, Beta, Theta, and Delta absolute power amplitudes across all regions (frontal, central, and posterior). Specifically, exercise significantly increased the power of Theta and Delta frequency ranges. Theta power increases stem from injury and pathophysiologic changes in the cerebral cortex [31]. As is known, concussion results in altered cerebral blood flow [98, 99], decreased energy metabolism [100], release of excitatory amino acids (EAA), and decreased post-synaptic function among other effects already mentioned. In the work by Nagata, they demonstrated that cortical blood flow (CBF) and oxygen (O_2) metabolism correlated negatively with Delta and Theta power [101]. The lack of specificity of this effect linked with a range of pathological conditions suggests that increases of slow waves (Delta/Theta frequencies) represent a typical response to any brain injury, pathology, and disruption of neural homeostasis.

The inclusion of EEG as a physiologic tool proves to have some worth in examining the recovering athlete and may provide clinicians with valuable data when making "Return to Activity" decisions. Furthermore, as demonstrated by this investigation, exercise may be an effective mechanism for uncovering residual abnormalities in recovering athletes.

Brain Lateralization Analysis, Psychological Symptoms, and the Evaluation of Both Using EEG

Brain lateralization has been a popular topic of research for many years and has been used to investigate neural processes in many different species. Specifically, brain lateralization describes the presence of asymmetrical signaling between the left and right hemispheres of the brain. The difference is seen in the power of the specific EEG waves mentioned in the *EEG Frequency Bands* section of this chapter. These differences in power can appear at various anatomical locations within the brain resulting in various outcomes, including differences in behavior, personality, and mood within a species as well as differences in developmental processes between different species [102]. To analyze the symmetrical components of the brain, one of the most commonly used tools is EEG. EEG has the ability to capture the difference in signaling between the two hemispheres in a practical, efficient manner, making it a leading tool in this field of study. Moreover, brain lateralization and EEG methods have been applied to research on many disorders, especially psychological disorders. These studies have shown promising results that have helped provide insight on the neurophysiological basis behind psychological disorders.

Depression is one of the most prevalent mental health disorders, with studies showing it affecting nearly 17.5 million people annually across the United States [103]. With the complex nature of the disease, the diagnostic and treatment processes have varying success depending on the individual. Since the late twentieth century, brain lateralization analysis through EEG has been a popular method for observing the differences between depressed and non-depressed brains. Pioneers of the topic had shown that individuals with depression present with alpha wave asymmetries in the frontal cortex of the brain [104, 105]. Specifically, studies have shown increased approach behavior in subjects with a relative increase in left frontal activation whereas an individual with a relative increase in right frontal activation demonstrated stronger inhibitory behavior [104]. Furthermore, EEG has even shown asymmetries in subjects who do not suffer from depression but have a family history of the disorder. A study by Bruder et al. investigated EEG differences between children with a family history of depression and children with no family history. Results supported noticeable EEG asymmetry present in the parietal brain region of the children who have at least one grandparent and one parent suffering from depression. More specifically, these individuals showed enhanced signaling in the right hemisphere relative to the left, resulting in asymmetrical readings [106]. There is still developing research for using brain lateralization on EEG as a diagnostic tool for depression; however, the progress made using this method to investigate psychological disorders is undeniable.

Depression is not only one of the most common psychological disorders throughout the world; it is also the most common psychological symptoms following a concussion or mTBI. The onset of depression following the injury has been shown to affect recovery time, performance, and overall self-efficacy, making it a popular topic of interest [107]. The greatest challenge when assessing an athlete for psychological symptoms following a concussion is the fact that these symptoms are invisible and often misconstrued by the athlete. However, EEG has potential to be a vital tool in assessing these symptoms objectively, by searching for brain asymmetries. Currently, our lab is conducting a study to explore the relationship between depression and concussion. Specifically, the study aims to investigate the physiological and functional differences between college-aged athletes who have depression, have a history of concussed, or have a combination of both. The physiological differences between groups will be measured using EEG while functional and cognitive performance will be assessed. The study hopes to increase knowledge about the complications following a concussion, especially in the realm of psychological symptoms, as well as show how EEG can be used in future practice as part of the complete assessment following a concussive injury.

References

1. McCrory P, Meeuwisse W, Dvořák J, Aubry M, Bailes J, Broglio S, et al. Consensus statement on concussion in sport-the 5th international conference on concussion in sport held in Berlin, October 2016. Br J Sports Med. 2017;51:838–47.
2. McCrea M, Hammeke T, Olsen G, Leo P, Guskiewicz K. Unreported concussion in high school football players: implications for prevention. Clin J Sport Med. 2004;14:13–7.
3. Torres DM, Galetta KM, Phillips HW, Dziemianowicz EMS, Wilson JA, Dorman ES, et al. Sports-related concussion. Neurol Clin Pract. 2013;3:279–87.
4. Miyashita TL, Timpson WM, Frye MA, Gloeckner GW. The impact of an educational intervention on college athletes' knowledge of concussions. Clin J Sport Med. 2013;23:349–53.
5. Bloodgood B, Inokuchi D, Shawver W, Olson K, Hoffman R, Cohen E, et al. Exploration of awareness, knowledge, and perceptions of traumatic brain injury among American youth athletes and their parents. J Adolesc Health. 2013;53:34–9.

6. Malinauskas R. College athletes' perceptions of social support provided by their coach before injury and after it. J Sports Med Phys Fitness. 2008;48:107–12.
7. Setnik L, Bazarian JJ. The characteristics of patients who do not seek medical treatment for traumatic brain injury. Brain Inj. 2007;21:1–9.
8. Guskiewicz KM, McCrea M, Marshall SW, Cantu RC, Randolph C, Barr W, et al. Cumulative effects associated with recurrent concussion in collegiate football players: the NCAA concussion study. JAMA. 2003;290:2549.
9. Gaetz M, Bernstein DM. The current status of electrophysiologic procedures for the assessment of mild traumatic brain injury. J Head Trauma Rehabil. 2001;16:386–405.
10. Choe MC, Babikian T, DiFiori J, Hovda DA, Giza CC. A pediatric perspective on concussion pathophysiology. Curr Opin Pediatr. 2012;24:689–95.
11. Giza CC, Hovda DA. The neurometabolic cascade of concussion. J Athl Train. 2001;36:228–35.
12. McCrory P, Johnston K, Meeuwisse W, Aubry M, Cantu R, Dvorak J, et al. Summary and agreement statement of the 2nd International Conference on Concussion in Sport, Prague 2004. Br J Sports Med. 2005;39:196–204.
13. Aubry M, Cantu R, Dvorak J, Graf-Baumann T, Johnston K, Kelly J, et al. Summary and agreement statement of the First International Conference on Concussion in Sport, Vienna 2001. Recommendations for the improvement of safety and health of athletes who may suffer concussive injuries. Br J Sports Med. 2002;36:6–10.
14. Giza CC, Kutcher JS, Ashwal S, Barth J, Getchius TSD, Gioia GA, et al. Summary of evidence-based guideline update: evaluation and management of concussion in sports: report of the Guideline Development Subcommittee of the American Academy of Neurology. Neurology. 2013;80:2250–7.
15. McCrory P, Meeuwisse W, Johnston K, Dvorak J, Aubry M, Molloy M, et al. Consensus statement on concussion in sport: the 3rd International Conference on Concussion in Sport Held in Zurich, November 2008. J Athl Train. 2009;44:434–48.
16. McCrory P, Meeuwisse WH, Aubry M, Cantu B, Dvorák J, Echemendia RJ, et al. Consensus statement on concussion in sport: the 4th International Conference on Concussion in Sport held in Zurich, November 2012. Br J Sports Med. 2013;47:250–8.
17. Halstead ME, Walter KD, Moffatt K, Council on Sports Medicine and Fitness. Sport-related concussion in children and adolescents. Pediatrics. 2018;142
18. Harmon KG, Drezner JA, Gammons M, Guskiewicz KM, Halstead M, Herring SA, et al. American Medical Society for Sports Medicine position statement: concussion in sport. Br J Sports Med. 2013;47:15–26.
19. Teasdale TW, Engberg AW. Suicide after traumatic brain injury: a population study. J Neurol Neurosurg Psychiatry. 2001;71:436–40.
20. Uryu K, Laurer H, McIntosh T, Praticò D, Martinez D, Leight S, et al. Repetitive mild brain trauma accelerates Abeta deposition, lipid peroxidation, and cognitive impairment in a transgenic mouse model of Alzheimer amyloidosis. J Neurosci. 2002;22:446–54.
21. Blaylock RL, Maroon J. Immunoexcitotoxicity as a central mechanism in chronic traumatic encephalopathy—A unifying hypothesis. Surg Neurol Int [Internet]. 2011 [cited 2020 Dec 22];2. Available from: https://www.ncbi.nlm.nih.gov/pmc/articles/PMC3157093/.
22. Barnes SM, Walter KH, Chard KM. Does a history of mild traumatic brain injury increase suicide risk in veterans with PTSD? Rehabil Psychol. 2012;57:18–26.
23. Arciniegas DB. Clinical electrophysiologic assessments and mild traumatic brain injury: state-of-the-science and implications for clinical practice. Int J Psychophysiol. 2011;82:41–52.
24. Bigler ED, Maxwell WL. Neuropathology of mild traumatic brain injury: relationship to neuroimaging findings. Brain Imaging Behav. 2012;6:108–36.
25. Berger H. Über das Elektrenkephalogramm des Menschen. Archiv f Psychiatrie. 1929;87:527–70.
26. Slobounov S, Bazarian J, Bigler E, Cantu R, Hallett M, Harbaugh R, et al. Sports-related concussion: ongoing debate. Br J Sports Med. 2014;48:75–6.

27. Williams D. The significance of an abnormal electroencephalogram. J Neurol Psychiatry. 1941;4:257–68.
28. Geets W, Louette N. Early EEG in 300 cerebral concussions. Rev Electroencephalogr Neurophysiol Clin. 1985;14:333–8.
29. Fenton GW. The postconcussional syndrome reappraised. Clin Electroencephalogr. 1996;27:174–82.
30. Tebano MT, Cameroni M, Gallozzi G, Loizzo A, Palazzino G, Pezzini G, et al. EEG spectral analysis after minor head injury in man. Electroencephalogr Clin Neurophysiol. 1988;70:185–9.
31. Montgomery EA, Fenton GW, McClelland RJ, MacFlynn G, Rutherford WH. The psychobiology of minor head injury. Psychol Med. 1991;21:375–84.
32. Pratap-Chand R, Sinniah M, Salem FA. Cognitive evoked potential (P300): a metric for cerebral concussion. Acta Neurol Scand. 1988;78:185–9.
33. Watson MR, Fenton GW, McClelland RJ, Lumsden J, Headley M, Rutherford WH. The postconcussional state: neurophysiological aspects. Br J Psychiatry. 1995;167:514–21.
34. Leon-Carrion J, Martin-Rodriguez JF, Damas-Lopez J, Martin JMBY, Dominguez-Morales MDR. A QEEG index of level of functional dependence for people sustaining acquired brain injury: the Seville Independence Index (SINDI). Brain Inj. 2008;22:61–74.
35. Nunez PL, Srinivasan R. A theoretical basis for standing and traveling brain waves measured with human EEG with implications for an integrated consciousness. Clin Neurophysiol. 2006;117:2424–35.
36. Whittingstall K, Logothetis NK. Frequency-band coupling in surface EEG reflects spiking activity in monkey visual cortex. Neuron. 2009;64:281–9.
37. Klem GH, Lüders HO, Jasper HH, Elger C. The ten-twenty electrode system of the International Federation. The International Federation of Clinical Neurophysiology. Electroencephalogr Clin Neurophysiol Suppl. 1999;52:3–6.
38. O'Neil BJ, Prichep L, Naunheim R, Chabot R. 92 can quantitative brain electrical activity aid in the triage of mild traumatic brain-injured patients. Ann Emerg Med. 2011;58:S208.
39. Shaw NA. The neurophysiology of concussion. Prog Neurobiol. 2002;67:281–344.
40. Bazanova OM, Vernon D. Interpreting EEG alpha activity. Neurosci Biobehav Rev. 2014;44:94–110.
41. Tallon-Baudry C, Bertrand O, Delpuech C, Permier J. Oscillatory gamma-band (30-70 Hz) activity induced by a visual search task in humans. J Neurosci. 1997;17:722–34.
42. Luu P, Tucker DM. Regulating action: alternating activation of midline frontal and motor cortical networks. Clin Neurophysiol. 2001;112:1295–306.
43. Schacter DL. EEG theta waves and psychological phenomena: a review and analysis. Biol Psychol. 1977;5:47–82.
44. Vogel W, Broverman DM, Klaiber EL. EEG and mental abilities. Electroencephalogr Clin Neurophysiol. 1968;24:166–75.
45. Slobounov S, Gay M, Johnson B, Zhang K. Concussion in athletics: ongoing clinical and brain imaging research controversies. Brain Imaging Behav. 2012;6:224–43.
46. Geets W, de Zegher F. EEG and brainstem abnormalities after cerebral concussion. Short term observations. Acta Neurol Belg. 1985;85:277–83.
47. Nuwer MR, Hovda DA, Schrader LM, Vespa PM. Routine and quantitative EEG in mild traumatic brain injury. Clin Neurophysiol. 2005;116:2001–25.
48. Koufen H, Dichgans J. Frequency and course of posttraumatic EEG-abnormalities and their correlations with clinical symptoms: a systematic follow up study in 344 adults (author's transl). Fortschr Neurol Psychiatr Grenzgeb. 1978;46:165–77.
49. Jacome DE, Risko M. EEG features in post-traumatic syndrome. Clin Electroencephalogr. 1984;15:214–21.
50. Cannon RL, Baldwin DR, Shaw TL, Diloreto DJ, Phillips SM, Scruggs AM, et al. Reliability of quantitative EEG (qEEG) measures and LORETA current source density at 30 days. Neurosci Lett. 2012;518:27–31.

51. Thornton KE, Carmody DP. Traumatic brain injury rehabilitation: QEEG biofeedback treatment protocols. Appl Psychophysiol Biofeedback. 2009;34:59–68.
52. Chen X-P, Tao L-Y, Chen ACN. Electroencephalogram and evoked potential parameters examined in Chinese mild head injury patients for forensic medicine. Neurosci Bull. 2006;22:165–70.
53. Coutin-Churchman P, Añez Y, Uzcátegui M, Alvarez L, Vergara F, Mendez L, et al. Quantitative spectral analysis of EEG in psychiatry revisited: drawing signs out of numbers in a clinical setting. Clin Neurophysiol. 2003;114:2294–306.
54. Korn A, Golan H, Melamed I, Pascual-Marqui R, Friedman A. Focal cortical dysfunction and blood-brain barrier disruption in patients with Postconcussion syndrome. J Clin Neurophysiol. 2005;22:1–9.
55. von Bierbrauer A, Weissenborn K, Hinrichs H, Scholz M, Künkel H. Automatic (computer-assisted) EEG analysis in comparison with visual EEG analysis in patients following minor cranio-cerebral trauma (a follow-up study). EEG EMG Z Elektroenzephalogr Elektromyogr Verwandte Geb. 1992;23:151–7.
56. McClelland RJ, Fenton GW, Rutherford W. The postconcussional syndrome revisited. J R Soc Med. 1994;87:508–10.
57. Fenton G, McClelland R, Montgomery A, MacFlynn G, Rutherford W. The Postconcussional syndrome: social antecedents and psychological sequelae. Br J Psychiatr. Cambridge University Press;. 1993;162:493–7.
58. Jordan BD. The clinical spectrum of sport-related traumatic brain injury. Nat Rev Neurol. 2013;9:222–30.
59. Thatcher RW. Maturation of the human frontal lobes: physiological evidence for staging. Dev Neuropsychol Routledge. 1991;7:397–419.
60. Thatcher R, North D, Curtin R, Walker R, Biver C, Gomez-Molina J, et al. An EEG severity index of traumatic brain injury. J Neuropsychiatry Clin Neurosci. 2001;13:77–87.
61. Thatcher RW, Walker RA, Gerson I, Geisler FH. EEG discriminant analyses of mild head trauma. Electroencephalogr Clin Neurophysiol. 1989;73:94–106.
62. Thornton K. Improvement/rehabilitation of memory functioning with neurotherapy/QEEG biofeedback. J Head Trauma Rehabil. 2000;15:1285–96.
63. Thatcher RW, Biver C, McAlaster R, Salazar A. Biophysical linkage between MRI and EEG coherence in closed head injury. NeuroImage. 1998;8:307–26.
64. Barr WB, Prichep LS, Chabot R, Powell MR, McCrea M. Measuring brain electrical activity to track recovery from sport-related concussion. Brain Injury Taylor & Francis. 2012;26:58–66.
65. Thornton K. The electrophysiological effects of a brain injury on auditory memory functioning. The QEEG correlates of impaired memory. Arch Clin Neuropsychol. 2003;18:363–78.
66. Theriault M, De Beaumont L, Tremblay S, Lassonde M, Jolicoeur P. Cumulative effects of concussions in athletes revealed by electrophysiological abnormalities on visual working memory. J Clin Exp Neuropsychol. 2011;33:30–41.
67. Schneider D, Hoffmann S, Wascher E. Sustained posterior contralateral activity indicates re-entrant target processing in visual change detection: an EEG study. Front Hum Neurosci [Internet]. Frontiers; 2014 [cited 2020 Dec 22];8. Available from: https://www.frontiersin.org/articles/10.3389/fnhum.2014.00247/full.
68. Corsi-Cabrera M, Solís-Ortiz S, Guevara MA. Stability of EEG inter- and intrahemispheric correlation in women. Electroencephalogr Clin Neurophysiol. 1997;102:248–55.
69. Pollock VE, Schneider LS, Lyness SA. Reliability of topographic quantitative EEG amplitude in healthy late-middle-aged and elderly subjects. Electroencephalogr Clin Neurophysiol. 1991;79:20–6.
70. Salinsky MC, Oken BS, Morehead L. Test-retest reliability in EEG frequency analysis. Electroencephalogr Clin Neurophysiol. 1991;79:382–92.
71. Harmony T, Fernández T, Rodríguez M, Reyes A, Marosi E, Bernal J. Test-retest reliability of EEG spectral parameters during cognitive tasks: II. Coherence. Int J Neurosci. 1993;68:263–71.

72. Nikulin VV, Brismar T. Long-range temporal correlations in alpha and beta oscillations: effect of arousal level and test-retest reliability. Clin Neurophysiol. 2004;115:1896–908.
73. Slobounov S, Sebastianelli W, Simon R. Neurophysiological and behavioral concomitants of mild brain injury in collegiate athletes. Clin Neurophysiol. 2002;113:185–93.
74. Thompson J, Sebastianelli W, Slobounov S. EEG and postural correlates of mild traumatic brain injury in athletes. Neurosci Lett. 2005;377:158–63.
75. De Beaumont L, Brisson B, Lassonde M, Jolicoeur P. Long-term electrophysiological changes in athletes with a history of multiple concussions. Brain Inj. 2007;21:631–44.
76. Maddocks D, Saling M. Neuropsychological deficits following concussion. Brain Inj. 1996;10:99–103.
77. Crabbe JB, Dishman RK. Brain electrocortical activity during and after exercise: a quantitative synthesis. Psychophysiology. 2004;41:563–74.
78. Moraes H, Ferreira C, Deslandes A, Cagy M, Pompeu F, Ribeiro P, et al. Beta and alpha electroencephalographic activity changes after acute exercise. Arq Neuropsiquatr. 2007;65:637–41.
79. Mh B, Dl A. Impact of activity and arousal upon spectral EEG parameters. Physiol Behav. 2001;74:291–8.
80. Cao C, Slobounov S. Alteration of cortical functional connectivity as a result of traumatic brain injury revealed by graph theory, ICA, and sLORETA analyses of EEG signals. IEEE Trans Neural Syst Rehabil Eng. 2010;18:11–9.
81. Conley AC, Cooper PS, Karayanidis F, Gardner AJ, Levi CR, Stanwell P, et al. Resting state electroencephalography and sports-related concussion: a systematic review. J Neurotrauma. 2018;
82. Slobounov S, Sebastianelli W, Moss R. Alteration of posture-related cortical potentials in mild traumatic brain injury. Neurosci Lett. 2005;383:251–5.
83. Cao C, Slobounov S. Application of a novel measure of EEG nonstationarity as 'Shannon entropy of the peak frequency shifting' for detecting residual abnormalities in concussed individuals. Clin Neurophysiol. 2011;122:1314–21.
84. Cao C, Tutwiler R, Slobounov S. Automatic classification of athletes with residual functional deficits following concussion by means of EEG signal using support vector machine. IEEE Trans Neural Syst Rehabil Eng. 2008;16:327–35.
85. Slobounov S, Sebastianelli W, Newell KM. Incorporating virtual reality graphics with brain imaging for assessment of sport-related concussions. Annu Int Conf IEEE Eng Med Biol Soc. 2011;2011:1383–6.
86. Smith ME, McEvoy LK, Gevins A. Neurophysiological indices of strategy development and skill acquisition. Brain Res Cogn Brain Res. 1999;7:389–404.
87. Corsi-Cabrera M, Sánchez A, Del-Río-Portilla Y, Villanueva Y, Pérez-Garci E. Effect of 38 h of total sleep deprivation on the waking EEG in women: Sex differences. Int J Psychophysiol. 2003;50:213–24.
88. Walter A, Finelli K, Bai X, Arnett P, Bream T, Seidenberg P, et al. Effect of Enzogenol® supplementation on cognitive, executive, and vestibular/balance functioning in chronic phase of concussion. Dev Neuropsychol. Routledge;. 2017;42:93–103.
89. Gosselin N, Thériault M, Leclerc S, Montplaisir J, Lassonde M. Neurophysiological anomalies in symptomatic and asymptomatic concussed athletes. Neurosurgery. 2006;58:1151–61; discussion 1151–1161.
90. Thériault M, De Beaumont L, Gosselin N, Filipinni M, Lassonde M. Electrophysiological abnormalities in well functioning multiple concussed athletes. Brain Inj. 2009;23:899–906.
91. Cancelliere C, Hincapié CA, Keightley M, Godbolt AK, Côté P, Kristman VL, et al. Systematic review of prognosis and return to play after sport concussion: results of the International Collaboration on Mild Traumatic Brain Injury Prognosis. Arch Phys Med Rehabil. 2014;95:S210–29.
92. Alla S, Sullivan SJ, McCrory P. Defining asymptomatic status following sports concussion: fact or fallacy? Br J Sports Med. 2012;46:562–9.
93. Ward AA. The physiology of concussion. Clin Neurosurg. 1964;12:95–111.

94. Echlin FA. Spreading depression of electrical activity in the cerebral cortex following local trauma and its possible role in concussion. Arch Neurol Psychiatr. 1950;63:830–2.
95. West M, Parkinson D, Havlicek V. Spectral analysis of the electroencephalographic response in experimental concussion in the rat. Electroencephalogr Clin Neurophysiol. 1982;53:192–200.
96. McCrea M, Prichep L, Powell MR, Chabot R, Barr WB. Acute effects and recovery after sport-related concussion: a neurocognitive and quantitative brain electrical activity study. J Head Trauma Rehabil. 2010;25:283–92.
97. Zhang K, Johnson B, Gay M, Horovitz SG, Hallett M, Sebastianelli W, et al. Default mode network in concussed individuals in response to the YMCA physical stress test. J Neurotrauma. 2012;29:756–65.
98. Len TK, Neary JP. Cerebrovascular pathophysiology following mild traumatic brain injury. Clin Physiol Funct Imaging. 2011;31:85–93.
99. Len TK, Neary JP, Asmundson GJG, Goodman DG, Bjornson B, Bhambhani YN. Cerebrovascular reactivity impairment after sport-induced concussion. Med Sci Sports Exerc. 2011;43:2241–8.
100. Vagnozzi R, Signoretti S, Cristofori L, Alessandrini F, Floris R, Isgrò E, et al. Assessment of metabolic brain damage and recovery following mild traumatic brain injury: a multicentre, proton magnetic resonance spectroscopic study in concussed patients. Brain. 2010;133:3232–42.
101. Nagata K. Metabolic and hemodynamic correlates of quantitative EEG mapping. Electroencephalogr Clin Neurophysiol. 1995;4:S49–50.
102. Halpern ME, Güntürkün O, Hopkins WD, Rogers LJ. Lateralization of the vertebrate brain: taking the side of model systems. J Neurosci. 2005;25:10351–7.
103. NIMH » Major Depression [Internet]. [cited 2020 Dec 22]. Available from: https://www.nimh.nih.gov/health/statistics/major-depression.shtml
104. Davidson RJ, Abercrombie H, Nitschke JB, Putnam K. Regional brain function, emotion and disorders of emotion. Curr Opin Neurobiol. 1999;9:228–34.
105. van der Vinne N, Vollebregt MA, van Putten MJAM, Arns M. Stability of frontal alpha asymmetry in depressed patients during antidepressant treatment. Neuroimage Clin. 2019;24:102056.
106. Bruder GE, Tenke CE, Warner V, Nomura Y, Grillon C, Hille J, et al. Electroencephalographic measures of regional hemispheric activity in offspring at risk for depressive disorders. Biol Psychiatry. 2005;57:328–35.
107. Iverson GL, Gardner AJ, Terry DP, Ponsford JL, Sills AK, Broshek DK, et al. Predictors of clinical recovery from concussion: a systematic review. Br J Sports Med. 2017;51:941–8.
108. Slobounov S, Cao C, Jaiswal N, Newell KM. Neural basis of postural instability identified by VTC and EEG. Exp Brain Res. 2009;199(1):1–16. https://doi.org/10.1007/s00221-009-1956-5.
109. Teel EF, Ray WJ, Geronimo AM, Slobounov SM. Residual alterations of brain electrical activity in clinically asymptomatic concussed individuals: an EEG study. Clin Neurophysiol. 2014;125(4):703–7. https://doi.org/10.1016/j.clinph.2013.08.027.
110. Barwick F, Arnett P, Slobounov S. EEG correlates of fatigue during administration of a neuropsychological test battery. Clin Neurophysiol. 2012;123(2):278–84. https://doi.org/10.1016/j.clinph.2011.06.027.
111. Slobounov S, Sebastianelli W, Newell KM. Incorporating virtual reality graphics with brain imaging for assessment of sport-related concussions. Conf Proc IEEE Eng Med Biol Soc. 2011;2011:1383–6.

Part II

Biomechanics and Motor Control Mechanisms of Concussion

Biomechanical Studies of Impact and Helmet Protection

Andrew S. Mcintosh

Introduction

Definitions of concussion have evolved over time and these definitions should inform our interpretation of past research. Studies on concussion in the not-too-distant past may have examined a constellation of brain injuries that are more severe than those currently considered as sport-related concussion (SRC). The current definition and signs and symptoms of SRC have been informed substantially by consensus statements [1]. SRC is defined as the outcome of a biomechanical load applied to the head directly or indirectly. Helmets have a well-proven role in managing loads applied directly to the head. However, we have been more successful in developing helmets to prevent moderate-to-severe head injuries, rather than SRC. For example, in August 2020, Riddell, a major supplier of helmets for American football, warned: "Contact in football may result in CONCUSSION-BRAIN INJURY which no helmet can prevent".

Developing effective helmets for sport is challenging. Intrinsic and extrinsic factors and the exposure profile of the inciting event all require consideration and realization in an affordable, lightweight and comfortable device that does not impede athletic performance or enjoyment. Intrinsic risk factors include age, gender, injury history, anatomy and behaviour. Extrinsic risk factors include the laws and rules of the game (especially around head contact), the environment (e.g. the playing surface from soft ground to ice) and the use of personal protective equipment and/or coaching strategies. The inciting event might be summarized into a small predictable pattern (e.g. in soccer head-to-head or arm-to-head impacts during the aerial contest

---

A. S. Mcintosh (✉)
McIntosh Consultancy and Research, Sydney, NSW, Australia

The Australian Centre for Research into Injury in Sport and its Prevention (ACRISP), School of Engineering, Edith Cowan University, Joondalup, WA, Australia

© Springer Nature Switzerland AG 2021
S. M. Slobounov, W. J. Sebastianelli (eds.), *Concussions in Athletics*,
https://doi.org/10.1007/978-3-030-75564-5_5

for the ball, also known as "elbowing"), be broad, or even unknown. Through the use of video and wearable head impact sensors, knowledge is being gained regarding exposure profiles across many sports and levels of play. In the context of SRC, this chapter describes current knowledge regarding helmet performance, consider helmet design characteristics and standards, human factors, research and development needs, and opportunities. A focus of the chapter is on padded or softshell headgear that is worn in sports such as rugby union, Australian football and combat sports.

Epidemiological Approaches – Effectiveness and Efficacy

Epidemiological studies in sport show that at present helmets cannot be relied upon as the primary method to prevent concussion [2–4]; Table 5.1. In a sporting team or organization, it is not possible to satisfy a duty of care by mandating helmet use. In some sports, for example, Australian rules football, rugby union, rugby league and soccer, there is no evidence that helmets, referring to padded headgear, may prevent concussion. In American football and ice hockey, the epidemiological evidence regarding the benefits of helmets in preventing concussion is inconclusive. In both these sports, there is inconsistent evidence that helmets are effective in preventing head injuries overall.

One of the major impediments to the use of epidemiological methods to assess the role of helmets in sports that have mandatory helmet use, for example, American football, is that comparisons can only be made between types of helmets, not

Table 5.1 Summary of effectiveness of helmets in preventing concussion

Sport	Concussion rate (games)	Proportion of injuries (%)	Helmet mandatory	Effective in reducing concussion
Rugby union	4.1–6.9 per 1000 player hours (all levels)	5–15	No	No
American football	0.5–5.3 per 1000 athletic exposures (high school and collegiate)	5	Yes	Inconclusive
Football (soccer)	0.06–1.08 per 1000 player hours	3	No	No
Ice hockey	0.2–6.5 per 1000 player hours (collegiate and professional)	2–19	Yes, including face shields in some competitions	Inconclusive
Bicycle riding	Not quantified	Depends on sample inclusion criteria	City, state and country dependent	Yes

There are variations in injury rate measures based on injury definitions, exposure measurements, chosen denominator, level of play and age groups assessed between athletes assigned randomly to a helmet group and a no helmet group. In 2013, McGuine's study reported no difference in concussion risk by helmet brand or year of manufacture amongst high school football players [5]. In an earlier study, Collins observed that a smaller proportion of high school football players wearing the then new Riddell Revolution® helmet were concussed (5.3%) than players wearing standard helmets (7.6%) [6]. A comparison between players wearing and not wearing a helmet is not possible. Thus, the overall benefit remains unclear. To this end, one American football helmet manufacturer advises the public that: "Scientists have not reached agreement on how the results of impact absorption tests relate to concussions. No conclusions about a reduction of risk or severity of concussive injury should be drawn from impact absorption tests", "No helmet system can prevent concussions or eliminate the risk of serious head or neck injuries while playing football", and "No helmet system can protect you from serious brain and/or neck injuries including paralysis or death. To avoid these risks, do not engage in the sport of football" [7].

Other issues, for example, non-compliance, confound the conduct, results and analysis of epidemiological studies. Non-compliance may arise in sports where helmet use is not mandatory and athletes are randomized to a helmet-wearing group but do not normally wear a helmet. In the largest randomized control trial of helmets in sport, the author and colleagues found actual helmet wearing compliance to be poor in each of the three study arms, which may have weakened the positive trend observed with the "modified" helmet for those players who stuck with wearing the helmet during the study [8]. In a compliance analysis, wearers of the "modified" headgear compared to non-wearers had a non-significant reduction of greater than 50% in the likelihood of concussion causing one missed game. Players reported that the "modified" helmet, which was thicker and heavier than the "standard" design, felt stiff and uncomfortable. Although helmets in rugby union are substantially lighter than in American football, the perception relative to the experience of an even lighter headgear or no headgear influenced compliance.

Bicycle helmets have been shown to reduce the likelihood of concussion when the injury patterns of helmet wearing bicycle riders are compared to non-wearers. In an analysis of admissions to a major metropolitan trauma centre bicycle riders wearing helmets were observed to have a 54% reduction in the likelihood of concussion and a 66% reduction in the likelihood of intracranial injury (including concussion) compared to bicycle riders not wearing a helmet [9]. In bicycle crashes with motor vehicles, a training hazard for professional and recreational sports cyclists, the majority of brain injuries (79%) were considered concussive or involved loss of consciousness [10]. Moderate concussive injuries were associated with a 46% reduction if a helmet was worn. Concussion cases in trauma admission data may be based on different diagnostic criteria, for example, the International Classification of Disease (ICD) or the Abbreviated Injury Scale (AIS), than those in many helmet studies in football where the sports concussion consensus guidelines have been applied.

Helmet Characteristics

The most important functional characteristic of a helmet in the context of concussion is impact energy attenuation; a characteristic that has also been referred to as acceleration management. Ideally, the impact will cause the helmet to deform a substantial proportion of its thickness, without fully deforming or "bottoming out". The liner of the helmet or, the entire helmet in the case of padded headgear worn in rugby union, largely determines the impact energy attenuation performance. In short, the greater the deformation of the helmet, the greater the reduction in impact force as well as in head acceleration. The helmet can also distribute the impact force over an area larger than the contact area. In helmets with a well-established role in transport and sport, for example, bicycle, equestrian and motorcycle helmets, the helmet is designed for a single crash event. In contrast, American football, rugby union and ice hockey helmets are intended to provide protection throughout a season or more of multiple head impact exposures. The general properties of helmets and their function have been addressed well by many authors, for example, Newman [11] and Hoshizaki and Brien [12].

The next most important functional characteristics of the helmet are the mass, mass distribution, fit, restraint system, vision and thermal comfort. Sports helmets need to be wearable during extreme physical activities; therefore, helmet mass must be minimized. The mass distribution of the helmet and attachments is important in reducing the flexion moment that the helmet may apply to the head and neck. A flexion moment will be counteracted by neck extensor activation leading to muscle fatigue and increased joint reaction forces. It is imperative to ensure that the helmet and all components are correctly selected and adjusted for the individual athlete. Providing a kit bag with a few helmets to fit all the team is not the best practice. Vision and the restraint system characteristics are usually addressed in sports helmet standards. Where faceguards (visors) are mounted to helmets to prevent projectile to face or head impacts, the adjustment of the faceguard is important as apertures may permit a projectile travelling at speed to strike the face directly. In recent history, the position of a faceguard or visor on a cricket helmet could be adjusted by the player. As a result, there was potential for injury due to misuse. Current cricket helmets have a fixed position mounting for the faceguard. Therefore, positive changes are possible.

Performance Requirements and Standards

Helmet performance is assessed in the laboratory by examining the capacity of the helmet to minimize headform acceleration in impact tests. These tests are conducted against set criteria, for example, a linear acceleration pass criterion, or to derive an injury risk estimate. During a test, a selected amount of impact energy is delivered to the helmet-headform system via a drop rig, pendulum or mechanical device. The headform's linear and, in some cases, angular acceleration is measured during the impact. The input characteristics of the tests, for example, energy, dimensions of impact interface and headform, have developed to reflect knowledge on impact exposures in specific sports. The output characteristics, for example, headform dynamic responses, have also developed to reflect knowledge on injury mechanisms and human tolerance. However, requirements in many helmet standards are not currently aligned to maximize the potential for standard compliant helmets to prevent concussion. This would require the lowering of pass levels, for example, headform acceleration, to well below 100 g, and consideration for angular acceleration criteria and related test methods. As will be presented in this section, more valid assessments of helmet performance are observed when the laboratory tests reflect the impact exposures in the specific sport (impact location, impact severity, interface characteristics and frequency) and the biofidelity of the head-neck system are considered. A range of headforms are used in research and standards testing: Hybrid III headforms, rigid ISO headforms and NOCSAE headforms. Each has a distinct influence on the test outcomes. In an otherwise equivalent impact, head acceleration will be greater with a rigid ISO headform in comparison to a Hybrid III headform.

The author and colleagues have conducted baseline tests on bare headforms. These reveal a clear risk of concussion related to linear head acceleration even in impacts equivalent to the head falling 0.5 m (3.13 m/s):

- Hybrid II dropped onto a flat rigid anvil at 3.13 m/s has a peak linear acceleration (PLA) of 282 g and head injury criterion of 906 [13].
- Projectile impacts (ice hockey puck, baseball and cricket ball) into a Hybrid III headform mean PLA were in the range of 233 to 316 g for 19 m/s impacts and 342 to 426 g for 27 m/s impacts [14].
- Hybrid III headform mean PLA in flat rigid anvil was in the range 241 to 261 g (HIC 493 to 741) at 3.13 m/s and 368 to 512 g (HIC 1620 to 2789) at 4.43 m/s [15].
- Hybrid III headform PLA and peak angular accelerations (PAA) were measured in 16 linear impactor tests at five sites at a speed of 4 m/s. The impactor mass was 4 kg with a Polyurethane 70A Duro (Shore hardness 65 to 70) head. The average PLA = 140 g (SD = 17 g) and PAA = 8400 rad/s^2 (SD = 2100 rad/s^2).

In the context of laboratory impact tests, helmets need to reduce both linear and angular headform acceleration. As a guide, the 15% likelihood of concussion for adult males is 45 g and the 50% likelihood is 75 g for resultant linear acceleration at the head's centre of gravity [16]. For the bare headform impacts described above helmets need to reduce the linear acceleration in the range of two to tenfold to prevent concussion. Angular acceleration tolerance thresholds vary; Rowson reported that the 75% likelihood of concussion for resultant angular acceleration is 6.9 krad/s^2 [17].

Testing of a commercially available padded headgear model in Australia under the conditions described above (4 m/s linear impactor tests with 4 kg mass) showed a large reduction in PLA with one model, average PLA = 70 g (SD = 12 g, n = 15) and PAA = 4600 rad/s^2 (SD = 700 rad/s^2), demonstrating a potential to reduce head accelerations to a level suggestive of a protective effect in an equivalent severity impact.

How Well Do Helmets Perform?

Rugby Padded headgear in rugby must comply with World Rugby's performance regulations [18]. The helmet properties are restricted to an undeformed thickness of 10 mm and a foam density of 45 kg/m^3. World Rugby's impact performance requirements state that in a 13.8 J rigid (EN 960) headform impact onto a rigid flat anvil the peak headform acceleration shall not be less than 200 g. The mandated performance requirements exclude headgear from preventing concussion due to the biomechanical criteria and are inconsistent with the philosophy of many helmet standards.

Impact tests on helmets meeting World Rugby's requirements ("standard") and a "modified" version were conducted by the author [19]. The modified headgear was 16 mm thick and made from 60 kg/m^3 polyethylene foam. The standard headgear was 10 mm thick and made from 45 kg/m^3 polyethylene foam. Tests using a rigid headform from a 0.3 m drop height produced peak accelerations in the range 276–689 g for standard headgear and 69–123 for modified headgear. At 0.4 m peak, accelerations for the modified headgear were 110–273 g. The performance of the modified headgear in laboratory tests identified a potential in low severity impacts for the headgear to reduce the linear acceleration to a tolerable range. In the epidemiological study, there was a greater than 50% non-significant reduction in missed game concussions based on a compliance analysis [8]. With greater compliance, this may have been a significant association.

Figure 5.1 shows the results of linear impactor testing of a range of more recent (2016/2017) padded headgears marketed for use in Rugby Union, Rugby League and Australian football superimposed onto PLA-based injury likelihood curves [16]. The linear impactor was similar to that described earlier, but with a different impactor head. The results showed the little benefit of then current commercial models and large potential benefit of prototype models with respect to bare headform tests.

Australian Football Data on head impact exposures in Australian Football have emerged over the last few years. We undertook studies of player cohorts using a combination of video and x-patch sensors to measure head impact exposures in unhelmeted players [20, 21]. One of the aims of this research has been to assist in the development of standards. Setting aside the challenges and disappointments with the x-patch sensors, we observed:

- In 53 male and female community-level players (mean age = 26 years), there were 118 head acceleration events (HAE) with PLA $\geq$ 30 g, 56% of which were verified on video [20]. The mean PLA for a definite direct head impact was 47.2 g ($n = 37$, range 30 to 102 g).
- In 210 male and female professional AFL players, there were 336 HAEs with PLA $\geq$ 30 g. The majority were distributed between 30 and 60 g, but there were a small number of impacts greater than 100 g [21].

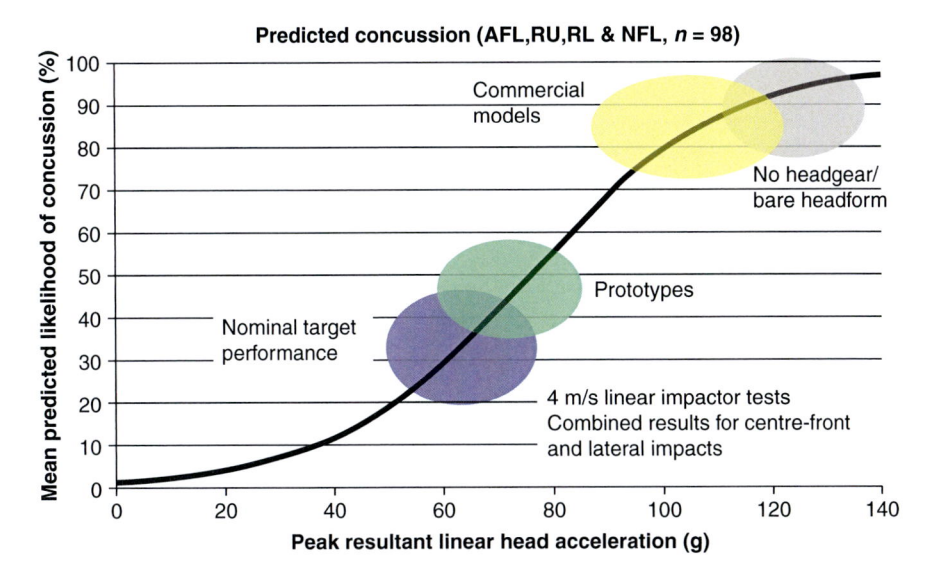

5 Biomechanical Studies of Impact and Helmet Protection

Fig. 5.1 Bare HIII headform and headgear performance in linear impactor tests superimposed onto an injury risk curve. PLA from impact tests and PLA-based concussion injury risk curve formed by pooling NFL and Australian (unhelmeted) football reconstructed injury and non-injury concussion cases

- These data indicate a role for headgear in reducing the severity of the less frequent direct head impacts that are associated with a concussion risk, for example, greater than 75 g on human heads, and managing the more common low severity impacts.

The Australian Football League (AFL) is working towards implementing performance standards for headgear. In short, the basic standard specifies drop tests at four sites, with three repeats, from 300 mm with PLA $\leq$ 150 g for the first impact and PLA $\leq$ 200 g on repeat impacts. The advanced specifies drop tests at four sites, with three repeats, from 300 mm with PLA $\leq$ 100 g for the first impact and PLA $\leq$ 140 g on repeat impacts and linear impactor tests as described above (4 m/s linear impactor tests with 4 kg mass) with PLA $\leq$ 75 g and PAA $\leq$ 7500 rad/s^2. Laboratory testing of prototype designs has demonstrated that these are achievable objectives. Ideally, once a model becomes available that is accepted by players, its effectiveness will be evaluated in a randomized controlled trial. The performance criteria reflect what is achievable currently and other factors, for example, the differences between the dynamic responses of the human head and a rigid headform, that is used in drop tests.

Combat sports A range of headgears intended for use in combat sports were evaluated using drop tests and linear impactor tests [22, 23]. The headgear models were selected because of their characteristics, that is, head coverage, density and thickness. Drop tests were performed with a rigid "M" headform (5.6 kg drop assembly) from 0.2, 0.4, 0.5 and 0.8 m with repeat tests at each site. Linear impactor tests were conducted at 4.11, 6.85 and 8.34 m/s with a Top Ten branded headgear designated for boxing; a glove/fist interface was used.

Some highlights of the drop tests were as follows:

- At 0.5 m drop height the lowest PLA was measured with the Macho Warrior headgear and the greatest was with the Adidas Taekwondo (TKW), 63 g and 546 g, respectively, for the mean of five repeat tests.
- Headgear "bottomed out" typically between 0.5 and 0.8 m drop heights; Macho Warrior would have bottomed out at a drop height greater than 0.8 m and Adidas TKW bottomed out between 0.2 and 0.3 m drop heights.
- There was a progressive reduction in impact performance at each drop height, even when the impact was well within the capacity of the material to attenuate energy.

The drop tests identified the expected differences based on material density and thickness. We wrote [22]:

> "The best performing headguards were either the heaviest—the Rival RHG 10 at 0.53 kg (average thickness 25 mm, density 140 kg/m^3)—or the thickest—the Macho Warrior at 37 mm (mass 0.3 kg, density 130 kg/m^3). The worst performing headguard was the Adidas Taekwondo model, which was the lightest and thinnest headguard. The two Macho brand headguard models had similar foam densities (125 kg/m^3), but the Warrior's average thickness was 37 mm compared with the Dyna's average thickness of 25 mm. The additional thickness explained the Warrior's superior performance. Comparatively, the Macho Warrior was between seven and eight times more effective in reducing headform acceleration compared with the Adidas Taekwondo model in rigid impacts, but with only a difference in mass of 0.09kg. The opportunities available to designers are to (1) maintain the thickness of the headguard and increase its density, (2) increase the thickness and maintain density or (3) do both".

The liner impactor results indicated that in simulated punches with speeds between 5 and 9 m/s, AIBA-approved boxing headgear, in combination with a glove, offers a large level of protection to the boxer's head. For example, in 6.85 m/s tests:

- PLA was greatly reduced from 86 and 89 g to 46 and 60 with headgear, respectively, means for lateral and centre front impacts.
- PAA was greatly reduced from 5200 and 5600 rad/s^2 to 2800 and 2900 rad/s^2 with headgear, respectively, means for lateral and centre front impacts.
- Under these punch loads, PLA was greater than a nominal concussion threshold of 75 g without headgear and reduced to less than the threshold with headgear; and, PAA was close to a nominal concussion threshold of 6000 rad/s^2 without headgear and halved with headgear.

In total, the testing of headgear for combat sports showed that the better performing models would offer protection during training and competition. Often, a false dichotomy is discussed regarding headgear, that is, the use of headgear results in poor defensive technique. There is no barrier to training with and without headgear to focus on technique and developing athletes with good technique and who also wear headgear. In motorsports, the pilots and riders adopt the best techniques and equipment.

Projectile sports (Cricket/Baseball) Helmets in cricket and baseball are intended to prevent head injury and provide a structure for mounting a faceguard or visor. The faceguard prevents facial and ocular injury, as well as other head injuries. Despite the similar hazards in the two sports, cricket helmets tend to have a thin relatively stiff liner in contrast to thick and compliant baseball liner. The success of helmets in managing the head impact acceleration in projectile impacts was assessed in a selection of helmets [14]. Standards for cricket helmets have developed in the intervening period and include a projectile test for the faceguard and neck protectors. Our work indicated little correlation between the magnitude of headform accelerations in equivalent impact energy tests conducted using drop tests onto a rigid anvil (as per the current standard) and projectile tests for cricket helmets. In contrast, there was a better correlation between projectile test results and drop tests onto a modular elastomeric programmer anvil for baseball and ice hockey helmets. This demonstrates that impact tests can be developed that do not necessarily resemble sports-specific impact characteristics but are indicative of helmet performance in sports-specific impacts. At that time, baseball helmets demonstrated a greater capacity to reduce headform acceleration than cricket helmets, although the results did not indicate that a baseball or cricket helmet would prevent concussion if the projectile struck the head in an impact directed radially (or centric) to the head's centre of gravity (Table 5.2). However, it is more common in match situations to observe a glancing ball-to-helmet impact.

Cycling Bicycle riding is a major sporting, recreational activity and means of transport. The hazards and injury risks in bicycle riding are broad and large. A cyclist may fall off while cycling and hit the road surface or in a more severe crash may collide with a moving car. As per American football, the initial rationale for bicycle helmets

Table 5.2 Cricket and baseball helmet projectile impact results

Ball speed (m/s)	Bare Hybrid III headform		HIII headform with helmet		Per cent reduction relative to bare headform (%)	
	Cricket PLA (g)	Baseball PLA (g)	Cricket PLA (g)	Baseball PLA (g)	Cricket	Baseball
19	278	316	67	72	76	77
27	347	426	160	139	54	67

Average of the maximum headform acceleration (PLA) is presented for all impact sites combined for bare headform and helmeted impacts with the appropriate ball

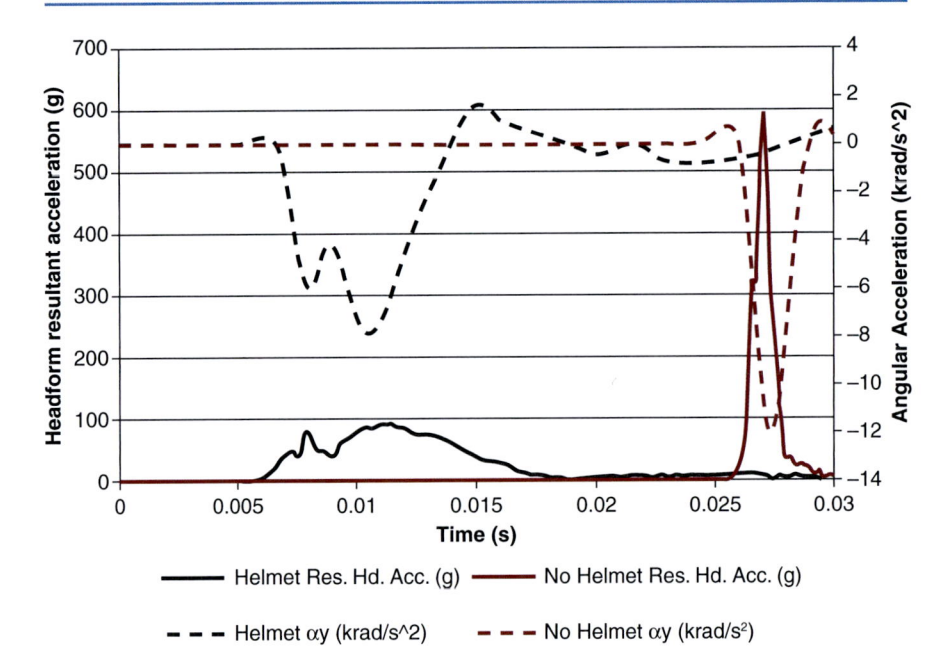

Fig. 5.2 Comparison of head linear and angular acceleration time histories in oblique impacts using a Hybrid III head and neck. Occipital impacts were conducted with a drop height of 1 m and striker (horizontal) speed of 15 km/h. The resultant headform acceleration was around 100 g for the bicycle helmet impact compared to 600 g for the bare headform impact. Peak angular acceleration in the helmet impact was almost half the bare headform impact

was to prevent a more severe spectrum of injury, including skull fracture, intracranial haemorrhage and penetrating wounds, rather than sports concussion. Recent comparative crash simulation tests have demonstrated that the laboratory performance of bicycle helmets is a reasonable predictor of the real-world performance [15]. In comparison to helmeted impacts across all impact configurations, mean maximum headform acceleration was 2.8–6.7 times greater without a helmet and angular accelerations were between 2.0 and 7.3 times greater without a helmet, depending on the exact impact characteristics (Fig. 5.2). An analysis of the oblique test results using biomechanical injury likelihood relationships again paralleled well the results of epidemiological studies. The analyses showed a significant effect of helmets on reducing the likelihood of severe head injury, but a potential for concussion to occur across a range of impacts. In contrast, the bare headform tests predicted a high risk of severe skull and brain injuries even in the more benign crash scenarios.

Heading in football/soccer: why current helmets are not needed Helmets are available and marketed for soccer. There are no convincing epidemiological or laboratory studies that demonstrate their effectiveness or efficacy. Although there is a risk of concussion in soccer, it is relatively low, compared to American football and/

or rugby. We measured PLA in a range of soccer skills from a shoulder collision to a finishing header [24]. For a range of heading drill events, we observed a mean PLA = 15.6 g (SD = 11.8 g) and in a limited number of training situations mean PLA = 20.7 g (SD = 10.6 g). These impacts are substantially lower in severity than in Australian Football. Despite concerns that heading itself may cause brain injury through a cumulative dose effect, the evidence suggests that during the aerial contest for the ball, head impacts causing immediate injury occur because of head-to-head impacts or arm-to-head impacts [25]. These intentional or accidental impacts can be controlled through the laws of the game. Arguably, helmets would reduce the ability of a player to head a ball and may lead to players compensating for the loss of ball rebound by changing their head-neck dynamics. This in turn might result in higher speed head-to-head impacts, although this is speculative. Unlike contact football where accidental head contact does occur frequently, soccer has other opportunities to prevent concussion through its laws, law enforcement, training and supervision. Considering a cumulative head acceleration dose, it is noteworthy that a dose component representing headers would be overwhelmed by PLA induced through non-contact general skills, for example, kicking a ball and re-directional running. The frequency of the non-contact general skills would be an order of magnitude greater than heading and the PLA magnitude associated with heading is not substantially greater than non-contact general skills. This could result in a very active player who experiences very few direct head contacts being considered "at risk" of developing a brain condition as a result of "sub-concussive impacts", when in fact there is no risk and the player's health, fitness and personal satisfaction are potentially compromised by their match and training exposure being reduced as a result of a falsely assessed risk.

Future Development

There is a need for general and sports-specific research and development to improve the protection offered by current helmets. Our understanding of the mechanisms of concussion generally and in specific sports, as well as human tolerance levels, continues to improve. Knowledge in these areas is consistent with established injury criteria for more severe head injuries. When this knowledge is applied to helmet test methods, standards and helmet design improvements in the ability of helmets to prevent concussion can be expected.

Correlations between biomechanical test data for helmets and epidemiological studies are generally high. The trends in improved impact energy attenuation are paralleled between the lab and field studies and absolute measures of head acceleration can predict on field helmet performance, albeit imperfectly. The strengths of the correlations are affected by intrinsic and extrinsic factors and the nature of the inciting event that influence injury likelihood and injury severity on field. These are not necessarily considered fully in laboratory test methods.

Current tolerance data treat concussion as one single pathology although the clinical symptoms and variation in cognitive and other impairments suggest differences within the umbrella term of concussion. Age-specific tolerance data are not available, for example, on children. It is also becoming clearer that impact direction and location influence concussion tolerance. In this context, the use of resultant head linear or angular acceleration criteria may not be optimal. Therefore, test methods will need to develop further.

The role of angular acceleration in concussion is gradually being resolved. It is rare for high angular acceleration to occur without high linear acceleration or impact force. Therefore, these characteristics are typically coupled. Despite the focus of helmet testing on linear acceleration management, helmets do reduce angular acceleration. Further improvements in this area are possible but require suitable test methods and standards, without compromising linear acceleration performance.

If a causal relationship between cumulative head impact exposure and brain injury is conclusively proven, that is, so-called sub-concussive impacts, then helmets in those sports that permit intentional head impact or have a high incidence of accidental head impact will need to offer even greater protection in comparison to protection against a single overload event. At present the objective should be to prevent concussion, because it is a known risk and there are known consequences of repeat concussions.

It is imperative that biomechanical laboratory studies and well-designed epidemiological and neuroimaging studies are conducted together. In comparison to epidemiological studies, laboratory studies are inexpensive and variations can be made and assessed rapidly. Confidence in laboratory studies that can be gained through validation through epidemiological studies assists in a cycle of improvement. Video analysis of games coupled with on-field monitoring of head impact biomechanics, behavioural surveys and usability studies further enhance knowledge gained from epidemiological studies, as these assist in the interpretation of the main epidemiological results.

As a final note, there has been an enormous expansion of biomechanical knowledge in the field of concussion and helmets in sport over the last 20 years. As research findings are translated into helmet design and as new helmet technologies develop, improvements in the ability of helmets to prevent concussion can be expected. This requires the support of the major sports, equipment manufacturers, research groups, public funding bodies, standards organizations and athletes.

Acknowledgement AM is a member of the Australian Centre for Research into Injury in Sport and its Prevention (ACRISP) at Edith Cowan University. ACRISP is one of the International Research Centres for the Prevention of Injury and Protection of Athlete Health supported by the International Olympic Committee (IOC).

References

1. McCory P, Meeuwisse W, Dvorak J, et al. Consensus statement on concussion in sport—the 5th international conference on concussion in sport held in Berlin, October 2016. Br J Sports Med. 2018;51:838–47.
2. Benson B, Hamilton G, Meeuwisse W, McCrory P, Dvorak J. Is protective equipment useful in preventing concussion? A systematic review of the literature. Br J Sports Med. 2009;43(1):i56–67.

3. Benson BW, McIntosh AS, Maddocks D, Herring SA, Raftery M, et al. What are the most effective risk reduction strategies in sport concussion? From protective equipment to policy. Br J Sports Med. 2013;47:321–6.
4. McIntosh AS, Andersen TE, Bahr R, Greenwald R, Kleiven S, et al. Sports helmets now and in the future. Br J Sports Med. 2011;45:1258–65.
5. McGuine BA, Hetzel S, Rasmussen J, McCrea M. The association of the type of football helmet and mouth guard with the incidence of sport related concussion in high school football players. In: Proceedings of the American Orthopedic Society for Sports Medicine Annual General Meeting. Chicago, USA; 2013.
6. Collins M, Lovell MR, Iverson GL, Ide T, Maroon J. Examining concussion rates and return to play in high school football players wearing newer helmet technology: a three-year prospective cohort study. Neurosurgery. 2006;58:275–86.
7. Shutt Helmets Website. http://www.schuttsports.com/Default.aspx. 2013.
8. McIntosh AS, McCrory P, Finch CF, Best JP, Chalmers DJ, et al. Does padded headgear prevent head injury in rugby union football? Med Sci Sports Exerc. 2009;41:306–13.
9. McIntosh AS, Curtis K, Rankin T, Cox M, Pang TY, et al. Associations between helmet use and brain injuries amongst injured pedal- and motor-cyclists: a case series analysis of trauma centre presentations. Australas Coll Road Saf. 2013;24:11–20.
10. Bambach MR, Mitchell RJ, Grzebieta RH, Olivier J. The effectiveness of helmets in bicycle collisions with motor vehicles: a case-control study. Accid Anal Pred. 2013;53:78–88.
11. Newman J. The biomechanics of head trauma: head protection. In: Nahum AM, Melvin JW, editors. Accidental Injury biomechanics and prevention. New York: Springer; 1993. p. 292–310.
12. Hoshizaki TB, Brien SE. The science and design of head protection in sport. Neurosurgery. 2004;55:956–67.
13. Benz G, McIntosh AS, Kallieris D, Daum R. A biomechanical study of bicycle helmet effectiveness in childhood. Eur J Pediatr Surg. 1993;3:259–63.
14. McIntosh AS, Janda D. Cricket helmet performance evaluation and comparison with baseball and ice hockey helmets. Br J Sports Med. 2003;37:325–30.
15. McIntosh AS, Lai A, Schilter E. Bicycle helmets: head impact dynamics in helmeted and unhelmeted oblique impact tests. Traffic Inj Prev. 2013;14(5):501–8.
16. McIntosh AS. Biomechanical considerations in the design of equipment to prevent sports injury, Proceedings of the Institution of Mechanical Engineers. Part P J Sports Eng Tech. 2012;226:193–9.
17. Rowson S, Duma S, Beckwith J, Chu JJ, Greenwald RM, et al. Rotational head kinematics in football impacts: an injury risk function for concussion. Ann Biomed Eng. 2012;40:1–13.
18. World Rugby, Headgear Performance Specification, 2019 Edition.
19. McIntosh AS, McCrory P, Finch C. Performance enhanced headgear—a scientific approach to the development of protective headgear. Br J Sports Med. 2004;38:46–9.
20. McIntosh AS, Willmott C, Patton DA, et al. An assessment of the utility and functionality of wearable head impact sensors in Australian football. J Sci Med Sport. 2019;22:784–9.
21. Reyes J, Mitra B, McIntosh AS, et al. An investigation of factors associated with head impact exposure in elite male and female Australian football. Am J Sports Med. 2020;48:1485–95.
22. McIntosh AS, Patton D. Boxing headguard performance in punch machine tests. Br J Sports Med. 2015;49:1108–12.
23. McIntosh AS, Patton D. The impact performance of headguards for combat sports. Br J Sports Med. 2015;49(17):1113–7.
24. Bahr Sandmo S, McIntosh AS, Andersen TE, Koerte IK, Bahr R. Evaluation of an in-ear sensor system for quantifying head impacts in youth football (Soccer). Am J Sports Med. 2019;47:974–81.
25. Andersen TE, Arnason A, Engebretsen L, Bahr R. Mechanisms of head injuries in elite football. Br J Sports Med. 2004;38:690–6.

Acute and Lingering Impairments in Post-Concussion Postural Control

6

Thomas A. Buckley, Kelsey N. Bryk, Katherine J. Hunzinger, and Alexander L. Enrique

Postural Control as a Concussion Biomarker

As discussed throughout this chapter, sports-related concussion has reached epidemic levels with estimates of up to 3.8 million concussions occurring annually in the United States [1]. However, some estimate that this may only reflect the tip of the iceberg as over half to three-quarters of all concussions may go unreported [2–4]. In order to appropriately manage sports-related concussions, accurate, sensitive, and specific diagnostic tools are required. Ideally, athletes would be forthcoming about symptoms following a potential injury, but many athletes are clearly unaware of common concussion symptoms or intentionally do not report suspected concussion [2–6]. While standard imaging technology (e.g., MRI and CT) is effective in identifying structural pathology, unfortunately these same procedures are not sensitive to the predominately physiological pathology of concussion [7, 8]. Recent imaging advances, including functional MRI, diffusion tensor imaging, MR spectroscopy, and others, hold promise for future utilization; however, they remain as research tools and are not recommended for routine clinical care [7–11]. Similarly, there have been multiple attempts at identifying a blood biomarker (e.g., S100B and UCH-L1) of concussion which, although promising, is likely not ready to move beyond research utilization [12–16]. While recent findings from the CARE consortium suggest that the 4-plex (GFAP, UCHL1, total tau, and NFL) can differentiate concussed versus controls, they conclude that the biomarkers do not correspond to clinical measurements or recovery [16]. Neuropsychological testing, while a valuable contribution to concussion management, has limitations including low to moderate test-retest reliability, low sensitivity, a small practice/learning effect, potential "sandbagging" of the test, and test administration differences [17–26]. Thus, a

T. A. Buckley (✉) · K. N. Bryk · K. J. Hunzinger · A. L. Enrique
Interdisciplinary Program in Biomechanics and Movement Science, Department of Kinesiology and Applied Physiology, University of Delaware, Newark, DE, USA
e-mail: TBuckley@UDel.edu; kbryk@udel.edu; khunzing@udel.edu; enriquea@udel.edu

© Springer Nature Switzerland AG 2021
S. M. Slobounov, W. J. Sebastianelli (eds.), *Concussions in Athletics*,
https://doi.org/10.1007/978-3-030-75564-5_6

robust, sensitive, and clinically feasible assessment of concussion recovery is needed to elucidate concussion recovery and prevent premature return to participation.

A systematic review with the current 5th Concussion in Sport (5th CIS) International Consensus Meeting concluded that physiological deficits persist despite apparent clinical recovery following a concussion [27]. Previously, the greatest risks were considered to be the rare, but potentially fatal, second impact syndrome as well as an elevated risk, as high as 3–6x, of recurrent concussion [28, 29]. This repeat concussion is likely to be more severe and have a prolonged recovery time [30, 31]. Recently, an elevated risk of post-concussion musculoskeletal injury has been identified [32–46] and preliminary evidence suggests that persistent impairments in postural control may be a contributing risk factor [43, 44]. Over the last decade, considerable attention has been paid to the potential association between concussions and later-life neuropathologies including mild cognitive impairment [47], clinically diagnosed depression [48], potentially earlier onset of Alzheimer's disease [47], chronic traumatic encephalopathy [49, 50], and amyotrophic lateral sclerosis [51]. Thus, it is clearly imperative for health-care providers to accurately identify concussions acutely as well as properly manage the condition post-injury. Therefore, this chapter explores the utilization of postural control as a biomarker of both concussion diagnosis and recovery.

Postural Control and Concussion

The phrases postural control, postural stability or instability, balance, and equilibrium are unfortunately frequently used interchangeably in both the lay vernacular and, occasionally, the professional literature [52, 53]. Postural control involves controlling the body's position in space for the dual purposes of stability and orientation, whereas postural stability is the ability to control the center of mass (COM) in relationship to the base of support [54]. The COM refers to the weighted average, in 3D space, of each of the body's segments and is generally considered to be the key variable in the postural control system [53–55]. The control of the COM during either static or dynamic tasks is generally categorized into three neurological components: (1) motor processes, (2) sensory processes, and (3) supraspinal or cognitive processes [54]. The motor processes include the organization of muscles throughout the body into neuromuscular synergies [54]. The sensory processes are comprised of three systems: (1) visual system, (2) vestibular system, and (3) somatosensory system [53]. The visual system is primarily involved in planning locomotion and avoiding obstacles, and the vestibular system, sometimes referred to as the body's gyro, senses linear and angular acceleration [53, 56]. Finally, the somatosensory system has multiple responsibilities including sensing the position and velocity of bodily segments, their contact with external objects, and the orientation of the body relative to gravity [53, 56]. The role of the cognitive processes in postural control is an emerging area of research with focus on "attentional resources" [54]. There are two primary theories underlying cognitive control of posture: (1)

"Capacity theory," which is based on the sharing of a limited set of neurological resources; and (2) "Bottleneck theory," which suggests that there is a competition between tasks for limited neurological resources and a prioritization occurs [54]. This challenge was noted with the "stops walking while talking" phenomenon that can occur in older adults [57]. Overall, postural control is the result of complex interactions between multiple body systems which have to work cooperatively to control the orientation and stability of the body [54].

Nearly all neuromuscular disorders result in some degeneration of the postural control systems and concussions are not an exception [53]. Indeed, the adverse effects of a concussion on postural control have been well elucidated in the literature [58, 59]. Briefly, a deficit in the interaction among the visual, vestibular, and somatosensory systems is generally considered the underlying post-concussion neuropathology [60]. Specifically, post-concussion it is believed that the individual is unable to appropriately integrate sensory input, ignore altered environmental conditions, and apply the appropriate motor control strategies to maintain precise postural control [60, 61]. Recently, an increased focus on vestibular considerations for post-concussion balance impairments had evolved and lead to recommendations for vestibular therapy in cases of delayed or prolonged recovery [62–65]. Finally, others have speculated that either diffuse axonal injury or the post-concussion neurometabolic cascade plays either a primary or secondary role in post-concussion impairments in postural control [66, 67].

Clinical Post-Concussion Postural Control Assessment Battery

The original assessment of postural control following a concussion incorporated the Romberg test which was developed in 1853 and was designed to subjectively assess somatosensory impairment in individuals with neurological conditions [68–70]. However, the Romberg test was criticized for failing to objectively identify subtle post-concussion balance deficits [61]. More recently, force plate measures have been developed to assess postural control and are valid and reliable, and numerous metrics have been investigated [52, 71–76]. One early utilized research system is the sensory organization test (SOT), which is both valid and reliable with impairments in postural control noted 3–5 days post-injury suggesting that the vestibular system of the sensory processing system is most commonly impaired [52, 58, 77–81]. However, both force plate (>$10,000) and sophisticated balance systems (SOT: >$75,000) are expensive, likely cost prohibitive for the overwhelming majority of sports medicine clinical sites, and may require extensive additional training or the addition of a biomechanist to the sports medicine staff. Indeed, even among NCAA Division I athletic trainers, less than 1% reported utilizing the SOT test and it was not utilized in lower NCAA Divisions [82, 83]. Thus, a cost-effective and practical postural control assessment paradigm is required to appropriately assess post-concussion impairments.

Current consensus of appropriate concussion management, whether on the sideline, during acute concussion assessment, or when tracking recovery, calls for a multifaceted assessment battery as no single test is highly sensitive [8, 21, 84–86]. The 5th CIS recommends a neurological screening which includes the modified balance error scoring system (mBESS) and a tandem gait for balance assessment [8]. The modified BESS (mBESS) consists of three stances (double, single, and tandem) on a single solid surface with the foam surface of the traditional BESS removed. Normal baseline/healthy scores range from 2 to 8 total errors with an increase of 2–3 errors acutely post-concussion (Fig. 6.1; [8, 87–89]). The mBESS has some similar limitations as the traditional BESS with low sensitivity and specificity acutely post-concussion [89, 90] as well as having demographic and anthropometric modifiers [91]. The tandem gait (TG) assessment consists of a heel-to-toe gait for 3 meters along a 38-mm-wide piece of tape, a 180 turn, and return along the same walkway. This is repeated four times and the best trial time is recorded as the individuals' score [92, 93]. Early results indicate that TG has a higher sensitivity (0.63) than either the BESS (0.45) or the mBESS (0.47) with a low minimal detectable change score of 0.38 s (Fig. 6.2; [94]). However, in the high school population, the previously applied cut-off of 14 s to complete the task appears inappropriate as over 75% of healthy athletes were unable to complete the task within this time frame [95]. Finally, emerging evidence, as discussed later in the gait section, suggests that dual-task TG, performing the TG trial while also completing a cognitive challenge, has strong potential as clinically feasible assessment, but requires further investigation [92, 96–99].

While the mBESS and TG are the current recommendations of the 5th CIS, the more commonly used postural control assessments post-concussion remain vital parts of the original BESS test [82, 83, 100, 101]. The original BESS consists of three stances (double, single, and tandem) on two surfaces (firm and foam) with errors being counted for deviations from the test position [78, 102]. The BESS appears sensitive to acute concussion with an increase of 6–8 errors post-injury being commonly reported [103–105] and is consistent with the SOT, which suggests that postural control recovers within 3–5 days post-concussion [60, 104]. The specificity of the BESS remains high (>0.91) through the first week post-injury; however, the sensitivity is low immediately post-injury (0.34), and continues to decrease to 0.16 over the first 3 days post-injury [89, 103, 106]. Unfortunately, the minimal detectable change values for the BESS test range from 7.3 (intra-rater) to 9.4 (inter-rater) at baseline and are even worse acutely post-concussion (intra-rater: 8.6; inter-rater: 11.3 errors) [90, 107]. Despite these psychometric limitations, a change of more than four errors in the firm components of the BESS was the second strongest predictor in a CART analysis of collegiate student athletes [108]. However, the BESS is also substantially limited by the practice effect associated with repeat administration [109–115], as well as fatigue, dehydration, functional ankle instability, neuromuscular training, and the testing environment [116–124]. Finally, the confounders of common sports injuries (e.g., ankle or knee sprains) which occur after baseline testing but prior to a post-concussion assessment have not currently been elucidated. Overall, the current utilization of the BESS test, despite being the most commonly used postural control assessment tool, is fundamentally flawed as there is scant evidence that critical test determinants are being considered [59].

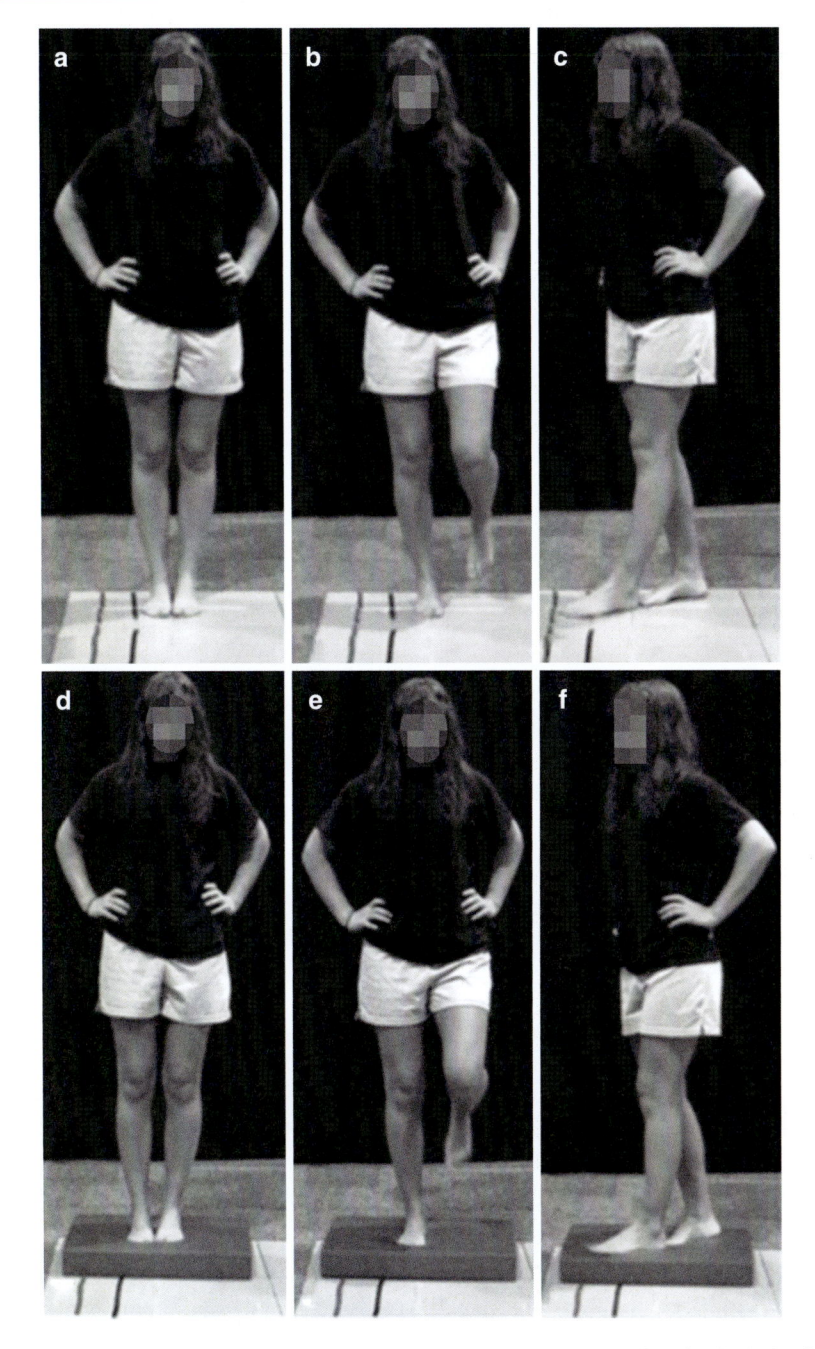

Fig. 6.1 The balance error scoring system. The six stances (**a**: double-leg firm; **b**: single-leg firm; **c**: tandem firm; **d**: double-leg foam; **e**: single-leg foam; and **f**: tandem foam) were performed for 20 s each. The BESS errors identified included: (1) the hands coming off of the iliac crest, (2) opening the eyes, (3) step, stumble, or fall, (4) moving the hip into greater than 30° of abduction, (5) lifting the forefoot or heel, and (6) remaining out of the test position longer than 5 s (Rahn et al. [226])

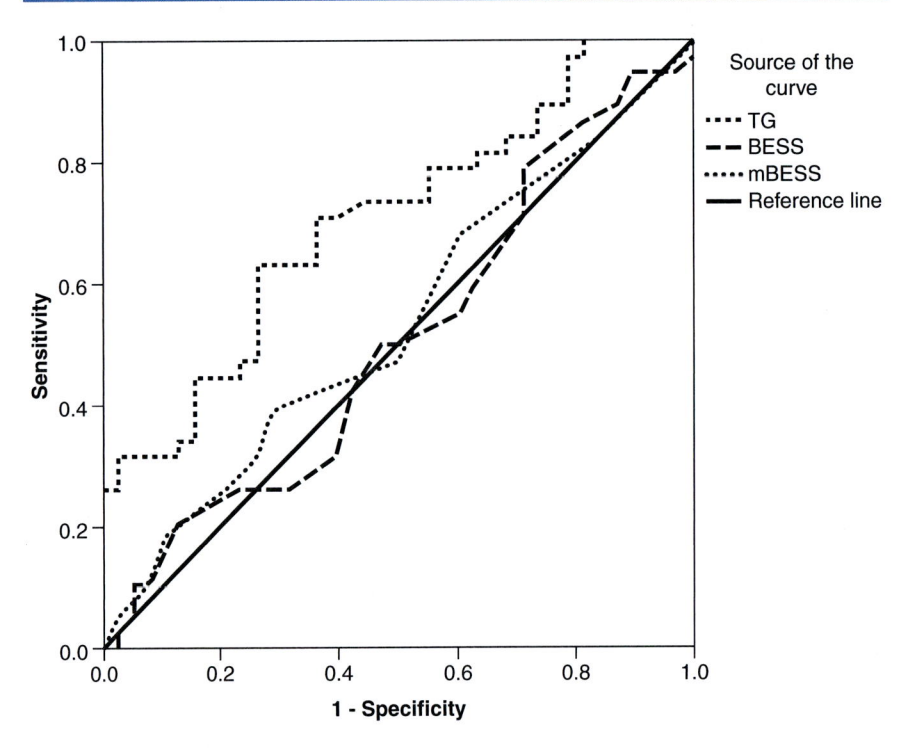

Fig. 6.2 Receiver operator characteristic curve for tandem gait (TG), balance error scoring system (BESS), and modified balance error scoring system (mBESS). The area under the curve was highest for TG (0.704) followed by mBESS (0.474) and the lowest was BESS (0.447) (Oldham et al. [94])

Instrumented Postural Control During Motor Tasks Post-Concussion

Early evidence of gait impairments following concussion was reported by McCrory and colleagues using video analysis of concussions sustained in the mid-1990s by competitors in Australian Rules Football [125]. Gait impairments, operationally defined as ataxic, stumbling, or unsteady gait, were noted post-injury in 41% of concussed athletes with the majority manifesting symptoms immediately post-injury; however, a small percentage (14%) had a minimal delay of 10–20 s prior to the onset of gait unsteadiness [125]. While not specifically studied, it was speculated that gait unsteadiness involved a brainstem pathology and was multifactorial including postural tone, and cerebellar and labyrinthine function [125]. This study, while limited to gross video observations without true biomechanical assessment, provided foundational evidence of post-concussion gait impairments. Compared to other commonly investigated neurological pathologies (e.g., Parkinson's disease, elderly falls, stroke, and amputee), investigations of gait to identify impairments in postural control post-concussion have only emerged in the last 15 years [126]. The majority of gait studies were performed at only a few laboratories, generally lacked within-subject pre-injury data, and have involved a variety of gait tasks including single-task gait, dual-task gait with working memory challenges, and obstacle avoidance tasks [44, 96, 126–158].

Single-Task Gait

Gait velocity has been termed the "Sixth Vital Sign" and in older adults decreases in velocity can be used to predict future health-related status, functional decline, fall risk, and decreased quality of life [159]. Furthermore, gait velocity is reliable, valid, sensitive, specific, and, as a critical activity of daily living, not associated with learning or practice effects from repeat test administration [159, 160].

Utilizing traditional clinical measures of balance (e.g., BESS), large cohort investigators have suggested that postural control returns to its baseline value within 3–5 days post-injury [103, 104]. The post-concussion gait studies which have been published are generally limited by lack of subjects' with baseline/pre-injury data; however, they are generally tightly matched to otherwise healthy control subjects. Within this context, gait velocity generally appears to return to a normal value by Day 5 or 6 post-injury despite individuals still experiencing concussion-related symptoms [96, 128–134, 143, 147, 153, 161], but some studies have also demonstrated deficits 1–2 months post-injury [130, 151, 162]. These and other similar findings need to be taken into context as either a practice effect or a Hawthorne effect [130, 151]. Similar findings were noted in the stepping characteristics (stride time, width, and length) and sagittal plane COM measurements (anterior displacement and velocity of the COM and the anterior COP-COM separation) [126, 129, 131]. Frontal plane kinematics may be a more revealing aspect post-concussion as there is a limited base of support during the single support phase of gait, thus requiring greater postural control [163]. During single-task gait, post-concussion participants demonstrated increases in the medial-to-lateral COM range of motion and velocity [128, 131, 134, 136]. These impairments appear to persist for up to 28 days post-injury despite apparent recovery on the traditional clinical assessment battery [131, 136]. Interestingly, in many of these studies, there was an apparent recovery on many dependent variables by Day 5 post-injury, but significant differences re-emerged 2–4 weeks later. These findings suggest either potential differences on Day 5 are not statistically significant due to small groups and the possibility of the study being underpowered, or some residual consequence of delayed impairment following a concussion. Overall, these gait studies suggest that a conservative gait strategy has been adopted post-concussion, although the rationale for these strategies remains unknown. Single-task gait has potential for clinical translation as simple timing devices can be utilized to track performance over known distances, similar to clinical evaluations used in older adults or those with neurological impairments. The use of cell phones or portable accelerometers to monitor gait in home living environments could considerably improve concussion management by identifying ongoing and lingering deficits.

Dual-Task Gait

These previous findings suggest that, acutely post-concussion, impairments in postural control are identified with single (motor)-task challenges; however, evidence over the last two decades suggests that reallocation of attentional resources and/or neural plasticity may allow the individual to overcome simple single-task challenges [75, 164, 165]. Typical dual-task (DT) challenges examine the effect of executing a secondary cognitive task (e.g., mental processing) on the concurrent performance of a primary motor task (e.g., walking), although other approaches (e.g., motor and motor: holding a full glass of water while walking) exist [165]. Even routine motor activities, such as sitting, standing quietly, or walking, require cognitive processing [166]. Previous investigations noted impaired postural control during both quiet stance and gait in healthy young adults under dual-task conditions [167, 168]. Simultaneous performance of a motor task and a cognitive task may interfere with the performance of one or both, probably due to competing demands for inherently limited attentional resources [169–171].

Adopting from methodologies utilized in studies of elderly or neurologically diseased state patients, the addition of a cognitive challenge to the motor task of gait has been explored post-concussion [126]. Both impairments in postural control and cognitive processing are known acute consequences of concussion and thus, not surprisingly, both are abnormal when tested within 24 h of the injury. Post-concussion gait studies utilizing a dual-task paradigm have largely focused on utilizing working memory challenges (e.g., reciting the months of the year backwards) from the mini-mental style examination to assess cognitive performance while performing either level overground gait or obstacle avoidance [92, 96, 126, 145, 149, 152, 153, 155, 172–182]. A recent systematic review and meta-analysis, using individualized participant data from 25 studies and on nearly 1000 concussed or control participants, demonstrated clear evidence of impaired DT gait up to 2 months post-concussion [126]. While a comprehensive set of outcome measures for clinical application was not able to be identified from the review, it is clear that both spatiotemporal characteristics (gait velocity) and kinematic variables (e.g., mediolateral COM velocity, anteroposterior COM displacement, and anteroposterior COM velocity) were persistently impaired well beyond clinical recovery. However, a considerable limitation in these studies was the cross-sectional design due to a lack of baseline/pre-injury data [126]. Previously, a pooled mean decrease of 0.13 m/s in DT gait velocity between acute concussion and control participants had been noted; however, a clinically meaningful difference value has not yet been determined [173]. Furthermore, DT gait has identified differences despite apparent recovery during clinical tests, including computerized neuropsychological assessments, suggesting these motor cognitive challenges may be more sensitive to recovery than even sophisticated neurocognitive assessments [155].

These results confirm that impairments persist beyond the generally accepted 2-week recovery. The clinical meaningfulness of these results remains to be determined; however, these deficits may be associated with the elevated risk of musculoskeletal (MSK) injury in the year following concussion. Specific supporting evidence was provided by Howell and colleagues who identified worsening DT cost (increased motor deficits during DT performance) in adolescent athletes who experienced subsequent MSK [43]. Further, Oldham recently identified slower DT gait speed (0.09 m/s) at return to participation, relative to baseline, in concussed athletes who experienced subsequent MSK [44]. Thus, it is clear that DT gait differences are prevalent following concussion, persist beyond clinical recovery, and emerging evidence suggests they are associated with subsequent MSK. Therefore, clinically feasible methods to assess gait performance could substantially improve clinical concussion management. Similar to single-task gait, the development of automated or smart phone-enabled assessments could dramatically improve concussion management.

Gait Initiation

The control of posture and locomotion are interdependent at several levels of the central nervous system [183]. Therefore, impaired posture and gait components may contribute to deficits in locomotion due to adaptive changes in neural control [183]. Many post-concussion balance assessments (e.g., BESS and SOT) are novel challenges and, as described, are subject to a substantial practice effect with repeat administration [109–112, 184]. Thus, "non-novel" tasks, tasks which are performed as regular activities of daily living and, therefore, not subject to a practice or learning effect, may elucidate deficits not otherwise noted. One task commonly utilized to investigate the interactions between posture and locomotion components is gait initiation (GI). Indeed, GI, the phase between motionless standing and steady-state locomotion requiring the generation of propulsive forces, has been shown to be a sensitive indicator of balance dysfunction [185]. GI challenges the postural control systems as it is a volitional transition from a large stable base of support to a smaller continuously unstable posture during gait [186]. From a motor control perspective, GI requires the central nervous system to regulate the spatial and temporal relationship between the position and motion of the COM [187]. Therefore, GI has been used to quantify impairments in postural instability among elderly, Parkinson's disease, stroke, and amputee patient groups and is generally considered more challenging than level overground gait [185–192].

During quiet stance, the center of pressure (COP) and center of mass (COM) are tightly coupled and located just anterior to the malleolus [193]. To initiate gait, they must decouple to generate forward momentum while maintaining upright balance [193, 194]. Initially, the COP moves posteriorly and laterally toward the initial swing limb (Fig. 6.3). This anticipatory postural adjustment (APA), likely controlled by the supplementary motor area and/or premotor area, involves bilateral tibialis anterior activation and soleus inhibition [195–197]. The initial posterior COP movement generates the forward momentum needed to separate the COP and COM while the lateral COP displacement, controlled by the gluteus medias, propels the COM toward the initial stance limb [198]. This momentum generation is necessary to achieve successful forward locomotion while

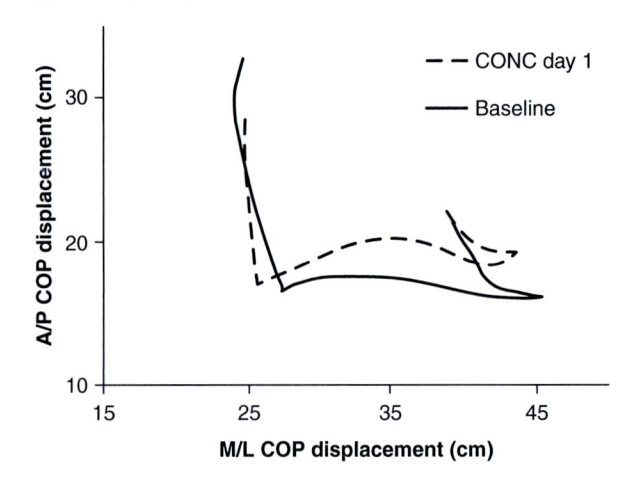

Fig. 6.3 Center of pressure (COP) displacement. Following movement initiation, the COP translates posterior and lateral toward the initial swing limb (S1 or APA phase). As the heel of the initial swing limb leaves the ground, the COP translates laterally toward the initial stance limb (S2 or transitional phase). Finally, as the initial stance limb leaves the ground to complete the initial step, the COP translates anteriorly (S3 or locomotor phase) (Buckley et al. [203])

maintaining upright balance. Thus, the initial posterior and lateral COP displacements are particularly sensitive indicators of balance dysfunction [191, 192, 199, 200].

Following a sports-related concussion, impairments in GI have been noted [201–205]. A typical healthy adult will displace their COP approximately 5–7 cm both posteriorly and laterally during the APA phase of GI. There are significant reductions in both the APA displacement and velocity acutely post-concussion, with large effect sizes (Cohen's $d > 1.0$), as compared to baseline/pre-injury performance. On an individual level, 97.6% (41/42) of post-concussion participants had reductions in the COP posterior displacement (Fig. 6.4; [202]). However, there were limited and small differences in the initial step characteristics suggesting that the motor planning of GI was impaired more than the task outcome [202]. Similarly, in a cross-sectional study, Doherty identified reductions in both COP and COM excursions within 10 days post-concussion which also suggests impaired motor planning and control [204]. Most recently, Buckley and colleagues identified deficits in motor planning during GI across concussion clinical milestones, including on the day the athlete returned to participation in sports after completing the 5th CIS recommended progressive protocol [205]. This finding suggests that persistent impairment in postural control is still present when the athlete returns to competition and may underlie the previously discussed increased risk of post-concussion musculoskeletal injury [38, 206]. While the longer term deficits have received limited attention, a continuum of performance was identified whereby athletes with ≥3 prior concussions demonstrated deficits

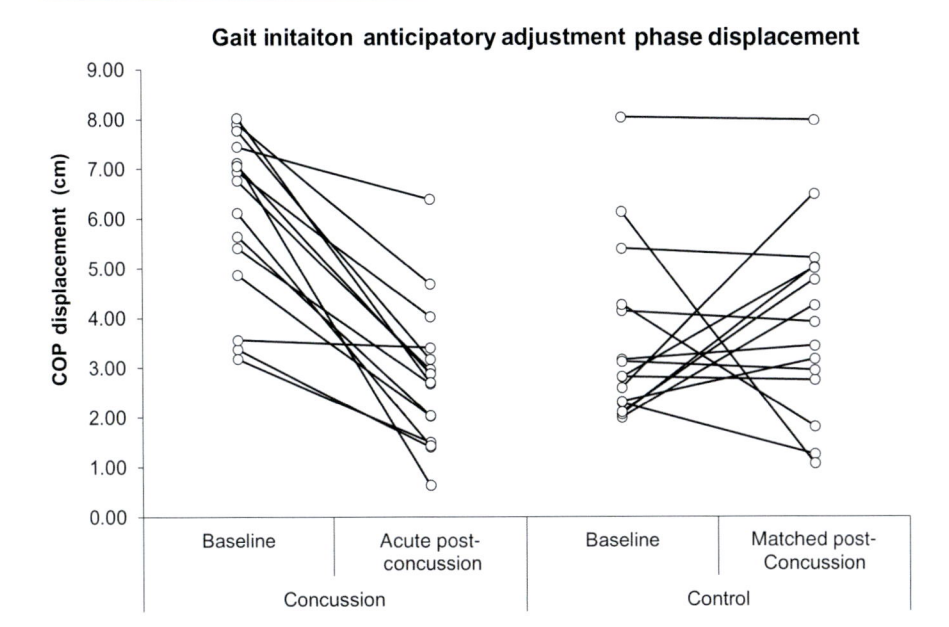

Gait initaiton anticipatory adjustment phase displacement

Fig. 6.4 Changes in COP posterior displacement. There was a significant reduction in the concussion group from baseline to acute post-concussion (5.7 ± 1.6 cm and 2.6 ± 2.1 cm, respectively, $p < 0.001$) but no difference in the control group (4.0 ± 1.6 cm and 4.0 ± 2.5 cm, respectively, $p = 0.921$). In the concussion group, 97.6% (41/42) participants had decreased COP posterior displacement acutely post-concussion (Buckley et al. [202]. This figure has not been previously published in this form, but is based on data from Fig. 2 in the archives paper – permission received)

relative to uninjured subjects, but far less than acute post-concussion subjects, which suggests the possibility of subtle deficits in motor planning in athletes who have experienced multiple concussions [203]. The underlying neurophysiological mechanisms and long-term consequences of these deficits remain to be elucidated.

Gait Termination

Gait termination (GT) is not a mirror image of GI [207]. Rather, GT is a process by which the central nervous system anticipates, controls, and arrests the forward momentum of the COM without exceeding the borders of the base of support [208, 209]. Further, GT has a known and invariant set of parameters that constrains the multiple degrees of freedom within the lower extremity [210–212]. However, GT poses a unique challenge to the postural control systems because the COM is often located outside the base of support at the onset of GT [194]. As a result, GT is an excellent model for investigating alterations in motor programming and neurologic dysfunction. The central neurophysiologic control of GT is more elusive than GI; however, fMRI studies have suggested that the prefrontal area, specifically the inferior frontal gyrus and the pre-supplementary motor area, likely control GT [207]. Mechanically, the termination of gait requires the coordinated activity of both legs. Indeed, force production is modulated bilaterally such that the lead limb (limb behind the COM) reduces foot push-off propulsive forces as the swing limb (limb in front of the COM) concurrently increases vertical and anteroposterior braking forces [210, 211, 213]. Reduced propulsive forces are caused by soleus inhibition and increased activation of the tibialis anterior while concurrent increases in braking forces are due to an increased soleus activity and inhibition of the tibialis anterior [214, 215]. Failure to reduce lead limb propulsive forces results in an increased reliance on a single limb stopping strategy and subsequently, longer termination times and a greater number of steps required to control the COM [216]. Therefore, increases in propulsive and braking forces have been identified as sensitive indicators of balance dysfunction and alterations in the cortical control of GT [211, 216, 217]. Indeed, GT has quantified impairments in postural control among the aging, people with Parkinson's disease, amputee groups, chronic ankle instability, and those with general balance disorders [211, 212, 214, 216–223].

There has been limited investigation into GT performance following concussion despite the potential for further understanding of neurophysiological impairments [224, 225]. When assessed acutely post-concussion, and on an individual level when compared to in their own healthy baseline data, there was a reduction in the braking and transitional phases of GT [224]. Similar to the GI studies, this would suggest impairments in motor planning during the task. These GT deficits appear to persist through the acute and sub-acute phases of concussion recovery for at least 10 days post-concussion as seen by altered force production gait despite apparent clinical recovery [225]. One would expect that the penultimate step during GT would produce a reduced propulsive force and the terminal step an increased braking force relative to normal gait. Conversely, post-concussion, the individual actually increases their propulsive force during the penultimate step and reduces their braking force during the termination step (Fig. 6.5; [225]). This highly inefficient pattern of performing GT is suggestive of a central deficit and the selection of an inappropriate motor program to perform the GT task. There presently are no investigations studying chronic deficits in GT performance.

6 Acute and Lingering Impairments in Post-Concussion Postural Control

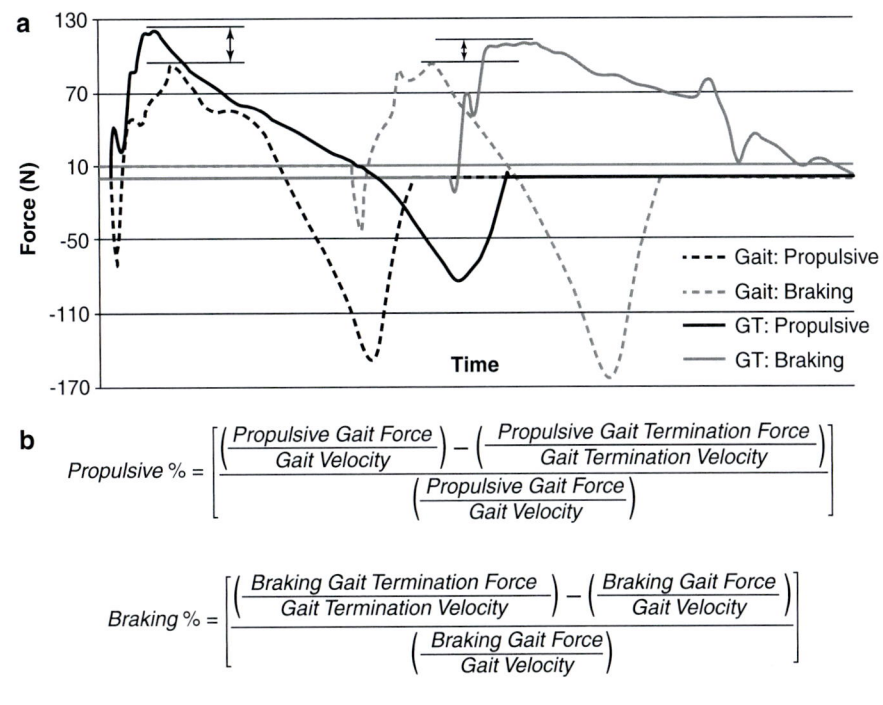

Fig. 6.5 (a) Representative propulsive and braking force curves. Peak propulsive (black lines) and braking forces (gray lines) from both standard gait and gait termination trials were identified (horizontal lines) and normalized to the trials gait velocity. Normalized gait termination forces were then expressed as a percentage of the normalized forces observed during standard gait trials. (b) The formulas used to calculate the propulsive and braking (Buckley et al. [225])

$$\text{Propulsive \%} = \left[\frac{\left(\frac{\text{Propulsive Gait Force}}{\text{Gait Velocity}}\right) - \left(\frac{\text{Propulsive Gait Termination Force}}{\text{Gait Termination Velocity}}\right)}{\left(\frac{\text{Propulsive Gait Force}}{\text{Gait Velocity}}\right)} \right]$$

$$\text{Braking \%} = \left[\frac{\left(\frac{\text{Braking Gait Termination Force}}{\text{Gait Termination Velocity}}\right) - \left(\frac{\text{Braking Gait Force}}{\text{Gait Velocity}}\right)}{\left(\frac{\text{Braking Gait Force}}{\text{Gait Velocity}}\right)} \right]$$

Conclusion

The 5th CIS suggests that most concussions resolve within a couple of weeks based on clinical measures; however, consistent findings of persistent deficits have been noted using more sophisticated measures. The SCAT-5 recommendation for postural control assessment is the BESS; however, this assessment suffers from numerous methodological limitations and may prematurely indicate recovery. Clinically, the tandem gait test has better psychometrics and fewer limitations than the BESS. Instrumented measures of postural control, including single- and dual-task gait, gait initiation, and gait termination, have all demonstrated impairments despite apparent clinical recovery. These noted deficits potentially provide insight into the supraspinal motor planning and control strategies activated following concussion. Furthermore, these deficits have been noted up to 2 months post-concussion and suggest that athletes are prematurely returning to athletic participation despite persistent neurological deficits. These deficits may underlie the recently identified elevated risk of post-concussion musculoskeletal injury. Moving forward, developing clinically feasible assessments of gait based upon postural control (e.g., single- and dual-task gait) utilizing smart phone technologies may critically improve current concussion management strategies and reduce the risk of premature return to participation.

References

1. Langlois JA, Rutland-Brown W, Wald MM. The epidemiology and impact of traumatic brain injury: a brief overview. J Head Trauma Rehabil. 2006;21(5):375–8.
2. McCrea M, Hammeke T, Olsen G, Leo P, Guskiewicz K. Unreported concussion in high school football players: implications for prevention. Clin J Sport Med. 2004;14(1):13–7.
3. Llewellyn TA, Burdette GT, Joyner AB, Buckley TA. Concussion reporting rates at the conclusion of an intercollegiate athletic career. Clin J Sport Med. 2014;24(1):76–9.
4. Meehan WP 3rd, Mannix RC, O'Brien MJ, Collins MW. The prevalence of undiagnosed concussions in athletes. Clin J Sport Med. 2013;23(5):339–42.
5. Kaut KP, DePompei R, Kerr J, Congeni J. Reports of head injury and symptom knowledge among college athletes: implications for assessment and educational intervention. Clin J Sport Med. 2003;13(4):213–21.
6. Players still willing to hide head injuries. Associated Press; 2011. Available from: http://espn.go.com/nfl/story/_/id/7388074/nfl-players-say-hiding-concussions-option.
7. Davis GA, Iverson GL, Guskiewicz KM, Ptito A, Johnston KM. Contributions of neuroimaging, balance testing, electrophysiology and blood markers to the assessment of sport-related concussion. Br J Sports Med. 2009;43(Suppl 1):i36–45.
8. McCrory P, Meeuwisse W, Dvorak J, Aubry M, Bailes J, Broglio S. Consensus statement on concussion in sport - the 5th international conference on concussion in sport held in Berlin, October 2016. Br J Sports Med. 2017;51(11):838–57.
9. Kutcher JS, McCrory P, Davis G, Ptito A, Meeuwisse WH, Broglio SP. What evidence exists for new strategies or technologies in the diagnosis of sports concussion and assessment of recovery? Br J Sports Med. 2013;47(5):299–303.
10. Dashnaw ML, Petraglia AL, Bailes JE. An overview of the basic science of concussion and subconcussion: where we are and where we are going. Neurosurg Focus. 2012;33(6):E5.
11. Dennis EL, Baron D, Bartnik-Olson B, Caeyenberghs K, Esopenko C, Hillary FG, et al. ENIGMA brain injury: framework, challenges, and opportunities. Hum Brain Mapp. 2020.
12. Unden J, Romner B. Can low serum levels of S100B predict normal CT findings after minor head injury in adults?: an evidence-based review and meta-analysis. J Head Trauma Rehabil. 2010;25(4):228–40.
13. Liu MC, Akinyi L, Scharf D, Mo JX, Larner SF, Muller U, et al. Ubiquitin C-terminal hydrolase-L1 as a biomarker for ischemic and traumatic brain injury in rats. Eur J Neurosci. 2010;31(4):722–32.
14. Papa L, Akinyi L, Liu MC, Pineda JA, Tepas JJ III, Oli MW, et al. Ubiquitin C-terminal hydrolase is a novel biomarker in humans for severe traumatic brain injury. Crit Care Med. 2010;38(1):138–44.
15. Jeter CB, Hergenroeder GW, Hylin MJ, Redell JB, Moore AN, Dash PK. Biomarkers for the diagnosis and prognosis of mild traumatic brain injury/concussion. J Neurotrauma. 2013;30(8):657–70.
16. Asken BM, Yang ZH, Xu HY, Weber AG, Hayes RL, Bauer RM, et al. Acute effects of sport-related concussion on serum glial Fibrillary acidic protein, ubiquitin C-terminal hydrolase L1, Total tau, and Neurofilament light measured by a multiplex assay. J Neurotrauma. 2020;37(13):1537–45.
17. Barr WB. Neuropsychological testing of high school athletes - preliminary norms and test-retest indices. Arch Clin Neuropsychol. 2003;18(1):91–101.
18. Broglio SP, Ferrara MS, Macciocchi SN, Baumgartner TA, Elliott R. Test-retest reliability of computerized concussion assessment programs. J Athl Train. 2007;42(4):509–14.

19. Randolph C. Baseline neuropsychological testing in managing sport-related concussion: does it modify risk? Curr Sports Med Rep. 2011;10(1):21–6.
20. Schatz P. Long-term test-retest reliability of baseline cognitive assessments using ImPACT. Am J Sports Med. 2010;38(1):47–53.
21. Register-Mihalik JK, Guskiewicz KM, Mihalik JP, Schmidt JD, Kerr ZY, McCrea MA. Reliable change, sensitivity, and specificity of a multidimensional concussion assessment battery: implications for caution in clinical practice. J Head Trauma Rehabil. 2013;28(4):274–83.
22. Iverson GL, Lovell MR, Collins MW. Interpreting change on ImPACT following sport concussion. Clin Neuropsychol. 2003;17(4):460–7.
23. Erdal K. Neuropsychological testing for sports-related concussion: how athletes can sandbag their baseline testing without detection. Arch Clin Neuropsychol. 2012;27(5):473–9.
24. Glatts C, Schatz P. "Sandbagging" baseline concussion testing on ImPACT is more difficult than it appears. Arch Clin Neuropsychol. 2012;27(6):621.
25. Moser RS, Schatz P, Neidzwski K, Ott SD. Group versus individual administration affects baseline neurocognitive test performance. Am J Sports Med. 2011;39(11):2325–30.
26. Resch J, Driscoll A, McCaffrey N, Brown C, Ferrara MS, Macciocchi S, et al. ImPact test-retest reliability: reliably unreliable? J Athl Train. 2013;48(4):506–11.
27. Kamins J, Bigler E, Covassin T, Henry L, Kemp S, Leddy JJ, et al. What is the physiological time to recovery after concussion? Systematic review. Br J Sports Med. 2017;51(12):935–40.
28. Zemper ED. Two-year prospective study of relative risk of a second cerebral concussion. Am J Phys Med Rehabil. 2003;82(9):653–9.
29. Guskiewicz KM, McCrea M, Marshall SW, Cantu RC, Randolph C, Barr W, et al. Cumulative effects associated with recurrent concussion in collegiate football players: the NCAA concussion study. JAMA. 2003;290(19):2549–55.
30. Collins MW, Lovell MR, Iverson GL, Cantu RC, Maroon JC, Field M. Cumulative effects of concussion in high school athletes. Neurosurgery. 2002;51(5):1175–9.
31. Eisenberg MA, Andrea J, Meehan W, Mannix R. Time interval between concussions and symptom duration. Pediatrics. 2013;132(1):8–17.
32. Fino PC, Becker LN, Fino NF, Griesemer B, Goforth M, Brolinson PG. Effects of recent concussion and injury history on instantaneous relative risk of lower extremity injury in division I collegiate athletes. Clin J Sport Med. 2019;29(3):218–23.
33. Lynall RC, Mauntel TC, Padua DA, Mihalik JP. Acute lower extremity injury rates increase following concussion in college athletes. Med Sci Sports Exerc. 2015;47(12):2487–92.
34. Lynall R, Mauntel T, Pohlig R, Kerr Z, Dompier T, Hall E, et al. Lower extremity musculoskeletal injury risk following concussion recovery in high school athletes. J Athl Train. 2017;52(11):1028–34.
35. Brooks MA, Peterson K, Biese K, Sanfilippo J, Heiderscheit BC, Bell DR. Concussion increases odds of sustaining a lower extremity musculoskeletal injury after return to play among collegiate athletes. Am J Sports Med. 2016;19(3):742–7.
36. Nordstrom A, Nordstrom P, Ekstrand J. Sports-related concussion increases the risk of subsequent injury by about 50% in elite male football players. Br J Sports Med. 2014;48(19):1447–50.
37. Herman DC, Jones D, Harrison A, Moser M, Tillman S, Farmer K, et al. Concussion may increase the risk of subsequent lower extremity musculoskeletal injury in collegiate athletes. Sports Med. 2017;47(5):1003–10.
38. McPherson A, Nagai T, Webster K, Hewett T. Musculoskeletal injury risk after sport-related concussion: a systematic review and meta-analysis. Am J Sports Med. 2018;47(7):1754–62.
39. Gilbert FC, Burdette GT, Joyner AB, Llewellyn TA, Buckley TA. Association between concussion and lower extremity injuries in collegiate athletes. Sports Health. 2016;8(6):561–7.
40. Cross M, Kemp S, Smith A, Trewartha G, Stokes K. Professional Rugby Union players have a 60% greater risk of time loss injury after concussion: a 2-season prospective study of clinical outcomes. Br J Sports Med. 2015;50(15):926–31.
41. Nyberg G, Mossberg KH, Lysholm J, Tegner Y. Subsequent traumatic injuries after concussion in elite ice hockey: a study over 28 years. Curr Res Concussion. 2015;2(3):109–12.

42. Buckley T, Howard C, Oldham J, Lynall R, Swanik C, Getchell N. No clinical predictors of postconcussion musculoskeletal injury in college athletes. Med Sci Sports Exerc. 2020;52(6):1256–62.
43. Howell D, Buckley T, Lynall R, Meehan W. Worsening dual-task gait costs after concussion and their association with subsequent sport-related injury. J Neurotrauma. 2018;35(14):1630–6.
44. Oldham JR, Howell DR, Knight CA, Crenshaw JR, Buckley TA. Gait performance is associated with subsequent lower extremity injury following concussion. Med Sci Sports Exerc. 2020;52(11):2279–85.
45. Pietrosimone B, Golightly YM, Mihalik JP, Guskiewicz KM. Concussion frequency associates with musculoskeletal injury in retired NFL players. Med Sci Sports Exerc. 2015;47(11):2366–72.
46. Kardouni JR, Shing TL, McKinnon CJ, Scofield DE, Proctor SP. Risk for lower extremity injury after concussion: a matched cohort study in soldiers. J Orthop Sports Phys Ther. 2018;48(7):533–40.
47. Guskiewicz KM, Marshall SW, Bailes J, McCrea M, Cantu RC, Randolph C, et al. Association between recurrent concussion and late-life cognitive impairment in retired professional football players. Neurosurgery. 2005;57(4):719–26; discussion 719–26.
48. Guskiewicz KM, Marshall SW, Bailes J, McCrea M, Harding HP Jr, Matthews A, et al. Recurrent concussion and risk of depression in retired professional football players. Med Sci Sports Exerc. 2007;39(6):903–9.
49. McKee AC, Cantu RC, Nowinski CJ, Hedley-Whyte ET, Gavett BE, Budson AE, et al. Chronic traumatic encephalopathy in athletes: progressive tauopathy after repetitive head injury. J Neuropathol Exp Neurol. 2009;68(7):709–35.
50. Schwartz A. Suicide reveals signs of a disease seen in N.F.L. New York Times. September 14, 2010; Sect. News.
51. McKee AC, Gavett BE, Stern RA, Nowinski CJ, Cantu RC, Kowall NW, et al. TDP-43 proteinopathy and motor neuron disease in chronic traumatic encephalopathy. J Neuropathol Exp Neurol. 2010;69(9):918–29.
52. Cavanaugh JT, Guskiewicz KM, Stergiou N. A nonlinear dynamic approach for evaluating postural control: new directions for the management of sport-related cerebral concussion. Sports Med. 2005;35(11):935–50.
53. Winter DA. Human balance and posture control during standing and walking. Gait Posture. 1995;3(4):193–214.
54. Shumway-Cook A, Woollacott MH. Motor control: translating research into clinical practice. 4th ed. Philadelphia: Lippincott Williams & Wilkins; 2012.
55. Scholz JP, Schoener G, Hsu WL, Jeka JJ, Horak F, Martin V. Motor equivalent control of the center of mass in response to support surface perturbations. Exp Brain Res. 2007;180(1):163–79.
56. Highstein SM, Holstein GR. The anatomical and physiological framework for vestibular prostheses. Anat Rec (Hoboken). 2012;295(11):2000–9.
57. LundinOlsson L, Nyberg L, Gustafson Y. "Stops walking when talking" as a predictor of falls in elderly people. Lancet. 1997;349(9052):617.
58. Guskiewicz KM. Balance assessment in the Management of Sport-Related Concussion. Clin Sports Med. 2011;30(1):89–102.
59. Buckley TA, Oldham JR, Caccese JB. Postural control deficits identify lingering postconcussion neurological deficits. J Sport Health Sci. 2016;5(1):61–9.
60. Guskiewicz KM. Postural stability assessment following concussion: one piece of the puzzle. Clin J Sport Med. 2001;11(3):182–9.
61. Ellemberg D, Henry LC, Macciocchi SN, Guskiewicz KM, Broglio SP. Advances in sport concussion assessment: from behavioral to brain imaging measures. J Neurotrauma. 2009;26(12):2365–82.
62. Chandrasekhar SS. The assessment of balance and dizziness in the TBI patient. NeuroRehabilitation. 2013;32(3):445–54.

63. Lei-Rivera L, Sutera J, Galatioto JA, Hujsak BD, Gurley JM. Special tools for the assessment of balance and dizziness in individuals with mild traumatic brain injury. NeuroRehabilitation. 2013;32(3):463–72.
64. Langevin P, Fait P, Fremont P, Roy JS. Cervicovestibular rehabilitation in adult with mild traumatic brain injury: a randomised controlled trial protocol. BMC Sports Sci Med Rehabil. 2019;11(1):25.
65. Schneider KJ, Meeuwisse WH, Nettel-Aguirre A, Barlow K, Boyd L, Kang J, et al. Cervicovestibular rehabilitation in sport-related concussion: a randomised controlled trial. Br J Sports Med. 2014;48(17):1294–U55.
66. Giza CC, Hovda DA. The neurometabolic cascade of concussion. J Athl Train. 2001;36(3):228–35.
67. Mouzon B, Chaytow H, Crynen G, Bachmeier C, Stewart J, Mullan M, et al. Repetitive mild traumatic brain injury in a mouse model produces learning and memory deficits accompanied by histological changes. J Neurotrauma. 2012;29(18):2761–73.
68. Jansen EC, Larsen RE, Olesen MB. Quantitative Romberg test - measurement and computer calculation of postural stability. Acta Neurol Scand. 1982;66(1):93–9.
69. Thyssen HH, Brynskov J, Jansen EC, Munsterswendsen J. Normal ranges and reproducibility for the quantitative Romberg test. Acta Neurol Scand. 1982;66(1):100–4.
70. Khasnis A, Gokula RM. Romberg's test. J Postgrad Med. 2003;49(2):169–72.
71. Riemann BL, Guskiewicz KM. Assessment of mild head injury using measures of balance and cognition: a case study. J Sport Rehabil. 1997;6(3):283–9.
72. Gao J, Hu J, Buckley T, White K, Hass C. Shannon and Renyi entropies to classify effects of mild traumatic brain injury on postural sway. PLoS One. 2011;6(9):e24446.
73. Slobounov S, Cao C, Sebastianelli W, Slobounov E, Newell K. Residual deficits from concussion as revealed by virtual time-to-contact measures of postural stability. Clin Neurophysiol. 2008;119(2):281–9.
74. Slobounov S, Sebastianelli W, Hallett M. Residual brain dysfunction observed one year post-mild traumatic brain injury: combined EEG and balance study. Clin Neurophysiol. 2012;123(9):1755–61.
75. Slobounov S, Tutwiler R, Sebastianelli W, Slobounov E. Alteration of postural responses to visual field motion in mild traumatic brain injury. Neurosurgery. 2006;59(1):134–9.
76. Cavanaugh JT, Guskiewicz KM, Giuliani C, Marshall S, Mercer V, Stergiou N. Detecting altered postural control after cerebral concussion in athletes with normal postural stability. Br J Sports Med. 2005;39(11):805–11.
77. Mrazik M, Ferrara MS, Peterson CL, Elliott RE, Courson RW, Clanton MD, et al. Injury severity and neuropsychological and balance outcomes of four college athletes. Brain Inj. 2000;14(10):921–31.
78. Riemann BL, Guskiewicz KM. Effects of mild head injury on postural stability as measured through clinical balance testing. J Athl Train. 2000;35(1):19–25.
79. Peterson CL, Ferrara MS, Mrazik M, Piland T, Elliott T. Evaluation of neuropsychological stability following cerebral domain scores and postural concussion in sports. Clin J Sport Med. 2003;13(4):230–7.
80. Cavanaugh JT, Guskiewicz KM, Stergiou N. Detecting altered postural control after cerebral concussion in athletes without postural instability. Lippincott Williams & Wilkins; 2004.
81. Register-Mihalik JK, Mihalik JP, Guskiewicz KM. Balance deficits after sports-related concussion in individuals reporting posttraumatic headache. Neurosurgery. 2008;63(1):76–80; discussion −2.
82. Kelly KA, Jordan EM, Burdette GT, Buckley TA. NCAA Division I athletic trainers concussion management practice patterns. J Athl Train. 2013;49(5):665–73.
83. Buckley T, Burdette G, Kelly K. Concussion-management practice patterns of National Collegiate Athletic Association Division II and III athletic trainers: how the other half lives. J Athl Train. 2015;50(8):879–88.
84. Broglio SP, Macciocchi SN, Ferrara MS. Sensitivity of the concussion assessment battery. Neurosurgery. 2007;60(6):1050–7.

85. Garcia G-GP, Broglio SP, Lavieri MS, McCrea M, McAllister T, Investigators CC. Quantifying the value of multidimensional assessment models for acute concussion: an analysis of data from the NCAA-DoD care consortium. Sports Med. 2018;48(7):1739–49.
86. Garcia G-GP, Lavieri MS, Jiang R, McAllister T, McCrea M, Broglio SP. A data-driven approach to unlikely, possible, probable, and definite acute concussion assessment. J Neurotrauma. 2019;36(10):1571–83.
87. Luoto TM, Silverberg ND, Kataja A, Brander A, Tenovuo O, Ohman J, et al. Sport concussion assessment tool 2 in a civilian trauma sample with mild traumatic brain injury. J Neurotrauma. 2014;31(8):728–38.
88. King LA, Horak FB, Mancini M, Pierce D, Priest KC, Chesnutt J, et al. Instrumenting the balance error scoring system for use with patients reporting persistent balance problems after mild traumatic brain injury. Arch Phys Med Rehabil. 2014;95(2):353–9.
89. Buckley TA, Munkasy BA, Clouse BP. Sensitivity and specificity of the modified balance error scoring system in concussed student-athletes. Clin J Sports Med. 2017;28(2):174–6.
90. Carlson CD, Langdon JL, Munkasy BA, Evans KM, Buckley TA. Minimal detectable change scores and reliability of the balance error scoring system in student-athletes with acute concussion. Athl Train Sports Health Care. 2020;12(2):67–73.
91. Iverson GL, Koehle MS. Normative data for the modified balance error scoring system in adults. Brain Inj. 2013;27(5):596–9.
92. Howell DR, Oldham JR, Meehan WP, DiFabio MS, Buckley TA. Dual task tandem gait and average walking speed in healthy collegiate athletes. Clin J Sports Med. 2019;29(3):238–44.
93. Oldham JR, DiFabio MS, Kaminski TW, DeWolf RM, Buckley TA. Normative tandem gait in collegiate athletes implications for clinical concussion assessment. Sports Health. 2016;9(4):305–11.
94. Oldham JR, DiFabio MS, Kaminski TW, DeWolf RM, Howell DR, Buckley TA. Efficacy of tandem gait to identify impaired postural control following concussion. Med Sci Sports Exerc. 2018;50(6):1162–8. PMID: 29315170.
95. Santo A, Lynall RC, Guskiewicz KM, Mihalik JP. Clinical utility of the sport concussion assessment tool 3 (SCAT3) tandem-gait test in high school athletes. J Athl Train. 2017;52(12):1096–100.
96. Howell DR, Oldham JR, DiFabio M, Vallabhajosula S, Hall EE, Ketcham CJ, et al. Single-task and dual-task gait among collegiate athletes of different sport classifications: implications for concussion management. J Appl Biomech. 2017;33(1):24–31.
97. Oldham JR, Howell DR, Bryk KN, Manois C, Koerte I, Meehan WP, et al. No differences in tandem gait performance between male and female athletes acutely post-concussion. J Sci Med Sport. 2020;23(9):814–9.
98. Howell DR, Brilliant AN, Meehan WP III. Tandem gait test-retest reliability among healthy child and adolescent athletes. J Athl Train. 2019;54(12):1254–9.
99. Howell DR, Berkstresser B, Wang F, Buckley TA, Mannix R, Stillman A, et al. Self-reported sleep duration affects tandem gait, but not steady-state gait outcomes among healthy collegiate athletes. Gait Posture. 2018;62:291–6.
100. Lynall RC, Laudner KG, Mihalik JP, Stanek JM. Concussion-assessment and -management techniques used by athletic trainers. J Athl Train. 2013;48(6):844–50.
101. Buckley T, Baugh C, Meehan W, DiFabio M. Concussion management plan compliance: a study of NCAA power 5 schools. Orthop J Sports Med. 2017;5(4):1–7.
102. Riemann BL, Guskiewicz KM, Shields EW. Relationship between clinical and forceplate measures of postural stability. J Sport Rehabil. 1999;8(2):71–82.
103. McCrea M, Barr WB, Guskiewicz K, Randolph C, Marshall SW, Cantu R, et al. Standard regression-based methods for measuring recovery after sport-related concussion. J Int Neuropsychol Soc. 2005;11(1):58–69.
104. McCrea M, Guskiewicz KM, Marshall SW, Barr W, Randolph C, Cantu RC, et al. Acute effects and recovery time following concussion in collegiate football players: the NCAA concussion study. JAMA. 2003;290(19):2556–63.

105. Caccese JB, Buckley TA, Kaminski TW. Sway area and velocity correlated with MobileMat balance error scoring system (BESS) scores. J Appl Biomech. 2016;32(4):329–34.
106. Mulligan IJ, Boland MA, McIlhenny CV. The balance error scoring system learned response among young adults. Sports Health. 2013;5(1):22–6.
107. Finnoff JT, Peterson VJ, Hollman JH, Smith J. Intrarater and interrater reliability of the balance error scoring system (BESS). PM R. 2009;1(1):50–4.
108. Broglio SP, Harezlak J, Katz B, Zhao S, McAllister T, McCrea M. Acute sport concussion assessment optimization: a prospective assessment from the CARE consortium. Sports Med. 2019;49(12):1977–87.
109. Hunt TN, Ferrara MS, Bornstein RA, Baumgartner TA. The reliability of the modified balance error scoring system. Clin J Sport Med. 2009;19(6):471–5.
110. McLeod TCV, Perrin DH, Guskiewicz KM, Shultz SJ, Diamond R, Gansneder BM. Serial administration of clinical concussion assessments and learning effects in healthy young athletes. Clin J Sport Med. 2004;14(5):287–95.
111. Valovich TC, Perrin DH, Gansneder BM. Repeat administration elicits a practice effect with the balance error scoring system but not with the standardized assessment of concussion in high school athletes. J Athl Train. 2003;38(1):51–6.
112. Burk JM, Munkasy BA, Joyner AB, Buckley TA. Balance error scoring system performance changes after a competitive athletic season. Clin J Sport Med. 2013;23(4):312–7.
113. Caccese J, Best C, Lamond L, DiFabio M, Kaminski T, Watson D, et al. Effects of repetitive head impacts on the concussion assessment battery. Med Sci Sports Exerc. 2019;51(7):1355–61.
114. Broglio SP, Katz BP, Zhao S, McCrea M, McAllister T. Test-retest reliability and interpretation of common concussion assessment tools: findings from the NCAA-DoD CARE consortium. Sports Med. 2018;48(5):1255–68.
115. Katz BP, Kudela M, Harezlak J, McCrea M, McAllister T, Broglio SP. Baseline performance of NCAA athletes on a concussion assessment battery: a report from the CARE consortium. Sports Med. 2018;48(8):1971–85.
116. Susco TM, McLeod TCV, Gansneder BM, Shultz SJ. Balance recovers within 20 minutes after exertion as measured by the balance error scoring system. J Athl Train. 2004;39(3):241–6.
117. Wilkins JC, McLeod TCV, Perrin DH, Gansneder BM. Performance on the balance error scoring system decreases after fatigue. J Athl Train. 2004;39(2):156–61.
118. Fox ZG, Mihalik JP, Blackburn JT, Battaglini CL, Guskiewicz KM. Return of postural control to baseline after anaerobic and aerobic exercise protocols. J Athl Train. 2008;43(5):456–63.
119. Onate JA, Beck BC, Van Lunen BL. On-field testing environment and balance error scoring system performance during preseason screening of healthy collegiate baseball players. J Athl Train. 2007;42(4):446–51.
120. Weber AF, Mihalik JP, Register-Mihalik JK, Mays S, Prentice WE, Guskiewicz K. Dehydration and performance on clinical concussion measures in collegiate wrestlers. J Athl Train. 2013;48(2):153–60.
121. Docherty CL, McLeod TCV, Shultz SJ. Postural control deficits in participants with functional ankle instability as measured by the balance error scoring system. Clin J Sport Med. 2006;16(3):203–8.
122. McLeod TCV, Armstrong T, Miller M, Sauers JL. Balance improvements in female high school basketball players after a 6-week neuromuscular-training program. J Sport Rehabil. 2009;18(4):465–81.
123. Erkmen N, Taskin H, Kaplan T, Sanioglu A. The effect of fatiguing exercise on balance performance as measured by the balance error scoring system. Isokinet Exerc Sci. 2009;17(2):121–7.
124. Caccese JB, Buckley TA, Tierney RT, Rose WC, Glutting JJ, Kaminski TW. Postural control deficits after repetitive soccer heading. Clin J Sport Med. 2021;31(3):266–72.
125. McCrory PR, Berkovic SF. Video analysis of acute motor and convulsive manifestations in sport-related concussion. Neurology. 2000;54(7):1488–91.

126. Buttner F, Howell DR, Ardern CL, Doherty C, Blake C, Ryan J, et al. Concussed athletes walk slower than non-concussed athletes during cognitive-motor dual-task assessments but not during single-task assessments 2 months after sports concussion: a systematic review and meta-analysis using individual participant data. Br J Sports Med. 2020;54(2):94–101.
127. Parker TM, Osternig LR, Chou L-S. Gait Stability in Athletes and Non-Athletes Following Concussion. Mcd Sci Sports Exerc. 2006;38(5):S2.
128. Parker TM, Osternig LR, Lee HJ, van Donkelaar P, Chou LS. The effect of divided attention on gait stability following concussion. Clin Biomech. 2005;20(4):389–95.
129. Parker TM, Osternig LR, van Donkelaar P, Chou L-S. Recovery of cognitive and dynamic motor function following concussion. Br J Sports Med. 2007;41(12):868–73.
130. Parker TM, Osternig LR, van Donkelaar P, Chou LS. Balance control during gait in athletes and non-athletes following concussion. Med Eng Phys. 2008;30(8):959–67.
131. Parker TM, Osternig LR, Van Donkelaar P, Chou LS. Gait stability following concussion. Med Sci Sports Exerc. 2006;38(6):1032–40.
132. Catena RD, van Donkelaar P, Chou L-S. The effects of attention capacity on dynamic balance control following concussion. J Neuroeng Rehabil. 2011;8:1–8.
133. Catena RD, van Donkelaar P, Chou L-S. Different gait tasks distinguish immediate vs. long-term effects of concussion on balance control. J Neuroeng Rehabil. 2009;6:1–7.
134. Catena RD, van Donkelaar P, Chou L-S. Altered balance control following concussion is better detected with an attention test during gait. Gait Posture. 2007;25(3):406–11.
135. Catena RD, van Donkelaar P, Chou LS. Cognitive task effects on gait stability following concussion. Exp Brain Res. 2007;176(1):23–31.
136. Catena RD, van Donkelaar P, Halterman CI, Chou LS. Spatial orientation of attention and obstacle avoidance following concussion. Exp Brain Res. 2009;194(1):67–77.
137. Fait P, McFadyen BJ, Swaine B, Cantin JF. Alterations to locomotor navigation in a complex environment at 7 and 30 days following a concussion in an elite athlete. Brain Inj. 2009;23(4):362–9.
138. Fait P, Swaine B, Cantin J-F, Leblond J, McFadyen BJ. Altered integrated locomotor and cognitive function in elite athletes 30 days postconcussion: a preliminary study. J Head Trauma Rehabil. 2013;28(4):293–301.
139. Parrington L, Fino PC, Swanson CW, Murchison CF, Chesnutt J, King LA. Longitudinal assessment of balance and gait after concussion and return to play in collegiate athletes. J Athl Train. 2019;54(4):429–38.
140. Fino PC, Nussbaum MA, Brolinson PG. Locomotor deficits in recently concussed athletes and matched controls during single and dual-task turning gait: preliminary results. J Neuroeng Rehabil. 2016;13:1–15.
141. Fino PC. A preliminary study of longitudinal differences in local dynamic stability between recently concussed and healthy athletes during single and dual-task gait. J Biomech. 2016;49(9):1983–8.
142. Fino PC, Nussbaum MA, Brolinson PG. Decreased high-frequency center-of-pressure complexity in recently concussed asymptomatic athletes. Gait Posture. 2016;50:69–74.
143. Berkner J, Meehan WP, Master CL, Howell DR. Gait and quiet-stance performance among adolescents after concussion-symptom resolution. J Athl Train. 2017;52(12):1089–95.
144. Brown LA, Hall EE, Ketcham CJ, Patel K, Buckley TA, Howell DR, et al. Turn characteristics during gait differ with and without a cognitive demand among collegiate athletes. J Sport Rehabil. 2019;12:1–20.
145. Howell DR, Osternig LR, Chou L-S. Dual-task effect on gait balance control in adolescents with concussion. Arch Phys Med Rehabil. 2013;94(8):1513–20.
146. Howell DR, Osternig LR, Koester MC, Chou L-S. The effect of cognitive task complexity on gait stability in adolescents following concussion. Exp Brain Res. 2014;232(6):1773–82.
147. Howell DR, Osternig LR, Chou L-S. Adolescents demonstrate greater gait balance control deficits after concussion than young adults. Am J Sports Med. 2015;43(3):625–32.
148. Howell D, Osternig L, Chou LS. Monitoring recovery of gait balance control following concussion using an accelerometer. J Biomech. 2015;48(12):3364–8.

149. Howell DR, Osternig LR, Chou L-S. Return to activity after concussion affects dual-task gait balance control recovery. Med Sci Sports Exerc. 2015;47(4):673–80.
150. Howell DR, Osternig LR, Chou LS. Consistency and cost of dual-task gait balance measure in healthy adolescents and young adults. Gait Posture. 2016;49:176–80.
151. Howell DR, Osternig LR, Christie AD, Chou LS. Return to physical activity timing and dual-task gait stability are associated 2 months following concussion. J Head Trauma Rehabil. 2016;31(4):262–8.
152. Howell DR, Stracciolini A, Geminiani E, Meehan WP 3rd. Dual-task gait differences in female and male adolescents following sport-related concussion. Gait Posture. 2017;54:284–9. https://doi.org/10.1016/j.gaitpost.2017.03.034.
153. Howell DR, Osternig LR, Chou LS. Single-task and dual-task tandem gait test performance after concussion. J Sci Med Sport. 2017;24(17):30256.
154. Howell DR, Beasley M, Vopat L, Meehan WP. The effect of prior concussion history on dual-task gait following a concussion. J Neurotrauma. 2017;34(4):838–44.
155. Howell DR, Osternig LR, Chou LS. Detection of acute and long-term effects of concussion: dual-task gait balance control versus computerized neurocognitive test. Arch Phys Med Rehabil. 2018;99(7):1318–24.
156. Powers KC, Kalmar JM, Cinelli ME. Dynamic stability and steering control following a sport-induced concussion. Gait Posture. 2014;39(2):728–32.
157. Baker CS, Cinelli ME. Visuomotor deficits during locomotion in previously concussed athletes 30 or more days following return to play. Physiol Rep. 2014;2(12):e12252.
158. Martini DN, Sabin MJ, DePesa SA, Leal EW, Negrete TN, Sosnoff JJ, et al. The chronic effects of concussion on gait. Arch Phys Med Rehabil. 2011;92(4):585–9.
159. Fritz S, Lusardi M. White paper: "walking speed: the sixth vital sign". J Geriatr Phys Ther. 2009;32(2):2–5.
160. Middleton A, Fritz SL, Lusardi M. Walking speed: the functional vital sign. J Aging Phys Act. 2015;23(2):314–22.
161. Howell DR, Mayer AR, Master CL, Leddy J, Zemek R, Meier TB, et al. Prognosis for persistent post concussion symptoms using a multifaceted objective gait and balance assessment approach. Gait Posture. 2020;79:53–9. https://doi.org/10.1016/j.gaitpost.2020.04.013.
162. Buckley TA, Vallabhajosula S, Oldham JD, Munkasy BA, Evans KM, Krazeise DA, et al. Evidence of a conservative gait strategy in athletes with a history of concussions. J Sport Health Sci. 2016;5(4):417–23.
163. van Donkelaar P, Osternig L, Chou LS. Attentional and biomechanical deficits interact after mild traumatic brain injury. Exerc Sport Sci Rev. 2006;34(2):77–82.
164. Chen JK, Johnston KM, Frey S, Petrides M, Worsley K, Ptito A. Functional abnormalities in symptomatic concussed athletes: an MRI study. NeuroImage. 2004;22(1):68–82.
165. Armieri A, Holmes JD, Spaulding SJ, Jenkins ME, Johnson AM. Dual task performance in a healthy young adult population: results from a symmetric manipulation of task complexity and articulation. Gait Posture. 2009;29(2):346–8.
166. Silsupadol P, Lugade V, Shumway-Cook A, van Donkelaar P, Chou LS, Mayr U, et al. Training-related changes in dual-task walking performance of elderly persons with balance impairment: a double-blind, randomized controlled trial. Gait Posture. 2009;29(4):634–9.
167. Kerr B, Condon SM, McDonald LA. Cognitive spatial processing and the regulation of posture. J Exp Psychol Hum Percept Perform. 1985;11(5):617–22.
168. Ebersbach G, Dimitrijevic MR, Poewe W. Influence of concurrent tasks on gait - a dual-task approach. Percept Mot Skills. 1995;81(1):107–13.
169. Shumway-Cook A, Woollacott M. Attentional demands and postural control: the effect of sensory context. J Gerontol A Biol Sci Med Sci. 2000;55(1):M10–6.
170. Plummer-D'Amato P, Altmann LJP, Saracino D, Fox E, Behrman AL, Marsiske M. Interactions between cognitive tasks and gait after stroke: a dual task study. Gait Posture. 2008;27(4):683–8.
171. Woollacott M, Shumway-Cook A. Attention and the control of posture and gait: a review of an emerging area of research. Gait Posture. 2002;16(1):1–14.

172. Bell R, Hall RCW. Mental status examination. Am Fam Physician. 1977;16(5):145–52.
173. Lee H, Sullivan SJ, Schneiders AG. The use of the dual-task paradigm in detecting gait performance deficits following a sports-related concussion: a systematic review and meta-analysis. J Sci Med Sport. 2013;16(1):2–7.
174. Howell DR, Stillman A, Buckley TA, Berkstresser B, Wang F, Meehan WP. The utility of instrumented dual-task gait and tablet-based neurocognitive measurements after concussion. J Sci Med Sport. 2018;21(4):358–62.
175. Howell D, Osternig L, Chou L-S. Return to physical activity following concussion affects recovery in balance control during dual-task walking. Brain Injury. 2014;28(5–6):606.
176. Howell DR, Brilliant A, Berkstresser B, Wang F, Fraser J, Meehan WP. The association between dual-task gait after concussion and prolonged symptom duration. J Neurotrauma. 2017;34(23):3288–94.
177. Chiu S-L, Osternig L, Chou L-S. Concussion induces gait inter-joint coordination variability under conditions of divided attention and obstacle crossing. Gait Posture. 2013;38(4):717–22.
178. Cossette I, Ouellet M-C, McFadyen BJ. A preliminary study to identify locomotor-cognitive dual tasks that reveal persistent executive dysfunction after mild traumatic brain injury. Arch Phys Med Rehabil. 2014;95(8):1594–7.
179. Cossette I, Gagne ME, Ouellet MC, Fait P, Gagnon I, Sirois K, et al. Executive dysfunction following a mild traumatic brain injury revealed in early adolescence with locomotor-cognitive dual-tasks. Brain Inj. 2016;30(13–14):1648–55.
180. Dorman JC, Valentine VD, Munce TA, Tjarks BJ, Thompson PA, Bergeron MF. Tracking postural stability of young concussion patients using dual-task interference. J Sci Med Sport. 2015;18(1):2–7.
181. Buckley TA, Oldham JR, Watson DJ, Murray NG, Munkasy BA, Evans KM. Repetitive head impacts in football do not impair dynamic postural control. Med Sci Sports Exerc. 2019;51(1):132–40.
182. Howell DR, Buckley TA, Berkstresser B, Wang F, Meehan WP. Identification of postconcussion dual-task gait abnormalities using normative reference values. J Appl Biomech. 2019;35(4):290–6.
183. Mille ML, Hilliard MJ, Martinez KM, Simuni T, Rogers MW. Acute effects of a lateral postural assist on voluntary step initiation in patients with Parkinson's disease. Mov Disord. 2007;22(1):20–7.
184. Pagnacco G, Carrick FR, Pascolo PB, Rossi R, Oggero E. Learning effect of standing on foam during posturographic testing preliminary findings. Biomed Sci Instrum. 2012;48:332–9.
185. Chang HA, Krebs DE. Dynamic balance control in elders: gait initiation assessment as a screening tool. Arch Phys Med Rehabil. 1999;80(5):490–4.
186. Hass CJ, Gregor RJ, Waddell DE, Oliver A, Smith DW, Fleming RP, et al. The influence of Tai Chi training on the center of pressure trajectory during gait initiation in older adults. Arch Phys Med Rehabil. 2004;85(10):1593–8.
187. Mille ML, Johnson ME, Martinez KM, Rogers MW. Age-dependent differences in lateral balance recovery through protective stepping. Clin Biomech. 2005;20(6):607–16.
188. Brunt D, Vanderlinden DW, Behrman AL. The relation between limb loading and control parameters of gait initiation in persons with stroke. Arch Phys Med Rehabil. 1995;76(7):627–34.
189. Halliday SE, Winter DA, Frank JS, Patla AE, Prince F. The initiation of gait in young, elderly, and Parkinson's disease subjects. Gait Posture. 1998;8(1):8–14.
190. Tokuno CD, Sanderson DJ, Inglis JT, Chua R. Postural and movement adaptations by individuals with a unilateral below-knee amputation during gait initiation. Gait Posture. 2003;18(3):158–69.
191. Vallabhajosula S, Buckley TA, Tillman MD, Hass CJ. Age and Parkinson's disease related kinematic alterations during multi-directional gait initiation. Gait Posture. 2013;37(2):280–6.
192. Hass CJ, Buckley TA, Pitsikoulis C, Barthelemy EJ. Progressive resistance training improves gait initiation in individuals with Parkinson's disease. Gait Posture. 2012;35(4):669–73.

193. Polcyn AF, Lipsitz LA, Kerrigan DC, Collins JJ. Age-related changes in the initiation of gait: degradation of central mechanisms for momentum generation. Arch Phys Med Rehabil. 1998;79(12):1582–9.
194. Jian Y, Winter DA, Ishac MG, Gilchrist L. Trajectory of the body COG and COP during initiation and termination of gait. Gait Posture. 1993;1(1):9–22.
195. Brunt D, Short M, Trimble M, Liu SM. Control strategies for initiation of human gait are influenced by accuracy constraints. Neurosci Lett. 2000;285(3):228–30.
196. Massion J. Movement, posture and equilibrium - interaction and coordination. Prog Neurobiol. 1992;38(1):35–56.
197. Chang W-H, Tang P-F, Wang Y-H, Lin K-H, Chiu M-J, Chen S-HA. Role of the premotor cortex in leg selection and anticipatory postural adjustments associated with a rapid stepping task in patients with stroke. Gait Posture. 2010;32(4):487–93.
198. Winter DA, Prince F, Frank JS, Powell C, Zabjek KF. Unified theory regarding A/P and M/L balance in quiet stance. J Neurophysiol. 1996;75(6):2334–43.
199. Hass CJ, Waddell DE, Fleming RP, Juncos JL, Gregor RJ. Gait initiation and dynamic balance control in Parkinson's disease. Arch Phys Med Rehabil. 2005;86(11):2172–6.
200. Hass CJ, Waddell DE, Wolf SL, Juncos JL, Gregor RJ. Gait initiation in older adults with postural instability. Clin Biomech. 2008;23(6):743–53.
201. Buckley TA. Concussion and gait. In: Li L, Holmes M, editors. Gait biometrics: basic patterns, role of neurological disorders and effects of physical activity. 1st ed. Hauppauge: Nova Science Publishers; 2014. p. 141–64.
202. Buckley T, Oldham J, Munkasy B, Evans K. Decreased anticipatory postural adjustments during gait initiation acutely post-concussion. Arch Phys Med Rehabil. 2017;98(10):1962–8. PMID: 28583462.
203. Buckley TA, Munkasy BA, Krazeise DA, Oldham JR, Evans KM, Clouse B. Differential effects of acute and multiple concussions on gait initiation performance. Arch Phys Med Rehabil. 2020;25(20):30218–5.
204. Doherty C, Zhao L, Ryan J, Komaba Y, Inomata A, Caulfield B. Concussion is associated with altered preparatory postural adjustments during gait initiation. Hum Mov Sci. 2017;52:160–9.
205. Buckley TA, Murray N, Munkasy BA, Oldham JR, Evans KM, Clouse BP. Impairments in Dynamic Postural Control Across Concussion Clinical Milestones. J Neurotrauma. 2020;38(1):86–93.
206. Howell DR, Lynall RC, Buckley TA, Herman DC. Neuromuscular control deficits and the risk of subsequent injury after a concussion: a scoping review. Sports Med. 2018;48(5):1097–115.
207. Wang JJ, Wai YY, Weng YH, Ng KK, Huang YZ, Ying LL, et al. Functional MRI in the assessment of cortical activation during gait-related imaginary tasks. J Neural Transm. 2009;116(9):1087–92.
208. Perry SD, Santos LC, Patla AE. Contribution of vision and cutaneous sensation to the control of centre of mass (COM) during gait termination. Brain Res. 2001;913(1):27–34.
209. Sparrow WA, Tirosh O. Gait termination: a review of experimental methods and the effects of ageing and gait pathologies. Gait Posture. 2005;22(4):362–71.
210. Bishop MD, Brunt D, Pathare N, Patel B. The interaction between leading and trailing limbs during stopping in humans. Neurosci Lett. 2002;323(1):1–4.
211. Bishop MD, Brunt D, Kukulka C, Tillman MD, Pathare N. Braking impulse and muscle activation during unplanned gait termination in human subjects with parkinsonism. Neurosci Lett. 2003;348(2):89–92.
212. O'Kane FW, McGibbon CA, Krebs DE. Kinetic analysis of planned gait termination in healthy subjects and patients with balance disorders. Gait Posture. 2003;17(2):170–9.
213. Crenna P, Cuong DM, Breniere Y. Motor programmes for the termination of gait in humans: organisation and velocity-dependent adaptation. J Physiol. 2001;537(3):1059–72.
214. Tirosh O, Sparrow WA. Age and walking speed effects on muscle recruitment in gait termination. Gait Posture. 2005;21(3):279–88.

215. Hase K, Stein RB. Analysis of rapid stopping during human walking. J Neurophysiol. 1998;80(1):255–61.
216. Bishop M, Brunt D, Marjama-Lyons J. Do people with Parkinson's disease change strategy during unplanned gait termination? Neurosci Lett. 2006;397(3):240–4.
217. Wikstrom EA, Bishop MD, Inamdar AD, Hass CJ. Gait termination control strategies are altered in chronic ankle instability subjects. Med Sci Sports Exerc. 2010;42(1):197–205.
218. Menant JC, Steele JR, Menz HB, Munro BJ, Lord SR. Rapid gait termination: effects of age, walking surfaces and footwear characteristics. Gait Posture. 2009;30(1):65–70.
219. Vrieling AH, van Keeken HG, Schoppen T, Otten E, Halbertsma JPK, Hof AL, et al. Gait termination in lower limb amputees. Gait Posture. 2008;27(1):82–90.
220. Vrieling AH, van Keeken HG, Schoppen T, Hof AL, Otten B, Halbertsma JPK, et al. Gait adjustments in obstacle crossing, gait initiation and gait termination after a recent lower limb amputation. Clin Rehabil. 2009;23(7):659–71.
221. Miff SC, Childress DS, Gard SA, Meier MR, Hansen AH. Temporal symmetries during gait initiation and termination in nondisabled ambulators and in people with unilateral transtibial limb loss. J Rehabil Res Dev. 2005;42(2):175–82.
222. Oates AR, Frank JS, Patla AE, VanOoteghem K, Horak FB. Control of dynamic stability during gait termination on a slippery surface in Parkinson's disease. Mov Disord. 2008;23(14):1977–83.
223. Cameron D, Murphy A, Morris ME, Raghav S, Iansek R. Planned stopping in people with Parkinson. Parkinsonism Relat Disord. 2010;16(3):191–6.
224. Oldham JR, Munkasy BA, Evans KM, Wikstrom EA, Buckley TA. Altered dynamic postural control during gait termination following concussion. Gait Posture. 2016;49:437–42.
225. Buckley T, Munkasy B, Tapia-Lovler T, Wikstrom E. Altered gait termination strategies following a concussion. Gait Posture. 2013;38(3):549–51. PMID: 23489951.
226. Rahn C, Munkasy BA, Joyner AB, Buckley TA. Sideline performance of the balance error scoring system during a live sporting event. Clinical Journal of Sport Medicine. 2015;25(3):248–53. PMID: 25098674.

The Role of the Playing Surface in Mitigating the Deleterious Effects of Head Impacts in Field Sports

Breana Cappuccilli, Nicolas Leiva-Molano, Thomas M. Talavage, and Eric A. Nauman

Motivation

It has been estimated that 1.1–1.9 million sports-related concussions occur in children under the age of 18 every year in the USA [1]. Common impact mechanisms in contact sports include player to player (76.7% in boy's lacrosse), surface to player (53.2% in boy's wrestling), and equipment to player contact (41.7% in girl's lacrosse) [2]. Kerr et al. conducted a study of 20 US high school sports from 2013 to 2018 [3–16] (Table 7.1) that found an average injury rate of diagnosed concussions to be 0.417 per 1000 athletic exposures (AE) across all sports. This injury rate was higher for girls (0.335 per 1000 AE) when compared to boys in sex-matched sports (0.151 per 1000 AE). The discrepancy between sex-matched sports and the overall average is due to American football for which there are no girls' teams, yet this group exhibits the highest concussion injury rate of 1.04 per 1000 AE. Concussions were more likely to be diagnosed during football competitions with an injury rate of 3.907 per 1000 AE.

B. Cappuccilli
School of Mechanical Engineering, Purdue University, West Lafayette, IN, USA

N. Leiva-Molano
Weldon School of Biomedical Engineering, Purdue University, West Lafayette, IN, USA

T. M. Talavage
Department of Biomedical Engineering, University of Cincinnati, Cincinnati, OH, USA

E. A. Nauman (✉)
School of Mechanical Engineering, Purdue University, West Lafayette, IN, USA

Weldon School of Biomedical Engineering, Purdue University, West Lafayette, IN, USA

Department of Basic Medical Sciences, Purdue University, West Lafayette, IN, USA
e-mail: enauman@purdue.edu

Table 7.1 Summary of web-based surveillance injury for a variety of sports, level of play, injury mechanism, body part affected by injury, and diagnosis during both practice and competition obtained from Kerr et al.

Sport (sex)	Level of play	Contact with surface (injury mechanism)		Head/face (body part)		Concussion (diagnosis)	
		Practice	Competition	Practice	Competition	Practice	Competition
Football (M)	High school	0.29	1.63	0.38	2.67	0.35	2.57
		12.80%	13.10%	16.70%	21.10%	15.50%	20.30%
	Collegiate	0.37	2.86	0.45	3.22	0.4	3.01
		8.20%	10.10%	10.20%	11.00%	9.10%	10.40%
Soccer (M)	High school	0.16	0.62	0.09	0.97	0.07	0.77
		15.20%	15.70%	9.10%	29.10%	6.70%	23.60%
	Collegiate	0.39	1.38	0.3	2.08	0.17	1.24
		8.60%	10.90%	7.90%	13.80%	4.80%	7.90%
Soccer (W)	High school	0.17	0.76	0.11	1.45	0.09	1.28
		19.20%	15.20%	9.30%	26.60%	8.10%	24.00%
	Collegiate	0.52	1.95	0.33	2.52	0.23	1.91
		13.00%	15.40%	7.90%	21.60%	5.80%	16.40%
Lacrosse (M)	High school	0.12	0.4	0.2	1.35	0.16	1.22
		10.80%	9.50%	16.80%	31.90%	13.80%	28.80%
	Collegiate	0.29	1.19	0.3	1.94	0.22	1.7
		8.40%	10.10%	8.40%	16.40%	6.30%	14.30%
Lacrosse (W)	High school	0.13	0.31	0.18	0.92	0.16	0.83
		13.30%	13.40%	17.90%	38.80%	15.20%	35.00%
	Collegiate	0.15	0.41	0.38	1.69	0.29	1.42
		5.60%	6.20%	13.40%	25.30%	10.20%	21.20%

Sports included were football [9], soccer [5, 8] and lacrosse [13, 14], where the latter two are further divided by sex (male and female). High school and collegiate levels are included for each sport. Due to the interest in head injury, contact with surface, head/face, and concussion were selected as the injury mechanism, body part, and diagnosis, respectively. Values summarized include the injury rates per 1000 athletic exposures and the percentage of injuries in sample. Each percentage represents the number of specific injury type (i.e., concussion) per total injury type (i.e., diagnosis) within event type per population. Example: 12.8% of all diagnosed injuries during high school football practice were from contact with surface

Quantifying Head Injury Severity

It is important not only to properly identify and treat head injuries when they occur, but to implement safety measures to mitigate the risk of sustaining these injuries. One way to ensure player safety is to mandate criteria, or *regulations,* for sport surface quality. The authority to enforce these regulations is assumed by sports governing bodies such as Fédération Internationale de Football Association (FIFA) and World Rugby (WR). Typically, these regulations are outlined alongside an assigned *testing standard* (a highly replicable in-lab or in situ protocol for testing). Each sports governing body adopts its own range of regulations and testing standards leading to ill-founded and conflicting criteria for surface attributes. The variations in regulations enforced across regions, sports, and levels of play highlight the lack of information available on optimal surface material properties (Table 7.2).

Table 7.2 Compilation of regulations established by testing standards for a series of surface attributes by sports governing bodies

Governing body (sport)	Surface attribute	Testing standard[a]	Regulation
FIFA			
Soccer (professional)	SA	1	60–70%
	VD	2	4–10 mm
	ER	3	–
Soccer (community)	SA	1	55–70%
	VD	2	4–11 mm
	ER	3	–
Futsal	SA	4	18–75%
	SR	5	80–155 mm
	VD	6	3–10 mm
World Rugby (WR)			
Rugby	SA	1	55–70%
	ER	3	20–50%
	HIC	7	<1000 @ 1.0 m
	VD	2	5.5–11 mm
International Hockey Federation (FIH)			
Multi-sport	SA	8	40–70%
	VD	8	4–10 mm
Football + Field Hockey (developmental)	SA	8	55–70%
	VD	8	4–12 mm
Hockey + Tennis	SA	8	>30%
	VD	8	2–9 mm
Field Hockey (elite)	SA	8	45–60%
	VD	8	4–9 mm
	ER	8	30–55%
National Rugby League Limited (NRL)			
Rugby (stadium)	HIC	8	1000 @ 1.3 m
	SA	9	50–65%
	VD	9	<11 mm
	ER	9	20–50%
Rugby (community)	HIC	8	1000 @ 1.3 m
	SA	9	50–70%
	VD	9	<11 mm
	ER	9	20–50%

Shock absorption (SA) is a measurement of force reduction of a surface given as a percentage compared to force reduction on concrete. Vertical deformation (VD) is an estimate of the displacement of the surface during impact. Energy restitution (ER) is a ratio of output to input kinetic energy given as a percentage. Slip resistance (SR) represents the frictional interaction between footwear and sports surface displayed as final shear displacement after impact. Head injury criterion (HIC) is a unitless impact severity index.

[a]Testing standards outlining the regulations and testing methodologies for surface attributes:
1. FIFA Test Method 04a [17]
2. FIFA Test Method 05a [17]
3. FIFA Test Method 13 [17]
4. FIFA Test Method Futsal01 [18]
5. EN 16837:2018
6. FIFA Test Method Futsal02 [18]
7. CEN 1177 [19]
8. CEN/TS 16717 [20]
9. AAA

Recurrent regulation attributes include shock absorption, vertical deformation, and energy restitution. These are outcomes of the sports surface system's properties, but not fundamentally related to injury risk. At the time of origination of these sports surface standards, classification of head injury and its severity was poorly defined. There is a clear need for regulation indices that are derived from injury risk including, but not limited to, head injuries. To develop a proper injury risk index, one that describes not just the intensity of the head impact but the injury outcome of that impact, biomechanical testing is required.

Quantifying impact severity and injury outcome of head impacts has been of interest in the field of biomechanics for over 60 years. Initial experiments were carried out by analyzing fracture patterns on human skulls [21, 22] with the main objective of these experiments to analyze a skull's resistance to fracture after impacts, most notably occurring in vehicle collisions. Subsequent studies began incorporating sensors to collect acceleration or pressure profiles occurring within the skull during experimental impacts [23–25]. Today, on-field measurement of head impacts in sports is commonly done by means of accelerometers attached to the player (either on the mastoid process, inner surface of the helmet/head band, or internally via mouthguard). These data, combined with mRI and other damage quantification approaches, have proven to be a powerful tool in defining thresholds of impact tolerance [26–28]. There is an apparent need for the current sports surface testing standards and regulations to be reinvented with what is currently known about head injury mechanisms.

Wayne State Tolerance Curve

One of the most foundational and promising efforts to define head injury risk was done by a research group at Wayne State University in the 1960s [25]. Four white, male human cadavers were attached to an upright, pendulum-like apparatus allowed to freely rotate until the forehead impacted the floor (Fig. 7.1). The brain material was extracted and replaced with a fluid gelatin assumed to mimic pressure transmission of the brain material. The artificial brain material also allowed for the insertion of an accelerometer within the skull cavity to measure impact accelerations within the fluid. Each cadaver was used repeatedly as long as it was deemed "undamaged" [25] by the researchers. If skull fracture occurred, the average acceleration and impulse time of the impact event were plotted (Fig. 7.2). These fractures occurred in acceleration events that had an effective average of ~112 g, with individual impact peaks observed as high as 200 g. In total, six of these skull fracture data points were used to generate the Wayne State Tolerance Curve (WSTC) [24, 25]. The WSTC set an initial threshold value of 42 g, stating that a human head can withstand an acceleration event of this magnitude for a "relatively long time" (~20 ms) without resulting in brain damage [24]. This threshold was later found to be exceeded during vehicle collisions without resulting injuries, increasing the proposed threshold for

Fig. 7.1 Testing apparatus used by researchers at Wayne State University. A human cadaver is fixed to a pendulum, allowing the forehead to impact a target object at a distance D. A is the length of the pendulum and H is the distance between the ground and the pendulum. (Schematic adapted from Lissner et al. [25])

Fig. 7.2 Experimental results obtained from testing cadavers at Wayne State University. Six data points were used to establish a relationship between the acceleration and time observed to fracture a skull from both free fall and guided pendulum apparatus. (Adapted from Lissner et al. [25])

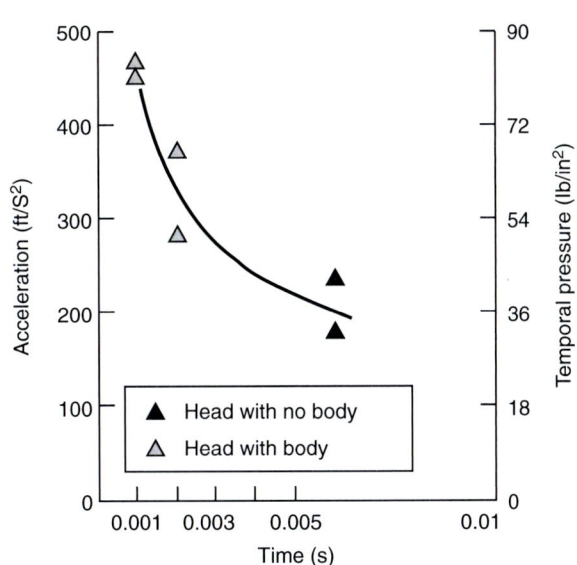

padded designs to 60–80 g [29]. To the author's knowledge, a data set of six points is the only published basis of the final WSTC [30].

The WSTC, though derived from a small number of tests, offered threshold criteria for fatal head injuries under specific parameters for the first time. However, application of this injury threshold to sports injury severity proved to be difficult. Since no biological brain material was present during the testing, the WSTC does not account for symptoms or indicators of mTBI resulting from concussive or subconcussive hits. Still, different severity indices were approximated from the original tolerance curve to predict lesser thresholds of risk through linear approximations.

Gadd Severity Index

Between 1962 and 1966, the Gadd Severity Index (GSI) became the next evolution of head injury indices and the most widely known severity index derived from the WSTC [31, 32]. Charles Gadd had the intention of quantifying the "dynamic response" [32] of the head (which indirectly leads to injury) prior to calculating biological material damage (which directly relates with injury). He proposed an integration of the impact acceleration profile rather than comparing peak or average acceleration in g's. This was novel for the decade considering that integration was still done by hand. "Modern curve readers and machine computation equipment" [32] were relatively inaccessible compared to opensource integration software available today. Still, the calculation for a severity index (I) is relatively straightforward:

$$I = \int a^n \, dt$$

where a is the acceleration profile (often reported in g's) integrated over the time length and n is a weighting factor. Since the slope of the logarithmic fit to the WSTC was approximately 2.5 (Fig. 7.3), this was selected as the weighting factor. A severity index of 1000 was chosen based on conversations with Prof. Patrick at Wayne State [32] when it was stated that select acceleration profiles along the WSTC "integrate to approximately 1000" [32]. The more common form of the GSI (with these chosen values for the weighting factor and severity index) is

$$1000 = T * A^{2.5}$$

where T is the time length of the impact event and A is the "effective acceleration". The severity index of 1000 acts as the threshold of acceptably injury, or the test's pass-fail criteria. A value greater than 1000 implies life-threatening injury and

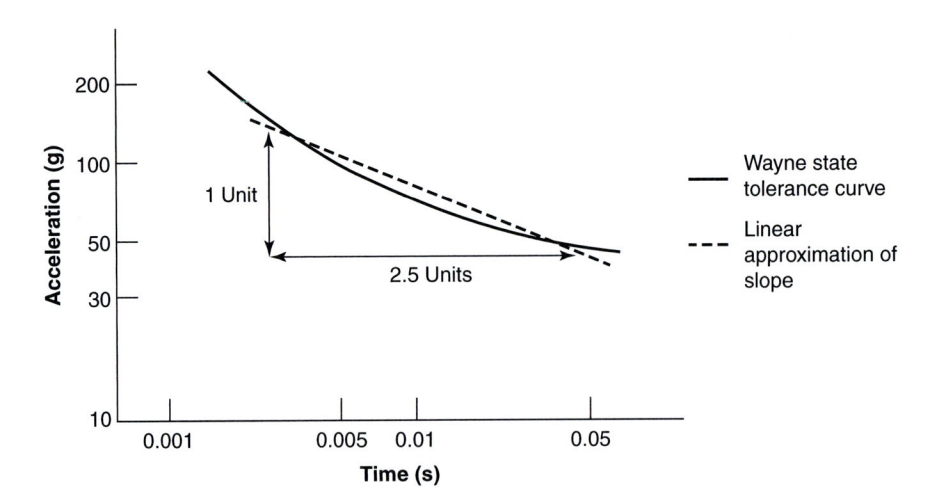

Fig. 7.3 Linear approximation of the WSTC used to determine a weighting factor of 2.5 used to define the Gadd Severity Index. (Adapted from Gadd [31, 32])

permanent damage. Any value less than 1000 is deemed an allowable amount of head injury. In regard to the original WSTC, any value less than 1000 only meant no noticeable, linear skull fracture occurred.

Much confusion has centered around the definition of the effective acceleration [33] and so it is useful to clarify its origination and interpretation. At the time the GSI was created, in-lab testing was restricted to highly controlled environments such as car crash simulations. The acceleration profiles of these tests were square or triangular waveforms with a single period. The effective acceleration of these profiles was intuitively the plateau of the square wave or 1/3rd the height of the triangular wave. For non-controlled acceleration profiles, as seen in on-field accelerometers or in-lab Hybrid III testing, the shape of the profile is parabolic (if not more complex), and thus the determination of effective acceleration is not easily visualized. The area under these acceleration profiles must be equated to that of a square wave occurring over the same time interval to determine the effective acceleration. Sometimes a true average of the acceleration data points is computed instead, though this value will vary slightly around the effective acceleration.

Head Injury Criterion

Mild adaptation of the GSI equation generated the head injury criterion (HIC) in 1970, the only accepted and applied injury risk index used within regulations applied to sports surfaces and equipment today [33]. The HIC equation is mathematically equivalent to the GSI equation with a more detailed explanation of effective acceleration:

$$\text{HIC} = (t_2 - t_1) \left(\frac{\int_{t_1}^{t_2} a\, dt}{t_2 - t_1} \right)^{2.5}$$

where t_1 and t_2 are time points during the pulse such that HIC is maximized and a is the acceleration profile in g's [33]. In this way, HIC carries units of $s \cdot g^{2.5}$ which are uniquely found within this application and do not appear within any kinematic or material-based model. HIC was eagerly accepted in the automotive and sports communities as it claimed to offer a means to scale head injury severity [34]. Since different injury mechanisms exhibit different pulses/waveforms, the interpretation of the data is not straightforward. By integrating the linear acceleration waveform and dividing by the time window, the impact event is equated to a square wave seen during controlled car impact tests. However, if the actual impulse time is not found from the event and used within the equation, the HIC equation deviates from GSI. Assigning time windows instead of measuring them per unique impact fixes the value for $(t_2 - t_1)$. This is the case for HIC-15 and HIC-36 where the time window is a fixed value of 15 ms or 36 ms, respectively, in advance of testing. These time windows are slightly larger than the 5.5 and 13.7 milliseconds head impact time windows observed in sports [35] and therefore, can underestimate true

HIC. Consequently, the dependence of severity on impulse time in the HIC equations is diminished, deviating further from the original design of the WSTC. Furthermore, HIC designates a maximum and minimum allowable time window that can be used, of 36 ms and 3 ms, respectively, which contradicts the original tests conducted by Lissner et al. where four of the six tests used to create the WSTC had time windows of <3 ms [25].

Testing Standards for Sport Surfaces

Because the equations for HIC are only dependent on a linear acceleration reading and a pre-assigned impulse time, various testing standards can be used to calculate this index. The National Operating Committee on Standards for Athletic Equipment (NOCSAE) has utilized drop tower tests as well as linear impact tests to calculate HIC as a predictor of head injury risk. Traditionally, these testing standards are used for helmet testing irrespective of surface types. For testing sports surfaces, the Advanced Artificial Athlete (AAA) is the common testing apparatus chosen since it is portable and can be used to measure HIC values along with shock absorption, vertical deformation, and energy restitution (Fig. 7.4). The AAA consists of a falling mass, spring, impact missile, and piezo-resistive accelerometer. The chosen mass of the impactor (20 kg) seems to be irrespective to any anatomical mass.

The testing standard consists of three consecutive impacts of the test foot on a 1 m × 1 m test specimen, while recording the acceleration [17]. The impact events are separated by 30-second intervals. Critical drop heights are calculated by

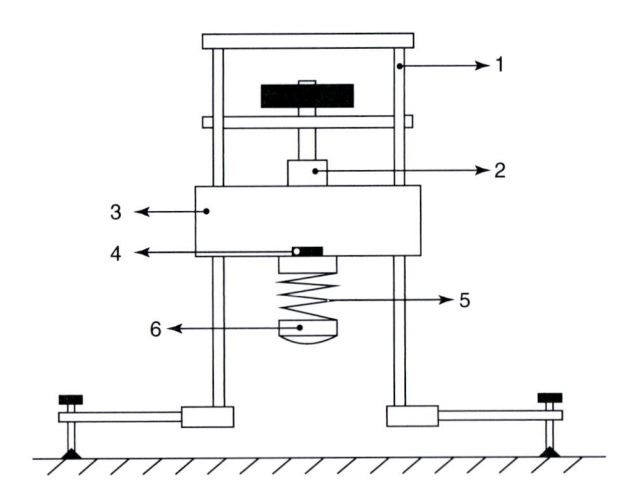

Fig. 7.4 Diagram of the Advanced Artificial Athlete where: (1) guide for the falling mass; (2) electric magnet used as a release system; (3) a falling mass that should have a total mass of 20 kg; (4) a piezo-resistive accelerometer; (5) a spiral steel spring; and (6) a test foot [17]. Used for in situ testing, the falling mass is released on specified AT field locations. Data recollection consists of three consecutive impacts, where the second and third impacts are averaged and utilized to calculate measures of AT surface performance

comparing maximum HIC values at different impact heights to the HIC threshold of 1000. This apparatus is used by FIFA, WR, and the British Standards Institution to certify natural and artificial surface systems. The limitations presented on the head injury criterion and other indices used to quantify safety will also have a deleterious effect on the intrinsic value of these testing metrics.

Limitations of Current Indices

There are several issues related to the data collected during the determination of the WTSC and subsequently, the determination of GSI and HIC. The main problem arises from the fact that the tolerance data were taken from a specific brain injury mechanism – acceleration events caused by height drops. This type of acceleration event may not be representative of other, more complex impacts experienced during sports play. More importantly, the WSTC and GSI were adjusted according to an ill-defined parameter of effective acceleration. Acceleration profiles from drop test in cadavers constrained the definition of the effective acceleration to the area under the acceleration waveform adjusted to the impact duration [23]. Patrick et al. claimed that the defined effective acceleration was restricted to a specific injury mechanism and that the value of 42 g was not realistic. Thus, a range of 60–80 g was proposed as the effective acceleration for "real people" [29]. Not having a clear definition of the effective acceleration that encompasses all injury mechanisms for the WSTC is an issue carried over to the GSI. The GSI formulates a pass/fail threshold for a level of acceleration that is inconsistent across different waveforms [33]. Versace stated that the form of effective acceleration should be defined prior to testing and not determined from a tolerance curve [33].

It is important to note that though HIC and GSI are claimed to be *injury risk indices,* they do not depend on any biological parameters. Furthermore, the determined thresholds are for risk of sustaining linear skull fractures, not closed-head, concussive injuries that are more commonly observed in sports. In this way, these metrics act more as *impact severity indices* with thresholds derived from simulated fatal head injuries. Alternatively, concussive impact thresholds have been theorized in the form of peak linear and angular accelerations of the center of mass of the head [36–40]. Furthermore, it has been found that structural [41] and functional [26, 28] changes in brain tissue are correlated with the accumulation of lower threshold impacts that do not result in a diagnosed concussion. However, these thresholds are not currently regarded in any testing standards or enforced regulation.

Modeling a Head Impact

An underlying issue with each of the available indices, including HIC, is that they are difficult to relate to an actual head impact event. For example, the most common HIC threshold of 1000 cannot be directly translated into the severity of a tackle during a football game. Instead, it is advantageous to approach these athletic impact events with dynamic models (Fig. 7.5a) as a way of relating input parameters (i.e., player mass, stance, forces) to output kinematics correlated with head injury (i.e., linear and rotational accelerations).

Single Particle Model

The single particle model is the most basic dynamic approach to modeling a head impact and has been used for decades. The entire head of the player is represented by a single point in space at its center of mass (COM; Fig. 7.5b). Position, velocity, and linear acceleration in each coordinate direction can be tracked for this point as it "experiences" an impact event. NOCSAE utilized this single particle model in their drop tower test (ND 001-M17B) [42] much like the on-field AAA testing device. However, in these cases, the model is simplified further by constricting the

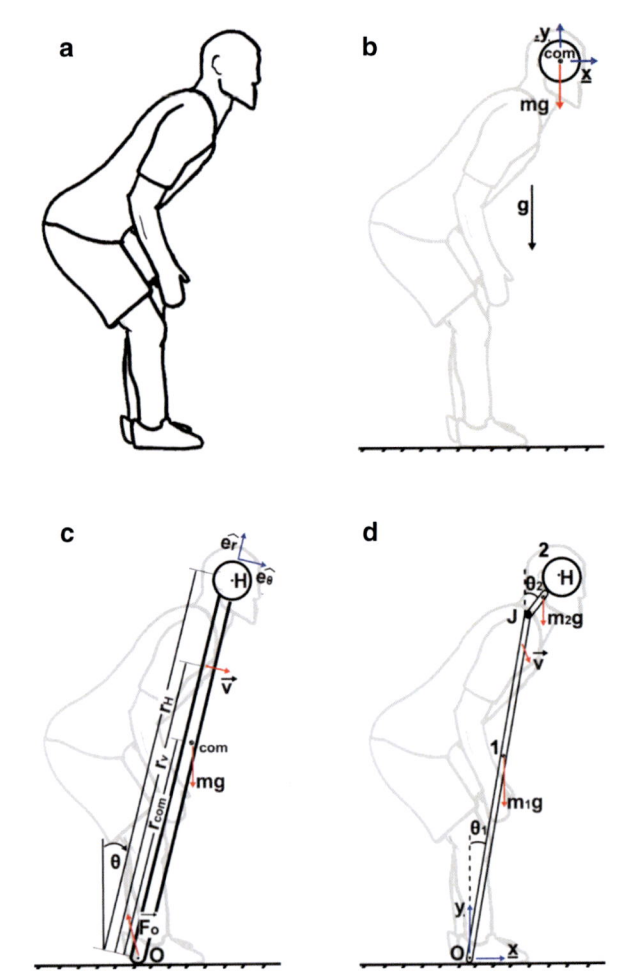

Fig. 7.5 Illustrations of biomechanics models based on an athlete before a fall. (**a**) Visual representation that will be used as a base throughout the different dynamic modeling approaches. (**b**) Single particle model, where the head of a player is represented by a single point in space with a mass m. (**c**) One-link model, where the link is a rigid body found between points O and H. (**d**) Two-link model, where link 1 is the rigid body connecting points O and J, while link 2 consists of the rigid body between points J and H

head forms to only move through a guided, one-dimensional fall. The pneumatic ram tests (ND 002-17M19A) [43] are another approach to validate helmets where the head form has additional degrees of freedom through a neck form constraint. Linear acceleration of the head form's COM is measured directly by means of accelerometers fixed within the testing apparatus. Measured acceleration waveforms for various heights in these tests are used to calculate HIC values. Still, there is little understanding as to what a HIC value of 50 means compared to 500. This kind of relativity is what is necessary to guide rational design strategy for protective equipment and sports surfaces.

Creating a single particle model, without sensor data to reference, is most easily accomplished with a work-energy approach. The basic model to determine the impacting speed (v_f) for a particle of any conceivable mass dropped from rest at player height (h) is

$$v_f = \sqrt{2gh} \qquad (7.1)$$

where g is the acceleration due to gravity (and in this case the maximum achievable acceleration). A single particle model, though simple in application, has many limitations in practice. Considering an in-game setting, it is hard to imagine a situation where gravity force alone will cause an athlete's head to fall directly downward into the surface. Even a tripping scenario, where no contact is made from another player, would require a more complex model to capture additional information such as player height and angular acceleration. Ultimately, the single particle model contains no useful biomechanical information that could be used to improve testing standards.

One-Link Model

Modeling an athlete as a rigid body as opposed to a single particle allows for basic anthropometric and kinetic information to be considered. Lissner et al. followed this approach in the design of their original cadaver experiments ultimately used to contrast the WSTC [25]. Considering the player's body and head as a single, rigid link will shift the COM away from the head and towards the torso (Fig. 7.5c). This rigid body assumption enforces the constraint that the head remain connected to the body (unlike the single particle model), and therefore its motion results from the kinematics of the body. Forces can be applied anywhere along the rigid body to set it into motion, however, for now we can represent this as an initial, applied velocity ($\overline{v_a}$). The player's mass (m) can be regarded as a force acting downward through the COM. We can assume the link is fixed to the ground at the feet (point O) and that the player's body falls forward until it hits the surface. A consequence of this "fixed pin" assumption for point O is the nonrealistic reaction force ($\overline{F_o}$) required to enforce the constraint. Tracking the position of the feet relative to the ground would create a better approximation; however, this data is not readily available.

This model requires Euler's Laws to balance a system of equations that solves for translational acceleration ($\vec{a}$) and velocity ($\vec{v}$) as well as the angular acceleration ($\vec{\alpha}$) and velocity ($\vec{\omega}$) of any point on the rigid body. The governing equations for the one-link model are as follows:

$$\sum \vec{M}_0 = \vec{r}_{COM} \times \overline{mg} = I_0 \vec{\alpha} + m\vec{r}_{COM} \times \vec{a}_O \tag{7.2}$$

$$\vec{a}_H = \vec{a}_O + \vec{\alpha} \times \vec{r}_H + \vec{\omega} \times (\vec{\omega} \times \vec{r}_H) \tag{7.3}$$

$$\vec{v}_V = \vec{v}_o + \vec{\omega} \times \vec{r}_V \tag{7.4}$$

where $\vec{r}_{COM}$ and $\vec{r}_H$ are position vectors from the fixed point O to the COM of the rigid body and head, respectively. The athlete's mass (m) and mass moment of inertia (I_0) are taken to be known constants for the system. It is important to note that the acceleration and velocity of fixed point O ($\vec{a}_o$ and $\vec{v}_o$) are always zero in this model. Equation (7.2) can be solved for $\vec{\alpha}$ resulting in

$$\vec{\alpha} = \frac{r_{COM} mg \sin(\theta)}{I_0} e_z, \tag{7.5}$$

where θ is the angle between the surface of impact and the forward falling link at any given time. Integration by parts of Eq. (7.5) allows us to solve for the angular velocity (ω) of the rigid body at any point during the fall before it impacts the ground,

$$\alpha = \frac{d(\dot{\theta})}{dt} = \frac{d(\dot{\theta})}{d\theta} \frac{d\theta}{dt} = \dot{\theta} \frac{d(\dot{\theta})}{d\theta} = \int_{\omega_i}^{\omega} \dot{\theta}\, d\dot{\theta} = \int_{\theta_i}^{\theta_f} \frac{r_{COM} mg \sin(\theta)}{I_0} d\theta. \tag{7.6}$$

Substituting from Eq. (7.4), $\omega_i = \frac{v}{r_V}$, yields

$$\omega = \sqrt{2\left(\frac{r_{COM} mg (\cos\theta_i - \cos\theta)}{I_0}\right) + \omega_i^2}, \tag{7.7}$$

where θ will always be $\leq 90°$ if the link lands on a horizontal impact surface and θ_i is representative of the starting stance of the athlete (i.e., 0° if completely vertical). Substituting Eqs. (7.4 and 7.6) into Eq. (7.2) to solve for the linear acceleration of the COM of the head ($\vec{a}_H$) provides

$$\vec{a}_H = -\omega^2 r_H e_r + \alpha r_H e_\theta. \tag{7.8}$$

For the COM of the head, this is useful information because it can be compared to acceleration thresholds observed in studies found to presage concussions [36–40]. However, it is likely that the deceleration event occurring once the player impacts the sport surface is much greater. This type of analysis requires material properties of the surface and will be shown in section "Hertz Contact Theory." A slight increase in model complexity from the single particle model to the one-link model has offered better impact visualization and control of input parameters. Nonetheless, a player has many additional joints that are unaccounted for in a single link system.

Two-Link Model

Adding a second link to the previous one-link model will allow us to simulate an impact event with additional degrees of freedom for the body. This joint can be placed anywhere along the body by adjusting the segment lengths of link one and link two. For example, it could be of benefit to move this joint toward the neck as to let the head whip in response to a hit. Or, this joint could be placed toward the knees to adjust the initial stance of the player to something more representative of game play (Fig. 7.5d).

Euler's approach can be used again to develop the system of equations for a system to capture the movement of each link throughout the falling motion. An equation of motion must be developed for each individual link, similar to Eqs. (7.2, 7.3, and 7.4) in the one-link model. The useful equations from summation of forces and moments are

$$\sum \vec{M}_{1/O} = \vec{r}_{1/O} \times \overrightarrow{m_1 g} + \vec{r}_{J/O} \times \overrightarrow{F_J} = I_{1/O} \vec{\alpha}_1 \tag{7.9}$$

$$\sum \vec{F}_2 = \vec{F}_J - \overrightarrow{m_2 g} = m_2 \vec{a}_2 \tag{7.10}$$

$$\sum \vec{M}_{2/J} = \vec{r}_{2/J} \times \overrightarrow{m_2 g} = I_{2/J} \vec{\alpha}_2 + m_2 \vec{r}_{2/J} \times \vec{a}_J \tag{7.11}$$

where $\vec{F}_J$ is the joint force between link 1 and link 2. The notation for positions ($\vec{r}_{i/k}$) and mass moments of inertia ($\bar{I}_{i/k}$) reads "the (parameter) of link i relative to position k." Equation (7.10) can be substituted into Eq. (7.9) to remove the unknown variable of joint force such that

$$I_{1/O} \ddot{\theta}_1 + m_1 g L_{1COM} \sin(\theta_1) - m_2 L_J \cos(\theta_1) a_{2x} + m_2 (g + a_{2y}) L_J \sin(\theta_1) = 0. \tag{7.12}$$

Since Eq. (7.9) results in only one equation in the $\hat{k}$ direction, the angular acceleration of each link is written in Eq. (7.12) as $\ddot{\theta}_i$. Similarly, the translational acceleration vectors can be broken into coordinate directions as a_{ix} for the x-direction and a_{iy} for the y-direction. Additional kinematic relationships are required for Eqs. (7.11 and 7.12) to be considered solvable equations of motion. The determination of the acceleration of each joint follows the form of Eq. (7.3) for the one-link model. These final kinematic relationships are as follows:

$$\vec{a}_J = \left[-L_J \cos(\theta_1) \ddot{\theta}_1 - L_J \sin(\theta_1) \dot{\theta}_1^2 \right] \hat{i} + \left[L_J \sin(\theta_1) \ddot{\theta}_1 - L_J \cos(\theta_1) \dot{\theta}_1^2 \right] \hat{j} \tag{7.13}$$

$$\vec{a}_2 = \left[a_{Jx} - L_{2COM} \cos(\theta_2) \ddot{\theta}_2 - L_{2COM} \sin(\theta_2) \dot{\theta}_2^2 \right] \hat{i} + \left[a_{Jy} - L_{2COM} \cos(\theta_2) \ddot{\theta}_2 + L_{2COM} \sin(\theta_2) \dot{\theta}_2^2 \right] \hat{j} \tag{7.14}$$

The lengths (and length to COM), masses, and mass moments of inertia for each link can be estimated with the help of anthropometric tables and NASA reports [44]. Using the kinematic Eqs. (7.13 and 7.14) within Eqs. (7.11 and 7.12) results in a system of second-order, homogenous differential equations written in matrix form as

$$[M]\begin{bmatrix}\ddot{\theta}_1\\ \ddot{\theta}_2\end{bmatrix}+[C]\begin{bmatrix}\dot{\theta}_1^{\,2}\\ \dot{\theta}_2^{\,2}\end{bmatrix}+\begin{bmatrix}(m_2 L_1 + m_1 L_{2COM})g\sin\theta_1\\ m_2 L_{2COM} g\sin\theta_2\end{bmatrix}=\vec{0}, \tag{7.15}$$

where the coefficient matrices are defined as

$$[M]=\begin{bmatrix} I_{1/0}+m_2 L_J^{\,2} & m_2 L_{2COM} L_J \cos(\theta_2-\theta_1)\\ m_2 L_{2COM} L_J \cos(\theta_2-\theta_1) & I_{2/J}\end{bmatrix} \tag{7.16}$$

$$[C]=\begin{bmatrix} 0 & m_2 L_{2COM} L_J \sin(\theta_2-\theta_1)\\ m_2 L_{2COM} L_J \sin(\theta_2-\theta_1) & 0\end{bmatrix}. \tag{7.17}$$

If the applied "tackling" force was introduced via an explicit, time-dependent forcing function $F(t)$ instead of an initial applied velocity, the system would be considered rheonomic and have a non-zero vector on the left-hand side of the equation. This type of system is left for future work since an acceptable forcing function representing a tackling force is currently undetermined.

It is important to note that the current two-link model does not account for any additional constraints due to muscle or skeletal forces. For example, the human spine will not allow hyperextension past a certain degree without damaging the skeletal structure. Whereas in the current, less constrained model, it is possible to apply initial conditions that lead to complete collapse of both links before they impact the surface. For future work, restricting the range of allowable values for neck extension and flexion to 70° and 80°, respectively, improves the possibility for realistic results [45]. Close attention should be given to the results of such a model before inferring any information about real-life falls and tackles.

Hertz Contact Theory

The models discussed thus far still do not include any material properties relating to the player or the surface and therefore cannot model any deceleration or deformation that occurs once the head impacts the surface. Contact theories such as the one proposed by Hertz can be used in conjunction with dynamic models to gain better insight into the maximum impact forces and deformations of the player's head [46]. Beginning with a particle model of the head (Fig. 7.6a), a simple work-energy approach yields

$$T_1 + V_1 + W_{1-2} = T_2 + V_2 \tag{7.18}$$

where T and V are the kinetic and potential energy of the COM of the head, respectively, and W_{1-2} is the nonconservative work done on the head as it impacts the ground. The subscripts for each term indicate a given time point of the impact. Time

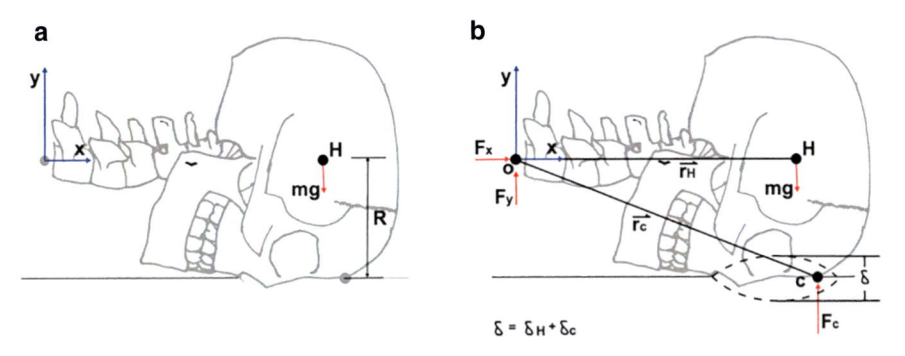

7 The Role of the Playing Surface in Mitigating the Deleterious Effects of Head...

Fig. 7.6 Schematic of a skull and partial cervical spine of a human impacting a surface. (**a**) Where the skull is modeled as a particle with mass m at a radius R. (**b**) Where point O is the origin of the neck joint, H is the COM of the head, and C is the point of contact with the head

point 1 is chosen to be right before the head contacts the surface. Time point 2 can be any point during the subsequent compression of the head/surface. Taking the surface level to be the datum line for potential energy provides the following expressions:

$$T_2 - T_1 = \frac{1}{2} m_H \left(v_{H2}^2 - v_{H1}^2 \right) \qquad (7.19)$$

$$V_2 - V_1 = m_H g \delta \qquad (7.20)$$

$$W_{1-2} = -\int_0^\delta F_c d\delta \qquad (7.21)$$

where m_H is the mass of the head, v_{H1} is the impacting velocity of the head determined previously, and F_c is the ground reaction force (GRF). A total deformation term δ represents the deformation of the head plus the deformation of the surface. Hertz contact theory defines GRF acting perpendicular to the area of contact, assuming that a sphere is contacting an infinitely long flat surface, as

$$F_c = \frac{4}{3} E^* R^{1/2} \delta^{3/2} \qquad (7.22)$$

where R is the radius of the head and E^* is the effective modulus of the system dependent on material properties of both the surface and the head [46]. Equation (7.22) can be substituted in Eq. (7.21) only as long as the direction of impact is considered such that

$$-\int_0^\delta k \delta^{\frac{3}{2}} d\delta = \frac{1}{2} m_H \left(v_{H2}^2 - v_{H1}^2 \right) + m_H g \delta \qquad (7.23)$$

where $k = \frac{4}{3} E^* R^{1/2}$ from Eq. (7.22). Maximum deformation occurs when final velocity of the head's COM is zero, and integration of Eq. (7.23) to this time point results in

$$\frac{2}{5}k\delta_{max}^{\frac{5}{2}} + m_H g\delta_{max} - \frac{1}{2}m_H v_{H1}^2 = 0. \tag{7.24}$$

This final substitution allows us to solve for δ_{max} and thereby maximum ground reaction force $F_{c,\,max}$ using Eq. (7.22). Equation (7.24), however, does not hold for the one-link and two-link system since angular velocity of the head about the neck joint (point N) is unaccounted for. In order to be consistent with the rigid body assumptions used earlier, the kinetic energy of the system must be modified as follows:

$$T_2 - T_1 = \frac{1}{2}m_H\left(v_{H2}^2 - v_{H1}^2\right) + \frac{1}{2}I_{H/N}\left(\dot{\theta}_{H2}^2 - \dot{\theta}_{H1}^2\right). \tag{7.25}$$

Angular velocity can again be related to translation velocity as $\dot{\theta}^2 = \dfrac{v}{r_{H/N}}$, simplifying Eq. (7.25). With this updated representation of kinetic energy for a rigid link, Eq. (7.18) now results in

$$\frac{2}{5}k\delta_{max}^{\frac{5}{2}} + m_H g\delta_{max} - \frac{1}{2}\left(m_H + \frac{I_{H/N}}{r_{H/N}^2}\right)v_{H1}^2 = 0. \tag{7.26}$$

Material properties for the sports surface and for an athlete's head (or protective headgear) can be applied within this model to obtain acceleration profiles and maximum ground reaction forces.

Model Comparison

In the theory presented thus far, increasing the degrees of freedom of the head impact model encompasses more input parameters that can influence impact severity. In order to understand the modeling potential of these approaches, we subjected the equations to a Monte Carlo sensitivity analysis. The aim of this analysis was to compare the three model types to determine if an increase in model complexity of sports surface regulations is warranted and how the model results depend on the properties of the surface. Furthermore, sensitivity indices are computed from a range of input parameters found in literature to assess the contribution of these input values on total impact severity outcomes. These outcomes are then related back to the head injury thresholds currently used in industry, namely, the WSTC and subsequent HIC.

Determination of Input Parameters

Distributions were assigned to each of the required inputs according to the principle of maximum entropy. A uniform distribution, $U(\alpha,\beta)$, was assigned to any variable where only a lower bound (α) and upper bound (β) of potential values was found (Table 7.3) [47]. This enforced an equal probability of any value within the observable range. The modulus of the sports surface (E_g) is not a widely available

7 The Role of the Playing Surface in Mitigating the Deleterious Effects of Head...

Table 7.3 Input parameters modeled with a uniform distribution

Parameter	Units	Required in model? Particle	1-Link	2-Link	Hertz	Lower bound	Upper bound	Ref.
θ_1	°		✓	✓		5	45	–
θ_2	°			✓		20	45	–
r_v	m	✓	✓	✓		0.5	1.3	–
v	m/s	✓	✓	✓		0.01	10	–
$^a E_G$	MPa				✓	6	52.7	Guisasola et al. [48]
μ_G	–				✓	0.05	0.49	Cole et al. [49]
μ_H	–				✓	0.2	0.5	Peterson and Dechow [47]

If the parameter is used in a specific model it is marked with a ✓. References for lower and upper limits are provided
^{a}This parameter distribution was used exclusively in sensitivity analysis

Table 7.4 Input parameters modeled with a normal distribution

Parameter	Units	Required in model? Particle	1-Link	2-Link	Hertz	Mean	Stdv	Ref.
m	kg	✓	✓	✓		88.7	15.6	CDC [52]
r_H	m	✓	✓	✓		1.759	0.0625	CDC [52]
R	m				✓	0.086	0.0027	Lacko et al. [50]
I_o	kg·m²		✓	✓		11.637	2.022	Santschi et al. [51]
$I_{2/J}$	kg·m²			✓		0.1418	0.0245	Dempster [53]
$^a E_G$	MPa				✓	6	0.3	Guisasola et al. [48]
E_H	MPa				✓	450	135	Boruah et al. [27]

If the parameter is used in a specific model it is marked with a ✓. References for mean and standard deviation values are provided
^{a}This parameter distribution was used exclusively in the simulations post-sensitivity analysis

measurement, and studies that do report its value have displayed at least a 3 orders of magnitude range [48, 49]. For this reason, a uniform distribution was chosen between two types of soils found in Guisasola et al. [48]

A normal distribution, $N(\mu,\sigma)$, was assigned to any variable where a mean (μ) and standard deviation (σ) was available in the literature (Table 7.4). This enforced an increased probability of the parameter taking values closer to the mean value. Much like the original WSTC studies, anthropometric parameters used in biomechanics analysis today frequently date to before the twenty-first century [51–55], and oftentimes result from a small subset of male cadaver data. For this reason, many of the normally distributed parameters apply to a simulated "male" model.

To reduce the likelihood of unrealistic combinations of anthropometric parameters, some inputs were chosen to be functions of other random variables (i.e., head mass is calculated as a percentage of total body mass). These parameters and their calculations can be found in Table 7.5 [27, 52].

Table 7.5 Input parameters that were chosen as percentages of primary inputs

Parameter	Required in model?				Calculation	Ref.
	Particle	1-Link	2-Link	Hertz		
m_2	✓	✓	✓	✓	8.26% of whole body mass	Plagenhoef et al. [54]
m_1			✓		91.74% of whole body mass	–
L_1			✓		80.4% of player height	Plagenhoef et al. [54]
L_2			✓		19.5% of player height	Plagenhoef et al. [54]
$L_{2,\,COM}$			✓	✓	10.75% of player height	Plagenhoef et al. [54]

If the parameter is used in a specific model it is marked with a ✓. References for % value calculations are provided

Sensitivity Analysis

A global sensitivity analysis (GSA) was performed to assess the influence of each input parameter to the linear acceleration of the head during surface impact per model type [56]. A variance-based method was utilized, in which the contribution of the individual parameter variability to the variability of the output was quantified. A Fourier Amplitude Sensitivity Test (FAST) was paired with a quasi-Monte Carlo algorithm. As found in Cannavó (2012), FAST approximates the functions of interest as a Fourier series and consequently quantifies Fourier coefficients through a Fourier analysis [56]. In order to obtain the sensitivity coefficients, a numerical integration of the Fourier coefficients is calculated through a probabilistic interpretation based on a quasi-Monte Carlo algorithm. A total of 9141 low-discrepancy sample points were selected, by calculating the Nyquist frequency and multiplying it by the number of discrete intervals chosen for the integration ($M = 10$). It is important to note that by calculating first-order sensitivity indices, the analysis only quantifies the contribution of individual input parameters to the variance of the output and disregards interaction terms between parameters [57].

Following the sensitivity analysis, a true Monte Carlo simulation with $N = 1000$ random samples was executed given the set of parameter distributions. This allows for better visualization of the modeled impacts and for comparison with the WSTC which is used to calculate HIC, and thereby determine safety regulations for sports surfaces.

Results

The sensitivity of peak translational acceleration (PTA) to the input variables is of interest since translational acceleration can be used to derive angular kinematics, GRF, and HIC values as presented previously as well as relate directly to on-field studies. The FAST sensitivity indices for each model type, with respect to the sensitivity threshold (1/# parameters), are given in Fig. 7.7. For the particle model, the modulus of the ground and the impacting mass had the largest contributions to PTA. Given this result, the modulus of the ground was further restricted to a single type of surface (clay-loam soil [48]) to reduce the variability in the outputs profiles after the Monte Carlo simulation.

Each model type also produced unique kinematic and impact severity outputs given the randomly distributed 1000 Monte Carlo sets of input parameters

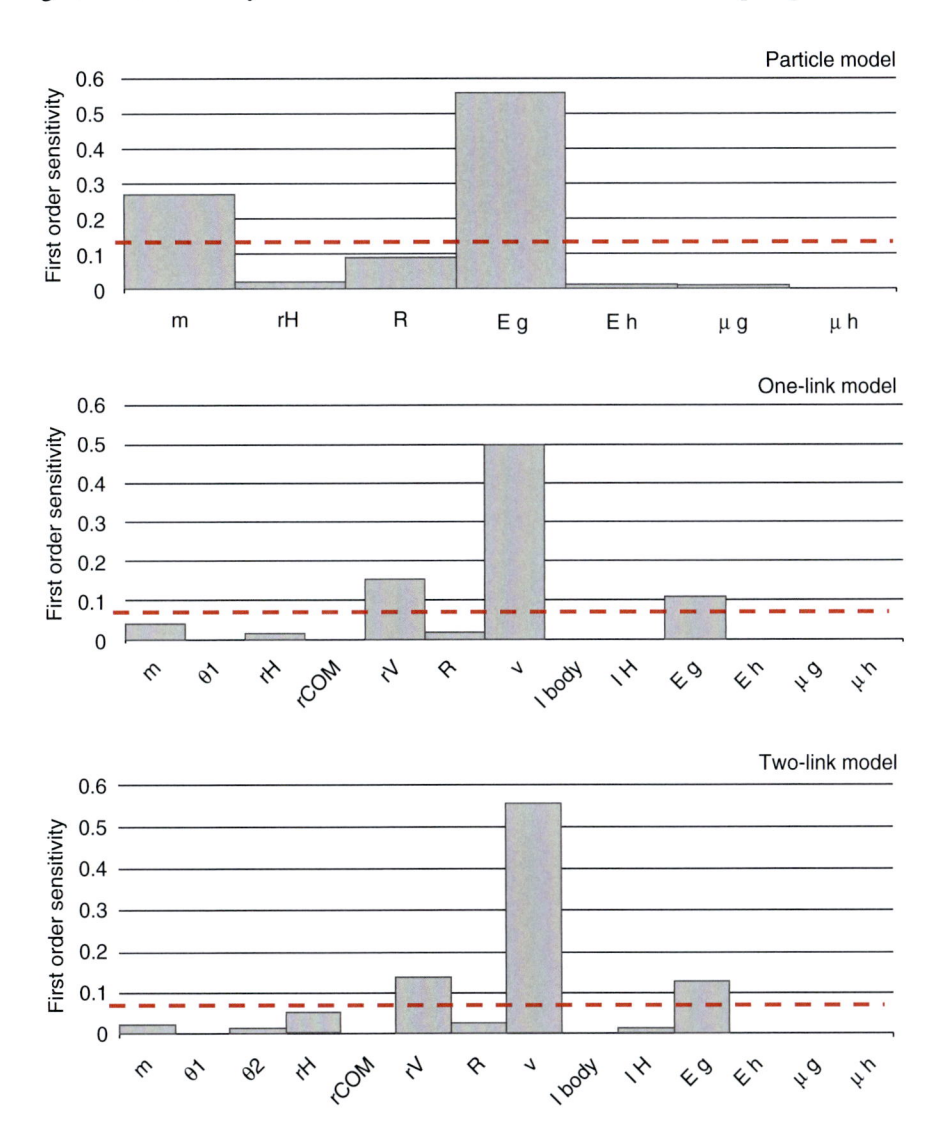

Fig. 7.7 First-order sensitivity indices determined using FAST for the particle, one-link, and two-link models independently. A red, dashed line indicates the model's threshold of sensitivity given the number of parameters

(Table 7.6). One of the random sets of inputs were found to produce a final velocity outside of the 99.7th percentile of the resultant population. For this reason, this set was selectively removed on the basis that it was unlikely to be a realistic combination of input parameters.

Translational acceleration profiles of the COM of the head during surface contact were determined by mirroring the start-to-peak profile (Fig. 7.8). The particle model was found to have a smaller range of modeling potential not only before impact, but during ground contact where PTA was only predicted in a small range of 56.6–106.9 g. The two-link model displayed the best range of potential outputs

Table 7.6 Calculated output metrics for each model type given $N = 999$ Monte Carlo simulations

	Particle		One-link		Two-link	
Before ground impact						
	Mean	Range	Mean	Range	Mean	Range
PTA (g)	1	–	13.1	2.8–69.0	49.4	2.3–236.5
PTV (m/s)	5.9	5.5–6.2	13.8	6.2–35.0	12.0	3.3–28.7
PAA (rad/s^2)	–	–	10.3	8.3–12.2	178.8	15.3–387.1
PAV (rad/s)	–	–	7.9	3.7–19.3	34.6	2.3–80.3
During ground impact						
	Mean	Range	Mean	Range	Mean	Range
PTA (g)	75.3	56.6–106.9	202.4	73.9–633.5	169.8	23.1–501.3
PAA (rad/s^2)	–	–	5768	2228–17658	4837	936–13971
GRF (kN)	5.3	3.3–7.3	16.8	4.96–57.0	14.1	2.3–44.8
Time to peak (ms)	14.5	10.1–18.4	13.2	9.5–18.3	13.6	9.9–19.3
HIC	316	200.–529	4698	352–44549	3020.	50.6–25810.
HIC-15	833	696–951	9607	980.–74159	6534	192–44986
HIC-36	224	187–256	2584	264–19946	1757	51.5–12099

The average, maximum, and minimum values for each metric is provided. Given metrics include peak translational acceleration (PTA), peak translational velocity (PTV), peak angular acceleration (PAA), peak angular velocity (PAV), ground reaction force (GRF), and head injury criterion (HIC)

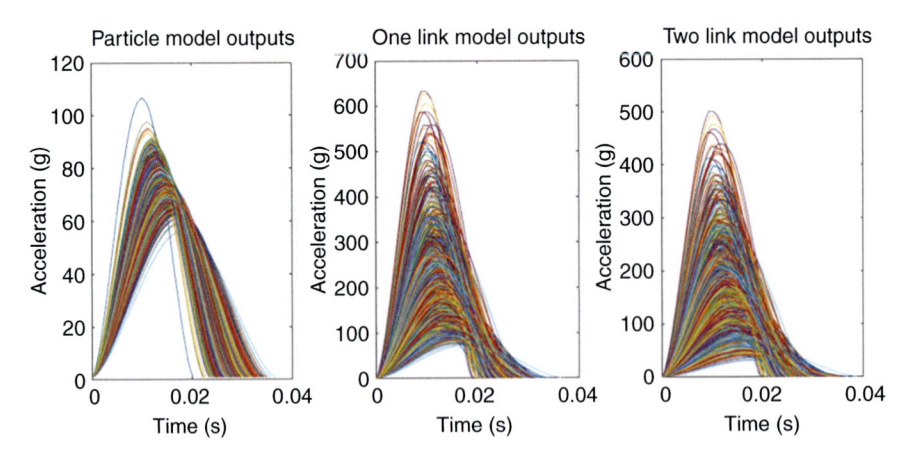

Fig. 7.8 Independent translational acceleration predictions during ground impact using Monte Carlo analysis ($N = 999$)

including a 23.1–501.3 g predictive range for PTA which encompasses the types of subconcussive and injury-causing hits seen in contact sports. This was a more conservative maximum prediction than that of the one-link model (118–996 g) implying that allowing the head (or second link) to whip backward mitigates the effect of the pin constraint at the ground.

From the predicted PTA profiles, the effective acceleration and total time of impact were determined as to compare these values to the original WSTC curve provided by Gurdjian et al. in 1964 [24] (Fig. 7.9). Special interest points were also determined using the particle model for the NOCSAE ND 001-17m17b [42] and FIFA football turf [17] testing standards. From this figure, the particle model only represents a family of impact types highly dependent on surface properties and impactor mass. A similar finding is that the current testing standards further reduce the modeling potential of the particle model by highly restricting impact velocity.

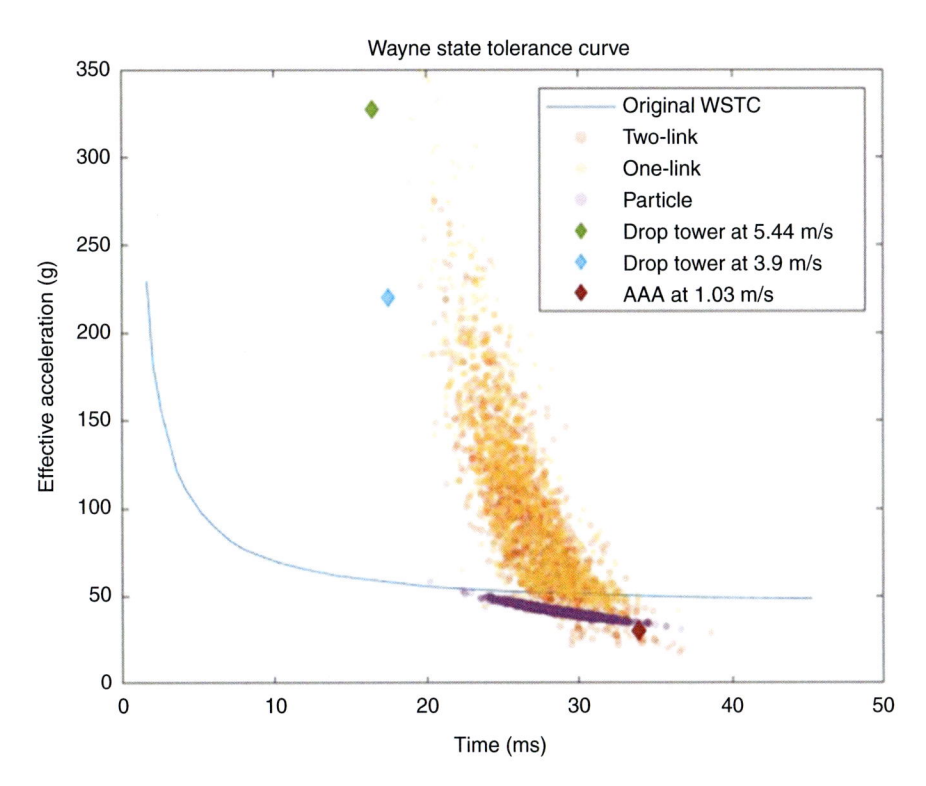

Fig. 7.9 Impact severity determination based on effective acceleration and total time of impact. The original curve-fit of the WSTC is provided as a reference along with special interest points from available sports testing standards. A drop tower test with impacting velocity of 5.44 m/s and 3.9 m/s is NOCSAE testing standard [42] while an AAA test with impacting velocity of 1.03 m/s is designated by FIFA [17]

Summary

The existing sports surface regulations are fundamentally derived from outdated definitions and modeling of head injury and, therefore, are not fulfilling their original purpose of mitigating player injury. With the recent progression of injury quantification research and focus on mTBI, there is an opportunity to modernize the way the industry approaches safety criteria. At the time the original Wayne State Tolerance Curve was generated, concussion was loosely defined as "unconsciousness after impact" and identified in cadavers as linear skull fracture. Even the Wayne State group acknowledged the ambiguity of this definition and repeatedly cautioned readers before broadly adopting their tolerance curve stating, "fracture and concussion are entirely different" [25] and "much more data must be obtained before valid conclusions can be drawn" [25].

Since the 1960s, not only has the definition of concussion evolved to encompass cognitive changes, but much research has proceeded these initial experiments that provide better indicators of head injury. Bari et al. [28] found a 50 g peak translational acceleration threshold to be indicative of the onset of metabolic changes in the brains of high school football athletes. This threshold is further supported by a similar study in female, high school soccer athletes that examined changes in blood flow [26]. Jang et al. [41] concluded that structural changes in white matter can be detected with peak linear accelerations as low as 20 g. This data is not accounted for with the tolerable HIC thresholds and has yet to be incorporated into any sports surface regulations. Furthermore, acceleration of this low magnitude is not obtainable with a guided particle approach, as with the AAA or drop tower. On the upper end of the spectrum, in order to reach HIC values larger than 1000 with a guided impactor test, the impactor mass must be larger than that of an average human head or drop heights taller than average human height.

Proposing peak linear acceleration thresholds on the order of tens of g's may seem virtually impossible for sport surface developers to design for. It is true that designing against skull fracture is much more attainable than to mitigate "subconcussive" impacts, which is potentially why HIC has been a firmly held metric for the last 50 years. However, the occurrence of the type of injury predicted by HIC is rarely observed within the area of sports biomechanics. Whereas, concussion and neurological changes are more prevalent and can arise from sports surface contact.

HIC and the WSTC do not have the capability of representing these types of sports-related injuries, yet they are continually used within sports surface regulations. Though HIC and NOCSAE testing standards claim to be correlated with head injury, their application to real-life scenarios falls short since they intrinsically model the entire player as a particle. The standard rigid-link dynamic models of player impact paired with Hertz contact theory better represents these types of injuries. Furthermore, these models paired with proposed linear and angular acceleration thresholds offer more insight into player safety than the available impact severity metrics. It is important to note that the current models are defined for unhelmeted sports. Future work will consider the interaction between helmets and the sports surface in a quantitative manner.

Despite their potential, improved models of head injury can be rendered ineffective without assessment of sport surface material properties. The sensitivity analysis presented for each model elucidated the paramountcy of sports surface properties on impact severity, irrespective of the number of degrees of freedom. Determination of true material properties of the sports surface should be fundamental to testing standards and regulations in the absence of injury metrics.

References

1. Bryan MA, Rowhani-Rahbar A, Comstock RD, Rivara F. Sports-and recreation-related concussions in US youth. Pediatrics. 2016;138:e20154635.
2. Baldwin GT, Breiding MJ, Dawn Comstock R. Epidemiology of sports concussion in the United States. In: Handbook of clinical neurology; 2018. https://doi.org/10.1016/B978-0-444-63954-7.00007-0.
3. Clifton DR, Hertel J, Onate JA, Currie DW, Pierpoint LA, Wasserman EB, Knowles SB, Dompier TP, Comstock RD, Marshall SW, Kerr ZY. The first decade of web-based sports injury surveillance: descriptive epidemiology of injuries in US high school girls' basketball (2005–2006 through 2013–2014) and National Collegiate Athletic Association women's basketball (2004–2005 through 2013–2014). J Athl Train. 2018;53:1037–48.
4. Clifton DR, Onate JA, Hertel J, Pierpoint LA, Currie DW, Wasserman EB, Knowles SB, Dompier TP, Marshall SW, Dawn Comstock R, Kerr ZY. The first decade of web-based sports injury surveillance: descriptive epidemiology of injuries in US high school boys' basketball (2005–2006 through 2013–2014) and National Collegiate Athletic Association men's basketball (2004–2005 through 2013–2014). J Athl Train. 2018;53:1025–36.
5. DiStefano LJ, Dann CL, Chang CJ, Putukian M, Pierpoint LA, Currie DW, Knowles SB, Wasserman EB, Dompier TP, Dawn Comstock R, Marshall SW, Kerr ZY. The first decade of web-based sports injury surveillance: descriptive epidemiology of injuries in US high school girls' soccer (2005–2006 through 2013–2014) and national collegiate athletic association women's soccer (2004–2005 through 2013–2014). J Athl Train. 2018;53:880–92.
6. Kerr ZY, Dawn Comstock R, Dompier TP, Marshall SW. The first decade of web-based sports injury surveillance (2004–2005 through 2013–2014): methods of the National Collegiate Athletic Association injury surveillance program and high school reporting information online. J Athl Train. 2018;53:729–37.
7. Kerr ZY, Gregory AJ, Wosmek J, Pierpoint LA, Currie DW, Knowles SB, Wasserman EB, Dompier TP, Dawn Comstock R, Marshall SW. The first decade of web-based sports injury surveillance: descriptive epidemiology of injuries in us high school girls' volleyball (2005–2006 through 2013–2014) and National Collegiate Athletic Association women's volleyball (2004–2005 through 2013–2014). J Athl Train. 2018;53:926–37.
8. Kerr ZY, Putukian M, Chang CJ, DiStefano LJ, Currie DW, Pierpoint LA, Knowles SB, Wasserman EB, Dompier TP, Dawn Comstock R, Marshall SW. The first decade of web-based sports injury surveillance: descriptive epidemiology of injuries in US high school boys' soccer (2005–2006 through 2013–2014) and National Collegiate Athletic Association men's soccer (2004–2005 through 2013–2014). J Athl Train. 2018;53:893–905.
9. Kerr ZY, Wilkerson GB, Caswell SV, Currie DW, Pierpoint LA, Wasserman EB, Knowles SB, Dompier TP, Dawn Comstock R, Marshall SW. The first decade of web-based sports injury surveillance: descriptive epidemiology of injuries in United States high school football (2005–2006 through 2013–2014) and National Collegiate Athletic Association football (2004–2005 through 2013–2014). J Athl Train. 2018;53:738–51.
10. Kroshus E, Utter AC, Pierpoint LA, Currie DW, Knowles SB, Wasserman EB, Dompier TP, Marshall SW, Dawn Comstock R, Kerr ZY. The first decade of web-based sports injury surveillance: descriptive epidemiology of injuries in US high school boys' wrestling (2005–2006 through 2013–2014) and National Collegiate Athletic Association men's wrestling (2004–2005 through 2013–2014). J Athl Train. 2018;53:1143–55.

11. Lynall RC, Gardner EC, Paolucci J, Currie DW, Knowles SB, Pierpoint LA, Wasserman EB, Dompier TP, Dawn Comstock R, Marshall SW, Kerr ZY. The first decade of web-based sports injury surveillance: descriptive epidemiology of injuries in US high school girls' field hockey (2008–2009 through 2013–2014) and National Collegiate Athletic Association women's field hockey (2004–2005 through 2013–2014). J Athl Train. 2018;53:938–49.
12. Lynall RC, Mihalik JP, Pierpoint LA, Currie DW, Knowles SB, Wasserman EB, Dompier TP, Comstock RD, Marshall SW, Kerr ZY. The first decade of web-based sports injury surveillance: descriptive epidemiology of injuries in US high school boys' ice hockey (2008–2009 through 2013–2014) and National Collegiate Athletic Association men's and women's ice hockey (2004–2005 through 2013–2014). J Athl Train. 2018;53:1129–42.
13. Pierpoint LA, Caswell SV, Walker N, Lincoln AE, Currie DW, Knowles SB, Wasserman EB, Dompier TP, Dawn Comstock R, Marshall SW, Kerr ZY. The first decade of web-based sports injury surveillance: descriptive epidemiology of injuries in US high school girls' lacrosse (2008–2009 through 2013–2014) and National Collegiate Athletic Association women's lacrosse (2004–2005 through 2013–2014). J Athl Train. 2019;54:42–54.
14. Pierpoint LA, Lincoln AE, Walker N, Caswell SV, Currie DW, Knowles SB, Wasserman EB, Dompier TP, Comstock RD, Marshall SW, Kerr ZY. The first decade of web-based sports injury surveillance: descriptive epidemiology of injuries in US high school boys' lacrosse (2008–2009 through 2013–2014) and National Collegiate Athletic Association men's lacrosse (2004–2005 through 2013–2014). J Athl Train. 2019;54:30–41.
15. Wasserman EB, Register-Mihalik JK, Sauers EL, Currie DW, Pierpoint LA, Knowles SB, Dompier TP, Dawn Comstock R, Marshall SW, Kerr ZY. The first decade of web-based sports injury surveillance: descriptive epidemiology of injuries in US high school girls' softball (2005–2006 through 2013–2014) and National Collegiate Athletic Association women's softball (2004–2005 through 2013–2014). J Athl Train. 2019;54:212–25.
16. Wasserman EB, Sauers EL, Register-Mihalik JK, Pierpoint LA, Currie DW, Knowles SB, Dompier TP, Comstock RD, Marshall SW, Kerr ZY. The first decade of web-based sports injury surveillance: descriptive epidemiology of injuries in US high school boys' baseball (2005–2006 through 2013–2014) and National Collegiate Athletic Association men's baseball (2004–2005 through 2013–2014). J Athl Train. 2019;54:198–211.
17. FIFA. FIFA quality programme for football turf: handbook of test methods. 2015. At: https://football-technology.fifa.com/media/1238/fqp-handbook-of-test-methods-v27.pdf
18. FIFA. FIFA quality programme for futsal surfaces handbook of test methods and requirements. 2019.
19. CEN. CEN 1177: impact attenuating playground surfacing – methods of test for determination of impact attenuation. 2017.
20. CEN. CEN 16717: surface for sports areas method of test for the determination of shock absorption, vertical deformation and energy restitution using the advanced artificial athlete. 2015.
21. Gurdjian ES, Webster JE, Lissner HR. The mechanism of skull fracture. Radiology. 1950;54:313–39.
22. Gurdjian ES, Webster JE, Lissner HR. Observations on prediction of fracture site in head injury. Radiology. 1953;60:226–35.
23. Gurdjian ES, Lissner HR, Evans FG, Patrick LM, Hardy WG. Intracranial pressure and acceleration accompanying head impacts in human cadavers. Surg Gynecol Obstet. 1961;113:185–90.
24. Gurdjian ES, Hodgson VR, Hardy WG, Patrick LM, Lissner HR. Evaluation of the protective characteristics of helmets in sports. J Trauma Inj Infect Crit Care. 1964;4:309–24.
25. Lissner HR, Lebow M, Gaynor Evans F. Experimental studies on the relation between acceleration and intercranial pressure changes in man. Surg Gynecol Obstet. 1960;111:329–38.
26. Svaldi DO, Joshi C, McCuen EC, Music JP, Hannemann R, Leverenz LJ, Nauman EA, Talavage TM. Accumulation of high magnitude acceleration events predicts cerebrovascular reactivity changes in female high school soccer athletes. Brain Imaging Behav. 2018;14:164–74.
27. Boruah S, Henderson K, Subit D, Salzar RS, Shender BS, Paskoff G. Response of human skull bone to dynamic compressive loading. Proc IRCOBI Conf. 2013;13:497.

28. Bari S, Svaldi DO, Jang I, Shenk TE, Poole VN, Lee T, Dydak U, Rispoli JV, Nauman EA, Talavage TM. Dependence on subconcussive impacts of brain metabolism in collision sport athletes: an MR spectroscopic study. Brain Imaging Behav. 2019;13:735–49.
29. Patrick LM, Lissner HR, Gurdjian ES. Sruvival by design – head protection. In: Proceedings: American Association for Automotive Medicine annual conference, vol. 7. Association for the Advancement of Automotive Medicine; 1963. p. 483–99.
30. Budson A, McKee AC, Cantu RC, Stern RA. Chronic traumatic encephalopathy. Boston: Elsevier; 2017. 198 pp.
31. Gadd C. Criteria for injury. Washington, DC; 1961.
32. Gadd C. Use of a weighted-impulse criterion for estimating injury hazard. SAE Technical Paper. 1966.
33. Versace J. A review of the severity index. 1971. https://doi.org/10.4271/710881.
34. McElhaney J. Head injury criteria. Polym Mech. 1976;12:411–29.
35. Greenwald R, Gwin J, Chu J, Crisco J. Head impact severity measures for evaluating mild traumatic brain injury risk exposure. Neurosurgery. 2008;62:798.
36. Zhang L, Yang KH, King AI. A proposed injury threshold for mild traumatic brain injury (Author Abstract). J Biomech Eng. 2004;126:226–36.
37. Brennan JH, Mitra B, Synnot A, McKenzie J, Willmott C, McIntosh A, Maller J, Rosenfeld J. Accelerometers for the assessment of concussion in male athletes: a systematic review and meta-analysis. Sports Med. 2017;47:469–78.
38. Broglio SP, Schnebel B, Sosnoff JJ, Shin S, Feng X, He X, Zimmerman J. Biomechanical properties of concussions in high school football. Med Sci Sport Exerc. 2010;42:2064–71.
39. Beckwith JG, Greenwald RM, Chu JJ, Crisco JJ, Rowson S, Duma SM, Broglio SP, Mcallister TW, Guskiewicz KM, Mihalik JP, Anderson S, Schnebel B, Brolinson PG, Collins MW. Head impact exposure sustained by football players on days of diagnosed concussion. Med Sci Sport Exerc. 2012;45:737–46.
40. Schnebel B, Gwin JT, Anderson S, Gatlin R. In vivo study of head impacts in football: a comparison of National Collegiate Athletic Association Division I versus high school impacts. Neurosurgery. 2007;60:490–6.
41. Jang I, Chun IY, Brosch JR, Bari S, Zou Y, Cummiskey BR, Lee TA, Lycke RJ, Poole VN, Shenk TE, Svaldi DO, Tamer GG, Dydak U, Leverenz LJ, Nauman EA, Talavage TM. Every hit matters: white matter diffusivity changes in high school football athletes are correlated with repetitive head acceleration event exposure. NeuroImage Clin. 2019;24:101930.
42. National Operating Committee on Standards for Athletic Equipment. Standard test method and equipment used in evaluating the performance characteristics of headgear/equipment – NOCSAE DOC (ND) 001-17m17b. 2017.
43. National Operating Committee on Standards for Athletic Equipment. Standard performance specification for newly manufactured football helmets – NOCSAE DOC (ND) 002-17m19a. 2019.
44. Reynolds H. The inertial properties of the body and its segments. 1978.
45. Swartz EE, Floyd RT, Cendoma M. Cervical spine functional anatomy and the biomechanics of injury due to compressive loading.(literature review) (Brief Article). J Athl Train. 2005;40:155–61.
46. Johnson KL. Contact mechanics. London: Cambridge University Press; 1985.
47. Peterson J, Dechow PC. Material properties of the human cranial vault and zygoma. Anat Rec. 2003;274A:785–97.
48. Guisasola I, James I, Llewellyn C, Stiles V, Dixon S. Quasi-static mechanical behaviour of soils used for natural turf sports surfaces and stud force prediction. Sports Eng. 2010;12:97–108.
49. Cole D, Forrester S, Fleming P. Mechanical characterization and numerical modelling of rubber Shockpads in 3G artificial turf. PRO. 2018;2:1–6.
50. Lacko D, Huysmans T, Parizel PM, De Bruyne G, Verwulgen S, Van Hulle MM, Sijbers J. Evaluation of an anthropometric shape model of the human scalp. Appl Ergon. 2015;48:70–85. https://doi.org/10.1016/j.apergo.2014.11.008. Epub 2014 Dec 6. PMID: 25683533.

51. Santschi W, Dubois J, Omoto C. Moments of inertia and centers of gravity of the living human body. Los Angeles; 1963.
52. Center for Health Statistics N. Vital Health Stat Ser. 2012;11(252):2007.
53. Dempster W. Space requirements of the seated operator. Wright-Patterson Air Force Base; 1995.
54. Plagenhoef S, Gaynor Evans F, Abdelnour T. Anatomical data for analyzing human motion. Res Q Exerc Sport. 1983;54:169–78.
55. Yoganandan N, Pintar FA, Zhang J, Baisden JL. Physical properties of the human head: mass, center of gravity and moment of inertia. J Biomech. 2009;42:1177–92.
56. Cannavó F. Sensitivity analysis for volcanic source modeling quality assessment and model selection. Comput Geosci. 2009;44:52–9.
57. Sobol I. Sensitivity estimates for nonlinear mathematical model. Math Model Comput Exp. 1993;1:407–14.

Part III

Physiology of Concussion and Subconcussive Injuries

Neuropathology of Mild Traumatic Brain Injury: Relationship to Structural Neuroimaging Findings

Erin D. Bigler

Introduction

The limits of neuroimaging technology specify what types of neuropathology can be detected in traumatic brain injury (TBI), especially if the injury is mild. Fortunately, tremendous advances in neuroimaging technologies, especially with magnetic resonance (MR) imaging (MRI), have been made in the last few years, even in detection of subtle pathology following mild TBI (mTBI). Most conventional MR studies configure anatomical images with millimeter resolution, meaning that structural MRI detects pathology at a similar level, although submillimeter resolution is now possible [1, 2]. However, the fundamental pathological changes that occur from mTBI happen at the micron and nanometer cellular level [3]. This means for brain injuries in the mild range, with the subtlest of neural injuries that the macroscopic lesions characteristic of more severe pathologies simply is not visible in most cases. For example, Fig. 8.1 is from Mayer et al. [4] that examined the frequency of visually objective findings in mild TBI in a large multisite sample of mTBI pediatric cases, initially identified and diagnosed in the emergency department but then followed up with MRI. As shown in Fig. 8.1, while visible abnormalities on MRI may be seen in cases of mTBI, they are only detected in a minority of the mTBI cases scanned and tend to be singular findings. Accordingly, there is a low yield in standard, routine clinical neuroimaging in detecting mTBI abnormalities. Fortunately, with contemporary advances in neuroimaging quantification and analysis, these advanced neuroimaging methods have provided improved insights into how underlying neuropathology associated with mTBI and how it can be detected [5, 6].

E. D. Bigler (✉)
Department of Psychology and Neuroscience Center, Brigham Young University, Provo, UT, USA

Departments of Psychiatry and Neurology, University of Utah, Salt Lake City, UT, USA
e-mail: erin_bigler@byu.edu

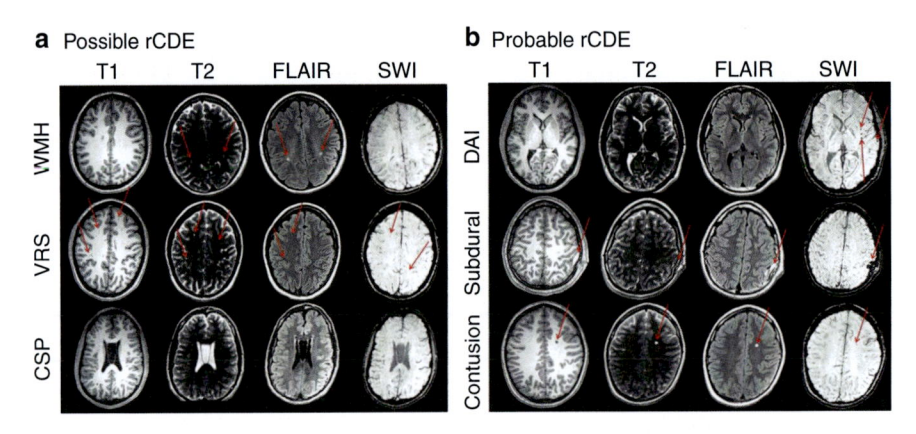

Fig. 8.1 (**a**) Selection of radiologic common data elements, or rCDEs, of possible (**a**) and probable (**b**) traumatic origin across four different MRI sequences. Cavum septum pellucidum (CSP), hematomas, and contusions were readily visible across T1-weighted, T2-weighted, fluid-attenuated inversion recovery (FLAIR), and susceptibility-weighted imaging (SWI) sequences. White matter hyperintensities (WMH) and prominent perivascular spaces (Virchow-Robin spaces [VRs]) were differentiated by their more conspicuous appearance on FLAIR and T2 sequences, respectively. In contrast, diffuse axonal injuries (DAI) were almost exclusively visible on SWI sequences. Note that abnormalities may only be observed on certain MRI sequences

From review of the images in Fig. 8.1, it is also evident that the location, size, and distribution of MRI abnormalities in mTBI are very heterogeneous. It is also evident that many of these visible abnormalities are small and sometimes rather inconspicuous. This is quite different from what may be observed in moderate-to-severe TBI. Straightforwardly, the contrast in gross visible detection of pathology from mild-to-severe TBI is demonstrated in Fig. 8.2.

In Fig. 8.2, all of the individuals with mTBI had a postresuscitation Glasgow Coma Scale [7] score of 15 and were part of the social outcomes of brain injury in kids [SOBIK] [8] investigation. Although all children in the SOBIK investigation who sustained mTBI had positive day-of-injury (DOI) computed tomography (CT), in the form of contusion, petechial hemorrhage, skull fracture, or edema, only about two-thirds of the 41 mTBI children had identifiable MRI abnormalities when followed up approximately a year or more postinjury. As demonstrated in the Bigler et al.'s [8] investigation, a number of children with subtle hemorrhage and/or localized edema on the DOI CT did not evidence visibly detectable abnormalities on follow-up MRI performed at least a year postinjury. While not possible in human mTBI studies, animal investigations that model mTBI where acute neuroimaging abnormalities become nondetectable over time nonetheless may show residual pathology at the histological level [9–11]. As such, it is safe to assume that DOI pathology like petechial hemorrhages that are not detected on follow-up imaging nonetheless indicates significant shear forces were present in the brain at the time of injury and likely do reflect where residual pathology may be present at the cellular level, just not detectable with contemporary neuroimaging methods.

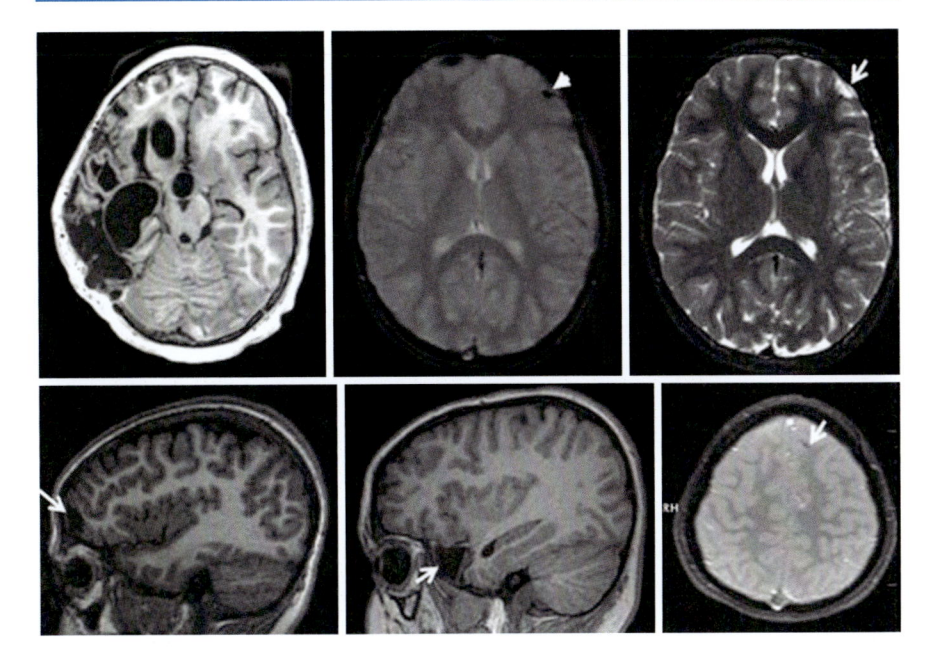

Fig. 8.2 The subtleness and diversity of MRI identified chronic (>6 months postinjury) brain lesions in four mTBI patients, all with a GCS of 15, compared to the massive structural pathologies associated with severe TBI presented in this figure. The mTBI case shown in the *top middle* and *right* shows characteristic area of small focal encephalomalacia with increased region of CSF (*arrow*) in the T2-weighted image (*top right*) associated with residual hemosiderin (*arrowhead*) in the gradient-recalled echo (GRE) sequence (*top middle*). These pathological changes were originally the result of a focal frontal contusion. In the sagittal image in the *bottom left*, focal frontal encephalomalacia is evident (*arrow*) and encephalomalacia in the temporal lobe (*arrow*) in the *middle* image with the *bottom right* image showing an axial scan with subtle hemosiderin right at the gray-white junction (*arrow*), all from different children. In contrast, the child with severe injury (axial view, *upper left*) has massive structural pathology. (From Bigler et al. [8]; used with permission)

The introduction above highlights the "visible" abnormalities in mTBI, but structural neuroimaging also provides other metrics to assess the pathoanatomical nature of injury. When abnormalities are detected, how does this assist the clinician or researcher in understanding outcome and treatment? In the last few years, a variety of both structural and functional neuroimaging techniques have led to a more informed approach for understanding brain networks, along with how network damage/dysfunction accompanies TBI [3, 12]. This is a particularly important neuroimaging and cognitive neuroscience advancement because the inference about location of the lesion or structural abnormality in mTBI may not be the most important factor associated with a traumatic injury, but how that traumatic pathology disrupts network functioning.

Figure 8.3 summarizes some of the network advances since the previous edition of this text [5]. In mathematics, graph theory provides metrics to examine pairwise relations between objects [13]. For brain structure, an "object" is defined as either a

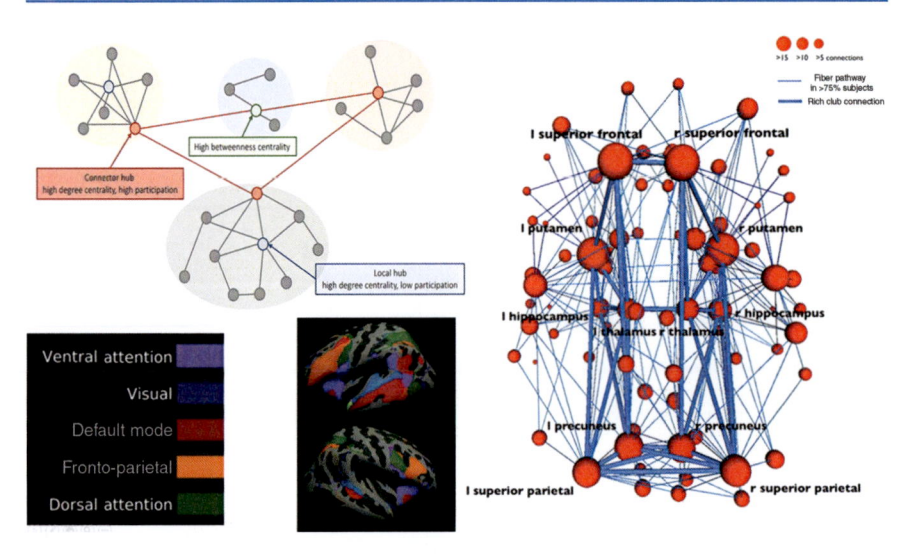

Fig. 8.3 (Top Left) The network schematic is from Arnatkeviciute and Fulcher [13], which shows different concepts of hubness in brain networks. A schematic representation of a modular network where nodes within a module (different background colors) show a relatively high degree of intramodular connectivity and a low degree of intermodular connectivity. High-degree nodes can be classified into (i) local hubs (blue) that have a high-degree centrality and low participation coefficient; and (ii) connector hubs (red) that have high degree and connect to nodes in other modules. Nodes with high betweenness centrality are located on shortest paths between nodes and can play an important role in linking different nodes, even if they have low degree (e.g., the green node supports communication between the yellow and orange modules). (Bottom Left) Adapted with permission from Bailey, Aboud [15] depicts several of the multicortical loci for different networks. Note how the regional representation is never in just one area, indicating the dependence of the network on white matter connectivity. The "Rich Club" network depicted to the right is from van den Heuvel and Sporns [16], used with permission. The schematic depicts the group connectome with rich-club connections marked in dark blue. Connections between rich-club regions (dark blue) and connections from rich-club nodes to the other regions of the brain network (light blue) link via hubs which vary in their strength of connection as reflected in their size. The figure shows that almost all regions of the brain have at least one link directly to the rich club

region of interest (ROI) or at a cellular level, how neuron A connects with neuron B, so on [3]. Connection strength is mathematically determined, where, as shown in Fig. 8.3, a graph matrix is generated by various vertices that connect two points or nodes which are connected by edges, forming linkage between those areas (see upper left, Fig. 8.3). Several important neuroimaging-derived networks are presented in Fig. 8.3 (bottom left). Note that each network has a rather diverse array of cortical representations, where each region of the network needs to be interconnected for a particular domain to function, meaning that connectivity is directly dependent on the health of axon integrity, ergo, and brain white matter. Accordingly, where traumatic pathology of any type may reside, the location of the pathology may not be as important as knowing how a particular network is affected. The importance of this point is that any focal TBI pathology has the potential to distally affect and disrupt the network far from the specific source of the pathology.

The image on the right of Fig. 8.3 provides a schematic of what is referred to as a "Rich Club" network, which euphemistically refers to the most critical parts of the network, including critical central hubs [14]. The importance of the network in this illustration is signified by the width of the connector lines and size of the hub icon. On the periphery of a network, minor connector points or nodes of a network probably have some redundancy with other aspects of the network where either via network adjustment or re-routing minimal to no damage to the network occurs, when that minor node is damaged. In this scenario of reworking the network, over time the effects of the injury may not be functionally detectable. On the other hand, if there is substantial pathology directly affecting a major hub, then more devastating effects occur, or if numerous peripheral nodes within a system get disrupted.

Because of these limitations with neuroimaging resolution in detecting abnormalities, a simple distinction in structural imaging may be developed between lesions or abnormalities visibly identified at the macroscopic level and those more empirically or quantitatively derived from scan metrics. This distinction between visible versus empirically derived quantitative metrics will be further explored in this chapter but first some mention of the role of CT in TBI will be discussed because it is the most common initial or emergently performed structural imaging modality performed in TBI, including mTBI [6, 17–19]. As such, typically, the first neuroimaging findings in TBI are CT based, providing important baseline information even when entirely negative. This chapter will not cover functional neuroimaging or magnetic resonance (MR) spectroscopy (MRS) as these techniques will be covered elsewhere and have previously been reviewed by Slobounov et al. [20]. Also, fundamentals of imaging will not be covered in this chapter as a variety of publications provide such information [21, 22].

Heterogeneity of mTBI

As already alluded to and shown in Figs. 8.1 and 8.2, no two head injuries are identical [23]. Even with the careful precision of animal models no two injuries can ever be identically replicated [24]. If one now adds to the complexity, individual differences in human development and experience (the brain is an experience/age-dependent organ), combined with genetic endowment and whatever unique circumstances that occur with each injury, an incredible mix of events and circumstance accompanies every injury. So, the pathology that is detectable via neuroimaging techniques will never be identical across individuals but there are common pathologies. As will be explained in greater detail throughout this chapter, particular vulnerability of white matter (WM) underlies much of the pathology associated with mTBI. The majority of axons are myelinated; with the vulnerability of WM damage from trauma, the WM designation infers that the axon element of the neuron is particularly susceptible in TBI. Interneuronal connection occurs via axons; thus, WM pathology in TBI may be considered a problem of neural connectivity, disruptive of the WM architecture that makes up neural networks as depicted in Fig. 8.3. With a neuron's cell body densely compacted within the gray matter neuropil and held tightly within this matrix of cell bodies, the axon extension becomes vulnerable because WM pathways course in multiple directions of various lengths creating a bend and interwoven lattice work of projecting axons. This makes WM especially vulnerable to stretch, strain, and tensile effects following mechanical deformation that occurs with impact injury [17, 18, 25, 26]. This is depicted in Fig. 8.4, which shows that only certain WM tracts are actually damaged within a particular biomechanical strain field (see [27]). Watanabe et al. [28] have shown how with each individual impact injury, unique influences occur from the biomechanical movement of the brain within the cranium in relation to body impact. In

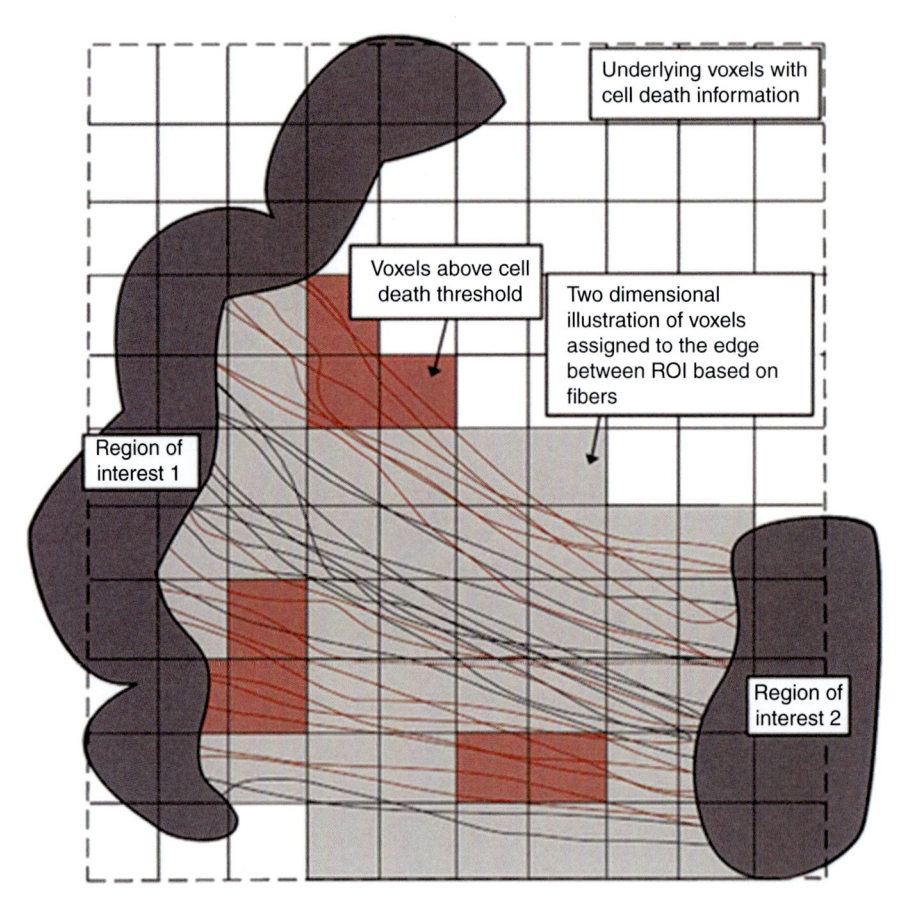

Fig. 8.4 This schematic shows how different axon trajectories may or may not be vulnerable to injury. As can be seen, there are only certain sectors where the biomechanical deformation sufficiently alters brain parenchyma to damage axons. *Lines* represent hypothetical axon projections from one gray matter structure to another. Note that even though all connect region of interest (ROI) 1 with ROI 2, and that out of all sectors where these hypothetical axons project, only eight of the sectors experienced sufficient deformation to damage axons because of the differences in crossing routes and trajectories numerous axons that were affected. (From Kraft et al. [27]; used with permission)

particular, Watanabe et al. show that with basic biomechanical modeling of injury that as the upper brainstem merges into the region of the base of the thalamus and internal capsular area, this also represents the center of parenchymal movement with simple acceleration and rotation. The point to make with this observation, is that some of the greatest strain occurs subcortically. However, the Watanabe et al. simulations also demonstrated that each injury produced unique brain displacement based on individual characteristics of impact biomechanics. These unique individual differences, when coupled with the fact that neural tissue has different elastic properties that are region and structure dependent [25], further reinforces the concept that no two injuries from mTBI will ever produce identical pathology detectable by neuroimaging. More about the biomechanics and regions of vulnerability will be reviewed at the end of the chapter.

Time Sequence of Neuropathology Associated with mTBI

There can be no dispute that an acute brain injury has occurred in a witnessed traumatic event associated with positive loss of consciousness (LOC) and obvious biomechanical forces. Therefore, such cases represent the best model for understanding the time sequence of symptom resolution and return to baseline function. The case shown in Fig. 8.5, which displays a negative DOI CT scan, provides such an example. This young adult female sustained an mTBI in an auto-pedestrian accident. She was struck by a passing car while standing next to her vehicle with family members nearby, but no other family member was struck or injured. She was thrown into the air striking her head on the curb, resulting in immediate LOC (no skull fracture), which lasted 2–3 min according to eyewitness family members present at the time of the accident. Emergency medical services were on the scene within 10 min, where they found her conscious but confused. She had orthopedic injuries to her legs (ligament knee injuries) and was stabilized and transported to the emergency department (ED) with a GCS of 15 noted on intake. During ED observation over the next couple of hours, GCS fluctuated between 13 and 15. With the head DOI CT being negative (see Fig. 8.5; top left), but given the severity of the impact, positive LOC, and fluctuating level of GCS she was monitored overnight and discharged the next day, with outpatient follow-up provided through the hospital concussion care program. Interestingly, her postconcussive symptoms (PCS) of headache, mental confusion, lethargy, and sleepiness increased in the days that followed. Some have speculated that PCS reaches its apex on the DOI and then dissipates. While true for some, peak symptoms following mTBI may occur hours to days postinjury [29, 30], which was the case with this patient. She was a student and attempted to go back to her studies approximately 3 weeks postinjury but experienced major cognitive challenges, especially problems with focused and sustained attention along with fatigue. Because of the persistence in symptoms and that MRI studies had not been done, several weeks postinjury an MRI was obtained which demonstrated residual hemosiderin deposition scattered in the right frontal region as shown in Fig. 8.5, which also corresponded to scattered WM hyperintensities. These abnormalities remained

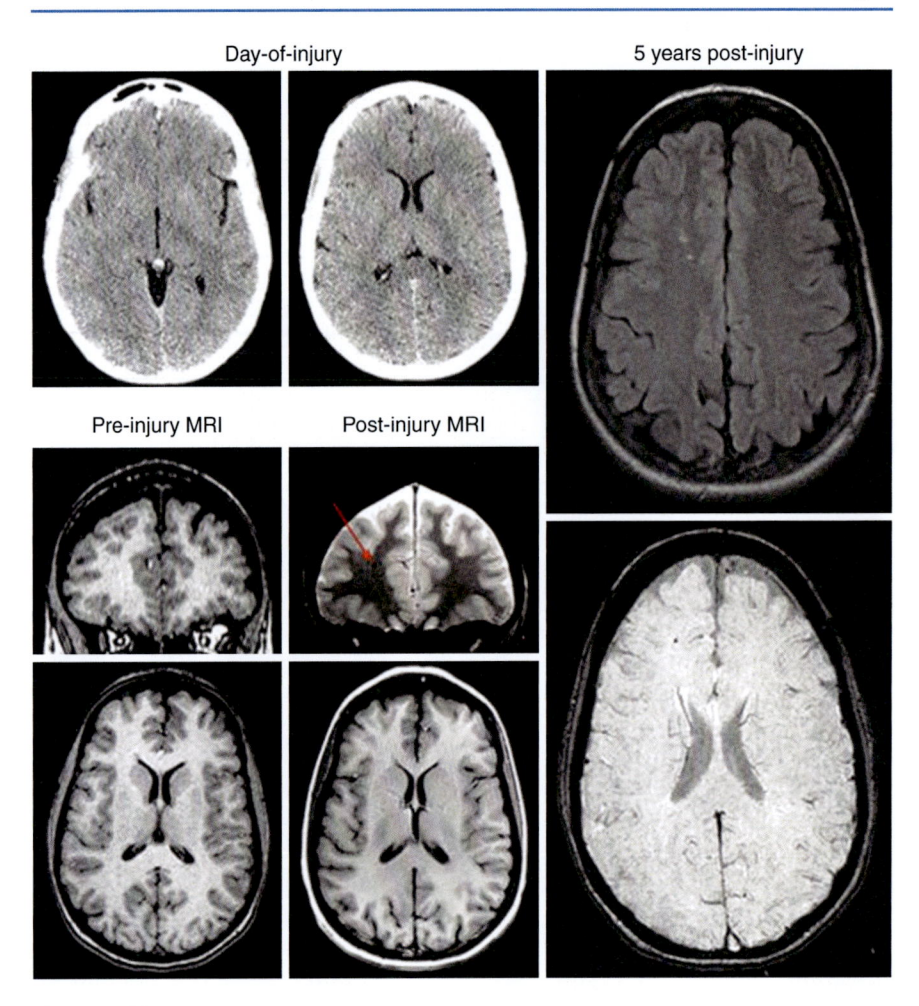

Fig. 8.5 This young adult sustained a significant mTBI in an auto-pedestrian injury where she had positive LOC, but the DOI CT revealed no abnormality. However, as symptoms persisted, this patient was assessed with MRI which revealed hemosiderin and focal white matter hyperintensities. Interestingly, this patient had participated as a research subject prior to the injury, confirming no prior brain abnormalities, as shown in the preinjury MRI, although only a T1-weighted MRI had been performed

stable over the next 5 years of follow-up and represent common neuroimaging sequelae associated with mTBI. The follow-up scans objectively document the damage from the mTBI and also demonstrate the insensitivity of CT in detecting some microhemorrhages and WM pathology associated with mild injury as well as other pathologies that undoubtedly, given the MRI findings, were present on the DOI but below the threshold for CT detection. With regard to the timeline of symptom onset, what is of particular interest as demonstrated in this case is that it took several days for the full effects of the mTBI to be manifested and weeks to diminish but chronic deficits remained as would be expected given the MRI findings, consistent with shear damage within the frontal lobes.

Although the positive LOC in mTBI is abrupt and an obvious indicator of TBI, by definition for mTBI it has to be brief and transient or, otherwise, the injury would no longer be considered "mild." LOC is also not a criterion for sustaining mTBI [31]. The evolution of symptoms/problems associated with the initial injury, regardless of whether there is alteration in level of consciousness, likely has much to do with complex cellular responses to the mechanical deformation of brain parenchyma following injury [32, 33]. Indeed, the fact that there may be an evolution of the pathophysiology of mTBI subsequent to the initial injury is well established [31, 34], as reviewed in the previous edition of *Concussion in Athletics*. Although mTBI is initiated by an event involving traumatic deformation of neural tissue, the event does not induce a singular, universal pathological event, but initiates the most complex array of structural and physiological changes in brain parenchyma. If the biomechanical deformation is minimal, only transient disruption in neuron integrity may occur [3, 26, 35]. This is depicted in the schematic presented in Fig. 8.6 [36], based on cultured neurons, that have been mechanically stretched to mimic injury, from minimal and transient to maximal with permanent damage. This illustration provides a nice heuristic, albeit simplistic, to visualize

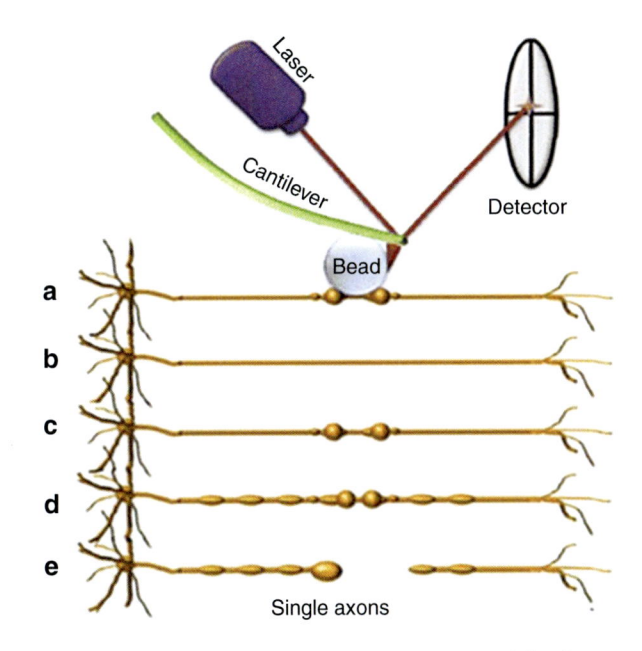

Fig. 8.6 This illustration depicts various potential axonal outcomes following stretch injury in an in vitro TBI model. (**a**) Shows stretch sufficient to create axon beading, which may have transient effect if minimal enough and as shown in (**b**) where axon morphology returns to baseline with no identifiable structural abnormality. However, initial beading may progress, as shown in (**c**) and (**d**), resulting in axon discontinuity and degeneration as shown in (**e**). (From Magdesian et al. [36]; used with permission)

what may occur following mTBI. Note, in this heuristic, transient injury may not lead to structural damage. In such a scenario, the injury did not reach a severity threshold where reparative influences could not overcome the initial cascade of potentially permanent damaging effects from the traumatic pathophysiological events. However, with more significant perturbation, the deformation may begin a process that results in irregular axon morphology and synaptic discontinuities to complete axonal degradation.

In Fig. 8.6, if structural neuroimaging is performed at point "b" in the illustration, there may be no structural neuroimaging counterpoint to show the injury or the damage that was initially induced. As such, the timing issue when neuroimaging is performed also relates to the complexity of what attends even a mild injury. Since when and what type of pathology is expressed further complicates what may be detected with neuroimaging techniques at any point in time postinjury, this underscores the importance of multimodality neuroimaging. For example, the pathobiological complexity mTBI based on severity and time postinjury can be readily demonstrated via in vitro models of stretch injury [37–39]. In their rodent model, Morrison et al. [38] used cultured cells, and then subjected them to stretch injury of different severity. Dependent on the severity of stretch and time postinjury, differences in damage occurred. For some cells, damage may be immediately sufficient to cause cell death, whereas other cells may just be rendered physiologically unstable but with the potential to return to baseline, whereas others progressively die or survive. Those who survive do so with the potential for altered physiological and structural properties.

Churchill and colleagues [40] (see also [41–43]) demonstrate this fluctuating change by plotting how dynamic influences in structural and functional pathologies may emerge in neuroimaging over time as depicted in Fig. 8.7. A take-home message from this illustration, as stated by Churchill et al. is that "Different physiologic aspects of the brain have different concussive recovery times, which can be observed by using MRI." How and when the physiological changes occur also influences when structural changes might be observed.

If a concussive injury is to be but a transient perturbation of physiological integrity, a large array of cellular functions must overtime return to homeostatic baseline. Translating this into what may occur in human mTBI, Fig. 8.8 shows how cognitive and neuroimaging findings change over time in mTBI during the first 8 days [44]. All of these mTBI patients had experienced an "uncomplicated" mTBI, meaning that no abnormalities were identified in the DOI CT scan, almost all with a GCS of 15 and all owing to the result of some type of motor vehicle accident. All subjects were assessed within 2 days of injury, and serially at days 3–4, 5–6, and 7–8 postinjury. Alternate forms of the Hopkins Verbal Learning Test-Recall (HVLT-R) were administered at each time point and, as can be seen in Fig. 8.8, memory performance typically dipped between days 3 and 6, suggesting the confluence of primary and secondary effects from mTBI reaching their apex at this point. Interestingly, these subjects were also assessed at each time point with MRI and diffusion tensor imaging (DTI), where the fractional anisotropy (FA) measurement was obtained on

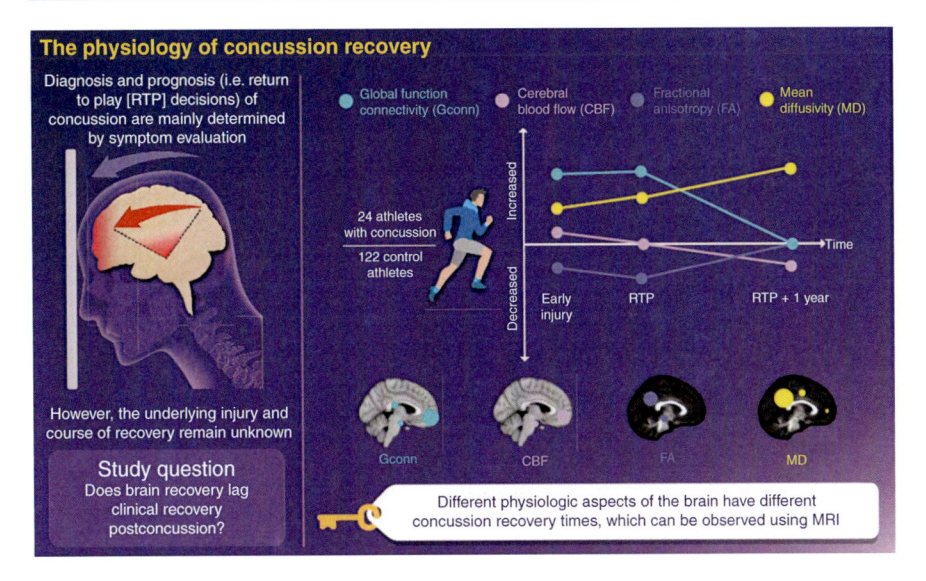

Fig. 8.7 This illustration is from Churchill et al. [40] and illustrates how different neuroimaging modalities detect changes over time in mild TBI. (Reproduced with permission from Neurology)

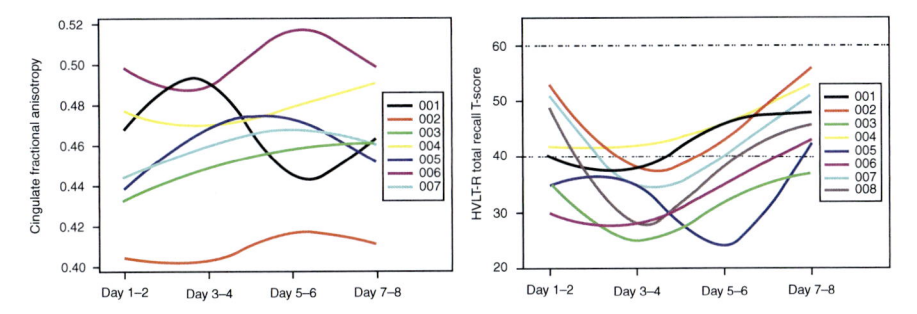

Fig. 8.8 Fractional anisotropy (FA) serial plots over the first 8 days postinjury for seven mTBI patients plotted with corresponding memory performance on the Hopkins Verbal Learning Test-Recall (HVLT-R) performed on the same day as the neuroimaging (note one patient did not have the serial neuroimaging performed). Note the fluctuation in FA, but also the general reduction in memory performance between days 3–4 and 7–8. (From Wilde et al. [44]; used with permission)

each occasion. As plotted in Fig. 8.8, FA exhibited variable fluctuations within each individual as did memory function over the first 8 days postinjury. In mTBI, acute increases in FA may reflect neuroinflammation [3] and, as seen in Fig. 8.8, several mTBI patients showed FA peaks between days 3–4 and 7–8. Decrease in FA may reflect axon damage but without preinjury neuroimaging to know precisely where each individual's FA baseline made it difficult to fully interpret these findings. However, from a memory performance perspective, almost all showed a decrease after day 1–2, with PCS symptoms reaching their peak around day 3. This does suggest that the variability in FA during this acute/subacute time frame may reflect instability of WM microstructure associated with the injury.

Computed Tomography in mTBI

CT imaging is especially rapid and, with contemporary technology, can be completed within seconds to minutes in the acutely injured individual. Since it uses X-ray beam technology, it is not influenced by paramagnetic objects like those which occur with MRI and, therefore, life support and other medical assist devices do not necessarily interfere with image acquisition or preclude its use. Likewise, metallic fragments from injury that may be paramagnetic can be imaged without concern about displacement by the strong magnetic fields generated by MRI, although image distortion occurs. Excellent contrast between bone and brain parenchyma can be achieved with CT, where CT clearly has the advantage over MRI in demonstrating the presence and location of skull fractures, common sequelae with head injury. CT also provides methods for examining cerebrovascular integrity, blood flow, and inflammation in TBI [45].

In mTBI, the commonly identified abnormalities that can be visualized using CT imaging are surface contusions typically at the brain-skull interface, petechial hemorrhages, and/or localized edema (see Fig. 8.1). The presence of petechial hemorrhage in TBI is considered a marker of DAI [3], two examples of which are shown in Fig. 8.9. Skull fracture is also readily identifiable with CT and must be considered as an indicator of potential brain injury because the distinct forces necessary to fracture bone are certainly sufficient to injure brain parenchyma. Often because of

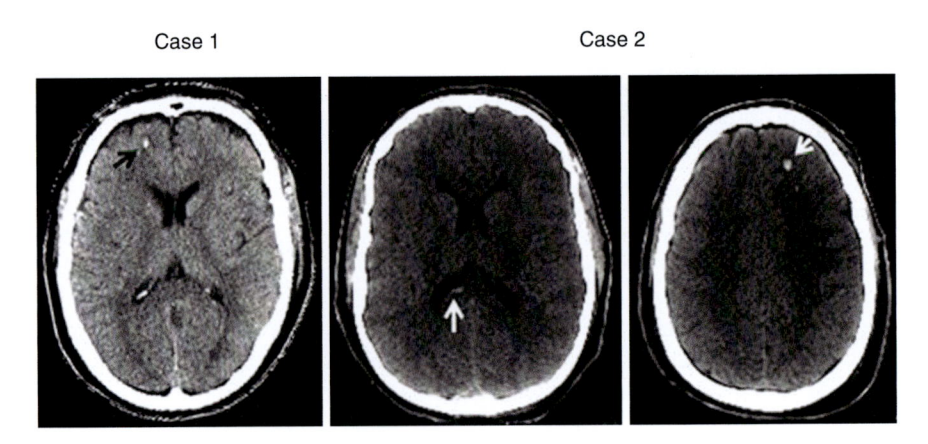

Fig. 8.9 CT appearance of petechial hemorrhage in two separate cases. Note the proximity of the lesion within the white matter but at the border of where the gray boundary is located. Both cases were adults and involved high-speed motor vehicle accidents. Note the *black arrow* in *Case 1* and the *top white arrow* in *Case 2* point to the hemorrhage which occurs right at the gray-white junction. In *Case 2* there is a contrecoup hemorrhagic lesion in the posterior corpus callosum, *bottom arrow*

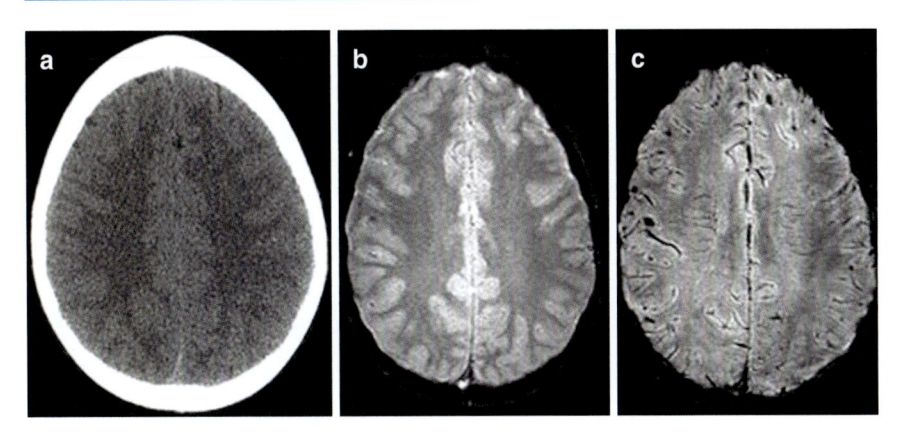

8 Neuropathology of Mild Traumatic Brain Injury: Relationship to Structural... 159

Fig. 8.10 The insensitivity of CT (**a**) and conventional gradient recalled echo (GRE, **b**) sequences to detect petechial hemorrhage are shown. The CT scan was interpreted to be within normal limits with no hemorrhage identified yet this individual agreed to participate in a research study and, therefore, was scanned with MRI procedures including susceptibility weighted imaging (SWI) as shown in (**c**) and magnetization transfer imaging (MTI, not shown), both show frontal abnormality and residual hemorrhage. (From Bigler [60]; used with permission)

the limited resolution of CT, even in the presence of some type of skull fracture in an individual with mTBI, parenchyma may appear normal on CT. Of course, just because neural tissue may appear "normal" does not mean normal microstructure and function because that is beyond the scope of what CT may detect [3, 11].

When an abnormality is present on the DOI CT, as stated earlier, criteria for the classification of "complicated mild TBI" are made. However, given contemporary advances that identify mTBI abnormalities that simply are not detected by CT imaging, this classification is mostly meaningless. Figure 8.5 demonstrated this point and another case is shown in Fig. 8.10. The presence of hemosiderin deposition is presumed to be the best marker for the existence of traumatic shear injury [3]. Currently, the superior MRI method for detecting hemorrhagic shear lesions in mTBI is susceptibility weighted imaging (SWI).

CT imaging readily identifies more serious acute injuries or evolving TBI pathologies that require neurosurgical intervention and is of critical importance in the initial triage and medical management of TBI, including mTBI [18, 46]. With that being said, however, it is of limited utility in mTBI [19].

Visible Macroscopic Abnormalities

To best understand what information may be gathered from MRI in TBI, it is important to appreciate that the abnormalities are, in part, as previously mentioned, time dependent and differ by primary as well as secondary injury effects. Bigler and Maxwell [47, 48] have outlined a time frame depicting the potential pathological changes that occur as presented in the schematic shown in Fig. 8.11, which depicts

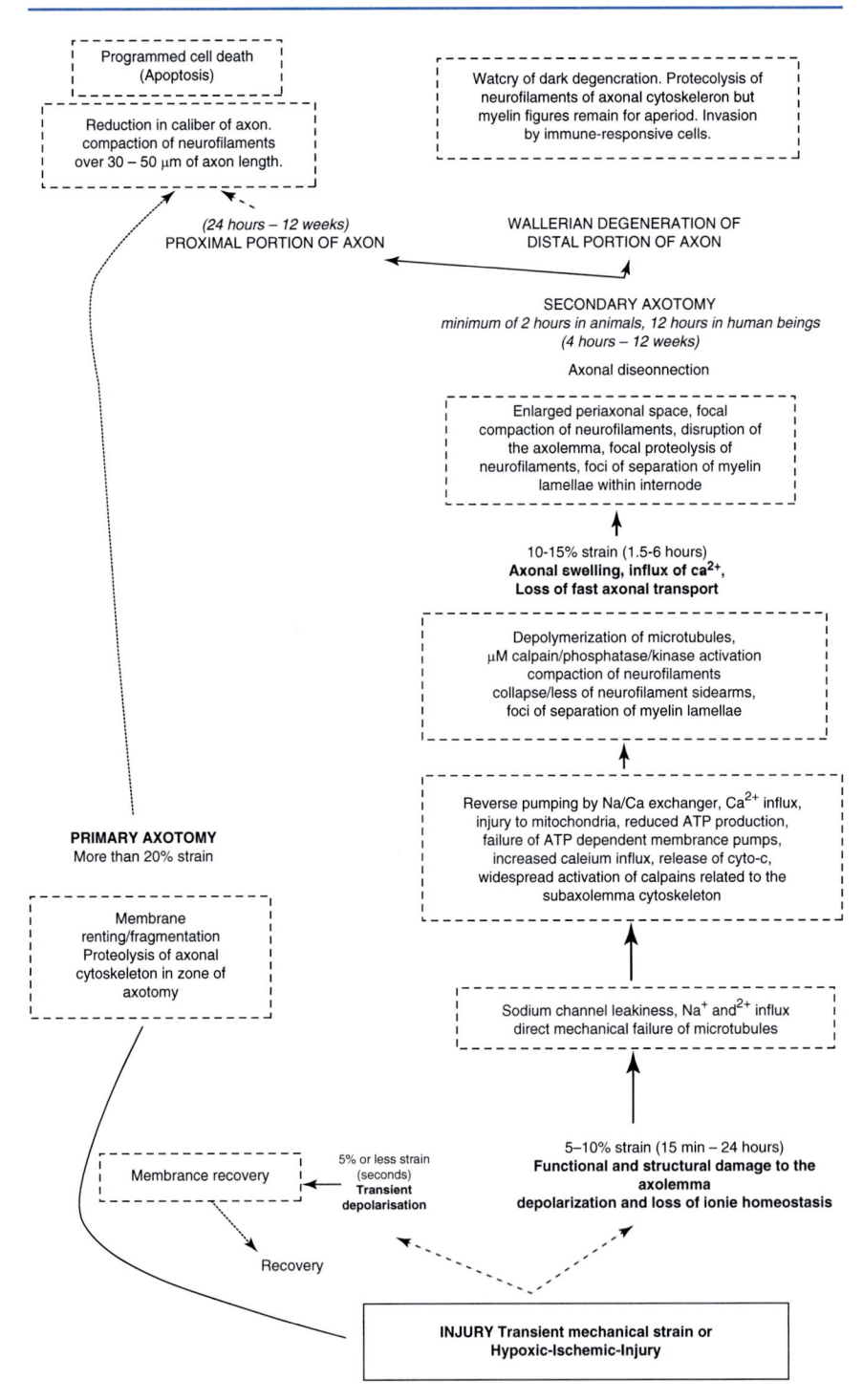

Fig. 8.11 Schematic overview of current thinking with regard to axonal injury in human DAI and animal diffuse traumatic brain injury. (Modified from Biasca and Maxwell [35] and from Bigler and Maxwell [47]; used with permission)

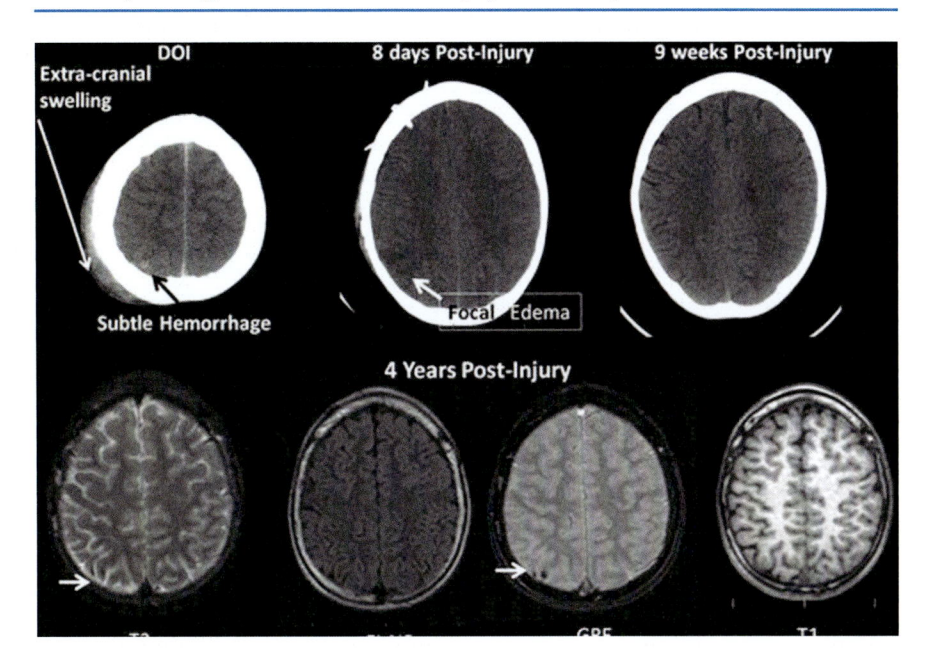

Fig. 8.12 Starting with the DOI CT scans, various lesion types are identified and using the DOI scan as baseline, changes from DOI to chronic state may be shown. The "lesion" starts off as a subtle subarachnoid hemorrhage, but by 8 days postinjury, it is seen as edema which appears to resolve by 9 weeks postinjury. However, with follow-up MRI, subtle hemosiderin deposition is identified

how visibly detectable lesions change over time. Characteristic primary and secondary pathologies can be readily defined when sequential imaging is performed, typically a combination of CT and MRI, as shown in Fig. 8.12.

In Fig. 8.12, the acute CT findings depict the faint appearance of blood, mostly likely indicative of a traumatic subarachnoid hemorrhage. The presence of hemorrhage in TBI, whether detected by CT or MRI, is commonly considered the best indicator of intracranial traumatic shear forces sufficient to produce traumatic axonal injury (TAI) [47, 48], since there was obvious biomechanical force to induce hemorrhage. However, even with the best of resolution that CT imaging provides, precise detection and localization of significant pathology is limited as demonstrated in Fig. 8.12. By 8 days postinjury, edema is identified, but the hemorrhage has basically resolved where phagocytosis has removed degraded blood by-products. By 2 months postinjury, CT imaging demonstrates what appears to be resolution. However, when scanned 4 years later with MRI, hemosiderin deposition is distinctly apparent not in the subarachnoid space, but within brain parenchyma. Imaging of the gyri where the hemorrhage was identified also distinctly demonstrates signal abnormality beyond the hemosiderin foci. When viewed with MRI and knowing the sequence of events, the initial impact forces in this region likely sheared both blood vessels and neural tissue, resulting in DAI and focal WM changes. However, the DOI CT mostly depicts subarachnoid hemorrhage, with little indication of underlying WM damage. Only through sequential imaging does the true clinical significance of this injury become apparent.

Combining information from Figs. 8.11 and 8.12, the primary and secondary effects of TBI can be inferred. At the point of impact, the primary injury occurs, and given the follow-up MRI findings there likely was traumatic shear injury resulting in primary axotomy. However, considerable secondary injury also likely occurred because of the edema, as well as vascular injury, and whatever local pathologic, metabolic, and neurotransmitter derangements and aberrations that occurred. Sheared blood vessels can no longer provide oxygenated blood to the neuropil resulting in additional neural tissue (both neurons and glial cells) compromise, degradation, and potential death. This becomes the source for focal atrophy. Neuronal degeneration ensues which cannot be detected by CT imaging but is revealed by MRI. This potential sequence of events and its adverse influence on the axon is depicted in Fig. 8.13 [35, 49].

Empirically Derived Quantitative MR Abnormalities

The common images generated from MR technology, like those shown in the various figures up to this point have all been generated by MR display metrics that form the basis for the image presentation. However, these quantitative MR metrics permit

Fig. 8.13 Evolving pathophysiology of traumatic injury in myelinated axons. In this figure, the author's attempts, in an abbreviated fashion, to illustrate some of the key events believed to be involved in the pathobiology of traumatic axonal injury and, thereby, identify potential therapeutic targets. Although framed in the view of primary nodal involvement (**a**), this focus does not preclude comparable change ongoing in other regions of the axon. Panels **b** and **c** show normal axonal detail including the paranodal loops and the presence of intraaxonal mitochondria, microtubules, and neurofilaments, together with the presence of multiple axolemmal channels localized primarily to the nodal domain. Mild-to-moderate traumatic brain injury in panel **d** is observed to involve a mechanical dysregulation of the voltage-sensitive sodium channels, which contribute to increased calcium influx via reversal of the sodium calcium exchanger and the opening of voltage-gated calcium channels. This also impacts on the proteolysis of sodium channel inactivation that contributes further to local calcium dysregulation. Microtubular loss, neurofilament impaction, and local mitochondrial damage can follow, which, if unabated, collectively alters/impairs axonal transport illustrated in panel **e**. Alternatively, if these abnormalities do not progress, recovery is possible (**f**). When progressive, these events not only impair axonal transport but also lead to rapid intraaxonal change in the paranodal and perhaps internodal domains that elicit the collapse of the axolemma and its overlying myelin sheath to result in lobulated and disconnected axonal segments (**g**) that, over the next 15 min–2 h, fully detach (**h**). The proximal axonal segment in continuity with the cell body of origin now continues to swell from the delivery of vesicles and organelles via anterograde transport while the downstream fiber undergoes Wallerian change (**i**). Finally, with the most severe forms of injury, the above identified calcium-mediated destructive cascades are further augmented by the poration of the axolemma, again primarily at the nodal region (**j**). The resulting calcium surge, together with potential local microtubular damage and disassembly, pose catastrophic intraaxonal change that converts anterograde into retrograde axonal transport, precluding continued axonal swelling, while the distal axonal segment fragments and disconnects (**k**), with Wallerian degeneration ensuing downstream (**l**). (From Smith et al. [49]; used with permission)

analyses separate from just the anatomical image display. For example, Fig. 8.14 shows the appearance of a DTI MR sequence with its associated color map. Two common metrics derived from DTI are referred to as fractional anisotropy or FA and apparent diffusion coefficient or ADC. Figure 8.14 provides a DTI schematic depicting the relationship of FA and ADC to axon integrity and what happens with axon

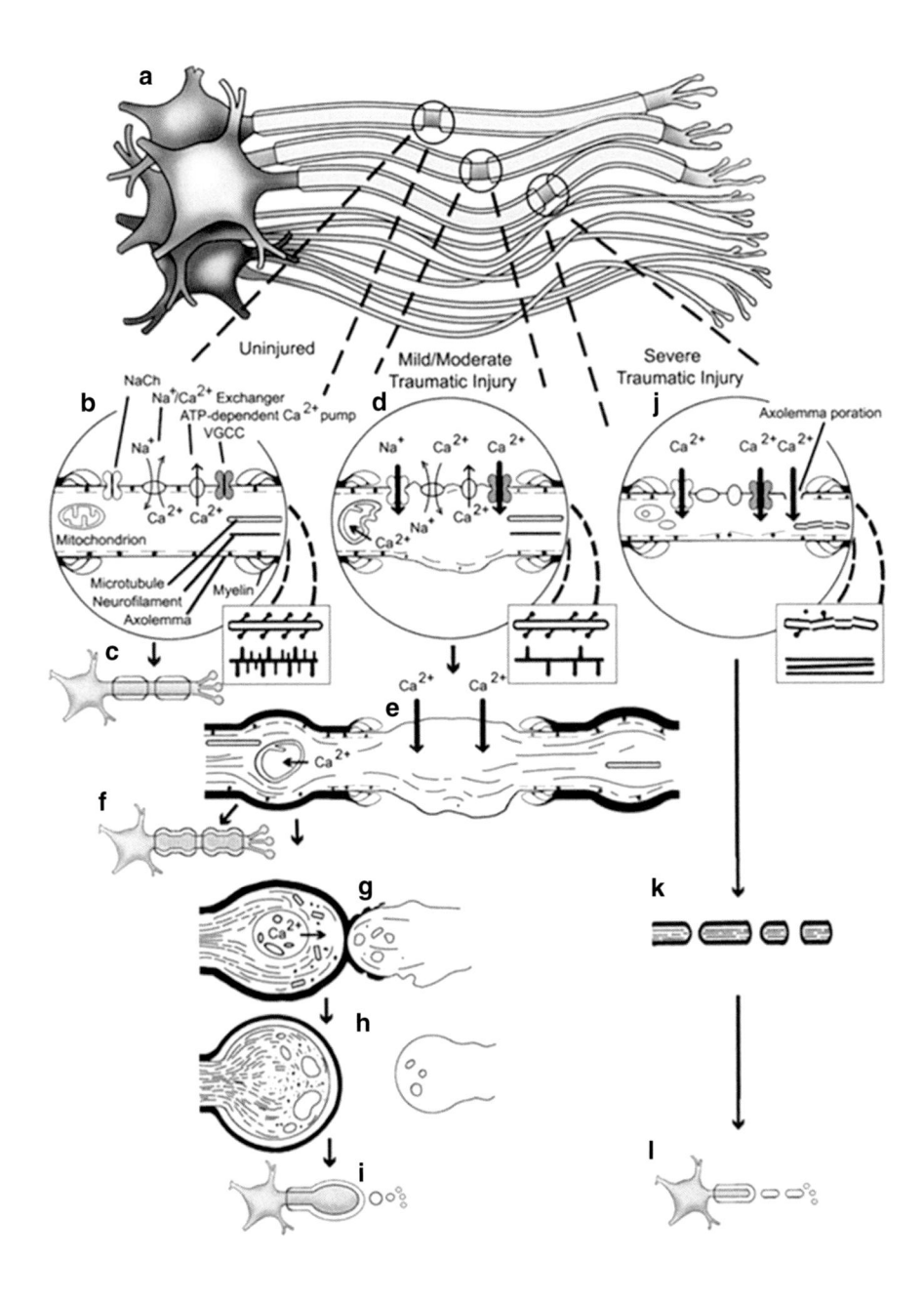

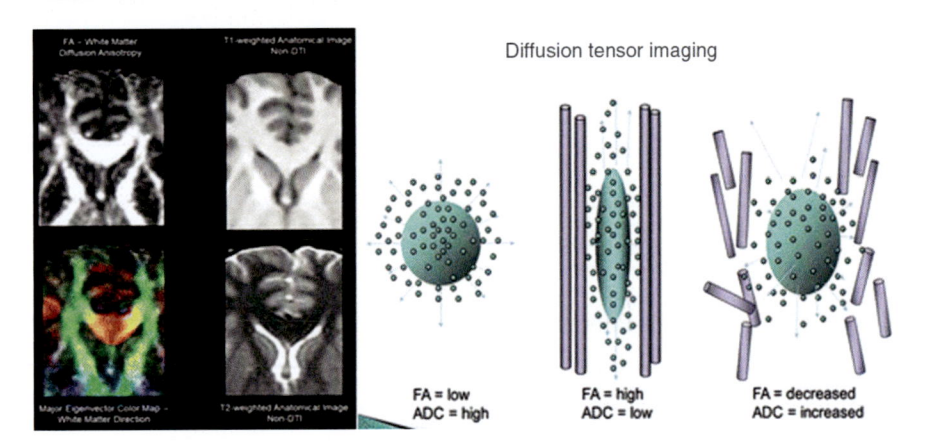

Fig. 8.14 [*Top*] The images on the *upper left* show the DTI acquisition image and the DTI color map (*middle left*) in comparison to the conventional T1 and T2. The cartoon on the *right* depicts the relationship of fractional anisotropy (FA) with the apparent diffusion coefficient (ADC) showing how normal conformity of membrane anatomy constrains water diffusion; however, if membrane dissolution occurs in any fashion, such as from TBI, water is freer to move and with lack of constraint, FA elevates and ADC declines. [*Bottom*] Results of voxel-wise meta-analysis findings of where DTI differences are most likely to occur based on the review by Hunter and Lubin [50]. Fractional anisotropy (FA) in those with TBI subjects demonstrated one cluster of high FA (red) in the right superior longitudinal fasciculus and seven clusters of low FA (blue), the largest two located in the corpus callosum

damage. These DTI metrics assess the microstructure of WM and are based on the characteristics of how myelin sheaths and cell membranes of WM tracts affect the movement of water molecules. Healthy axonal membranes constrain the free movement and direction of movement of water. Consequently, water molecules tend to move faster in parallel to nerve fibers rather than perpendicular to them. This characteristic, which is referred to as anisotropic diffusion and is measured by FA, is determined by the thickness of the myelin sheath and of the axons. FA ranges from 0 to 1, where 0 represents maximal isotropic diffusion (e.g., free diffusion in perfect sphere) and 1 represents maximal anisotropic diffusion, that is, diffusion in one direction (e.g., a long cylinder of minimal diameter). Diffusion anisotropy varies across WM regions, putatively reflecting differences in fiber myelination, fiber diameter, and directionality.

The aggregate fiber tracts of an entire brain can be derived from DTI, as shown in Fig. 8.15. In TBI, DTI may demonstrate a loss of fiber tract integrity, reflected as a thinning out of the number of aggregate tracts. This is also demonstrated in Fig. 8.15, where a patient with TBI is compared to a similar aged individual with typical development. The loss of aggregate tracts in the TBI whole-brain network analysis demonstrates an overall reduction in WM connectivity. DTI methods provide various techniques to view the pathological effects of TBI within the context of WM network connectivity.

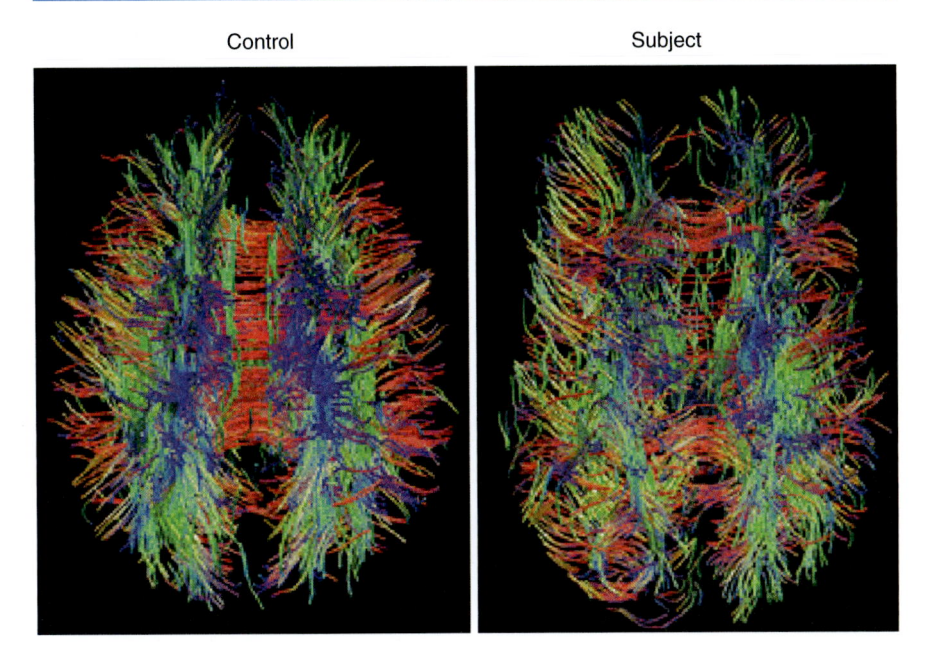

Fig. 8.15 DTI-derived aggregate tracts of the brain can be visualized where in a healthy adult, the dorsal view of the control participant on the left depicts the dense organization of fiber tracts where green streamlines show tract orientation (red/orange = laterally projecting tracts, blue = vertically orientated tracts and green = anterior-posterior projections). In the TBI subject on the right who had sustained a severe TBI, thinning of the tracts is visibly obvious implicating widespread loss of white matter integrity

When DTI metrics are applied to milder injuries, the dramatic changes as visualized in Fig. 8.15 are typically not observed but at a group level, a variety of characteristic changes in WM integrity may be detected. For example, returning to Fig. 8.14, the illustration from Hunter and Lubin [50] summarizes DTI findings involving an mTBI review and meta-analysis of quantitative DTI findings, where the most overlapping abnormalities have been reported. As shown in Fig. 8.14 (bottom), the most common FA changes are consistently observed in mild TBI that occurs within the corpus callosum.

Trauma-induced edematous reactions in the brain compress parenchyma, which in turn, may influence water diffusion potentially detected by DTI. Using the FA metric, increases in FA beyond some normal baseline may signify neuroinflammation, whereas low FA may occur when axon degradation and membrane abnormalities increase water diffusion or when actual degeneration has occurred, which increases extracellular water [3]. Since TBI may induce dynamic changes over time, differences in FA over acute, subacute, and chronic time frames postinjury may differ as well. When axons degenerate, the increased space frees extracellular water, resulting in lower FA. Thus, in mTBI, low FA may reflect WM degeneration with increased FA beyond normative baseline, and may indicate neuroinflammation [51, 52].

Heterogeneity Visible mTBI Lesions

Bigler et al. [8] examined a sample of 41 children with complicated mTBI. When assessed with MRI at least 6 months postinjury, regardless of whether the residual lesion was an area of focal encephalomalacia, hemosiderin deposit, or WM hyperintensity, *none* of the lesions perfectly overlapped, although the majority were distributed within the frontal and temporal lobes. Just from the randomness of the lesions, this would indicate that each mTBI produced its own unique injury and with unique injury this would indicate the likelihood that mTBI sequelae would likely be rather idiosyncratic to the individual as well.

Cellular Basis of mTBI Neuropathology

Based on the position statement by the International and Interagency Initiative toward Common Data Elements for Research on Traumatic Brain Injury and Psychological Health, the definition of traumatic brain injury is "… an alteration in brain function, or other evidence of brain pathology, caused by an external force [31]." External force induces brain injury via deformation of neural tissue that surpasses tolerance limits for normal displacement or strain that accompanies movement such as jumping, rapid turning of the head, and simple bumps to the head. So, at the most fundamental level of injury, cellular deformation disrupts anatomy and physiology sufficient to at least transiently impair function when the threshold for mTBI has been reached.

Too often, neural cells are viewed schematically as an artist's rendition of what a neural cell looks like, such as that shown in Fig. 8.16, but artistic schematics detract from the true complexity and delicate nature of what really constitutes neural tissue. For example, Fig. 8.16 depicts two cortical pyramidal cells identified in the rat cerebral cortex based on their physiological response and their appearance via electron microscopy. Note how small these structures are and that these views are merely two dimensional of a three-dimensional structure and note that the axon is but a few microns in thickness. Additionally, note the numerous dendritic spines and how the axon intertwines with the spines. Understanding this delicate balance of what generates brain parenchyma makes it easier to understand why deformation of neural tissue may be injurious.

As the definition implies, TBI occurs from some external force, which in turn must deform brain parenchyma such that a sufficient distortion of the typical shape of cellular tissue no longer lines up and/or connects as it should. Returning to Fig. 8.16, note again the complex intertwining of dendritic spines with axon segments where any misalignment would likely affect synaptic integrity. Likewise, if the axon membrane is disrupted, membrane permeability will directly impact neuronal function and propagation of axon potentials. Only one axon segment needs to be affected to disrupt neural transmission for the entire axon. A variety of finite elements and various methods for recreating the motion that displaces brain parenchyma that results in concussive injury have been performed, mostly using sports

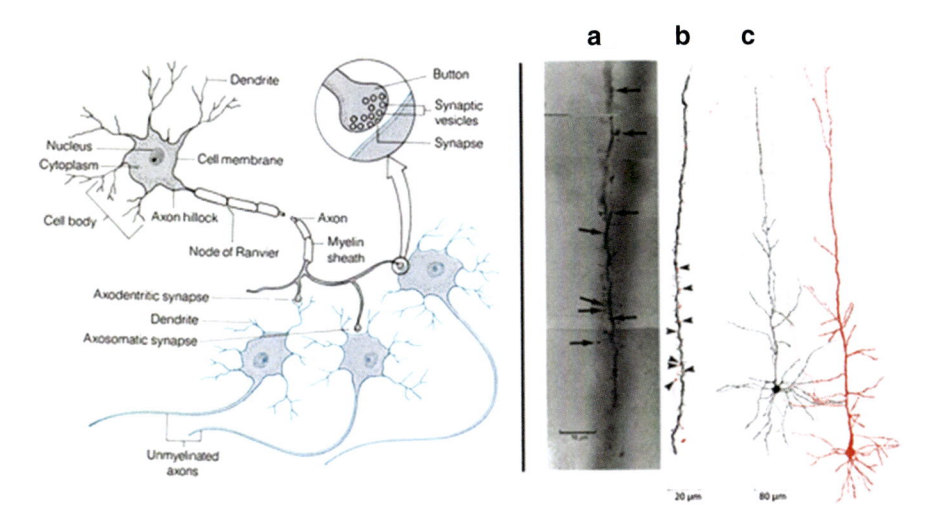

Fig. 8.16 (*Left*) The schematic of a neuron shows a hypothetical neuron with what appears to be a bulky, sturdy axon protruding from the cell body and interfacing with other neurons. However, the reality is something quite different. (From Pinel [61]; used with permission). (*Right*) Two cortical cells in a rat cortex that have been isolated. Note the micron level of the axon—it is infinitesimally small. Note also how the single axon intertwines the dendrite and the dendritic spines as highlighted in the photomicrograph. When thinking about TBI, one must view the potential neuropathological effects at this microscopic level. (From Deuchars et al. [62]; used with permission)

concussion models. For example, Viano et al. [53] showed on average in the typical sports-related concussion that the brain displaces between 4 and 8 mm in regions like the corpus callosum, midbrain, medial temporal lobe, and fornix. Viewing Fig. 8.16 from the perspective of this amount of deformation, noting that the photomicrograph depicts an axon that is about 0.1 mm in length, would reflect a massive distortion of neurons of this size.

Blood vessels are just as delicate as neural tissue, especially at the capillary level. Each neuron is dependent on receiving a continuous source of glucose and oxygen with the smallest capillaries large enough for just a single red blood cell to traverse the capillary to deliver its oxygen and glucose [47, 48]. As such, blood vessels are just as susceptible to the shear–strain biomechanics of head injury as are neurons [54].

Deformation Biomechanics and the Most Vulnerable Areas for Brain Injury

From the above discussion, all deformation in mTBI must be viewed at the cellular level, but biomechanical schematics are typically presented at the whole brain level. Ropper and Gorson [55] provided a schematic of where the greatest deformations have been modeled in mTBI and this is provided in Fig. 8.17. This illustration clearly depicts the known frontotemporal regions for cortical surface compression, but also WM tracts of the upper brainstem corpus callosum and cingulum. In mTBI,

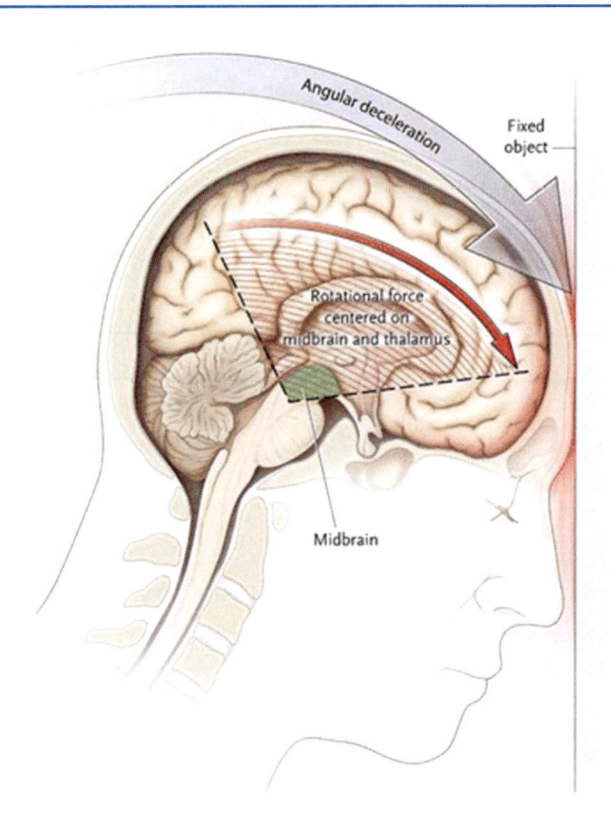

Fig. 8.17 The mechanism of concussion is outlined in this illustration. Biomechanical investigations dating back to the beginning of the twentieth century suggest that concussion results from a rotational motion of the cerebral hemispheres in the anterior-posterior plane, around the fulcrum of the fixed-in-place upper brain stem. If the neck is restrained, concussion is difficult to produce. Concussions as portrayed in movies and cartoons, in which the back of the head is struck with a blunt object and no motion is transferred to the brain, are implausible. The modern view is that there is disruption of the electrophysiological and subcellular activities of the neurons of the reticular activating system that are situated in the midbrain and diencephalic region, where the maximal rotational forces are exerted. Alternative mechanisms for concussive LOC, such as self-limited cortical seizures or a sudden increase in intracranial pressure, have also been proposed, but with limited supporting evidence. An animated version of this figure is available with the full text of the article at www.nejm.org. (From Ropper and Gorson [55]; used with permission)

as already mentioned by definition of what constitutes a TBI, the WM abnormalities at the brainstem level could not represent major pathology because LOC must be brief to meet mTBI criteria. Likewise, alteration in mental status that would result in prolonged posttraumatic amnesia would also disqualify someone for mTBI classification. So while subtle brainstem pathology may persist in the mTBI patient, as Heitger et al. [56] have shown, as well as frontotemporal pathology, as numerous investigators have shown, major pathologies at these levels are unlikely because if major pathology persisted in these regions during the acute phase, the individual likely would not meet criteria for mTBI. Nonetheless, the one that is depicted in

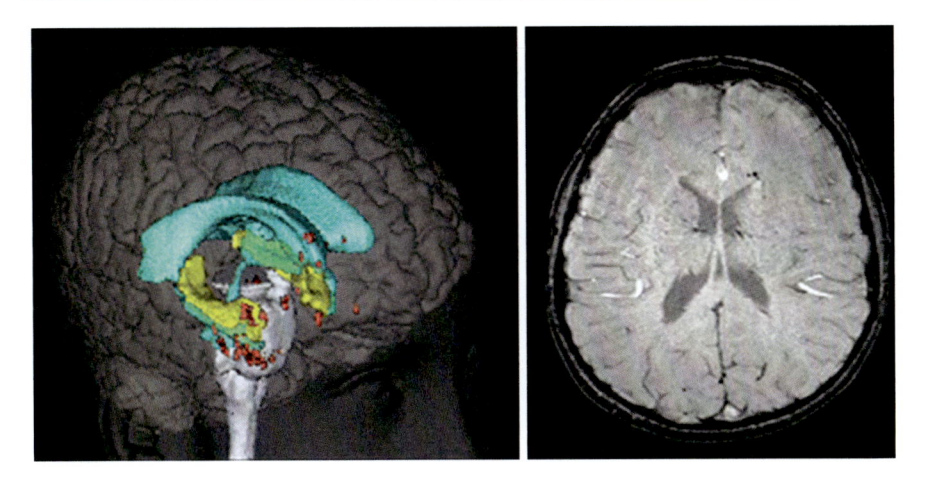

Fig. 8.18 This preadolescent child sustained an mTBI in a ski accident. When symptoms persisted, MRI demonstrated multiple regions of hemosiderin deposition. Note the frontotemporal distribution and location of hemosiderin in the forceps minor region of the corpus callosum on the susceptibility weighted image on the *right*. In the three-dimensional image, the ventricle is shown in aquamarine to provide landmark points with the *red* signifying where hemosiderin was identified, and the *yellow* indicates the hippocampus

Fig. 8.17 from Ropper and Gorson provides a wonderful heuristic for where likely changes in mTBI will be observed in neuroimaging studies.

For example, Fig. 8.18 is from a child with mTBI from a skiing accident who sustained an mTBI. When symptoms persisted, this child, who had a negative DOI CT, was scanned with MRI. The follow-up MRI revealed hemosiderin deposition in frontotemporal areas and anterior corpus callosum, as would be predicted from the schematic in Fig. 8.17. Likewise, note from Fig. 8.14 that the corpus callosum is a common area of DTI defined WM pathology from mTBI.

Volumetry Findings in mTBI

As shown in Fig. 8.17, if atrophic changes associated with mTBI were to occur, they would most likely be found within those regions associated with the greatest likelihood for shear/strain and deformation injury. Indeed, several studies that have prospectively examined mTBI subjects have demonstrated this regional atrophy [3, 57, 58]. For example, Zhou et al. [59] demonstrated that by establishing a baseline in mTBI patients within the acute to early subacute time frame that when assessed with various volumetric techniques 1 year later that significant volume loss was observed in the anterior cingulum, cingulate gyrus, and scattered regions within the frontal lobes. Interestingly, they observed volume loss in the cuneus and precuneus regions as well. The volume loss with the cuneus and precuneus, posterior brain regions, may actually be the result of Wallerian degeneration from the more focal frontal loss disrupting long-coursing frontoparietal connections particularly vulnerable to stretching and shearing effects [3]. Sussman and da Costa [58] applied volumetric analyses to assess cortical morphometry in those with mTBI and concluding the following: "… a single concussive episode induces measurable changes in brain structure manifesting as diffuse and local patterns of altered neuromorphometry (p. 650)."

Conclusion

Structural neuroimaging provides a variety of methods to detect underlying neuropathology that results from mTBI. The most common visible abnormalities are in the form of focal encephalomalacia, hemosiderin deposition, and/or WM hyperintensity. A variety of quantitative MRI methods have demonstrated techniques for the detection of underlying pathology associated with mTBI, which differ depending on the time postinjury that the scan is performed.

References

1. Fidan E, et al. Metabolic and structural imaging at 7 tesla after repetitive mild traumatic brain injury in immature rats. ASN Neuro. 2018;10:1759091418770543.
2. Schweser F, et al. Visualization of thalamic calcium influx with quantitative susceptibility mapping as a potential imaging biomarker for repeated mild traumatic brain injury. NeuroImage. 2019;200:250–8.
3. Victoroff J, Bigler ED. Concussion and traumatic encephalopathy. New York: Cambridge University Press; 2019.
4. Mayer AR, et al. Radiologic common data elements rates in pediatric mild traumatic brain injury. Neurology. 2020;94(3):e241–53.
5. Bigler ED. Systems biology, neuroimaging, neuropsychology, neuroconnectivity and traumatic brain injury. Front Syst Neurosci. 2016;10:55.
6. Bigler ED. Structural neuroimaging in sport-related concussion. Int J Psychophysiol. 2018;132(Pt A):105–23.
7. Teasdale G, Knill-Jones R, van der Sande J. Observer variability in assessing impaired consciousness and coma. J Neurol Neurosurg Psychiatry. 1978;41(7):603–10.
8. Bigler ED, et al. Heterogeneity of brain lesions in pediatric traumatic brain injury. Neuropsychology. 2013;27(4):438–51.
9. Perez-Polo JR, et al. A rodent model of mild traumatic brain blast injury. J Neurosci Res. 2015;93(4):549–61.
10. Hylin MJ, et al. Behavioral and histopathological alterations resulting from mild fluid percussion injury. J Neurotrauma. 2013;30(9):702–15.
11. Hoogenboom WS, et al. Diffusion tensor imaging of the evolving response to mild traumatic brain injury in rats. J Exp Neurosci. 2019;13:1179069519858627.
12. Raizman R, et al. Traumatic brain injury severity in a network perspective: a diffusion MRI based connectome study. Sci Rep. 2020;10(1):9121.
13. Arnatkeviciute A, Fulcher BD, Fornito A. Uncovering the transcriptional correlates of hub connectivity in neural networks. Front Neural Circuits. 2019;13:47.
14. Sporns O. Structure and function of complex brain networks. Dialogues Clin Neurosci. 2013;15(3):247–62.
15. Bailey SK, et al. Applying a network framework to the neurobiology of reading and dyslexia. J Neurodev Disord. 2018;10(1):37.

16. van den Heuvel MP, Sporns O. Rich-club organization of the human connectome. J Neurosci. 2011;31(44):15775–86.
17. Bigler ED, et al. Structural neuroimaging findings in mild traumatic brain injury. Sports Med Arthrosc Rev. 2016;24(3):e42–52.
18. Douglas DB, et al. Neuroimaging of traumatic brain injury. Med Sci (Basel). 2018;7(1):2.
19. Suri AK, Lipton ML. Neuroimaging of brain trauma in sports. Handb Clin Neurol. 2018;158:205–16.
20. Slobounov S, et al. Concussion in athletics: ongoing clinical and brain imaging research controversies. Brain Imaging Behav. 2012;6(2):224–43.
21. Griauzde J, Srinivasan A. Advanced neuroimaging techniques: basic principles and clinical applications. J Neuroophthalmol. 2018;38(1):101–14.
22. Wilde EA, Hunter JV, Bigler ED. A primer of neuroimaging analysis in neurorehabilitation outcome research. NeuroRehabilitation. 2012;31(3):227–42.
23. Post A, Hoshizaki B, Gilchrist MD. Finite element analysis of the effect of loading curve shape on brain injury predictors. J Biomech. 2012;45(4):679–83.
24. Statler KD, et al. Traumatic brain injury during development reduces minimal clonic seizure thresholds at maturity. Epilepsy Res. 2008;80(2–3):163–70.
25. Smith D, et al. Multi-excitation MR elastography of the brain: wave propagation in anisotropic white matter. J Biomech Eng. 2020;142(7):0710051.
26. Okamoto RJ, et al. Insights into traumatic brain injury from MRI of harmonic brain motion. J Exp Neurosci. 2019;13:1179069519840444.
27. Kraft RH, et al. Combining the finite element method with structural connectome-based analysis for modeling neurotrauma: connectome neurotrauma mechanics. PLoS Comput Biol. 2012;8(8):e1002619.
28. Watanabe R, et al. Research of the relationship of pedestrian injury to collision speed, car-type, impact location and pedestrian sizes using human FE model (THUMS version 4). Stapp Car Crash J. 2012;56:269–321.
29. Prichep LS, et al. Time course of clinical and electrophysiological recovery after sport-related concussion. J Head Trauma Rehabil. 2013;28(4):266–73.
30. Duhaime AC, et al. Spectrum of acute clinical characteristics of diagnosed concussions in college athletes wearing instrumented helmets: clinical article. J Neurosurg. 2012;117(6):1092–9.
31. Menon DK, et al. Position statement: definition of traumatic brain injury. Arch Phys Med Rehabil. 2010;91(11):1637–40.
32. Hammad A, Westacott L, Zaben M. The role of the complement system in traumatic brain injury: a review. J Neuroinflammation. 2018;15(1):24.
33. Stahel PF, Morganti-Kossmann MC, Kossmann T. The role of the complement system in traumatic brain injury. Brain Res Brain Res Rev. 1998;27(3):243–56.
34. Kamins J, et al. What is the physiological time to recovery after concussion? A systematic review. Br J Sports Med. 2017;51(12):935–40.
35. Biasca N, Maxwell WL. Minor traumatic brain injury in sports: a review in order to prevent neurological sequelae. Prog Brain Res. 2007;161:263–91.
36. Magdesian MH, et al. Atomic force microscopy reveals important differences in axonal resistance to injury. Biophys J. 2012;103(3):405–14.
37. Rosas-Hernandez H, et al. Characterization of uniaxial high-speed stretch as an in vitro model of mild traumatic brain injury on the blood-brain barrier. Neurosci Lett. 2018;672:123–9.
38. Morrison B 3rd, et al. An in vitro model of traumatic brain injury utilising two-dimensional stretch of organotypic hippocampal slice cultures. J Neurosci Methods. 2006;150(2):192–201.
39. Dolle JP, et al. Newfound sex differences in axonal structure underlie differential outcomes from in vitro traumatic axonal injury. Exp Neurol. 2018;300:121–34.
40. Churchill NW, et al. Mapping brain recovery after concussion: from acute injury to 1 year after medical clearance. Neurology. 2019;93(21):e1980–92.
41. Churchill NW, et al. Scale-free functional brain dynamics during recovery from sport-related concussion. Hum Brain Mapp. 2020;41(10):2567–82.

42. Di Battista AP, et al. The relationship between symptom burden and systemic inflammation differs between male and female athletes following concussion. BMC Immunol. 2020;21(1):11.
43. Churchill NW, et al. Baseline vs. cross-sectional MRI of concussion: distinct brain patterns in white matter and cerebral blood flow. Sci Rep. 2020;10(1):1643.
44. Wilde EA, et al. Serial measurement of memory and diffusion tensor imaging changes within the first week following uncomplicated mild traumatic brain injury. Brain Imaging Behav. 2012;6(2):319–28.
45. Creeden S, et al. Interobserver agreement for the computed tomography severity grading scales for acute traumatic brain injury. J Neurotrauma. 2020;37(12):1445–51.
46. Bonfante E, Riascos R, Arevalo O. Imaging of chronic concussion. Neuroimaging Clin N Am. 2018;28(1):127–35.
47. Bigler ED, Maxwell WL. Neuropathology of mild traumatic brain injury: relationship to neuroimaging findings. Brain Imaging Behav. 2012;6(2):108–36.
48. Bigler ED, Maxwell WL. Neuroimaging and neuropathology of TBI. NeuroRehabilitation. 2011;28(2):63–74.
49. Smith DH, Hicks R, Povlishock JT. Therapy development for diffuse axonal injury. J Neurotrauma. 2013;30(5):307–23.
50. Hunter LE, et al. Comparing region of interest versus voxel-wise diffusion tensor imaging analytic methods in mild and moderate traumatic brain injury: a systematic review and meta-analysis. J Neurotrauma. 2019;36(8):1222–30.
51. Narayana S, et al. Neuroimaging and neuropsychological studies in sports-related concussions in adolescents: current state and future directions. Front Neurol. 2019;10:538.
52. Schneider DK, et al. Diffusion tensor imaging in athletes sustaining repetitive head impacts: a systematic review of prospective studies. J Neurotrauma. 2019;36(20):2831–49.
53. Viano DC, et al. Concussion in professional football: brain responses by finite element analysis: part 9. Neurosurgery. 2005;57(5):891–916; discussion 891–916.
54. Madri JA. Modeling the neurovascular niche: implications for recovery from CNS injury. J Physiol Pharmacol. 2009;60(Suppl 4):95–104.
55. Ropper AH, Gorson KC. Clinical practice. Concussion. N Engl J Med. 2007;356(2):166–72.
56. Heitger MH, et al. Impaired eye movements in post-concussion syndrome indicate suboptimal brain function beyond the influence of depression, malingering or intellectual ability. Brain. 2009;132(Pt 10):2850–70.
57. Bigler ED. Volumetric MRI findings in mild traumatic brain injury (mTBI) and neuropsychological outcome. Neuropsychol Rev. 2021; https://doi.org/10.1007/s11065-020-09474-0.
58. Sussman D, et al. Concussion induces focal and widespread neuromorphological changes. Neurosci Lett. 2017;650:52–9.
59. Zhou Y, et al. Mild traumatic brain injury: longitudinal regional brain volume changes. Radiology. 2013;267(3):880–90.
60. Bigler ED. Neuropsychology and clinical neuroscience of persistent post-concussive syndrome. J Int Neuropsychol Soc. 2008;14(1):1–22.
61. Pinel JPJ. Biopsychology. Boston: Allyn & Bacon; 1990.
62. Deuchars J, West DC, Thomson AM. Relationships between morphology and physiology of pyramid-pyramid single axon connections in rat neocortex in vitro. J Physiol. 1994;478(3):423–35.

Advanced Neuroimaging of Mild Traumatic Brain Injury

9

Zhifeng Kou and E. Mark Haacke

Introduction

Traumatic brain injury (TBI) affects 1.7 million Americans each year [1–3] and most of them are considered mild TBI (mTBI) [4]. In fact, over 1.2 million Americans suffer from an mTBI annually, making it a major public healthcare burden that has been overlooked for decades [1, 2]. Despite its name, the impact of mTBI to the patients and their family is not mild at all [4]. A significant percentage of mTBI patients may develop a constellation of physical, cognitive, and emotional symptoms, collectively known as post-concussive syndrome (PCS), that significantly impact the quality of their lives. The direct cost of mTBI in the United States is approximately $16.7 billion each year and this does not include the indirect costs to society and families [4–6].

The major causes of TBI are motor vehicle crash (MVC) accidents, falls, assaults, and participation in sport. MVC has been thought as the major contributor to diffuse axonal injury (DAI) or traumatic axonal injury (TAI), which is more devastating than focal injury and tends to result in long-term neurocognitive sequelae in patients [7]. Among the 1.7 million TBI patients each year, over 1.2 million (70%) of them visit the emergency department for treatment, and among them, mTBI accounts for over one million of those emergency visits [8]. Meanwhile, most mTBI patients stay in the emergency department for a few hours and then are discharged home due to their negative computed tomography (CT) findings. Therefore, an emergency department could be a major battlefield in mTBI detection and outcome prediction.

Z. Kou (✉)
Departments of Biomedical Engineering and Radiology, Wayne State University School of Medicine, Detroit, MI, USA
e-mail: zhifeng_kou@wayne.edu

E. M. Haacke
Department of Radiology, Wayne State University School of Medicine, Detroit, MI, USA

Up to 50% of mTBI patients develop persistent neurocognitive symptoms that last about up to 3 months, and 5–15% of mTBI patients develop symptoms that last about 1 year [8, 9]. Meanwhile, among the 1.8 million American troops who have served in Iraq and Afghanistan, it is estimated that at least 20% of returning troops have suffered at least one mTBI. This means up to 360,000 veterans may have brain injuries after discharge [10]. However, most *symptomatic* mTBI patients have normal anatomical findings on clinical CT and conventional magnetic resonance imaging (MRI) [11, 12]. In addition to neuroimaging, clinical indices of severity, such as the Glasgow Coma Scale (GCS) and duration of posttraumatic amnesia (PTA), are lacking sensitivity in mTBI and are not useful in predicting outcome [13]. In summary, using currently available clinical instruments is difficult to determine which mTBI patients will have prolonged or even permanent neurocognitive symptoms.

It has been recognized that mTBI is not a single disease; mTBI has a full spectrum of pathophysiologic conditions. After the initial biomechanical insult to neurons, axons, glia, and the neural vascular system, the brain will undergo a complicated biochemical process, called secondary injury. As a result, the brain may manifest disturbed cerebral blood flow and metabolism, intracranial hemorrhage, edema, and even elevated intracranial pressure, as part of the cascade. Over time, the injured axons may suffer Wallerian degeneration or neurons may suffer cell loss, manifested as brain atrophy. There is no single "silver bullet" which could capture the full spectrum of injury. However, with both hardware advances and pulse sequence design advances, newer MRI methods have demonstrated the ability to detect and localize, with high resolution, *several* of the pathologic and pathophysiologic consequences of mTBI. These advanced MR technologies include susceptibility-weighted imaging (SWI) for hemorrhage detection [14]; MR spectroscopy (MRS) for metabolite measurement [15]; diffusion-weighted and diffusion tensor imaging (DWI/DTI) for edema quantification [16] and axonal injury detection [17]; perfusion-weighted imaging (PWI) and arterial spin labeling (ASL) to measure blood flow to brain tissue [18]; and functional MRI (fMRI) which measures changes in blood oxygen level locally in response to neuronal activity [19]. Having a set of imaging biomarkers, all of which are obtained in a single scanning session (or multiple for longitudinal study), and are sensitive to different consequence of traumatic injury, offers great advantages: (1) enhanced sensitivity, (2) ability to study interrelationships among these biomarkers and between the biomarkers and clinical/neurocognitive deficits, (3) improved clinical management resulting from more precise characterization of injuries, and (4) enhanced power of clinical interventional studies. In this chapter, we will focus on neuroimaging of traumatic vascular and axonal injury of mild TBI by using two advanced MRI techniques.

Imaging Traumatic Vascular Injury

DAI or TAI has been reported as an important pathology in mTBI. To date, limited data exist on neural vascular injury after trauma despite the fact that the neural vascular system is tightly meshed into the neuronal, glial cell, and white matter tracts.

Despite the fact that only a small percentage of patients have microhemorrhages in mTBI, the vascular system is certainly not immune to injury during an insult to neurons and/or axons.

Depending on the magnitude of insult, traumatic vascular injury (TVI) may manifest itself at different levels. During a relatively lighter impact, the tight junction of endothelia cells may undergo direct stretch and temporal opening that results in a leaky blood-brain barrier (BBB) [20–22]. As a consequence, red blood cells (RBCs) will leak into extravascular space [23], and other central nervous system (CNS)-specific proteins will get into the blood stream, which makes serum-based biomarkers detectable as well [24]. At this stage, however, the injury may not be visible on routine structural MRI scanning. When the biomechanical load at the regional level gets more severe, the damaged vascular system may suffer dysregulated cerebral blood flow, or even thrombosis, which manifests as reduced blood oxygenation in the venous system. It will manifest as prominent veins with higher contrast than regular veins on SWI images. If the vascular damage is more significant to cause direct rupture of the vessel wall, it will cause a hemorrhagic bleeding at the local level that is visible on routine MRI and CT scans, if the size or volume is big enough.

Susceptibility-Weighted Imaging of Hemorrhagic Lesions

In diagnostic radiology, intracranial hemorrhage has been sought as a biomarker of mTBI. The confirmation of bleeding in mTBI will automatically categorize a patient into "complicated mild TBI," whose outcome tends to be worse than those without any intracranial bleeding of mTBI and even close to moderate TBI [25]. A most recent study of 135 mTBI patients, scanned at 12 days after injury, demonstrated that one or more brain contusions on structural MRI and ≥4 foci of hemorrhagic axonal injury on MRI were each independently associated with poorer 3-month outcomes [26]. Some investigators have suggested that the presence of hemorrhage in DAI is predictive of poor outcome in moderate to severe TBI as well [27]. SWI was developed by Haacke et al. [28] as a high-resolution venography method and has been used to evaluate moderate to severe TBI patients since 2003 in work by Tong et al. [14]. Tong and colleagues have shown that SWI is three to six times more sensitive than conventional T2* gradient echo imaging (GRE) for detecting suspected DAI lesions in children [14, 29]. SWI has been shown to detect tiny hemorrhages that may be the only abnormal finding that can confirm the presence of brain injury and change clinical management of the patient. In addition, lesion number and volume identified by SWI are negatively associated with the patients' outcome [29] and neuropsychological functions [30] in moderate to severe TBI patients.

After brain injury, the hemorrhagic bleed may undergo a temporal transformation: from oxyhemoglobin to de-oxyhemoglobin in the acute stage, from intra- to extracellular methemoglobin in the subacute stage, and finally to hemosiderin in the chronic stage [31–33]. SWI is sensitive to deoxyhemoglobin in the acute stage as well as extracellular methemoglobin in the subacute stage and hemosiderin in the chronic stage [31].

Therefore, positive results on SWI could provide a biomarker for hemorrhagic brain injury at any stage. However, very few studies have been reported regarding the possible role of SWI as a tool for improving detection of microhemorrhages and its use in predictive value of a patient's outcome after mTBI. Unlike DTI, which requires complex post-processing and comparison with proper control subjects, SWI is readily available for radiological reading right after completion of MRI scans. This makes SWI more likely to have a direct impact on radiological diagnosis. In fact, many medical centers have already begun to use SWI as a prime sequence for the detection of intracranial hemorrhages in clinical radiology. Figure 9.1 demonstrates an exemplary case to show SWI detection of brain hemorrhages in mTBI in the acute stage in comparison with the usual clinical T2* GRE.

Quantitative Susceptibility Mapping of Bleeding and Blood Oxygenation

Despite its improved sensitivity in the detection of microhemorrhages, SWI is still a qualitative, rather than quantitative, approach. Theoretically, blood product at different stages, from deoxyhemoglobin, to extracellular methemoglobin and then hemosiderin, has different susceptibilities. As a natural extension, susceptibility-weighted

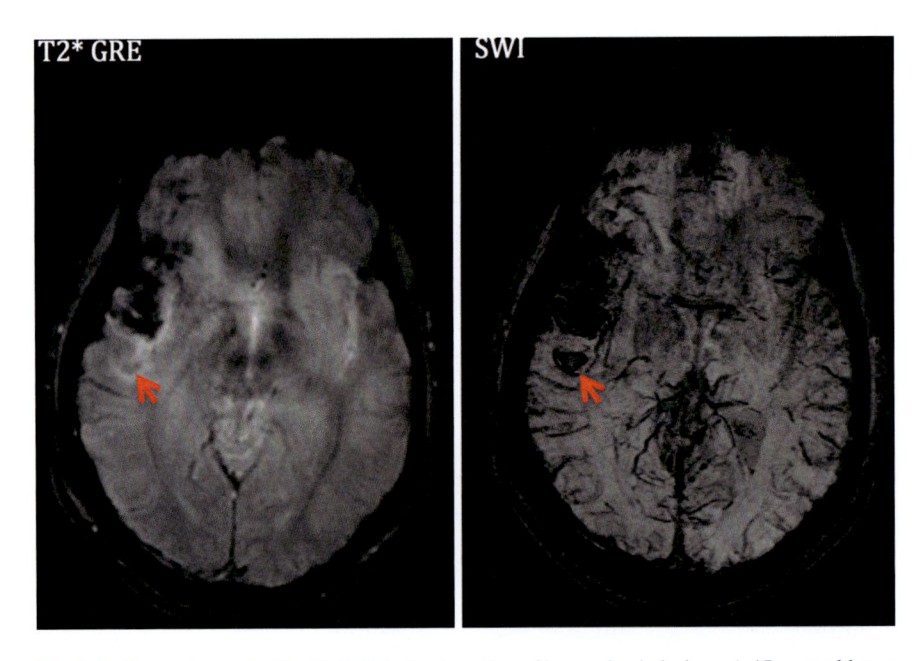

Fig. 9.1 Comparison of T2* with SWI in the detection of hemorrhagic lesions. A 45-year-old man fell down from a staircase and then visited ER with a severe headache. Both T2* GRE and SWI detected hemorrhages on the right side of inferior temporal lobe. However, in a small area with mixed blood and edema signal, T2* GRE only detected edema (bright signal) and SWI detected hemorrhage (dark signal) (see arrow), which suggests methemoglobin at the acute stage

imaging and mapping (SWIM), also called quantitative susceptibility mapping (QSM), is the next generation of SWI development, which could quantify the susceptibility values of blood products. Ideally SWIM/QSM could have the following potential usage in mTBI:

(a) Differentiating new from old hemorrhage. Fresh blood at the acute stage of injury with deoxyhemoglobin has relatively low susceptibility, subacute blood with extracellular methemoglobin has relatively higher susceptibility, and chronic blood with hemosiderin has the highest susceptibility. Therefore, the susceptibility signal intensity will be able to differentiate the stage of the bleeding.
(b) Improving detection of microhemorrhages. One difficulty in clinical radiology is to differentiate microbleeds from veins, especially at the cortical surface, where the brain is enriched with a venous structure and therefore prone to bleeding. A cross section of a cortical vein or pial vein could be easily misinterpreted as a microhemorrhage, and a microhemorrhage buried in the surrounding venous structure could be easily overlooked as a vein. By using minimal intensity projection (mIP), the dark venous signal on adjacent slices can be projected onto one slice to see the continuity of the venous structure. Even so, a radiologist still needs to navigate through several slides to check the morphology, including the continuity of the black dots and smoothness of a potential vessel wall, to verify whether it is a vein or bleed. With the addition of SWIM, chronic bleeds (hemosiderin) have a much higher susceptibility than the surrounding veins. The high signal intensity would easily distinguish itself from the veins (see Fig. 9.2 for a chronic bleeding case).

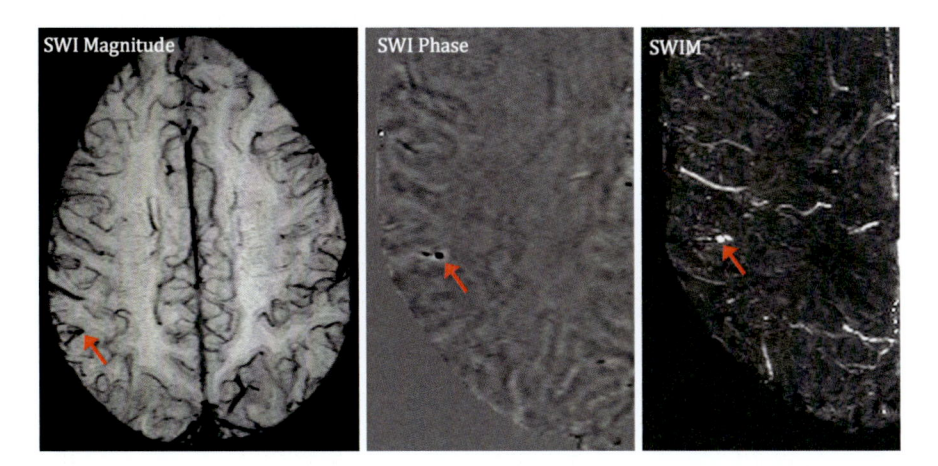

Fig. 9.2 Quantitative susceptibility mapping of chronic bleeding after mTBI. A chronic mTBI case with a microbleed embedded into surrounding pial vein on cortical surface. SWI phase image demonstrates that its shape more looks like a pial vein. SWIM signal demonstrates very high susceptibility value (2200 ppm), which is much higher than a normal vein (usually around 200, no more than 250), suggesting chronic bleeding in the form of hemosiderin instead of venous structure

Another challenge in clinical radiology is to differentiate hemorrhage from calcification. Empirically, calcification tends to happen in a symmetrical manner in the basal ganglia and choroid plexus in the lateral ventricles. However, it could be misinterpreted as a bleed if it is in the brain parenchyma because both calcification and hemorrhage have low signal on SWI images. From a physics point of view, hemorrhage and calcification have opposite susceptibility behaviors: hemorrhage is paramagnetic and shows high signal on SWIM images in contrast with the low signal of calcification, which is diamagnetic. With SWIM, they can be easily differentiated [34].

(c) Quantifying blood oxygenation. After injury, the damaged cerebral vascular structure may present with reduced cerebral blood flow, venous stenosis or even venous thrombosis. Both animal data and recently reported clinical data identify venous thrombosis after TBI [35]. There is even an ongoing clinical trial for venous thrombolysis after TBI [35]. Reduced blood oxygenation or thrombosis will manifest itself as an increased susceptibility signal on SWIM images. As a result, we have developed SWIM technique to quantify susceptibility value as a means to estimate blood oxygenation in major veins [36]. With SWIM, researchers could quantify the degree and extent of venous blood oxygenation. See Fig. 9.3 as an example to show quantitative susceptibility signal of a transmedullary vein after blast induced TBI.

(d) Quantify disease progression or treatment effect. The availability of quantitative signal would allow researchers to track the progression of blood product over time, which could be a biomarker for disease progression. This could be

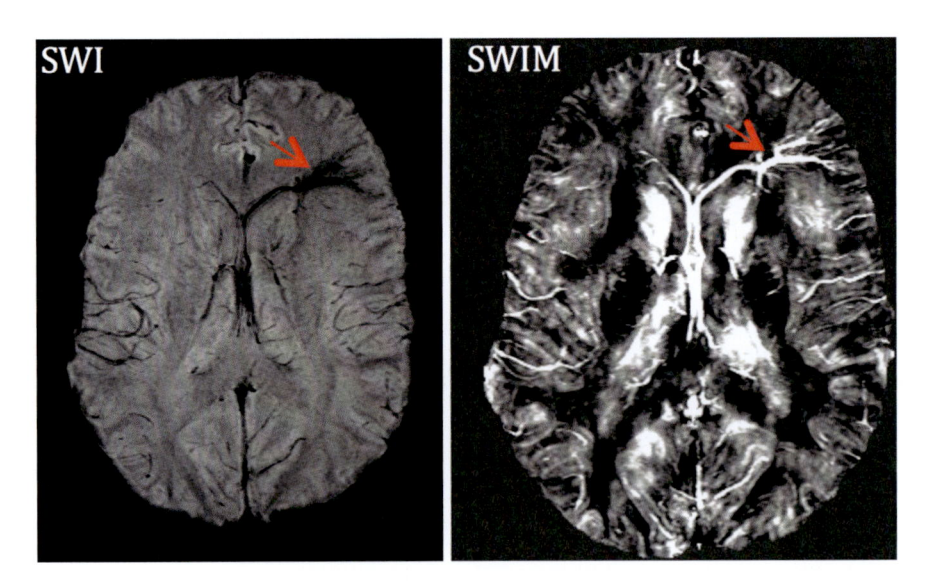

Fig. 9.3 Decreased venous blood oxygenation in septal vein after blast-induced TBI. SWI image (left) shows abnormal signal on left anterior septal vein but short of quantitation. SWIM (right) shows the decreased blood oxygenation on the vein with signal intensity linearly proportional to the concentration of deoxyhemoglobin

very useful for bleeding and re-bleeding cases. Chronically, the hemosiderin deposit after hemorrhage may stay in the brain tissue for a long time and become toxic to the brain by inducing edema [37] or hydrocephalus [38, 39]. Iron chelation drug treatment could be a treatment to remove these iron deposits and is being reported in correlation with outcome improvement in animal models of intracerebral hemorrhage [40, 41]. The availability of SWIM will certainly provide a means for in vivo assessment of iron chelation treatment.

In summary, there is still a need to further investigate the traumatic vascular injury in a large number of mTBI patients by using SWI/SWIM and these sequences may represent a promising direction for mTBI research in the coming years.

Diffusion Tensor Imaging (DTI) of Axonal Injury

Diffusion imaging sequences are sensitive primarily to traumatic axonal injury (TAI) and secondarily to stretch and shear forces. DTI measures the bulk motion of water molecular diffusion in biological tissues. It is most useful when tissues are anisotropic, that is, when diffusion is not equivalent in all directions, such as in skeletal muscle or axons in the white matter of the central nervous system. Histological correlates have validated DTI's sensitivity to brain injury for both focal [42] and diffuse axonal injury [43] models. The apparent diffusion coefficient (ADC) and fractional anisotropy (FA) [44, 45] are two parameters derived from DTI that have been extensively studied in TBI. ADC is an estimate of the average *magnitude* of water movement in a voxel (regardless of direction), while FA is an index of the *directional non-uniformity,* or anisotropy, of water diffusion within a voxel.

FA has been used to detect alterations in directional diffusion resulting from tissue damage. FA in white matter is highest when fibers are long (relative to voxel dimension) and oriented uniformly (collinear) within a voxel and lowest when fibers are not collinear (e.g., "crossing fibers") or have been damaged. When axons are injured, as in acceleration/deceleration injuries (such as MVCs), diffusion anisotropy typically decreases. Loss of diffusion anisotropy is the result of a number of axonal changes after injury including the following: (1) increased permeability of the axonal membrane; (2) swelling of axons; (3) decreased diffusion in the axial (long axis) direction; and (4) degeneration and loss of axons in the chronic stage. In general, any pathological alteration of white matter fibers will result in FA decrease, since one or more of these axonal changes occurs in disorders of white matter. Not surprisingly, most clinical studies of moderate and severe TBI have shown FA to be more sensitive than ADC to traumatic injury. On the other hand, ADC, FA, and directionally selective diffusivities (principal, intermediate, and minor components of diffusion) can help to better characterize brain injury pathologies. Trace and mean diffusivity are two other measurements similar to ADC and vary similarly. Changes in FA in association with ADC changes can differentiate the type of edema. For example, in the acute stage, decreased FA in association with increased ADC suggests vasogenic edema, while increased FA in association with decreased ADC suggests cytotoxic edema. Decreased FA in association with decreased ADC and decreased longitudinal (parallel to the long axis of the axons) water diffusivity suggests axonal transport failure as occurs in degenerative neurological diseases like ALS.

Regarding the location of brain lesions detected by DTI, Niogi et al. [46] summarized that the frontal association pathways, including anterior corona radiata, uncinate fasciculus, superior longitudinal fasciculus, and genu of corpus callosum (CC), are the mostly frequently injured WM structures in mTBI patients. Single subject results were not reported, but it can be assumed that significant inter-individual variability for location and extent of WM injury exists due to varying injury mechanisms (and forces) and biological (neural and non-neural) differences across patients.

Imaging at Different Pathological Stages

Interestingly, despite the higher incidence of milder TBI compared with more severe TBI in western countries, there are much fewer mTBI imaging studies reported in the literature. One reason is the fact that recruitment of mTBI patients is more difficult, since they are typically outpatients. Another reason is the common conception that mTBI is a transient functional disorder from which virtually all who are afflicted will recover fully and spontaneously. Therefore, some question the clinical importance of studying mTBI. Certainly, insurance reimbursement for MRI scanning of mTBI is rare, and even rarer in the acute setting, so that "adding on research sequences" is not feasible and/or realistic.

With these limitations in mind, a growing literature on DTI in mTBI has begun to address the DTI findings at different stages (See Fig. 9.4 as an example of axonal injury).

Acute stage: There are conflicting findings for FA and ADC reported in mTBI. Chu et al. [47] and Wilde et al. [48, 49] from Baylor College of Medicine scanned 10–12 adolescents with mTBI within 6 days of injury and reported *increased FA, reduced ADC and reduced radial (short axis) diffusivity* in WM regions and the left thalamus. Similarly, Bazarian et al. [50] studied six mTBI patients within 72 h and reported *increased* FA in the posterior CC and *reduced* ADC in the anterior limb of the internal capsule (IC). Similar to Chu et al. [47] and Wilde et al. [48, 49], Mayer et al. [51] studied 22 mTBI patients within 12 days of injury and reported *FA increase* and *reduced radial* diffusivity in the CC and left hemisphere tracts.

Inglese et al. [52], in contrast to Chu et al. [47], Wilde et al. [48, 49], Bazarian et al. [50] and Mayer et al. [51], found *reduced FA* in the splenium of CC and posterior limb of IC in 20 mTBI patients imaged up to 10 days after injury (mean = 4 days). Manually drawn regions of interest were used to assess the genu and splenium of the CC, the centrum semiovale and the posterior limb IC bilaterally. In the same line as

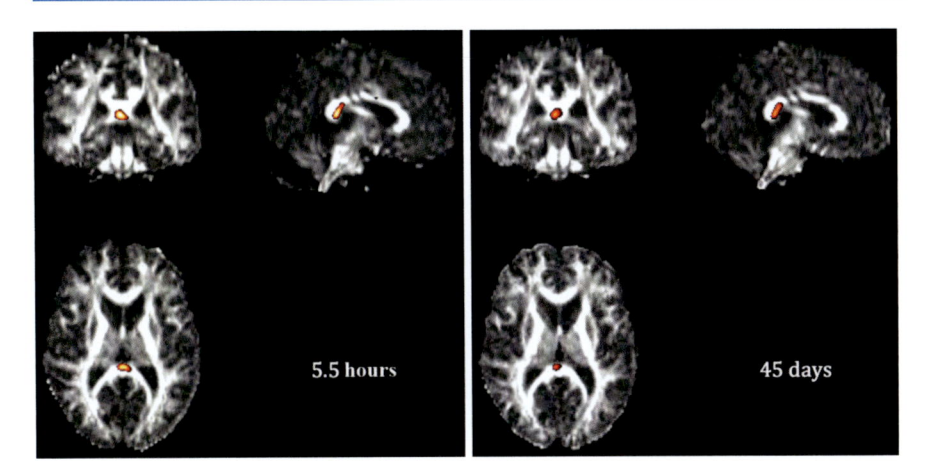

Fig. 9.4 DTI analysis of an mTBI patient scanned on the day of injury (5.5 h after injury) and 6 weeks later. A 31-year-old male fell 10 ft. off a ladder striking the back of his head with brief loss of consciousness and confusion. The patient developed persistent mild cognitive symptoms after 6 weeks of injury. Note the same location of reduced FA in left corona radiata. Global WM FA mean was within normal

Inglese et al., Arfanakis and colleagues [53] studied a handful of mTBI patients at the acute stage and reported FA *decrease* in major WM tracts.

Most recent data on sports-related injury further reported that DTI FA changes could be bidirectional, which means the coexistence of both increased and decreased FA in different locations of the same brain [54]. Kou et al. also demonstrated this bidirectional change of FA in mTBI patients in the acute setting (within 24 h after injury) [55].

Subacute stage: Most studies reported *reduced FA* and/or *increased diffusivity*, that is, ADC, trace or mean diffusivity (MD), at this stage. Messe et al. [56] studied 23 mTBI at the subacute stage and found significantly *increased MD* in mTBI patients with poor outcome [56]. The authors did not find significant changes of FA values. Lipton et al. [57] scanned 20 mTBI patients in the subacute stage and demonstrated *reduced FA* and *increased MD* in frontal subcortical WM. Miles et al. [58] studied 17 acute and subacute mTBI patients and found *reduced FA and increased MD*. All of these studies at the subacute stage reported a similar profile of DTI measures except for different locations of injury.

Chronic stage: Three studies report either *reduced* FA or *increased* diffusivity or both and one study reported *increased* FA at this stage. Cubon et al. [59] studied 10 collegiate athletes with concussion at the chronic stage and found *MD increases* in left WM tracts, internal capsule, and thalamic acoustic radiations. Lo et al. studied 10 mTBI patients and reported *reduced FA* and *increased ADC* in the left genu of the CC and *increased FA* in internal capsule bilaterally [60]. Niogi et al. [61] studied

43 chronic mTBI and reported *reduced FA* in a large number of WM tracts. In contrast, Lipton et al. [62] reported bidirectional changes (both increases and decreases) of FA in chronic mTBI patients.

All DTI studies of moderate to severe TBI patients [17, 63–65] and most subacute/ chronic mTBI patients [52, 61, 66–68] report FA *decreases* which are correlated with clinical or neuropsychological measures. However, there are seemingly contradictory findings in mild TBI in the acute stage (within 1 week after injury) in the literature: Inglese [52] and Arfanakis [53] both reported FA *decreases,* while Wilde [49] and Bazarian [50] reported FA *increases* and decreased radial diffusivity.

It has been suggested that in the acute phase decreased FA may reflect vasogenic edema. In contrast, increased FA acutely may reflect cytotoxic edema [49], which would shunt extracellular fluid into swollen cells. This could have the effect of reducing inter-axonal free water and therefore increasing anisotropy. The bidirectional changes of FA in recent studies further suggest the coexistence of both types of edema, and therefore, clinical data could be much more complicated than we thought [54, 55].

Longitudinal studies: Only a few studies have followed FA over time in the same patients. Sidaros et al. [69] studied 23 severe TBI patients at 8 weeks and again at 12 months and found that partial recovery of initially depressed FA values in the internal capsule and centrum semiovale predicted a favorable outcome. Kumar et al. [70] studied 16 moderate to severe TBI patients at 2 weeks or less, 6 months, and 2 years and found persistently reduced FA except in the genu of the corpus callosum where there was partial normalization by 2 years. Recently, two studies by Mayer et al. [51] and Rutgers et al. [67] reported that FA may partially normalize, reflecting recovery from injury. This evidence suggests that a systematic investigation of a large number of mTBI patients at acute, subacute, and chronic stages is warranted to reveal the evolution of pathophysiology of mTBI.

Correlation Between DTI-Derived WM Injury Topography and Neuropsychological Deficits

Mild TBI patients often develop a constellation of physical, cognitive, and emotional symptoms after injury that can manifest, and change, over their injury. In terms of neurocognitive symptoms, there are four key domains implicated in chronic neuropsychological impairment after mTBI. These domains include the following: (1) higher order attention, (2) executive function, (3) episodic memory, and (4) speed of information processing. To date, several studies have demonstrated typical mTBI cognitive profiles and association with DTI findings. Niogi et al. summarized the topographic and neurocognitive deficits [46]. Kou et al. gave a systemic review of susceptible WM tracts due to injury and their related functional and cognitive deficits in patients, based on the reported findings [71].

Damage to the frontal WM has been reported to be associated with impaired executive function. Lipton et al. [57] studied 20 acute to subacute patients and reported that reduced FA in WM of dorsolateral prefrontal cortex (DLPRC) is correlated with worse executive function. Frontal WM injury is also associated with attention deficits. Niogi et al. [72] reported that reduced FA in the left anterior corona radiata is correlated with attention control problems in chronic mTBI patients. Injury at the temporal WM tracts or cingulum bundle may cause memory problems. Niogi et al. reported that reduced FA in uncinate fasciculus correlated with memory tasks performance [72]. Furthermore, Wu et al. [48] reported that reduced FA measures of left cingulum bundle correlated with delayed recall.

Injury of the callosal fibers has been reported to be associated with PCS scores. Wilde et al. [49] studied 10 adolescent mTBI patients in the acute stage and reported that increased FA and decreased ADC and MD in the corpus callosum were correlated with patients' PCS scores. Bazarian et al. [50] studied six mild TBI patients in the acute stage and reported that a lower mean trace in the left anterior IC and a higher FA in the posterior CC correlated with patients' 72 h PCS score and visual motor speed and impulse control.

The overall burden, or extent, of WM injury is associated with both speed of information processing and overall functional outcome. Niogi et al. [61] studied 34 subacute to chronic mTBI patients and reported that FA decreased in several WM regions, including anterior corona radiata, uncinate fasciculus, CC genu, and cingulum bundle. Furthermore, the number of damaged WM regions correlated with patient's reaction time. Miles et al. [58] studied 17 mTBI patients at the acute stage and followed them up to 6 months after injury. They reported that, in the acute stage, the increased mean diffusivity (MD) in the central semiovale, the genu and splenium of CC, and the posterior limb of IC correlated with a patient's response speed at 6 months after injury. Regarding the overall outcome, Messe et al. [56] divided mTBI patients into two outcome groups: poor outcome (PO) versus good outcome (GO). PO patients showed significantly higher mean diffusivity (MD) values than both controls and GO patients in the corpus callosum, the right anterior thalamic radiations, the superior longitudinal fasciculus, the inferior longitudinal fasciculus, and the fronto-occipital fasciculus bilaterally.

Interestingly, injury or reduced blood supply in the thalamus, which is the relay station of neuronal pathways, may cause a constellation of symptoms affecting the speed of information processing, verbal memory, and executive function. Grossman et al. studied 22 subacute to chronic mTBI patients by using diffusion kurtosis imaging, which is a more advanced form of diffusion analysis, and demonstrated that overall cognitive impairment is associated with the diffusion measurement in the thalamus and internal capsule [73]. This work is along the same line of a perfusion study by the same group, which demonstrated that reduced blood flow in the thalamus correlated with patient's overall neurocognitive function [74].

In summary, significant progress has been made by researchers in recent years regarding the prognostic value of DTI in the form of FA for mTBI patients' neurocognitive outcome. However, more recent evidence suggests that tensor model may not be the ideal approach to the complicated pathophysiological process in

TBI. Particularly, despite its high sensitivity, DTI suffers low specificity to trauma. Numerous medical reasons could cause water diffusivity changes and lead to changed FA including neurodegenerative diseases, stroke, cancer, multiple sclerosis, hypertension, and diabetes, to name a few. Any pre-existing conditions in the brain could affect the diffusivity and FA changes. Conflicting data on FA changes at the acute stage suggest that the field needs a better approach to characterizing the injury pathology than the current DTI model. This approach should be more specific to a TBI pathological process and could be used to evaluate the neural basis of patients' injury to recovery process in longitudinal studies over a large number of patients.

Connectomic Assessment of mTBI

With advancement of neuroscience research, largely stimulated by advanced biomedical imaging, the neuroscience community recognized that the brain works by a concerted effort of functional networks, particularly on a large scale. Though the white matter fibers provide physical infrastructure of these functional networks, the study of brain structure itself alone is not enough to explain the puzzle the community face. Researchers have to study the brain from a network perspective, particularly in large-scale brain networks or connectome, for the assessment of both structural and functional networks. As a result, the connectome approach to brain injury draws new interest of the field [75]. Based on this concept, the brain consists of many small networks, both structurally and functionally, working together to perform daily functions. Due to the fine granularity of these small networks, one key aspect is the choice of seed region or regional of interest (ROI) for each small network. Due to individual variation, it will be a challenge to choose group-wise consistent and individual-specific ROIs in large network analysis. A slight variation of a small ROI may migrate to other networks. Based on the connectional finger print concept in neuroscience [76], the same brain networks across individuals should also share similar structural connectivity in support of their functional connectivity. Therefore, their fiber tracts should be very similar. As a result, the seed region of a network in an individual subject may slightly different from others; however, the individual's fiber connectivity or fiber tract shape should be very similar to the group. By using this concept, Iraji et al. investigated a cohort of 40 mTBI patients at the acute stage of injury in comparison with 50 healthy controls [75]. By using a framework of a network atlas with 358 networks, Iraji et al. identified 41 networks that show significant group difference. By using these 41 ROIs to do fiber tractography, we can see a sharp difference between controls and patients. Because these ROIs are widely spread over the brain, using these 41 ROIs in controls would be able to track the whole brain white matter fibers. In contrast, these ROIs in patients cannot track the whole brain fibers because they are not well connected to the rest of the brain network (see Fig. 9.5). By further using the 317

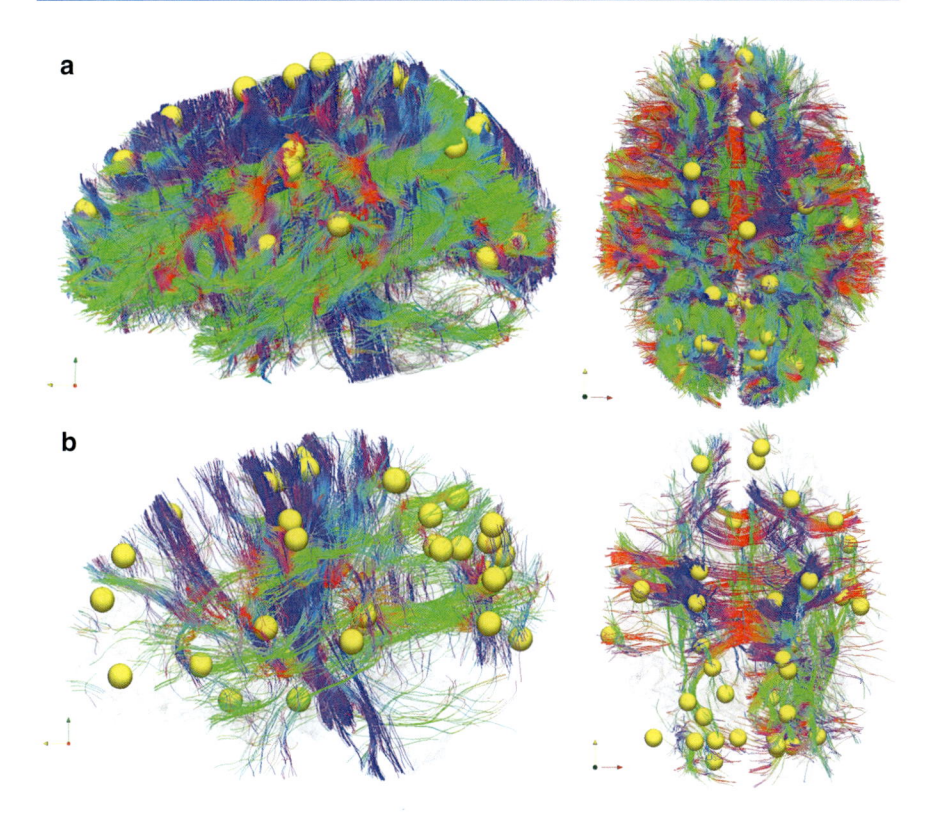

Fig. 9.5 Comparison of white matter fiber tractography between a randomly selected patient and control by using the 41 seed regions that show group difference in network connectivity. Fiber tractography by using these 41 regions in a control (panel **a**) can track the whole brain fibers as these 41 networks are well connected with other brain networks across the whole brain. However, fiber tractography using these 41 regions in a patient brain (panel **b**) can only show very sparse connectivity as the 41 brain networks defined by these seed regions already demonstrated group difference and are not well connected with other networks

common ROIs that do not show structural disruption as functional network nodes, we can also see 60 out of 385 functional connectivities as the most distinctive and discriminative between groups (see Fig. 9.6). This further confirms the community's belief that the network alterations after mTBI are far more complex than we initially thought.

One challenge associated with connectomic assessment of brain networks is its neurocognitive or neuropsychological correlations. Questions remaining to be answered include what brain networks or network aspects account for subjects' neurocognitive or neuropsychological deficits or post concussive syndrome? and what brain networks suffer physical damage and what brain networks try to compensate and how they are related with patients' functional performance?

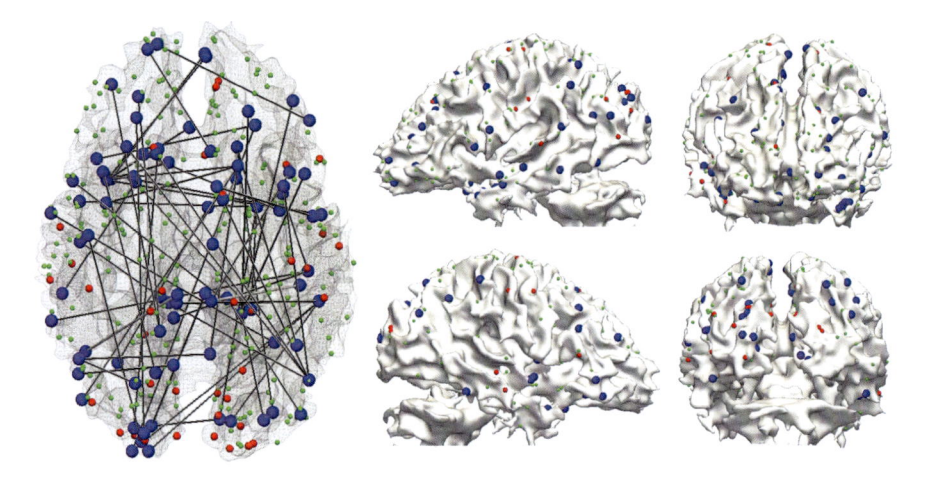

Fig. 9.6 Group differences in functional connectivity. The red bubbles are seed regions that show group difference between structural connectivity. The blue bubbles are seed regions that show group difference between functional connectivity. The green bubbles are seed regions that do not show either structural or functional difference between groups. This demonstrates that a network without structural damage can still have functional alterations

Deliver the Impact to mTBI Care

Despite the fact that the emergency department (ED) sees the majority of mTBI patients [77], most of them stay in the ED for only a few hours and then are discharged home. After that, most patients fail to be followed up. The acute stage, within 24 h after injury, is the critical time point for imaging to deliver a real impact to medicine [78]. Either an improved detection or outcome prediction will greatly help emergency physicians to better determine referral pattern or management plans for the patient and family.

However, most mTBI patients at the acute stage do not get an MRI scan due to the high cost and improper imaging techniques. Furthermore, to date, very few imaging studies are designed to target this critical time point. There is an urgent need for a comprehensive use of advanced MRI techniques to evaluate patients across all stages of injury. In the future, the availability of MR magnets in EDs and reduced costs for MRI scanning will make acute stage imaging possible. However, to determine who will need an MRI scan in ED is another important research question to be addressed. One avenue of this has been the use of serum blood biomarkers. Kou et al. was the first one reporting a complementary use of both MRI and blood biomarkers [79]. Their study pilot data suggest that mTBI patients with intracranial hemorrhage on SWI have significantly higher glial fibrillary acidic protein (GFAP) levels than those without hemorrhage. This implies that GFAP could serve as a screening tool for intracranial hemorrhage (see Fig. 9.7 as an example). The interaction of imaging and blood biomarker data

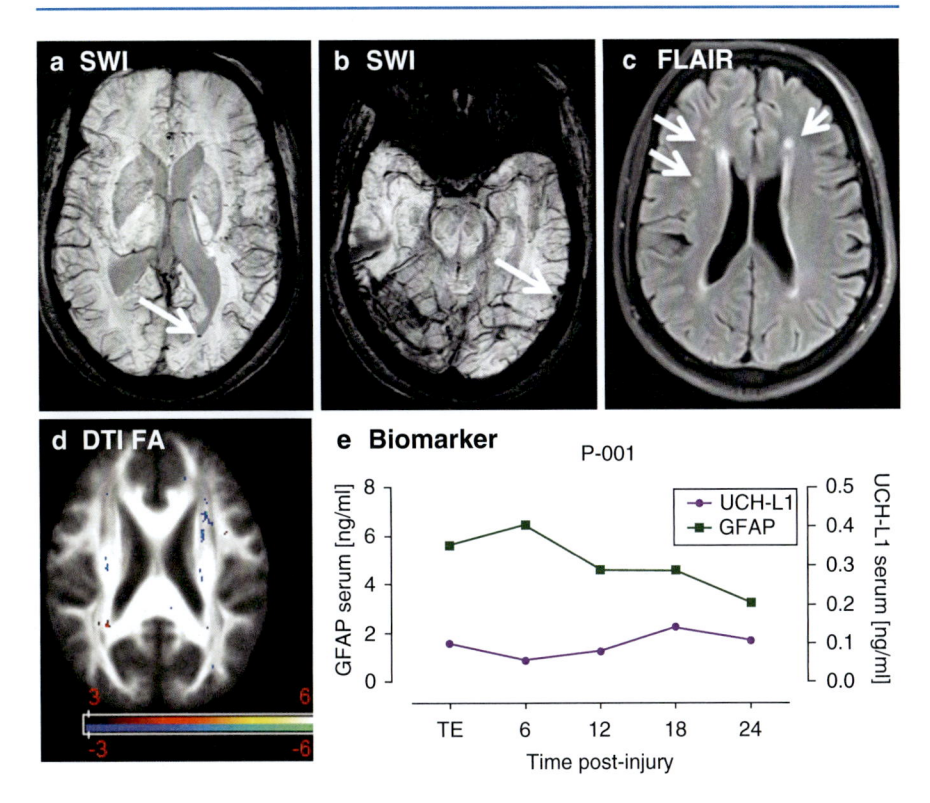

Fig. 9.7 MRI and biomarker profile in a patient with intraventricular hemorrhage missed by CT. Panels (**a**) and (**b**) are SWI images at different locations of the brain showing intra-ventricular blood and left lingual gyrus blood product (see arrows); panel (**c**) FLAIR image showing nonspecific white matter hyperintensities (see arrows); panel (**d**) DTI FA map showing the coexistence of voxels with increased and decreased FA measures (red color means FA decrease and blue color FA increase in comparison with controls, $t > 3$ for t-test); panel (**e**) blood biomarker temporal profile, exhibiting extraordinarily high GFAP levels over time in comparison with controls (median 0.004, interquartile range 0.004–0.015). Despite being missed by CT, the patient's case was still detected by both blood biomarker and MRI

might represent an important future direction for mTBI clinical diagnosis and additional information about the utilization of blood biomarkers can be found in this textbook.

Conclusions

MRI has demonstrated superior capabilities over CT in the detection of subtle changes in the brain after mTBI. As an advanced MRI technique, diffusion tensor imaging can detect white matter abnormalities that are overlooked in structural MRI and further correlate it with the patients' specific domain of neuropsychological symptoms. In conjunction with functional MRI, it can reveal the connectome brain networks on a large scale after brain injury. Susceptibility-weighted imaging and mapping can improve the detection and quantification of traumatic hemorrhage and blood oxygenation after vascular injury. In the future, these advanced MRI techniques should be used in a comprehensive way in a large cohort of patients to provide a panoramic view of brain pathologies. MRI investigations during the acute stage, within 24 h after injury, will most likely impact emergency medicine, which is at the forefront of mTBI care. Assessment of large brain networks or brain connectome holds promise of the brain complexity investigation. Furthermore, the use of serum biomarkers may help identify TBI patients who need advanced MRI imaging in the acute setting in order to prognosticate evolution of injury.

References

1. Kay T. Neuropsychological treatment of mild traumatic brain injury. J Head Trauma Rehabil. 1993;8:74–85.
2. National Institutes of Health. NIH consensus development panel on rehabilitation of persons with traumatic brain injury. JAMA. 1999;282:974–83.
3. Faul MXL, Wald MM, Coronado VG. Traumatic brain injury in the United States: emergency department visits, hospitalizations, and deaths. Atlanta: Centers for Disease Control and Prevention, National Center for Injury Prevention and Control; 2010.
4. CDC. Report to congress on mild traumatic brain injury in the United States: steps to prevent a serious public health problem. Atlanta: Centers for Disease Control and Prevention, National Center for Injury Prevention and Control; 2003.
5. Bazarian JJ, McClung J, Shah MN, Cheng YT, Flesher W, Kraus J. Mild traumatic brain injury in the United States, 1998-2000. Brain Inj. 2005;19(2):85–91.
6. Ruff R. Two decades of advances in understanding of mild traumatic brain injury. J Head Trauma Rehabil. 2005;20(1):5–18.
7. Gennarelli TA. Mechanisms of brain injury. J Emerg Med. 1993;11:5–11.
8. Bazarian JJ, Wong T, Harris M, et al. Epidemiology and predictors of post-concussive syndrome after minor head injury in an emergency population. Brain Inj. 1999;13:173–89.
9. Alves W, Macciocchi SN, Barth JT. Postconcussive symptoms after uncomplicated mild head injury. J Head Trauma Rehabil. 1993;8(3):48–59.
10. Warden D. Military TBI during the Iraq and Afghanistan wars. J Head Trauma Rehabil. 2006;21(5):398–402.
11. Belanger HG, Vanderploeg RD, Curtiss G, Warden DL. Recent neuroimaging techniques in mild traumatic brain injury. J Neuropsychiatry Clin Neurosci. 2007;19(1):5–20.
12. National Academy of Neuropsychology. Mild traumatic brain injury-an online course. Denver: National Academy of Neuropsychology; 2002.
13. Tellier A, Della Malva LC, Cwinn A, Grahovac S, Morrish W, Brennan-Barnes M. Mild head injury: a misnomer. Brain Inj. 1999;13:463–75.
14. Tong KA, Ashwal S, Holshouser BA, Shutter LA, Herigault G, Haacke EM, Kido D. Hemorrhagic shearing lesions in children and adolescents with posttraumatic diffuse axonal injury: improved detection and initial results. Radiology. 2003;27(2):332–9.
15. Holshouser BA, Tong KA, Ashwal S, Oyoyo U, Ghamsary M, Saunders D, Shutter L. Prospective longitudinal proton magnetic resonance spectroscopy imaging in adult traumatic brain injury. J Magn Reson Imaging. 2006;24:33–40.
16. Marmarou A, Signoretti S, Fatouros PP, Portella G, Aygok GA, Bullock MR. Predominance of cellular edema in traumatic brain swelling in patients with severe head injuries. J Neurosurg. 2006;104(5):720–30.

17. Benson RR, Meda SA, Vasudevan S, Kou Z, Govindarajan KA, Hanks RA, et al. Global white matter analysis of diffusion tensor images is predictive of injury severity in TBI. J Neurotrauma. 2007;24(3):446–59.
18. Kim J, Whyte J, Patel S, Avants B, Europa E, Wang J, Slattery J, Gee JC, Coslett HB, Detre JA. Resting cerebral blood flow alterations in chronic traumatic brain injury: an arterial spin labeling perfusion FMRI study. J Neurotrauma. 2010;27(8):1399–411.
19. McAllister TW, Saykin AJ, Flashman LA, Sparling MB, Johnson SC, Guerin SJ, Mamourian AC, Weaver JB, Yanofsky N. Brain activation during working memory 1 month after mild traumatic brain injury: a functional MRI study. Neurology. 1999;53(6):1300–8.
20. Rinder L, Olsson Y. Studies on vascular permeability changes in experimental brain concussion, part 2. Duration of altered permeability. Acta Neuropathol. 1968;11:201–9.
21. Povlishock JT, Kontos HA, Rosenblum WI, et al. A scanning electron microscope analysis of the intraparenchymal brain vasculature following experimental hypertension. Acta Neuropathol. 1980;51:203–12.
22. Povlishock JT, Kontos HA. The pathophysiology of pial and intraparenchymal vascular dysfunction. In: Grossman RG, Gildenberg PL, editors. Head injury, basic and clinical aspects. New York: Raven Press; 1982. p. 15–30.
23. Maxwell WL, Irvine A, Adams JH, et al. Response of cerebral microvasculature to brain injury. J Pathol. 1988;155:327–35.
24. Manley GT, Diaz-Arrastia R, Brophy M, Engel D, Goodman C, Gwinn K, Veenstra TD, Ling G, Ottens AK, Tortella F, Hayes RL. Common data elements for traumatic brain injury: recommendations from the biospecimens and biomarkers working group. Arch Phys Med Rehabil. 2010;9(11):1667–72.
25. Williams DH, Levin HS, Eisenberg HM. Mild head injury classification. Neurosurgery. 1990;217(3):442–8.
26. Yuh EL, Mukherjee P, Lingsma HF, Yue JK, Ferguson AR, Gordon WA, Valadka AB, Schnyer DM, Okonkwo DO, Maas AI, Manley GT, TRACK-TBI investigators. Magnetic resonance imaging improves 3-month outcome prediction in mild traumatic brain injury. Ann Neurol. 2013;73(2):224–35.
27. Paterakis K, Karantanas AH, Komnos A, Volikas Z. Outcome of patients with diffuse axonal injury: the significance and prognostic value of MRI in the acute phase. J Trauma. 2000;49:1071–5.
28. Reichenbach JR, Venkatesan R, Schillinger DJ, Kido DK, Haacke EM. Small vessels in the human brain: MR venography with deoxyhemoglobin as an intrinsic contrast agent. Radiology. 1997;204:272–7.
29. Tong KA, Ashwal S, Holshouser BA, Nickerson JP, Wall CJ, Shutter LA, Osterdock RJ, Haacke EM, Kido D. Diffuse axonal injury in children: clinical correlation with hemorrhagic lesions. Ann Neurol. 2004;56:36–50.
30. Babikian T, Freier MC, Tong KA, Nickerson JP, Wall CJ, Holshouser BA, Burley T, Riggs ML, Ashwal S. Susceptibility weighted imaging: neuropsychologic outcome and pediatric head injury. Pediatr Neurol. 2005;33(3):184–94.
31. Kou Z, Benson RR, Haacke EM. Susceptibility weighted imaging in traumatic brain injury. In: Gillard J, Waldman A, Barker P, editors. Clinical MR Neuroimaging. 2nd ed. Cambridge: Cambridge University; 2010.
32. Thulborn KR, Sorensen AG, Kowall NW, McKee A, Lai A, McKinstry RC, Moore J, Rosen BR, Brady TJ. The role of ferritin and hemosiderin in the MR appearance of cerebral hemorrhage: a histopathologic biochemical study in rats. AJNR Am J Neuroradiol. 1990;11:291–7.
33. Bradley WG. MR appearance of hemorrhage in the brain. Radiology. 1993;189:15–26.
34. DA Schweser F, Lehr BW, Reichenbach JR. Differentiation between diamagnetic and paramagnetic cerebral lesions based on magnetic susceptibility mapping. Med Phys. 2010;37(10):5165–78.
35. Jamjoom AAJA. Safety and efficacy of early pharmacological thromboprophylaxis in traumatic brain injury: systematic review and meta-analysis. J Neurotrauma. 2013;30(7):503–11.

36. Haacke EM, Tang J, Neelavalli J, Cheng YCN. Susceptibility mapping as a means to visualize veins and quantify oxygen saturation. J Magn Reson Imaging. 2010;32:663–76.
37. Dong MXG, Keep RF, Hua Y. Role of iron in brain lipocalin 2 upregulation after intracerebral hemorrhage in rats. Brain Res. 2013;1505:86–92.
38. Okubo SSJ, Keep RF, Hua Y, Xi G. Subarachnoid hemorrhage-induced hydrocephalus in rats. Stroke. 2013;44(2):547–50.
39. Wang LXG, Keep RF, Hua Y. Iron enhances the neurotoxicity of amyloid β. Transl Stroke Res. 2012;3(1):107–13.
40. Okubo SXG, Keep RF, Muraszko KM, Hua Y. Cerebral hemorrhage, brain edema, and heme oxygenase-1 expression after experimental traumatic brain injury. Acta Neurochir Suppl. 2013;118:83–7.
41. Keep RFHY, Xi G. Intracerebral haemorrhage: mechanisms of injury and therapeutic targets. Lancet Neurol. 2012;11(8):720–31.
42. Mac Donald CL, Dikranian K, Song SK, Bayly PV, Holtzman DM, DL B. Detection of traumatic axonal injury with diffusion tensor imaging in a mouse model of traumatic brain injury. Exp Neurol. 2007;205(2007):116–31.
43. Kou Z, Shen Y, Zakaria N, Kallakuri S, Cavanaugh JM, Yu Y, et al. Correlation of fractional anisotropy with histology for diffuse axonal injury in a Rat Model. Joint Annual Meeting ISMRM-ESMRMB; May 19–25, 2007; Berlin, Germany, 2007.
44. Shimony JS, McKinstry RC, Akbudak E, Aronovitz JA, Snyder AZ, Lori NF, et al. Quantitative diffusion-tensor anisotropy brain MR imaging: normative human data and anatomic analysis. Radiology. 1999;212:770–84.
45. Conturo TE, McKinstry RC, Akbudak E, Robinson BH. Encoding of anisotropic diffusion with tetrahedral gradients: a general mathematical diffusion formalism and experimental results. Magn Reson Med. 1996;35:399–412.
46. Niogi SN, Mukherjee P. Diffusion tensor imaging of mild traumatic brain injury. J Head Trauma Rehabil. 2010;25(4):241–55.
47. Chu Z, Wilde EA, Hunter JV, McCauley SR, Bigler ED, Troyanskaya M, Yallampalli R, Chia JM, Levin HS. Voxel-based analysis of diffusion tensor imaging in mild traumatic brain injury in adolescents. AJNR Am J Neuroradiol. 2010;31(2):340–6.
48. Wu TC, Wilde EA, Bigler ED, Yallampalli R, McCauley SR, Troyanskaya M, Chu Z, Li X, Hanten G, Hunter JV, Levin HS. Evaluating the relationship between memory functioning and cingulum bundles in acute mild traumatic brain injury using diffusion tensor imaging. J Neurotrauma. 2010;27(2):303–7.
49. Wilde EA, McCauley SR, Hunter JV, Bigler ED, Chu Z, Wang ZJ, et al. Diffusion tensor imaging of acute mild traumatic brain injury in adolescents. Neurology. 2008;70(12):948–55.
50. Bazarian JJ, Zhong J, Blyth B, Zhu T, Kavcic V, Peterson D. Diffusion tensor imaging detects clinically important axonal damage after mild traumatic brain injury: a pilot study. J Neurotrauma. 2007;24(9):1447–59.
51. Mayer AR, Ling J, Mannell MV, Gasparovic C, Phillips JP, Doezema D, et al. A prospective diffusion tensor imaging study in mild traumatic brain injury. Neurology. 2010;74(8):643–50.
52. Inglese M, Makani S, Johnson G, Cohen BA, Silver JA, Gonen O, et al. Diffuse axonal injury in mild traumatic brain injury: a diffusion tensor imaging study. J Neurosurg. 2005;103:298–303.
53. Arfanakis K, Haughton VM, Carew JD, Rogers BP, Dempsey RJ, ME M. Diffusion tensor MR imaging in diffuse axonal injury. Am J Neuroradiol. 2002;23:794–802.
54. Bazarian JJZT, Blyth B, Borrino A, Zhong J. Subject-specific changes in brain white matter on diffusion tensor imaging after sports-related concussion. Magn Reson Imaging. 2012;30(2):171–80.
55. Zhifeng Kou RG, Kobeissy F, Welch R, O'Neil B, Woodard J, Ayaz SI, Kulek A, Kas'shamoun R, Mika V, Zuk C, Haacke EM, Hayes R, Tomasello F, Mondello S. Combining biochemical and imaging markers to improve diagnosis and characterization of mild traumatic brain injury in the acute setting: results from a pilot study. PLoS ONE. 2013;8(11):e80296.
56. Messé A, Caplain S, Paradot G, Garrigue D, Mineo JF, Soto Ares G, Ducreux D, Vignaud F, Rozec G, Desal H, Pélégrini-Issac M, Montreuil M, Benali H, Lehéricy S. Diffusion tensor

imaging and white matter lesions at the subacute stage in mild traumatic brain injury with persistent neurobehavioral impairment. Hum Brain Mapp. 2011;32(6):999–1011.
57. Lipton ML, Gulko E, Zimmerman ME, Friedman BW, Kim M, Gellella E, Gold T, Shifteh K, Ardekani BA, Branch CA. Diffusion-tensor imaging implicates prefrontal axonal injury in executive function impairment following very mild traumatic brain injury. Radiology. 2009;252(3):816–24.
58. Miles L, Grossman RI, Johnson G, Babb JS, Diller L, Inglese M. Short-term DTI predictors of cognitive dysfunction in mild traumatic brain injury. Brain Inj. 2008;22(2):115–22.
59. Cubon VA, Putukian M, Boyer C, Dettwiler A. A diffusion tensor imaging study on the white matter skeleton in individuals with sports-related concussion. J Neurotrauma. 2011;28(2):189–201.
60. Lo C, Shifteh K, Gold T, Bello JA, Lipton ML. Diffusion tensor imaging abnormalities in patients with mild traumatic brain injury and neurocognitive impairment. J Comput Assist Tomogr. 2009;33(2):293–7.
61. Niogi SN, Mukherjee P, Ghajar J, Johnson C, Kolster RA, Sarkar R, et al. Extent of microstructural white matter injury in postconcussive syndrome correlates with impaired cognitive reaction time: a 3T diffusion tensor imaging study of mild traumatic brain injury. AJNR Am J Neuroradiol. 2008;29(5):967–73.
62. Lipton ML, Kim N, Park YK, Hulkower MB, Gardin TM, Shifteh K, Kim M, Zimmerman ME, Lipton RB, Branch CA. Robust detection of traumatic axonal injury in individual mild traumatic brain injury patients: intersubject variation, change over time and bidirectional changes in anisotropy. Brain Imaging Behav. 2012;6(2):329–42.
63. Newcombe VF, Williams GB, Nortje J, Bradley PG, Harding SG, Smielewski P, et al. Analysis of acute traumatic axonal injury using diffusion tensor imaging. Br J Neurosurg. 2007;21(4):340–8.
64. Levin HS, Wilde EA, Chu Z, Yallampalli R, Hanten GR, Li X, et al. Diffusion tensor imaging in relation to cognitive and functional outcome of traumatic brain injury in children. J Head Trauma Rehabil. 2008;23(4):197–208.
65. Kou Z, Gattu R, Benson RR, Raz N, Haacke EM, editors. Region of interest analysis of DTI FA histogram differentiates mild traumatic brain injury from controls. In: Proceedings of International Society for Magnetic Resonance in Medicine, Toronto, Canada, 2008.
66. Wozniak JR, Krach L, Ward E, Mueller BA, Muetzel R, Schnoebelen S, et al. Neurocognitive and neuroimaging correlates of pediatric traumatic brain injury: a diffusion tensor imaging (DTI) study. Arch Clin Neuropsychol. 2007;22(5):555–68.
67. Rutgers DR, Fillard P, Paradot G, Tadié M, Lasjaunias P. Diffusion tensor imaging characteristics of the corpus callosum in mild, moderate, and severe traumatic brain injury. AJNR Am J Neuroradiol. 2008;29(9):1730–5.
68. Kraus MF, Susmaras T, Caughlin BP, Walker CJ, Sweeney JA, DM L. White matter integrity and cognition in chronic traumatic brain injury: a diffusion tensor imaging study. Brain. 2007;130:2508–19.
69. Sidaros A, Engberg AW, Sidaros K, Liptrot MG, Herning M, Petersen P, Paulson OB, Jernigan TL, Rostrup E. Diffusion tensor imaging during recovery from severe traumatic brain injury and relation to clinical outcome: a longitudinal study. Brain. 2008;131(Pt2):559–72.
70. Kumar R, Saksena S, Husain M, Srivastava A, Rathore RK, Agarwal S, Gupta RK. Serial changes in diffusion tensor imaging metrics of corpus callosum in moderate traumatic brain injury patients and their correlation with neuropsychometric tests: a 2-year follow-up study. J Head Trauma Rehabil. 2010;25(1):31–42.
71. Kou Z, VandeVord PJ. Traumatic white matter injury and glial activation. Glia. 2014;62(11):1831–55.
72. Niogi SN, Mukherjee P, Ghajar J, Johnson CE, Kolster R, Lee H, Suh M, Zimmerman RD, Manley GT, McCandliss BD. Structural dissociation of attentional control and memory in adults with and without mild traumatic brain injury. Brain. 2008;131(12):3209–21.

73. Grossman EJ, Ge Y, Jensen JH, Babb JS, Miles L, Reaume J, Silver JM, Grossman RI, Inglese M. Thalamus and cognitive impairment in mild traumatic brain injury: a diffusional kurtosis imaging study. J Neurotrauma. 2011;29(13):2318–27.
74. Ge Y, Patel MB, Chen Q, Grossman EJ, Zhang K, Miles L, Babb JS, Reaume J, Grossman RI. Assessment of thalamic perfusion in patients with mild traumatic brain injury by true FISP arterial spin labelling MR imaging at 3T. Brain Inj. 2009;23(7):666–74.
75. Iraji ACH, Wiseman N, Zhang T, Welch R, O'Neil BJ, Kulek A, Ayaz S, Wang X, Zuk C, Haacke EM, Liu T, Kou Z. Connectome-scale assessment of structural and functional connectivity in mild traumatic brain injury at the acute state. Neuroimage Clin. 2016;12:100–15.
76. Passingham RE, Stephan KE, Kötter R. The anatomical basis of functional localization in the cortex. Nat Rev Neurosci. 2002;3(8):606–16.
77. Bazarian JJ, McClung J, Cheng YT, Flesher W, Schneider SM. Emergency department management of mild traumatic brain injury in the USA. Emerg Med J. 2005;22:473–7.
78. Jagoda AS, Bazarian JJ, Bruns JJ Jr, Cantrill SV, Gean AD, Howard PK, et al. Clinical policy: neuroimaging and decisionmaking in adult mild traumatic brain injury in the acute setting. Ann Emerg Med. 2008;52(6):714–48.
79. Zhifeng Kou PV. Traumatic glial and white matter injury: review. Glia. 2013; Accepted.

Analytical Monitoring of Brain Metabolism: Not a Research Tool for Elite Academy but an Essential Issue for Return to Play Following Concussion

10

Stefano Signoretti, Francesco Saverio Pastore, Barbara Tavazzi, Giuseppe Lazzarino, and Roberto Vagnozzi

Introduction

Traumatic brain injury (TBI) has been referred to as a "silent epidemic" [1, 2]. The overall incidence of TBI, independent of cause and severity, was recently calculated to account for up to more than 900 cases per 100,000 people globally (95% CI: 874–1005). Thus, an estimated 69 million (95% CI: 64.2–73.8 million) people suffer a TBI each year worldwide [3].

According to the classic Glasgow Coma Scale (GCS) classification, the "mild" form of TBI (mTBI) represents the vast majority of cases, totaling almost 56 million cases per year. Recent systematic reviews acknowledged that the sports contexts are

---

Stefano Signoretti and Francesco Saverio Pastore contributed equally with all other contributors.

S. Signoretti
Division of Emergency-Urgency, UOC of Neurosurgery, S. Eugenio Hospital, Rome, Italy
e-mail: stefano.signoretti@aslroma2.it

F. S. Pastore · R. Vagnozzi
Institute of Neurosurgery, Department of System's Medicine, University of Rome Tor Vergata, Rome, Italy
e-mail: pastore@uniroma2.it; vagnozzi@uniroma2.it

B. Tavazzi (✉)
Department of Basic Biotechnological Sciences, Intensive and Perioperative Clinics, Section of Biochemistry, Catholic University of Rome, Rome, Italy

Fondazione Policlinico Universitario Agostino Gemelli IRCCS, Rome, Italy
e-mail: barbara.tavazzi@unicatt.it

G. Lazzarino (✉)
Department of Biomedical and Biotechnological Sciences, Division of Medical Biochemistry, University of Catania, Catania, Italy
e-mail: lazzarig@unict.it

accountable for up to one-third of all TBIs (1.5–30.3%) [4] and are so frequent as an etiologic factor that they generated a distinct subset, namely, sports-related (SR) TBI. Due to the lack of specific data, classification of SR-TBI ranges widely. Some authors reported that 97.6% of SR-TBIs are encompassed in the mild category while other studies divided them according to a different distribution such as: 67.3% of mild, 25% of moderate, and 7.7% of severe TBI [4, 5].

Whatever the statistics are it is then unquestionable that, among the many benefits of participating in sports and recreational activities, a substantial risk of experiencing TBI is present, although preponderantly of the "mild" type. *Mildness*, however, lacks biological specificity or predictive validity, just indicating a subjective state of illness. In the case of brain functions, this gives raise to unspecific, poorly defined, difficult to objectively quantify, and slightly altered (or non-altered at all) levels of consciousness that provide no insights into the actual post-injury brain cell dysfunction. In any emergency department, during hectic everyday practice, the label "mild" still represents the less severe end of the brain injury spectrum and typically reflects no neurosurgical and/or neuro-intensivist significance [6–8].

Mixed into the vast world of SR-TBI lies the "concussion," ultimately labeled sports-related concussion (SRC). Independently of the causes producing the impact, all concussions fall, undoubtedly, and by definition, within the category of mTBI [9]. Certainly, most symptoms recover spontaneously in the initial days and weeks following trauma, but not in every case. Compelling evidence exists that a substantial number of people (reported with percentage peaks up to 15%) [10, 11]) experiencing SRC continue suffering chronic symptoms, including cognitive deficits and balance difficulties, headaches, emotional disturbances, and sleep difficulties. In some cases, longer-term disorders might occur, particularly in those players experiencing multiple SRC [12, 13], uncovering the presence of a further subcohort of patients, suffering persistent psychiatric and severe cognitive dysfunction.

According to a PubMed inquiry (obtained by typing "concussion" as the keyword, at the beginning of May 2020), more than 12,300 papers have been published during the last decade, including 1609 reviews and 259 clinical trials. By querying "Sports-Related Concussion," 2216 articles were found, including 461 reviews and 43 clinical trials. These numbers indicate fervent research activity, peculiarly paralleled by an urgent need to constantly review the "state of science," revealing scattered lines of research, and continuous introduction of new classifications and management protocols, mostly based on retrospective data, frustrating the definition of rigid inclusion criteria to be used in clinical trials.

A periodic attempt to summarize the current state of knowledge has been made by the Concussion in Sport Study Group, who recently published the sixth consensus statement, following the Berlin 2017 conference meeting, the last of a series initiated in Wien in 2001 [14, 15]. The main announcement of the latest document, however, appears weak, stating that: *"although agreement exists on the principal messages delivered, the authors acknowledge that the science of concussion is incomplete and therefore management and return-to-play decisions lie largely in the realm of clinical judgment on an individualized basis."* The 2018 conclusion is very similar to that written after the Wien meeting, almost 20 years ago: *"research is essential in contributing to the science of concussion and will potentially provide valuable information for such important issues as clinical management, return to play guidelines, and long-term outcome."*

In the view of increasing the efficiency and effectiveness of clinical research studies, by ameliorating data quality of SRC publications, the U.S. National Institute of Neurological Disorders and Stroke (NINDS), in partnership with the National Institutes of Health (NIH) and the Department of Defense (DOD), created in 2016 a panel of experts named Sports Concussion Common Data Elements (CDE) Working Group [16]. The aim of this team was to identify sets of CDEs for SRC research and to support the right documentation to assist investigators. To provide an example, within the first 72 h, to evaluate neuropsychological function, examiners are strongly suggested to use one of the following tests identified as "Core" from the panel, namely: Automated Neuropsychological Assessment Metrics (ANAM), Axon Sports Computerized Cognitive Assessment Tool (CCAT), CNS Vital Signs, and Immediate Post-Concussion Assessment and Cognitive Testing (ImPACT).

Although systematized approaches are methodologically helpful, it is very clear at present that true SRC prognosis could be inaccurate by only using symptoms-based diagnostic tools, since they do not measure any objective biomolecular parameter capable to determine the underhand, yet crucial, alterations of the post-concussed brain tissue. Many studies have in fact raised the strong and founded suspicion that suffering from a "concussive" injury shortly after a previous one increases symptom persistence delaying the recovery. Most importantly, this may have catastrophic consequences in individuals who recovered from clinical disturbances and symptoms, but not from a still altered brain metabolism [17, 18]. Therefore, even though SRC has typically a benign evolution in the majority of cases, with full spontaneous recovery overtime, a well-documented "miserable minority" will experience a very slow, or never-reaching, complete recovery; fairly, these patients claim for more than just "symptoms-based" diagnostics.

Undoubtedly, besides quick, reliable, and cost-effective testing, accompanied by a whole-time course monitoring tools, there is a need for objective parameters allowing to evaluate fine brain changes, before stating clearance (also forensic) from the post-traumatic state. The finalization of these tests relies on quantitative analyses, faithfully reflecting molecular and microstructural cerebral damages, at subcellular, cellular, and tissue levels, in relation to different kinds of concussion and their specific, unique evolution.

Understanding Biomechanics

According to the last definition of the Berlin Consensus, SRC is: *"… a traumatic brain injury induced by biomechanical forces transmitted to the head."* The "physical" response of the brain and the related post-traumatic sequelae are then strictly linked to the kinematics of the event. However, there is often uncertainty in describing the exact "mechanical patterns" of a concussive injury. One primary component of such scarce accuracy stems from the many different motions occurring when the forces (of variable entities) involved in the impact are transferred to the head, unavoidably generating a great range of unevenness in the eventual post-concussive syndromes and correlated damages. Moreover, our current understanding of brain kinematics comes predominantly from "helmeted collisions"; the final kinematic of the traumatic event, therefore, ought to necessarily account for the helmet intrinsic features. This complex helmet-skull-brain interaction contributes to making each injury-causing event nearly unique and practically irreproducible [19].

Most of the modern literature indeed seems to refute a finite concussive-threshold and current research has focused on the concept of "individual-specific thresholds" [20]. This "tailored" approach should account for the many aforementioned unlearned factors playing a role in ones' ability to tolerate concussive impact forces transmitted to the head. No link between biomechanical input and SRC symptoms and outcome has been established to date. Certainly, investigating relationships between objective parameters measured during impacts (linear and rotational accelerations) and patient-reported presentation, duration, and resolution of symptoms can be prone to several confounding factors: firstly, an underreporting issue. Reasons for underreporting injuries have been described as: "not thinking the injury was serious" or "not wanting to be removed from competition." Some athletes might report less severe (or no) symptoms in hopes to return to competition and play sooner [20].

In one recent study, a concussive event was associated with accelerations of 66 g and 2611 rad/s^2, while hundreds of other measured impacts with accelerations greater in magnitude did not result in concussion. Interestingly, this value (66 g) was the second highest magnitude impact for that subject. Another case from the same cohort showed an individual sustaining a concussion associated with an impact to the side of the helmet equaling 53 g and 2885 rad/s^2. This is not a "remarkable" value but corresponded to the highest magnitude side impact that the subject ever sustained in the season. The overall results showed that out of 319 athletes who sustained an impact, 297 were not "concussively" injured. However, of the 22 athletes reporting symptoms, 90% experienced one of the top five highest magnitude accelerations [21]. This work strongly supports the "individual-specific-threshold" concept.

Further predisposing intrinsic variables might contribute to this puzzling relation, including age, genetics, epigenetics, cerebrospinal fluid levels, randomly associated extrinsic factors, such as muscular strength, sport position, impact velocity, and, as already stated, helmet type [22]. Additionally, and most importantly, a history of subconcussive impacts or prior SRC may possibly affect an individual's threshold for an indefinable future period of time [23].

The critical moment of the concussive injuries lies in the mechanical energy transfer process of forces discharged on impact; more specifically, in how much these forces move and deform the brain tissues. Brain is one of the softest biologic materials, defined as a viscoelastic body, acting simultaneously as a solid and a liquid, obeying the physical laws of both matters' state, and showing non-linear behavior in changing its properties in response to the applied loading rate [24, 25]. Brain tissue deforms easily when shearing forces are applied but reveals considerable resistance to changing its shape when subjected to pressures. Inertial (linear and rotational) accelerations underwent intense scrutiny during the last decade, but less has been studied about pressure gradients, which of course poses formidable challenges for in vivo laboratory reproduction. Even in cultured cells, the effects of pressure are studied much less than the effects of deformation. Interestingly, applying rapid pressure changes to a fluid-filled chamber, containing either a brain slice or primary cell cultures, can lead to typical biochemical changes and subsequent neural impairment [26]. What is known, however, is that linear acceleration causing brain deformation will in turn generate smaller pressure gradients throughout the brain, even at considerable distance. Consequently, even if the shearing linear force does not reach the hypothetical shear-damage threshold, the contribution in generating a smaller gradient of pressure can cause exquisite biochemical dysregulation and no shearing-related symptoms [27]. As far as rotational forces are concerned, it is well established that rapid head spins generate angular accelerations, having an associated high energy potential to cause shear-induced tissue damage. Introducing or allowing a rotational component during impact, substantially increases the likelihood of an unconscious episode.

The principle of directionally dependent brain damage is confirmed in a series of studies across different species and is a critical factor in understanding the human tolerance to injuries such as concussion [28–31]. The ventricular system, for example, may have an important damping effect on the strains that appear during rotational motions as well as the membranes that partition the cerebral hemispheres and the cerebellum from the cerebrum might influence the patterns on deformation that appear for a given head motion [32, 33]. These basic anatomical differences could explain variability in symptoms and damage among concussed subjects of increasing ages. To date, our understanding of concussion biomechanics is theoretical and mainly focused on prevention and the precise process describing *how* the mechanical energy of motion and/or impact transfers to the brain tissue remains to be fully understood and described.

The net result is a sudden, wide, non-specific increase in plasma membrane permeability of brain cells, causing extra-intracellular ionic movements and immediate neuronal transmission imbalance [34]. Also, a direct mechanical solicitation activates membrane receptors and alters voltage-dependent channels, a phenomenon coupled with a sudden release of neurotransmitters, particularly excitatory amino acids [35], further contributing to derangement of neuronal ionic homeostasis. Transmission and synaptic signaling are then impaired just a few minutes after trauma [36], as reported in many clinical observations. However, this is just the initiation of a much more complex series of chained biochemical pathways giving origin to the so-called neurometabolic cascade, extensively portrayed in the recent literature [37]. Beside this cascade, a well-established phenomenon implying unidirectional chain reactions, a competition between complex cellular processes having opposite purposes, also develops following concussion. The prevalence of damaging or protective mechanisms will determine the destiny of cerebral cells and axons involved and the overall outcome [38].

The Biomolecular Network and the Post-Concussion Brain "Vulnerability"

One of the most important direct consequences of the aforementioned ionic disorder is the mitochondrial calcium overloading, a pivotal event that negatively impacts the main organelle function, namely, the electron transport chain (ETC) coupled with oxidative phosphorylation (OXPHOS) for energy production (ATP). The results are energy imbalance, oxidative/nitrosative stress, and further macromolecular damages such as ROS and RNS-induced lipid peroxidation [39, 40].

Mitochondrial dysfunction and the inevitable imbalance between ATP consumption and production is the reason for a third fundamental observable fact: neurons are obligated to work overtime via the more rapid, but less efficient, oxygen-independent glycolysis. It has been experimentally demonstrated that brain tissue after concussion-like mTBI undergoes a biphasic period of initial general metabolic depression with decreased glycolytic rate (when mitochondria are dysfunctional), followed by an increase in the glycolytic rate when mitochondria recovered their metabolic activity [41].

It is noteworthy to recall that the brain meets its energy requirements by completely coupling glucose consumption with oxygen consumption. To ensure this pairing, fundamental metabolic steps are mandatory: the pyruvate produced via glycolysis is converted to acetyl-CoA by the multienzymatic complex of pyruvate dehydrogenase (PDH); the tricarboxylic acid (TCA) cycle and PDH will generate the correct number of NADH and $FADH_2$ molecules, the ETC will efficiently transfer NADH and $FADH_2$ electrons to molecular oxygen, while pumping the right number of protons into the mitochondrial inter-membrane space; ultimately, protons will be efficiently utilized by ATP-synthase to generate ATP molecules. Under these conditions, glucose consumption almost coincides with glucose oxidation.

In a research carried out in our laboratories, we evaluated the effects of graded head impacts (including a concussion-like mTBI) on the genes and protein expressions of PDH, as well as on that of major enzymes of TCA, in whole brain homogenates of post-injured rats [42]. Gene expressions of PDH were analyzed from 6 h up to 5 days post injury, along with those of kinases and phosphatases (PDK1–4 and PDP1–2, respectively) regulating PDH activity, citrate synthase (CS), isocitrate dehydrogenase (IDH), oxoglutarate dehydrogenase (OGDH), succinate dehydrogenase (SDH), succinyl-CoA synthase (SUCLG), and malate dehydrogenase (MDH). Results of this research indicated that, after concussion-like mTBI, PDH and TCA gene expressions underwent general transient decreases followed by significant increases, showing no change in acetyl-CoA and free CoA-SH concentrations. The picture was clearly and dramatically different in the case of severe TBI, where permanent PDH and TCA downregulation occurred, caused by PDP1–2 downregulations and PDK1–4 overexpression. As known, the TCA cycle requires continuous supply of acetyl-CoA [43], a reaction catalyzed by the PDH complex, through oxidative decarboxylation of pyruvate. It is important to underline that glycolysis-derived pyruvate represents almost the only source of acetyl-CoA. Therefore, brain

PDH activity and TCA cycle are strictly connected and represent an indirect gauge to assess mitochondrial function devoted to energy production [44].

Following concussion-like mTBI, an increase in the gene expressions of all subunits of the PDH complex and of the PDP1 and 2 isoforms (activating PDH) occurred at 48 h and, more evidently, at 120 h post injury, and were accompanied by a downregulation of the genes encoding for the PDK1–4 isoforms (inhibiting PDH). It then appears that brain cells adjusted to overall conditions, regulating the activity of the PDH complex early (inhibiting) or late (activating) post injury, that is, when mitochondria were, respectively, inappropriately or correctly functioning [45–47]. Data for the gene and protein expressions of the TCA cycle indicate coherent transient mitochondrial "inefficiency," confirming previous findings evidencing a "gene strategy" activating a sort of neuroprotection program adopted by "mildly" injured cerebral cells [48]. These data collectively endorse the hypothesis that mitochondria are particularly sensitive to mechanical forces delivered at the time of impact. These subcellular organelles, following concussion-like mTBI may be defined as transiently dormant, and are not yet truly dysfunctional – unless some other event will occur and frustrate this protection strategy. In other words, the mildly injured cells lie in a condition of "metabolic debt"; as long as this condition will not be overcome, cerebral cells and potentially the whole brain can be defined "vulnerable."

Another cellular homeostasis deeply disturbed by the traumatic insult is the metabolism of free amino acids (FAA) and amino group containing compounds (AGCC), molecules exerting fundamental roles in numerous neurochemical functions [49]. Within this relatively small group of substances, some are involved in the following:

- Neurotransmission, such as glutamate (Glu), γ-aminobutyrric acid (GABA), D-serine (D-Ser), and glycine (Gly)
- Indirect control of neurotransmission, such as glutamine (Gln), aspartate (Asp), tryptophan (Trp), phenylalanine (Phe), and tyrosine (Tyr)
- Cellular energy metabolism, indirectly, such as leucine (Leu), isoleucine (Ile), and valine (Val)
- Specific metabolic pathways (the so-called methyl cycle), such as methione (Met), cystathionine (L-Cystat), and S-adenosylhomocysteine (SAH) [50–55].

In a recent original experimental study from our laboratories, the influence of different levels of TBI (including concussion-like mTBI) on the time course changes of FAA and ACCG was investigated for the first time, highlighting previously unknown connections between alterations in N-acetylasparte (NAA) homeostasis and changes of amino acids directly or indirectly linked to post-injury excitotoxic phenomena [56]. Understanding NAA alterations is of inestimable importance, since this represents a copious, almost esclusively neuronal-specific, compound that is easily detectable, non-invasively, in human brains via proton magnetic resonance spectroscopy (^{1}H-MRS). These and other modifications (i.e., dysfunction of the methyl-cycle, increased nitrosative stress) are clearly reversible and of limited magnitude in concussion-like mTBI, thereby corroborating the hypothesis of the existence of a post-traumatic period of time characterized by generalized metabolic sufferance, involving main cell biological pathways and functions, even after a concussive-like episode.

A complex and interrelated mechanism connecting energy imbalance, glucose dysmetabolism, oxidative/nitrosative stress, NAA, and amino acid levels is then jeopardized by the concussive trauma. These "networked" biochemical modifications confirm, unequivocally, the crucial role of mitochondria in maintaining the biomolecular milieu of brain cells [57, 58].

Being one of the most involved subcellular organelles following a mechanical insult, it is becoming necessary to deepen our interest in understanding mitochondrial dynamics, since little has been reported in the available literature in the field of TBI [59]. Mitochondrial dynamics are regulated by a complex system of proteins representing the mitochondrial quality control (MQC). MQC balances antagonistic forces of fusion and fission determining mitochondrial wellness and cell fates. Either physiologically or pathologically, the life of mitochondria is maintained by a complex network of proteins, inter-connected by their activity and regulated by post-translational modifications involved in the control of mitochondrial fusion, fission, and autophagy [60, 61]. The continuous process of fusion and fission is a physiologic turnover, part of the usual mitochondrial network dynamics, causing macroscopic changes to the organelle morphology, and is considered to be the mitochondrial quality control (MQC) system for eukaryotic cells [62].

A recent study from our group provided, for the first time, a satisfactory vision of the (dys)regulation of the main components supervising fusion, fission, and mitophagy following graded TBI (including concussion-like mTBI) [63]. According to the data obtained in our trauma model, which mostly produces a gradable diffuse brain injury [64, 65], it is possible to postulate that cerebral cells after concussion-like mTBI are committed to increase fusion and to concomitantly decrease fission and mitophagy. Conversely, brain cells after sTBI are more prone to activate fission and mitophagy, the two phenomena being paralleled by a remarkable downregulation of fusion. Activation of fusion, in this study, resulted in a net increase in cerebral mitochondrial mass at later time points post concussion-like mTBI injury. This should not only induce the prevention of apoptosis [66, 67], but also mitochondrial cristae remodeling [68, 69], with improvement of ETC coupled to OXPHOS, thanks to the increased expression in optical dominant atrophy-1 (OPA1) protein [70]. Activation of mitochondrial fusion following concussion-like mTBI was accompanied by a significant inhibition of fission. As revealed by the gene analysis, the downregulation of the DRP1 gene (by almost 3 times) should have had remarkable beneficial effects; this hypothesis is sustained by data demonstrating that inhibiting DRP1 using the mitochondrial division inhibitor-1 (Mdivi-1) reduces cell death in different cellular and animal models [71–74]. Moreover, it has very recently been shown that Mdivi-1 reduces cortical cell loss and improves spatial memory after TBI in mice [75]. The sum of fusion stimulation and fission inhibition in our concussion-like mTBI animals has had the cumulative effect of producing no activation of mitophagy, as indicated by the unchanged (or modest change of) expressions of the genes encoding for PINK1 and PARK2, that is, the two genes regulating the PINK1/PARK2 pathway of mitophagy [76, 77]. The slight increase of PINK1, only late post injury, might be related to the additional PINK1 biochemical activities rather than activators of mitophagy, including regulators of complex I function and promoters of cell survival via interaction of calcium homeostasis [78]. Combining the data on citrate synthase, the indication is that concussion-like mTBI induces only a transitory increase in the number of "dysfunctional" mitochondria.

Putting together all of these findings, it is possible to depict a complex network of evolving molecular events, triggered by the traumatic insult, modifying cellular metabolism and metabolites, altering enzymatic activities, and influencing gene and protein expressions. How and to what degree of reversibility these modifications will progress mainly depends on the net TBI severity. All of these changes are deeply interconnected and encompass mitochondria as either main players or main targets. This has serious repercussions on the destiny and survival not only of the mitochondrion itself, but even on the cell, determining which processes contributing to the MQC (fusion, fission, mitophagy) will prevail. According to these unique reported data, following experimental concussion-like mTBI, the process will have a spontaneous benign evolution during a defined period of time, during which fusion prevails over fission and mitophagy. A schematic representation of some of the main the biochemical/metabolic/molecular targets affected by concussive brain injuries is depicted in Fig. 10.1.

The number of "disturbed" biochemical tasks during this window of time is so evidently increasing as a consequence of additional research reports that biometabolic parameters should strictly accompany the clinical assessment in the management of concussed athletes. Whatever the clinical situation could be, it is fairly conceivable to state that during a variable and scarcely foreseeable post-injury period of time, brain cells must be defined as biochemically, metabolically, and genetically vulnerable. A second injury, even milder, occurring within this window of time might have early or late disastrous consequences. The aforementioned findings might be relevant to explain why repeated concussions, taking place during this period of "biomolecular vulnerability," at least causes a disproportion between the severity of the second impact and the time of normalization of brain metabolism and resolution of symptoms [61]. But they may also explain why, in a minority of cases, repeated concussions may give raise to the catastrophic second impact syndrome [79–83], leading to malignant brain edema and intracranial hypertension.

It is also easily possible that repeated mTBIs may cause enduring impairment of the aforementioned biochemical networked systems causing "chronic" mitochondrial malfunctioning and imbalance of the MQC, up to a point of no return, given a permanent damage of complex organogram of the subcellular biomolecular "apparatuses." This phenomenon might potentially be involved in the development of chronic traumatic encephalopathy (CTE) observed, for instance, in athletes with a long history of multiple concussions [84].

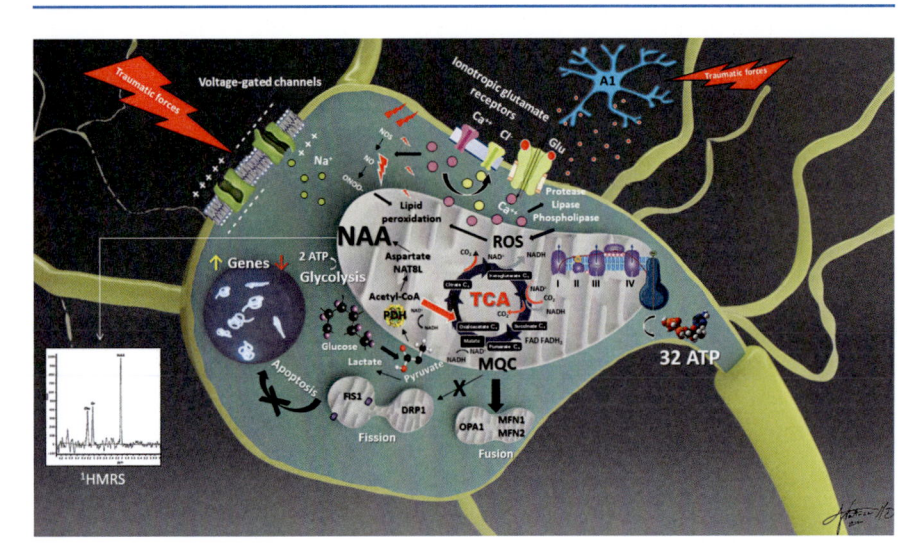

Fig. 10.1 Schematic representation of the main biochemical/metabolic/molecular targets of the energy associated with the forces acting at the time of impact (linear, rotational, causing acceleration-deceleration phenomena of the brain) and discharged to the cerebral tissue on occurrence of concussive episodes. Dysregulation of ionic homeostasis triggers a series of molecular events, affecting multiple pathways and cycles of neuronal metabolism, in which mitochondria are the main "players." At early stages post-concussion, mitochondria are transiently dysfunctional, showing decreased supply of reducing equivalents (NADH and FADH$_2$) for ETC coupled to OXPHOS functioning as well as diminished rate of ATP synthesis. During this period (named window of metabolic brain vulnerability), there is a well-orchestrated change in various gene expressions to optimize energy production and consumption and aimed to neuroprotection, by avoiding mitochondria to work at their maximal capacity while dysfunctional, thus inhibiting/limiting insurgence of oxidative/nitrosative stress cause by increased production of ROS and RNS

The reduction in energy availability alters the physiologic rate of NAA biosynthesis with a net decrease in its cerebral levels, clearly evident in post-concussed athletes when measured using ^{1}H-MRS. In the recovery phase, genes controlling the mitochondrial quality control (MCQ) system promote fusion (via OPA1, MFN1 and MFN2) and inhibit fission (via FIS1 and DRP1), thus preventing cytochrome c release, induction of mitophagy, and apoptosis. The concomitant upregulation and activation of key enzymes of glycolysis (hexokinase, phosphofructokinase, pyruvate kinase), of the pyruvate dehydrogenase (PDH) complex, of the TCA cycle allow to increase ATP production and overcome the energy crisis. This is accompanied by increased acetyl-CoA availability that ensures restoration of the NAA level, also thanks to the concomitant upregulation of the NAA biosynthetic enzyme NAT8L. Monitoring NAA levels in post-concussed athletes by ^{1}H-MRS can therefore incorporate precious information related to the time course of these biochemical/metabolic/molecular processes in the post-concussive period and it is of invaluable relevance to forecast the metabolic state of this complex network, an essential condition for safer return of concussed athletes to play

Clinical Implications: The Return-to-Play Dilemma

In the previous edition of this chapter [85], we presented a robust set of experimental and clinical data (either retrospective or prospective trials) questioning the validity of the clinical criteria (such as: neuropsychological tests, and balance tests) as the sole diagnostic and prognostic way to determine the safe return of athletes to play. We have been able to demonstrate in fact that recovery of the altered brain metabolism certainly happens significantly later than the disappearance of symptoms and/or normalization of other currently used clinical tests. Signs and symptoms are fundamental both in the diagnosis of concussion and in the early post-concussive phase management. Notwithstanding, our conclusions strongly sustain the evidence of a desperate need to "biologically" grade the "severity" of concussions.

It is the authors' belief that attempts of classification should include objective, quantifiable, and measurable "biological" parameters. After all, approaching a concussed athlete means determining their full recovery, for a safe return to play. This translates into monitoring the post-injury course and establishing the normalization of any biochemical/metabolic/molecular objective measures, demonstrating the closure of the window of brain vulnerability, a dynamic and time-based condition that is individually variable and therefore poorly liable to accurate forecasting. It should be considered hazardous (if not unethical) to allow the return to play after a concussion without having established the "healing" of biochemical/molecular parameters related to various biological brain processes as well as the normalization of eventual ultrastructural brain modifications.

The possibility of having a second concussive injury within this interval (i.e., days or weeks) has been reported to be even fatal, a phenomenon that Saunders and Harbaugh [79] called "the second-impact syndrome of catastrophic head injury" (SIS), first described by Schneider [80]. Subsequently, a handful of published cases have been reported, describing patients (mostly involved in sports-related activities) who, while still having symptoms from a previous concussive injury, experienced a second concussion that led to sustained intracranial hypertension and catastrophic outcomes, albeit the second blow might had been remarkably minor [86–88].

Several authors have asserted skepticism about SIS [89, 90], and a recent study no less questioned its "diagnostic credibility" [91]. The key concern declared by the authors of this report is that SIS seems to be a rather uncommon clinical condition, lacking a "unique presentation scheme" to support a standardized World Health Organization definition and International Classification of Disease (ICD) coding. In our opinion, it is not without a sense of irony that the most important features of SIS happen to be the main cause for questioning its own very existence.

The experimental timeline of the exquisitely metabolic nature of the "brain vulnerability" is certainly difficult to be directly translated to humans; furthermore, many other uncontrolled variables will render each second impact different from every other individual. It is then rather unlikely that SIS will ever show a fixed, clinically "unique presentation scheme," since its adverse pathophysiology (yet to be fully understood) is influenced over time by multiple variables. Paradoxically, if these authors' arguments were correct, even concussion itself (not to mention moderate and severe TBI) should be questioned, since there is no one TBI equaling another. For example, a person suffering from moderate TBI would range from GCS 13 to 9. However, this taxonomy is confusing since a GCS 13 patient lies 1 point below to eventual discharge; a GCS 9 patient lies 1 point above potential intubation.

This is the reason why in the ICD-9-CM TBI is represented by six major coding-blocks (800.0, 801.9, 803.0, 804.9, 850.0, 854.1), each one including many other subspecifications, resulting in literally hundreds of codes. Although SIS is indeed an uncommon event, a conventional code would not certainly be the most inappropriate. The unquestionable facts are that several deaths occurred to athletes receiving a second concussion at a short time from the previous one and that most of these athletes died because of refractory intracranial hypertension [92].

However, according to data obtained following experimental repeated concussions from our and other research groups [45, 93–97], it is our strong opinion that the concept of SIS should be widened and applied to those many cases (non-catastrophic) in which a clear disproportion between the entity of the second trauma and the time for recovery (in terms of clearance of clinical symptoms and normalization of brain metabolism) is present [98].

To support these notions, we briefly summarize data we obtained in our last 10 years of research using ^{1}H-MRS to determine recovery from concussion in over 200 adults (both athletes and non-athletes). According to what the patients declared on anamnesis, none of them had a previous history of concussion. In 35% of cases, the decrease in NAA was accompanied by a decrease in Cr [99], revealing different times of recovery and showing no priority patterns of metabolite normalization. In these singly concussed adults, symptoms lasted 11.2 ± 6.4 days, while recovery of brain metabolism was fulfilled after 34.5 ± 9.7 days. Worth of note is that to date, ^{1}H-MRS evaluation never showed either false positive (subjects with no concussion and with altered brain metabolite levels) or false negative (clinically concussed subjects with normal brain metabolite levels).

The aforementioned results not only almost overlap with results we previously published [17, 100], but most importantly are singularly coincident with data reported in a study published in 2020 [101]. In this paper, the advanced neuroradiological technique, Diffusion Kurtosis Imaging (DKI), was used to monitor the effects of SRC on the brain and the curve of recovery in 96 concussed American football players, at <48 h, 8, 15, and 45-days post injury. All clinical symptoms cleared by the eighth day post injury. In the concussed group, axial kurtosis was found significantly higher compared to the control group at 48 h, increased in extent and magnitude at 8 days, receded at 15 days, and returned to the normal levels by 45 days. Kurtosis Fractional Anisotropy exhibited a delayed response, with a consistent increase by days 15 and 45. In this study, changes detected in the acute period appeared to be prolonged compared to clinical recovery, and additional changes, not observable acutely, appeared to progress.

To further support all the aforementioned evidence, we here present preliminary data from a small set of 14 adolescent patients (Table 10.1). Symptoms in this cohort persisted for 25.9 ± 8.6 days, a duration 3.1 times longer than in adults, while brain metabolism recovered within 90 days from concussion, that is, metabolic vulnerability lasted 3 times longer than in adults. This summary is prodromal to introduce and describe three peculiar cases that are useful to answer to those authors who sustain that SIS is inexistent, that is, the pure fantasy birth of those who described SIS.

Table 10.1 Clinical features of the cohort of 14 adolescents studied by ¹HMRS to evaluate recovery of brain metabolism following concussion

Case number	Age (years)	Sex	Category	Cause of injury	LOC	Main symptoms	Duration of symptoms (days)
1	14	M	Athlete	Head-to-head (soccer)	N	Confusion, vision disturbances, hyperactivity	19
2	15	M	Athlete	Knee to head (soccer)	N	Nausea, vision disturbances, mood disorders	28
3	14	F	Athlete	Back bottom to the ground (horse riding)	N	Retrograde amnesia, insomnia, cognitive deficit	24
4	17	M	Athlete	Head-to-head (soccer)	Y	Headache, insomnia, dizziness, vision disturbances, cognitive deficit	41
5	16	M	Non-athlete	Scooter accident	Y	Confusion, headache, nausea, hyperactivity, cognitive deficit	26
6	18	M	Athlete	Foot-to-head (martial arts)	Y	Retrograde amnesia, vision disturbances, cognitive deficit	22
7	13	F	Athlete	Back bottom to the ground (skiing)	N	Headache, confusion, anxiety	14
8	16	M	Athlete	Head-to-head (soccer)	Y	Retrograde amnesia, dizziness, cognitive deficit	37
9	17	M	Non-athlete	Scooter accident	N	Insomnia, nausea, retrograde amnesia, cognitive deficit	26
10	14	M	Athlete	Head-to-head (soccer)	N	Headache, vision disturbances, cognitive deficit	15
11	15	M	Athlete	Rough contrast (soccer)	Y	Retrograde amnesia, headache, sleep disorders, cognitive deficit	33
12	14	M	Athlete (repeat concussions)	Foot-to-head (martial arts)	Y	Confusion, headache, retrograde amnesia, insomnia, vision disturbances, cognitive deficit	>120

(continued)

Table 10.1 (continued)

Case number	Age (years)	Sex	Category	Cause of injury	LOC	Main symptoms	Duration of symptoms (days)
13	18	M	Athlete (repeat concussions)	Punches-to-head (boxer)	Y	Confusion, headache, retrograde amnesia, insomnia, vision disturbances, cognitive deficit	>120
14	18	M	Athlete (repeat concussions)	Unknown (rugby)	Y	Confusion, headache, retrograde amnesia, insomnia, vision disturbances, anxiety, cognitive deficit	>120

Patients with number 12, 13, and 14 suffered from two repeat concussions and are fully described in the text

Case 1

A 16-year-old male, practicing martial arts, sparred with an older and heavier companion to better prepare for an upcoming tournament, receiving many blows – much more than usual. He experienced headache the same evening that persisted in the next days. Parents talked to the trainer who told them that mild headache could be due to intensive, heavy training, and was confident about his tournament participation, to be held 4 days later. During the official match, in the second round, the patient received a very modest kick on the neck, and still standing, started to reveal ataxia and slowed reflexes. Less than a minute after, he fell down experiencing 1 min of LOC. Immediately transported to hospital, he reached the ER still conscious, but a tonic crisis followed by convulsions occurred, causing a comatose state. A CT scan revealed severe brain swelling and a thin (less than 1 cm) right hemispheric subdural hematoma with 3–4 mm midline shift (Fig. 10.2a). To measure intracranial pressure and following an ICP-guided approach, an intraventricular catheter was introduced (ventriculostomy) (Fig. 10.2b). Opening pressure was above 30 mmHg, but CSF prompt escaping lowered this value to 16 mmHg, normalizing on day 3. On the sixth day, spontaneous wake up occurred, followed by gradual pharmacology intensity level weaning, up to discharge. Glasgow Outcome Scale at 30 days was classified as "good recovery." However, the player experienced typical post-concussive symptoms lasting 4 months. Serial ^{1}H-MRS were performed starting from 40 days after the second concussion. Brain metabolism recovered in 10 months, with NAA preceding Cr retrieval.

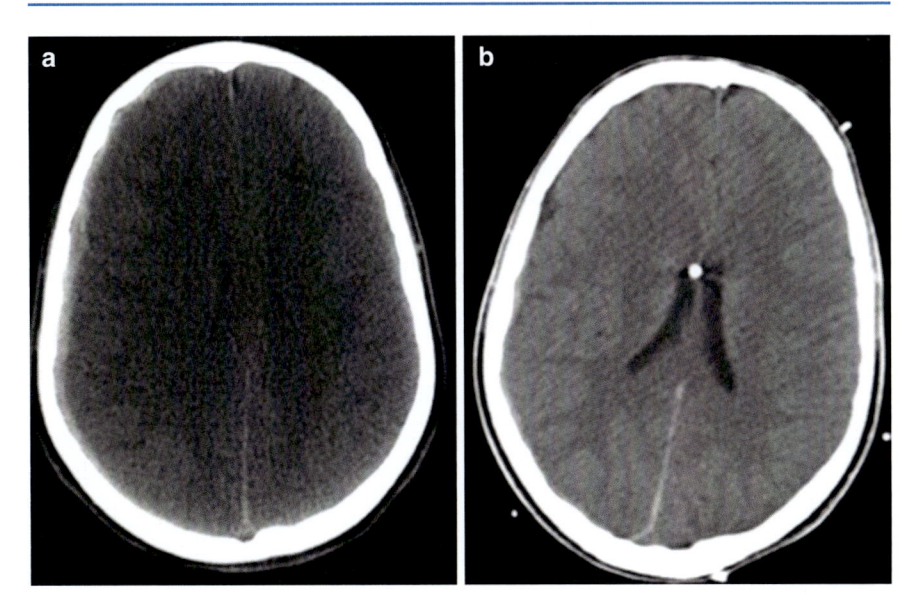

Fig. 10.2 Panel (**a**) Admission CT scan of Case 1 showing massive bilateral swelling, slightly more represented in the right hemisphere, where it was associated with a "typical" subdural hematic collection, causing minimum midline shift. Panel (**b**): Post ventriculostomy CT scan showing complete disappearance of the subdural hematoma and early amelioration of brain swelling

Case 2

An 18-year-old male was involved in a semi-professional federal boxing tournament. Sparring with a boxer of a heavier category during a pre-match training, he receives a series of punches to the head, with no particular consequences at first. On the way to the hotel, he began to suffer from headache, lasting overnight, mildly persisting for 3 days and fully cleared the morning of the fourth day where he returned to spar in the afternoon. After a few minutes of routine sparring, he asked to stop the training for recurrence of headache. It is worthy to note that he received only minor and warming-up hits during this brief period. On the bus to the hotel, he reported a sudden, rapidly increasing headache. No LOC had occurred so far. Immediately transported to the ER, he arrived comatose. A CT scan showed massive brain swelling and left, hemispheric subdural hematoma, causing more than 1 cm midline shift (Fig. 10.3a). Transferred to the neurosurgery department, he underwent an urgent fronto-temporal left craniotomy (Fig. 10.3b). The very next day, he was weaned from mechanical ventilation and was conscious, with no gross neurological impairment. However, post-concussive symptoms lasted 3 months and metabolic recovery was completed at 8 months from the second impact. In this case, levels of both Cr and NAA during this observational period were lower than the reference values of age- and sex-matched healthy controls, with Cr recovering faster than NAA.

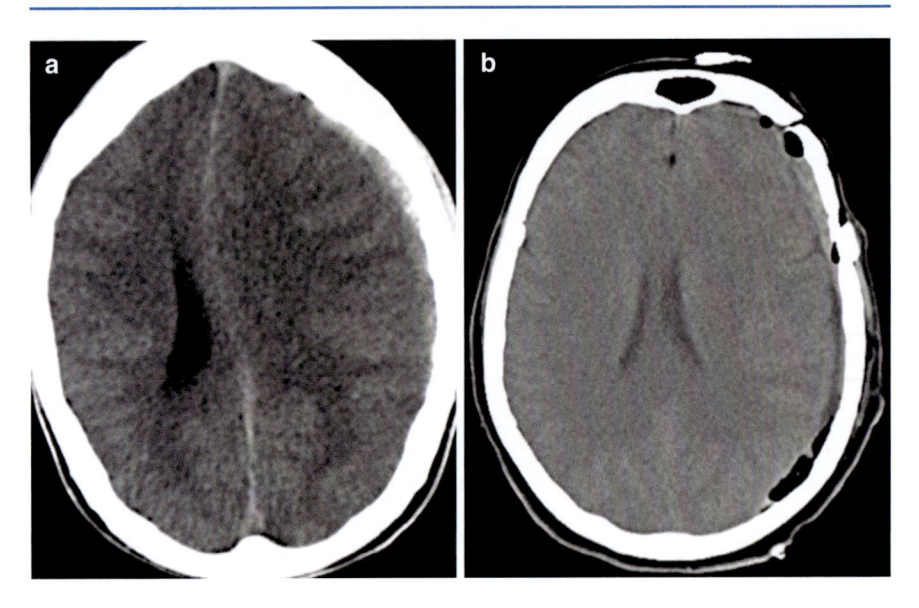

Fig. 10.3 Panel (**a**): Admission CT scan of Case 2 showing predominant left hemispheric swelling and an ipsilateral small subdural hematoma. A significant midline shift is present, not entirely accountable to the subdural collection, but mainly due to asymmetric swelling. Panel (**b**): Immediate post-operative CT scan showing resolution of the midline shift and a net amelioration of swelling, confirmed by the re-visualization of the lateral ventricles. It is worthy to notice that, as a general occurrence following any craniotomy, the subdural collection is still visible, however causing no compressive phenomena

The astonishing analogies between these two cases are intuitive, as well as the comparison of their CTs with two further examples of SIS reported in the literature, one of them almost 15 years ago (Fig. 10.4a–d).

Case 3

An 18-year-old semi-professional rugby player experienced a first concussive episode in April 2017 and did not play in any other game until next December, when he suffered from two significant hits in the same match. That evening he reported nausea, vomiting, persistent headache, and insomnia, which then were present for 2 months, when the player also started suffering from slight cognitive deficits during scholar activities. A decreased capacity to concentrate was constant with frequent insurgence of headache even for bumps while going by car, symptoms protracting until April of the following year (2018). Neuropsychological tests for the evaluation of attention, working memory, short-term memory, and episodic memory (Visual Search, Dual Task, P.A.S.A.T. – Paced Auditory Serial Addition Task, and Rey Auditory Verbal Learning Test) showed modest impairment in the verbal short-term memory. MRI resulted in no gross signal alteration, whilst ^{1}H-MRS showed persistent lower values of brain metabolites. Symptoms cleared at 6 months following the

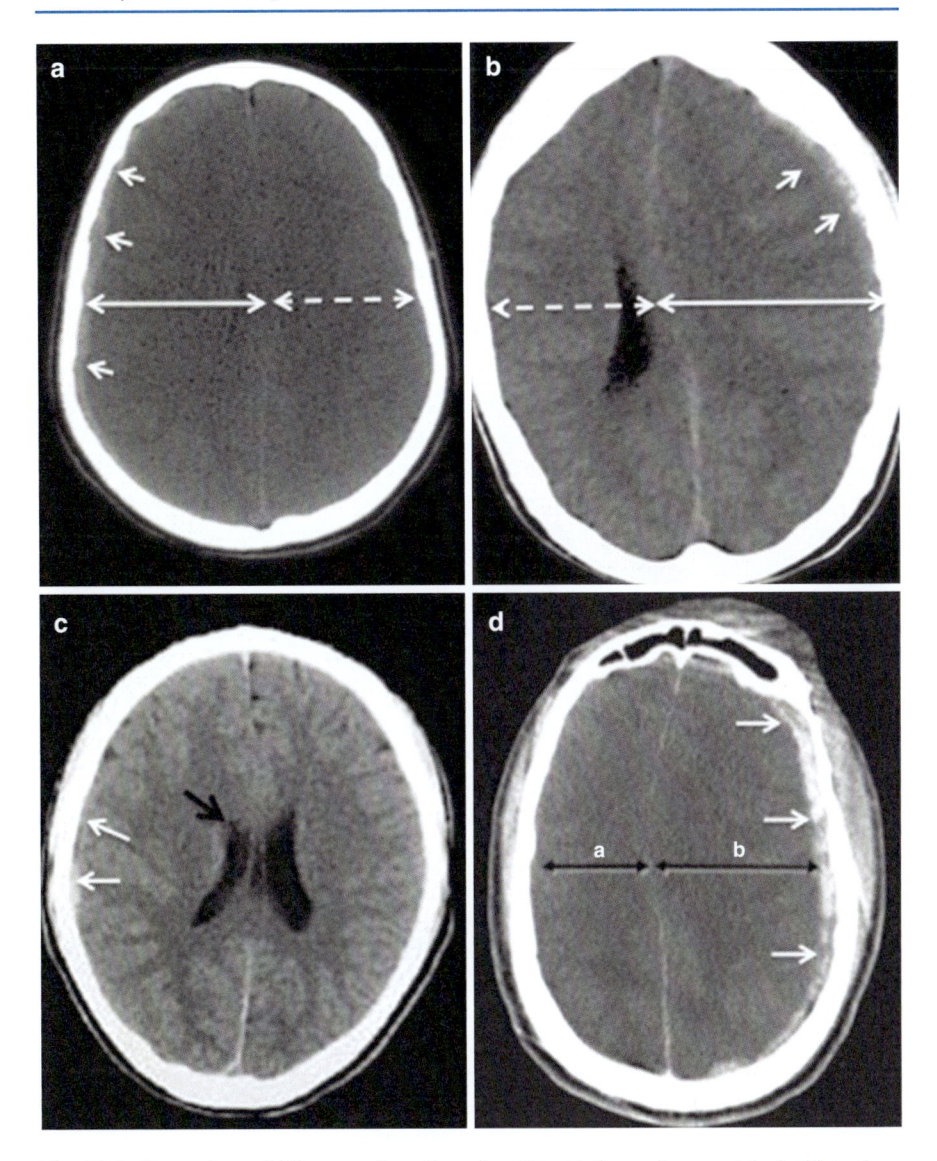

Fig. 10.4 Comparison of CT scans of our Cases 1 and 2 with those of age-matched athletes (previously published in the literature and suffering from SIS) with different dynamics but very similar clinical course and radiological presentation. Panel (**a**): Admission CT scan of Case 1 showing right hemispheric subdural hematoma (short white arrows), with midline shift and asymmetric brain swelling (long white full and dotted arrows). Panel (**b**): Admission CT scan of Case 2 showing massive left hemisphere swelling (long white arrows), causing midline shift, associated with a small left subdural hematoma (short white arrows). Panel (**c**): Admission CT scan of an athlete who experienced a second impact at 4 days from the first, revealing cerebral swelling of the right hemisphere and lateral ventricle compression (black arrow). A thin rim of subdural hematoma (white arrows) in the right fronto-temporal convexity is also visible (From Mori et al. [83]). Panel (**d**): Admission CT scan of an athlete who experienced a second impact at 4 weeks from the previous, showing a left hemispheric subdural hematoma (white arrows) associated to ipsilateral brain swelling (**b**), right hemisphere compression (**a**), and severe midline shift (black arrows). (From Cantu and Gean [87])

second concussion, but brain metabolism recovered at 9 months. In this case, NAA recovered faster than Cr.

SIS is currently defined as "the presence of malignant brain swelling occurring in a subject receiving repeat concussions minutes, days or weeks after the initial one." However, as clearly shown by the three above-described clinical cases, SIS does not necessarily result in "fatal" or "catastrophic" outcome. A broad definition of SIS is advisable, including the frequent disproportion among the entity of the second concussion and the severity of following symptoms, the time for symptom clearance after the second trauma, and the time necessary for metabolic restoration.

From a pathophysiologic point of view, SIS takes place when a subject receives the second concussion before symptoms from an earlier one have subsided. We believe that even in this case the concept needs to be broadened by stating that SIS might occur every time that a second concussion will fall within the temporal window of metabolic/biochemical/molecular brain vulnerability state. The degree of "severity" of SIS, including fatality, will depend on which phase of the metabolic recovery the brain is in at the time of the second blow.

At present, it is unpredictable how long the period of brain vulnerability will last. Our experience with the cohort of 232 athletes, confirming the previous bench data obtained and using the theoretical translation of the "rat time" into "human time" [95], strongly suggests that, in the case of subjects with no prior history of concussion, the duration of this period ranges between 20- and 45-days post injury, with a mean value of 35 days. It is worth noting that only the observation that brain metabolism has fully recovered will demonstrate the closure of the temporal window of brain vulnerability and that a new concussive episode will not develop into SIS (either fatal or non-fatal).

From Diagnosis to Prognosis: Magnetic Resonance Applications and "Deep Structural Neuroimaging"

Traditional structural neuroimaging techniques are normal in athletes who sustain SRC, particularly when referring to MRI. A prospective, large-scale study was recently published, stating that less than 1% of SRCs are associated with acute injury findings on qualitative structural MRI, thus providing empirical support for clinical guidelines not recommending the use of MRI following SRC [102]. This notion was well acknowledged by emergency physicians, neurologists, neurosurgeons, and intensivists.

Not even in severe TBIs MRI can find application during the early phases, given the complex management of an intubated and mechanically ventilated, multi-invasively monitored patient. Indication apart, the logistic issue is enormous. In this clinical setting, CT technology rules unchallenged, and MR investigations are taken generally in the subacute period having lost its "native" diagnostic role, revealing instead an important prognostic function. Interestingly, the prospective evidence of the above-cited study showed that SRC was indeed associated with a higher incidence of non-specific MRI findings, yet requiring clinical follow-up. Sinus disease, heterotopia, tumor, aneurysm, and pineal cyst are described examples of clearly non-trauma-related findings; white matter hyperintensity, chronic microhemorrhages, and pituitary abnormalities are examples accountable to prior head trauma. In other words, MRI not only lacks SRC specificity, but also carries "unnecessary" sensitivity. Is it then "inconvenient" to perform MRIs given the risk of facing occasional brain abnormalities that, regardless, would require discontinuing an athlete activity?

Approximately 640 papers were published in the last 10 years specifically addressing concussion and various advanced MRI applications in mTBI; as far as SRC is concerned, 290 studies were found, 280 of which entirely focused on advanced MRI.

The modern growing interest in advanced MRI is mainly dedicated to developing "biomarkers of brain connectivity," from resting-state functional (rs-fMRI) to diffusion tensor imaging (DTI), with the purpose of aiding objective data useful in the diagnosis and management of concussion. A systematic review identified 1351 citations, but with only 14 studies meeting the review inclusion criteria (5 rs-fMRI and 10 DTI; 680 patients with mTBI vs. 436 controls) including those where advanced MRI was performed from less than 12 h [103]. The most common clinical outcome measure used in these studies was symptom burden, namely, the Rivermead Post-Concussion Questionnaire. The most frequently studied brain connectivity biomarkers evaluated by advanced MRI were global functional connectivity, default-mode network, and fractional anisotropy (FA). Although the rigid selection reduced the amount of available data, the conclusion indicated that brain connectivity biomarkers (measurable by advanced MRI), obtained within 1 month of injury, are useful in predicting outcome.

As reported in another paper, however, studies are typically cross-sectional (CS) comparing groups of concussed and uninjured athletes, while it would be important to determine whether these findings are consistent with longitudinal (LNG) changes at the individual level, relative to their own pre-injury baseline [104]. Among concussed athletes, abnormalities were identified for white matter FA and mean diffusivity, along with gray matter cerebral blood flow, using both CS and LNG approaches. Comparing data with uninjured matched controls equally studied (to have a longitudinal control group), patterns of abnormality for CS and LNG were distinct, with significant differences in the percentage of abnormal voxels. These results highlighted the importance of using pre-injury individual baseline data when evaluating concussion-related abnormalities and the return to play issue.

In the future, more clarifying data about symptoms and recovery patterns are expected to come from "connectomics" [105]. Indeed, this new field of innovative MRI enables researchers to conduct a much deeper analysis, combining anatomical neural network data with actual DTI fiber tractography to reconstruct a reliable map of damaged connections. In addition, using T1-weighted surface-based morphometry (SBM), it is possible to perform distinct exploration of cortical surface, area, thickness, and volume alterations over the entire cortex [106]. By means of a combination of DTI fiber tractography and graph-theoretical network analysis, brain complexity is mapped as a widely distributed network of nodes and edges. Therefore, the strength of the anatomical link is measured as the total number of interconnecting fibers, thus enabling to quantify the post-injury disrupted network efficiency [107].

At present, however, there is an urging "clinical," not hypothetical, need for more sophisticated, non-invasive imaging capable of detecting changes in neurophysiology after injury. Concussion is associated with prognostic neurometabolic changes, impairing axonal-network functions. Proton magnetic resonance spectroscopy (^{1}H-MRS) is nowadays capable of measuring and monitoring brain biochemistry and identifying and quantifying adverse physiologic changes after concussion [108]. A systematic review of articles published in the English language up to February 2013, including observational, cohort, correlational, cross-sectional, and longitudinal studies revealed that only 11 publications satisfied the inclusion criteria, comprising data on 200 athletes and 116 controls [109]. Nine of the 11 studies reported an MRS abnormality consistent with an alteration in neurochemistry, far beyond the resolution of symptoms. Many more and larger, prospective, longitudinal studies are needed, rather than periodic reviews of the literature. This is probably the reason why, notwithstanding the uniformity of the clinical data with results of laboratory studies, several researchers involved in SRCs still consider ^{1}H-MRS merely as a sophisticated, possibly superfluous, "research tool" of no clinical utility.

The long-term neurobiological effects of concussion were recently assessed in youths, to determine the association between a history of concussion and NAA levels in the dorsolateral prefrontal cortex (DLPFC) [110]. Two and half years post injury, lower levels of NAA were measured in the right DLPFC in school athletes with past concussion compared to controls. The effect of lower NAA concentrations in the right DLPFC was primarily driven by youth with a single prior concussion versus those with multiple concussions. NAA in the left DLPFC, but not in right DLPFC, was associated with worse emotional symptoms in youth with concussion.

A ^{1}H-MRS investigation in symptomatic former NFL players was carried out to address long-term neurologic consequences of exposure to repetitive head impacts (RHI) [111]. The sample included 77 symptomatic former NFL players and 23 asymptomatic individuals without a head trauma history. NAA, glutamate/glutamine, choline, myo-inositol, creatine, and glutathione were measured in the posterior (PCG) and anterior (ACG) cingulate gyrus, and parietal white matter (PWM). PWM NAA was lower among the former NFL players, showing a direct effect between RHI and reduced cellular energy metabolism (i.e., lower Cr).

A longitudinal ^{1}H-MRS study to determine deviations in the neurometabolic profile of patients with mTBI from healthy controls at different stages of mTBI, and the associations between acute neurometabolic findings and chronic neurocognitive performance, was published in 2014 [112]. The CS comparison revealed decreasing trends of NAA/Cr at the early subacute stages in the thalamus and centrum semiovale (CSV), recovering over time. Most interestingly, within the trauma group, absolute concentration of Cr measured in the CSV at early subacute stages (5 ± 3 days), showed a positive correlation with chronic cognitive impairment.

Strictly linked to metabolism is the intrinsic neuronal activity appearing as spontaneous fluctuations in the blood oxygen level-dependent (BOLD) functional MRI (fMRI) signal, exhibiting synchrony within neuroanatomically and functionally related brain regions. Intrinsic neuronal signaling accounts for most of the brain's energy expenditure. Many established methods, each with its own advantages and disadvantages, are available for characterizing synchrony in intrinsic neuronal activity (functional connectivity) [113]. Changes in functional connectivity have been reported in various neurological and psychiatric diseases, and such alterations might have potential as clinical biomarkers in the long-term post-concussive effects [114].

Much of the progress that has been made in our basic science understanding neuronal metabolism can be applied to neuronal network activity, as detected by fMRI, aiding in the interpretation of clinical changes during concussive-damage evolution. Among these networks, the default-mode network (DMN) is of particular interest [115]. The DMN is a definite network that is active at rest and abolished when activities implying attention and decision-making are in function. Essential components of DMN are the posterior cingulate cortex (PCC), precuneus, inferior parietal, and medial prefrontal cortex (MPFC) nodes. A key cognitive role is assigned to these networks as memory encoding and consolidation, and space orientation for PCC. MPFC appears involved in self-consideration, rapid error identification, and social functions. In patients with concussion, these high-level cognitive functions are often negatively affected.

Finally, pre-injury connectivity and NMDA receptor subtype composition (NR2A and NR2B content) are considered important predictors of node loss and remodeling [116]. Mechanistically, stretch injury, causing a reduction in voltage-dependent Mg^{2+} and blocking the NR2B-containing NMDA receptors, will further impair the network function and plasticity. Given the demonstrated link between the NR2B-NMDA complex and mitochondrial dysfunction, it does not appear surprising that ultimately neuronal de-integration from the network is again mediated through mitochondrial signaling [117].

Conclusion

Even if classified as an mTBI, concussion is directly responsible for sudden biochemical changes occurring at the time of impact but spreading over time in a chained-reactive fashion. These complex biochemical derangements, involving not only metabolic changes but also down- or up-regulations of a vast number of protein and gene expressions, can result in a dangerous state for the brain, generating a situation of metabolic vulnerability, a condition that is imperative to assess before allowing a safe return to play of a concussed athlete. Following single, double, or repeated concussions, cellular and subcellular dysfunctions might be responsible for changes of supreme importance at an ultra-structural level, far beyond the resolution of current non-invasive technologies. Currently, management of concussed athletes and their return to play are only based on presence of symptoms and neuropsychologic test score, none of them being capable of measuring any objective biological parameter connected to the hundreds of biochemical/molecular nervous cell modifications triggered by concussions. This is probably why, paradoxically, "the mildest" of all TBIs is, to date, the least understood.

At present, determination of different brain metabolites by proton ^{1}H-MRS (including NAA, Cr, and Cho) represents a rapid, easy-to-perform, non-invasive instrument to accurately and dynamically quantify the most important modification of cerebral biochemistry. This technique shows that alterations of brain metabolism last much longer than symptom clearance and neuropsychologic test normalization in post-concussed athletes. One of the biggest challenges of the next years will be to expand the application of MR technology, and to achieve a clearer picture of post-concussive neurobiology, by reliably identifying biological objective parameters to corroborate the initial clinical management. Further advances in this domain will tremendously improve our comprehension of what is occurring to the neuronal network and the possible evolution of a concussion. To date, since there is not even one preclinical study showing that concussive-like injuries leave brain metabolism and functions equal to those observable before impact, it is clear that these changes are intrinsic and typical of concussions and that, if found in laboratory animals, they certainly occur to nervous cells of human beings after a concussion. In light of this, also considering the availability of the different advanced neuroimaging techniques (^{1}H-MRS, DTI, fMRI, etc.), it is becoming challenging that concussed athletes are allowed to return to play without undergoing objective analyses capable of determining whether fine biochemical, molecular, metabolic, ultra-structural brain parameters are equal to those of healthy controls. Coupling such data with those related to clinical follow-up cannot be considered just a research speculation matter, since it would enable a far more accurate and conscientious understanding to cure and prevent short- and long-term consequences of this truly peculiar form of traumatic brain injury.

Acknowledgement We wish to thank Dr. G. Natuzzi M.D. for his help in realizing the illustration of this chapter.

References

1. Dewan MC, Rattani A, Gupta S, Baticulon RE, Hung YC, Punchak M, et al. Estimating the global incidence of traumatic brain injury. J Neurosurg. 2018:1–18. https://doi.org/10.3171/2017.10.JNS17352.
2. Rusnak M. Traumatic brain injury: giving voice to a silent epidemic. Nat Rev Neurol. 2013;9:186–7.
3. Rubiano AM, Carney N, Chesnut R, Puyana JC. Global neurotrauma research challenges and opportunities. Nature. 2015;527:S193–7.
4. Theadom A, Mahon S, Hume P, et al. Incidence of sports-related traumatic brain injury of all severities: a systematic review. Neuroepidemiology. 2020;54:192–9. https://doi.org/10.1159/000505424.
5. Gardner AJ, Zafonte R. Neuroepidemiology of traumatic brain injury. Handb Clin Neurol. 2016;138:207–23. https://doi.org/10.1016/B978-0-12-802973-2.00012-4.

6. Kristman VL, Borg J, Godbolt AK, Salmi LR, Cancelliere C, Carroll LJ, et al. Methodological issues and research recommendations for prognosis after mild traumatic brain injury: results of the international collaboration on mild traumatic brain injury prognosis. Arch Phys Med Rehabil. 2014;95(3 Suppl):S265–77.
7. Roozenbeek B, Maas AI, Menon DK. Changing patterns in the epidemiology of traumatic brain injury. Nat Rev Neurol. 2013;9:231–6.
8. Coronado VG, Xu L, Basavaraju SV, et al. Surveillance for traumatic brain injury-related deaths--United States, 1997-2007. MMWR Surveill Summ. 2011;60:1–32.
9. McCrory P, Johnston K, Meeuwisse W, et al. Summary and agreement statement of the 2nd international conference on concussion in sport, Prague 2004. Br J Sports Med. 2005;39:196–204. https://doi.org/10.1136/bjsm.2005.018614.
10. Signoretti S, Vagnozzi R, Tavazzi B, Lazzarino G. The pathophysiology of concussive brain injury. In: Victoroff J, Bigler E, editors. Textbook of concussion and traumatic encephalopathy. Cambridge: Cambridge University Press; 2019. p. 138–52.
11. De Koning ME, Scheenen ME, Van Der Horn HJ, Spikman JM, Van Der Naalt J. From 'miserable minority' to the 'fortunate few': the other end of the mild traumatic brain injury spectrum. Brain Inj. 2018;32:540–3. https://doi.org/10.1080/02699052.2018.1431844.
12. Manley G, Gardner AJ, Schneider KJ, Guskiewicz KM, Bailes J, Cantu RC, et al. A systematic review of potential long-term effects of sport-related concussion. Br J Sports Med. 2017;51:969–77. https://doi.org/10.1136/bjsports-2017-097791.
13. McAllister T, McCrea M. Long-term cognitive and neuropsychiatric consequences of repetitive concussion and head-impact exposure. J Athl Train. 2017;52:309–17. https://doi.org/10.4085/1062-6050-52.1.14.
14. McCrory P, Meeuwisse W, Dvořák J, Aubry M, Bailes J, Broglio S, et al. Consensus statement on concussion in sport-the 5th international conference on concussion in sport held in Berlin, October 2016. Br J Sports Med. 2017;51:838–47. https://doi.org/10.1136/bjsports-2017-097699.
15. Aubry M, Cantu R, Dvorak J, Graf-Baumann T, Johnston KM, Kelly J, Concussion in Sport (CIS) Group, et al. Summary and agreement statement of the 1st international symposium on concussion in sport, Vienna 2001. Clin J Sport Med. 2002;12:6–11.
16. Broglio SP, Kontos AP, Levin H, Schneider K, Wilde EA, Cantu RC, et al. National Institute of Neurological Disorders and Stroke and Department of Defense Sport-Related Concussion Common Data Elements Version 1.0 Recommendations. J Neurotrauma. 2018;35:2776–83. https://doi.org/10.1089/neu.2018.5643.
17. Vagnozzi R, Signoretti S, Tavazzi B, Floris R, Ludovici A, Marziali S, et al. Temporal window of metabolic brain vulnerability to concussion: a pilot ^{1}H-magnetic resonance spectroscopic study in concussed athletes. Part III. Neurosurgery. 2008;62:1286–96. https://doi.org/10.1227/01.neu.0000333300.34189.74.
18. Wojtys EM, Hovda D, Landry G, Boland A, Lovell M, McCrea M, et al. Current concepts. Concussion in sports. Am J Sports Med. 1999;27:676–87. https://doi.org/10.1177/03635465990270052401.
19. Post A, Blaine Hoshizaki T, Gilchrist MD, Brien S, Cusimano MD, Marshall S. The influence of acceleration loading curve characteristics on traumatic brain injury. J Biomech. 2014;47:1074–81. https://doi.org/10.1016/j.jbiomech.2013.12.026i.
20. Rowson S, Duma SM, Stemper BD, Shah A, Mihalik JP, Harezlak J, et al. Correlation of concussion symptom profile with head impact biomechanics: a case for individual-specific injury tolerance. J Neurotrauma. 2018;35:681–90. https://doi.org/10.1089/neu.2017.5169.
21. Rowson S, Bland ML, Campolettano ET, Press JN, Rowson B, Smith JA, et al. Biomechanical perspectives on concussion in sport. Sports Med Arthrosc Rev. 2016;24:100–7.
22. Romeu-Mejia R, Giza CC, Goldman JT. Concussion pathophysiology and injury biomechanics. Curr Rev Musculoskelet Med. 2019;12:105–16. https://doi.org/10.1007/s12178-019-09536-8.

23. Beckwith JG, Greenwald RM, Chu JJ, Crisco JJ, Rowson S, Duma SM, et al. Timing of concussion diagnosis is related to head impact exposure prior to injury. Med Sci Sports Exerc. 2013;45:747–54.
24. Guskiewicz KM, Mihalik JP. Biomechanics of sport concussion. Exerc Sport Sci Rev. 2011;39:4–11.
25. Caccese JB, Buckley TA, Tierney RT, Arbogast KB, Rose WC, Glutting JJ, et al. Head and neck size and neck strength predict linear and rotational acceleration during purposeful soccer heading. Sports Biomech. 2017;3141:1–15.
26. Magou GC, Pfister BJ, Berlin JR. Effect of acute stretch injury on action potential and network activity of rat neocortical neurons in culture. Brain Res. 1624;2015:525–35.
27. Yap YC, Dickson TC, King AE, Breadmore MC, Guijt RM. Microfluidic culture platform for studying neuronal response to mild to very mild axonal stretch injury. Biomicrofluidics. 2014;8:044110.
28. Sullivan S, Eucker SA, Gabrieli D, Bradfield C, Coats B, Maltese MR, et al. White matter tract-oriented deformation predicts traumatic axonal brain injury and reveals rotational direction-specific vulnerabilities. Biomech Model Mechanobiol. 2015;14:877–96.
29. Ahmadzadeh H, Smith DH, Shenoy VB. Viscoelasticity of tau proteins leads to strain rate-dependent breaking of microtubules during axonal stretch injury: predictions from a mathematical model. Biophys J. 2014;106:1123–33.
30. Pan Y, Sullivan D, Shreiber DI, Pelegri AA. Finite element modeling of CNS white matter kinematics: use of a 3D RVE to determine material properties. Front Bioeng Biotechnol. 2013;1:19. https://doi.org/10.3389/fbioe.2013.00019.
31. Prange MT, Meaney DF, Margulies SS. Defining brain mechanical properties: effects of region, direction, and species. Stapp Car Crash J. 2000;44:205–13.
32. Ivarsson J, Viano DC, Lovsund P. Influence of the lateral ventricles and irregular skull base on brain kinematics due to sagittal plane head rotation. J Biomech Eng. 2002;124:422–31.
33. Ivarsson J, Viano DC, Lovsund P, Aldman B. Strain relief from the cerebral ventricles during head impact: experimental studies on natural protection of the brain. J Biomech. 2000;33:181–9.
34. Geddes DM, Cargill RS 2nd, Laplaca MC. Mechanical stretch to neurons results in a strain rate and magnitude-dependent increase in plasma membrane permeability. J Neurotrauma. 2003;20:1039–49.
35. Yi JH, Hazell AS. Excitotoxic mechanisms and the role of astrocytic glutamate transporters in traumatic brain injury. Neurochem Int. 2006;48:394–403.
36. Spaethling JM, Klein DM, Singh P, Meaney DF. Calcium-permeable AMPA receptors appear in cortical neurons after traumatic mechanical injury and contribute to neuronal fate. J Neurotrauma. 2008;25:1207–16.
37. Giza CC, Hovda DA. The neurometabolic cascade of concussion. J Athl Train. 2001;36:228–35.
38. Signoretti S, Vagnozzi R, Tavazzi B, Lazzarino G. Biochemical and neurochemical sequelae following mild traumatic brain injury: summary of experimental data and clinical implications. Neurosurg Focus. 2010;29:E1. https://doi.org/10.3171/2010.9.FOCUS10183.
39. Tavazzi B, Vagnozzi R, Signoretti S, Amorini AM, Belli A, Cimatti M, et al. Temporal window of metabolic brain vulnerability to concussions: oxidative and nitrosative stresses. Part II. Neurosurgery. 2007;61:390–6. https://doi.org/10.1227/01.neu.0000255525.34956.3f.
40. Di Pietro V, Yakoub KM, Caruso G, Lazzarino G, Signoretti S, Barbey AK, et al. Antioxidant therapies in traumatic brain injury. Antioxidants. 2020;9:260. https://doi.org/10.3390/antiox9030260.
41. Amorini AM, Lazzarino G, Di Pietro V, Signoretti S, Lazzarino G, Belli A, et al. Metabolic, enzymatic and gene involvement in cerebral glucose dysmetabolism after traumatic brain injury. Biochim Biophys Acta. 1862;2016:679–87. https://doi.org/10.1016/j.bbadis.2016.01.023.
42. Lazzarino G, Amorini AM, Signoretti S, Musumeci G, Lazzarino G, Caruso G, et al. Pyruvate dehydrogenase and tricarboxylic acid cycle enzymes are sensitive targets of traumatic brain

injury induced metabolic derangement. Int J Mol Sci. 2019;20:5774. https://doi.org/10.3390/ijms20225774.
43. Shi L, Tu BP. Acetyl-CoA and the regulation of metabolism: mechanisms and consequences. Curr Opin Cell Biol. 2015;33:125–31.
44. Lapel M, Weston P, Strassheim D, Karoor V, Burns N, Lyubchenko T, et al. Glycolysis and oxidative phosphorylation are essential for purinergic receptor-mediated angiogenic responses in vasa vasorum endothelial cells. Am J Physiol Cell Physiol. 2017;312:C56–70.
45. Vagnozzi R, Tavazzi B, Signoretti S, Amorini AM, Belli A, Cimatti M, et al. Temporal window of metabolic brain vulnerability to concussions: mitochondrial-related impairment. Part I. Neurosurgery. 2007;61:379–89. https://doi.org/10.1227/01.NEU.0000280002.41696.D8.
46. Tavazzi B, Signoretti S, Lazzarino G, Amorini AM, Delfini R, Cimatti M, et al. Cerebral oxidative stress and depression of energy metabolism correlate with severity of diffuse brain injury in rats. Neurosurgery. 2005;56:582–9. https://doi.org/10.1227/01.neu.0000156715.04900.e6.
47. Signoretti S, Di Pietro V, Vagnozzi R, Lazzarino G, Amorini AM, Belli A, et al. Transient alterations of creatine, creatine phosphate, N-acetylaspartate and high-energy phosphates after mild traumatic brain injury in the rat. Mol Cell Biochem. 2010;333:269–77.
48. Amorini AM, Di Pietro V, Amorini AM, Tavazzi B, Hovda DA, Signoretti S, et al. Potentially neuroprotective gene modulation in an in vitro model of mild traumatic brain injury. Mol Cell Biochem. 2013;375:185–98.
49. Lazzarino G, Di Pietro V, Signoretti S, Lazzarino G, Belli A, Tavazzi B. Severity of experimental traumatic brain injury modulates changes in concentrations of cerebral free amino acids. J Cell Mol Med. 2017;21:530–42.
50. Gundersen V, Storm-Mathisen J, Bergersen LH. Neuroglial transmission. Physiol Rev. 2015;95:695–726.
51. Meunier CN, Dallérac G, Le Roux N, Levasseur G, Amar M, Pollegioni L, et al. D-serine and glycine differentially control neurotransmission during visual cortex critical period. PLoS One. 2016;11:e0151233. https://doi.org/10.1371/journal.pone.0151233.
52. Sekine A, Okamoto M, Kanatani Y, Sano M, Shibata K, Fukuwatari T. Amino acids inhibit kynurenic acid formation via suppression of kynurenine uptake or kynurenic acid synthesis in rat brain in vitro. Springerplus. 2015;4:48. https://doi.org/10.1186/s40064-015-0826-9.
53. Olsen GM, Sonnewald U. Glutamate: where does it come from and where does it go? Neurochem Int. 2015;88:47–52.
54. Shnitko TA, Taylor SC, Stringfield SJ, Zandy SL, Cofresí RU, Doherty JM, et al. Acute phenylalanine/tyrosine depletion of phasic dopamine in the rat brain. Psychopharmacology. 2016;233:2045–54.
55. De Simone R, Vissicchio F, Mingarelli C, De Nuccio C, Visentin S, Ajmone-Cat MA, et al. Branched-chain amino acids influence the immune properties of microglial cells and their responsiveness to pro-inflammatory signals. Biochim Biophys Acta. 1832;2013:650–9.
56. Di Pietro V, Amorini AM, Tavazzi B, Vagnozzi R, Logan A, Lazzarino G, et al. The molecular mechanisms affecting N-acetylaspartate homeostasis following experimental graded traumatic brain injury. Mol Med. 2014;20:147–57.
57. Ruszkiewicz J, Albrecht J. Changes in the mitochondrial antioxidant systems in neurodegenerative diseases and acute brain disorders. Neurochem Int. 2015;88:66–72.
58. Kaminskyy VO, Zhivotovsky B. Free radicals in cross talk between autophagy and apoptosis. Antioxid Redox Signal. 2014;21:86–102.
59. Fischer TD, Hylin MJ, Zhao J, Moore AN, Neal Waxham M, Dash PK. Altered mitochondrial dynamics and TBI pathophysiology. Front Syst Neurosci. 2016;10:29. https://doi.org/10.3389/fnsys.2016.00029.
60. Lehmann S, Martins LM. Insights into mitochondrial quality control pathways and Parkinson's disease. J Mol Med. 2013;91:665–71.
61. Twig G, Elorza A, Molina AJA, Mohamed H, Wikstrom JK, Walzer G, et al. Fission and selective fusion govern mitochondrial segregation and elimination by autophagy. EMBO J. 2008;27:433–46.

62. Bohovych I, Chan SS, Khalimonchuk O. Mitochondrial protein quality control: the mechanisms guarding mitochondrial health. Antioxid Redox Signal. 2015;22:977–94.
63. Di Pietro V, Lazzarino G, Amorini AM, Signoretti S, Hill LJ, Porto E, et al. Fusion or fission: the destiny of mitochondria in traumatic brain injury of different severities. Sci Rep. 2017;7:9189. https://doi.org/10.1038/s41598-017-09587-2.
64. Marmarou A, Foda MA, van den Brink W, Campbell J, Kita H, Demetriadou K. A new model of diffuse brain injury in rats. Part I: pathophysiology and biomechanics. J Neurosurg. 1994;80:291–300.
65. Foda MA, Marmarou A. A new model of diffuse brain injury in rats. Part II: Morphological characterization. J Neurosurg. 1994;80:301–13.
66. Frezza C, Cipolat S, Martins de Brito O, Micaroni M, Beznoussenko GV, Rudka T, et al. OPA1 controls apoptotic cristae remodeling independently from mitochondrial fusion. Cell. 2006;126:177–89.
67. Jahani-Asl A, Pilon-Larose K, Xu W, MacLaurin JG, Park DS, McBride HM, et al. The mitochondrial inner membrane GTPase, optic atrophy 1 (Opa1), restores mitochondrial morphology and promotes neuronal survival following excitotoxicity. J Biol Chem. 2011;286:4772–82.
68. Kao S, Yen M, Wang A, Yeh Y, Lin A. Changes in mitochondrial morphology and bioenergetics in human lymphoblastoid cells with four novel OPA1 mutations. Invest Ophthalmol Vis Sci. 2015;56:2269–78.
69. Kumar R, Bukowski MJ, Wider JM, Reynolds CA, Calo L, Lepore B, et al. Mitochondrial dynamics following global cerebral ischemia. Mol Cell Neurosci. 2016;76:68–75.
70. Mishra P, Carelli V, Manfredi G, Chan DC. Proteolytic cleavage of Opa1 stimulates mitochondrial inner membrane fusion and couples fusion to oxidative phosphorylation. Cell Metab. 2014;19:630–41.
71. Cassidy-Stone A, Chipuk JE, Ingerman E, Song C, Yoo C, Kuwana T, et al. Chemical inhibition of the mitochondrial division dynamin reveals its role in bax/bak-dependent mitochondrial outer membrane permeabilization. Dev Cell. 2008;14:193–204.
72. Rappold PM, Cui M, Grima JC, Fan RZ, de Mesy-Bentley KL, Chen L, et al. Drp1 inhibition attenuates neurotoxicity and dopamine release deficits in vivo. Nat Commun. 2014;5:5244. https://doi.org/10.1038/ncomms6244-.
73. Grohm J, Kim SW, Mamrak U, Tobaben S, Cassidy-Stone A, Nunnari J, et al. Inhibition of Drp1 provides neuroprotection in vitro and in vivo. Cell Death Differ. 2012;19:1446–58. https://doi.org/10.1038/cdd.2012.18.
74. Zhao Y, Cui M, Chen S, Dong Q, Liu X. Amelioration of ischemic mitochondrial injury and Bax-dependent outer membrane permeabilization by Mdivi-1. CNS Neurosci Ther. 2014;20:528–38.
75. Wu Q, Xia SX, Li QQ, Gao Y, Shen X, Ma L, et al. Mitochondrial division inhibitor 1 (Mdivi-1) offers neuroprotection through diminishing cell death and improving functional outcome in a mouse model of traumatic brain injury. Brain Res. 1630;2016:134–43.
76. Alavi MV, Fuhrmann N. Dominant optic atrophy, OPA1, and mitochondrial quality control: understanding mitochondrial network dynamics. Mol Neurodegener. 2013;8:32. https://doi.org/10.1186/1750-1326-8-32.
77. Ashrafi G, Schwarz TL. PINK1- and PARK2-mediated local mitophagy in distal neuronal axons. Autophagy. 2015;11:187–9.
78. Voigt A, Berlemann LA, Winklhofer KF. The mitochondrial kinase PINK1: functions beyond mitophagy. J Neurochem. 2016;139(Suppl 1):232–9.
79. Saunders RL, Harbaugh RE. Second impact in catastrophic contact-sports head trauma. JAMA. 1984;252:538–9.
80. Schneider RC. Head and neck injuries in football: mechanisms, treatment and prevention. Baltimore: Williams & Wilkins; 1973.
81. Cobb S, Battin B. Second-impact syndrome. J Sch Nurs. 2004;20:262–7.
82. Logan SM, Bell GW, Leonard JC. Acute subdural hematoma in a high school football player after 2 unreported episodes of head trauma: a case report. J Athl Train. 2001;36:433–6.

83. Mori T, Katayama Y, Kawamata T. Acute hemispheric swelling associated with thin subdural hematomas: pathophysiology of repetitive head injury in sports. Acta Neurochir Suppl. 2006;96:40–3.
84. Singla A, Leineweber B, Monteith S, Oskouian RJ, Tubbs RS. The anatomy of concussion and chronic traumatic encephalopathy: a comprehensive review. Clin Anat. 2019;32:310–8. https://doi.org/10.1002/ca.23313.
85. Signoretti S, Tavazzi B, Lazzarino G, Vagnozzi R. The relevance of assessing cerebral metabolic recovery for a safe return to play following concussion. In: Slobounov SM, Sebastianelli WJ, editors. Concussions in athletics. From Brain to Behavior. New York: Springer Science+Business Media; 2014. p. 89–112. https://doi.org/10.1007/978-1-4939-0295-8_6.
86. May T, Foris LA, Donnally CJ III. Second impact syndrome. In: StatPearls. Treasure Island: StatPearls Publishing; 2020.
87. Cantu RC, Gean AD. Second-impact syndrome and a small subdural hematoma: an uncommon catastrophic result of repetitive head injury with a characteristic imaging appearance. J Neurotrauma. 2010;27:1557–64. https://doi.org/10.1089/neu.2010.1334.
88. Stovitz SD, Weseman JD, Hooks MC, Schmidt RJ, Koffel JB, Patricios JS. What definition is used to describe second impact syndrome in sports? A systematic and critical review. Curr Sports Med Rep. 2017;16:50–5. https://doi.org/10.1249/JSR.0000000000000326.
89. McLendon LA, Kralik SF, Grayson PA, Golomb MR. The controversial second impact syndrome: a review of the literature. Pediatr Neurol. 2016;62:9–17.
90. Mccrory P, Davis G, Makdissi M. Second impact syndrome or cerebral swelling after sporting head injury. Curr Sports Med Rep. 2012;11:21–3.
91. Hebert O, Schlueter K, Hornsby M, Van Gorder S, Snodgrass S, Cook C. The diagnostic credibility of second impact syndrome: a systematic literature review. J Sci Med Sport. 2016;19:789–94. https://doi.org/10.1016/j.jsams.2015.12.517.
92. Tator C, Starkes J, Dolansky G, Quet J, Michaud J, Vassilyadi M. Fatal second impact syndrome in rowan stringer, a 17-year-old Rugby player. Can J Neurol Sci. 2019;46:351–4. https://doi.org/10.1017/cjn.2019.14.
93. Vagnozzi R, Signoretti S, Tavazzi B, Cimatti M, Amorini AM, Donzelli S, et al. Hypothesis of the postconcussive vulnerable brain: experimental evidence of its metabolic occurrence. Neurosurgery. 2005;57:164–71. https://doi.org/10.1227/01.NEU.0000163413.90259.85.
94. Longhi L, Saatman KE, Fujimoto S, Raghupathi R, Meaney DF, Davis J, et al. Temporal window of vulnerability to repetitive experimental concussive brain injury. Neurosurgery. 2005;56:364–74.
95. Fehily B, Fitzgerald M. Repeated mild traumatic brain injury: potential mechanisms of damage. Cell Transplant. 2017;26:1131–55. https://doi.org/10.1177/0963689717714092.
96. Hubbard WB, Joseph B, Spry M, Vekaria HJ, Saatman KE, Sullivan PG. Acute mitochondrial impairment underlies prolonged cellular dysfunction after repeated mild traumatic brain injuries. J Neurotrauma. 2019;36:1252–63. https://doi.org/10.1089/neu.2018.5990.
97. Mountney A, Boutté AM, Cartagena CM, Flerlage WF, Johnson WD, Rho C, et al. Functional and molecular correlates after single and repeated rat closed-head concussion: indices of vulnerability after brain injury. J Neurotrauma. 2017;34:2768–89. https://doi.org/10.1089/neu.2016.4679.
98. Signoretti S, Lazzarino G, Tavazzi B, Vagnozzi R. The pathophysiology of brain concussion. PM R. 2011;3(10 Suppl 2):S359–68. https://doi.org/10.1016/j.pmrj.2011.07.018.
99. Vagnozzi R, Signoretti S, Floris R, Marziali S, Manara M, Amorini AM, et al. Decrease in N-Acetylaspartate following concussion may be coupled to decrease in Creatine. J Head Trauma Rehabil. 2012;28:284–92. https://doi.org/10.1097/HTR.0b013e3182795045.
100. Vagnozzi R, Signoretti S, Cristofori L, Alessandrini F, Floris R, Isgrò E, et al. Assessment of metabolic brain damage and recovery following mild traumatic brain injury: a multicenter, proton magnetic resonance spectroscopy study in concussed athletes. Brain. 2010;133:3232–42. https://doi.org/10.1093/brain/awq200.

101. Muftuler LT, Meier T, Keith M, Budde MD, Huber DL, McCrea M. A serial diffusion kurtosis MRI study during acute, subacute and recovery periods after sport-related concussion. J Neurotrauma. 2020;37(19):2081–92. https://doi.org/10.1089/neu.2020.6993.
102. Klein AP, Tetzlaff JE, Bonis JM, et al. Prevalence of potentially clinically significant magnetic resonance imaging findings in athletes with and without sport-related concussion. J Neurotrauma. 2019;36:1776–85. https://doi.org/10.1089/neu.2018.6055.
103. Klein AP, Tetzlaff JE, Bonis JM, Nelson LD, Mayer AR, Huber DL, et al. Magnetic resonance imaging biomarkers of brain connectivity in predicting outcome after mild traumatic brain injury: a systematic review. J Neurotrauma. 2019;36:1776–85. https://doi.org/10.1089/neu.2018.6055.
104. Churchill NW, Hutchison MG, Graham SJ, Schweizer TA. Baseline vs. cross-sectional MRI of concussion: distinct brain patterns in white matter and cerebral blood flow. Sci Rep. 2020;10:1643. https://doi.org/10.1038/s41598-020-58073-9.
105. Churchill NW, Hutchison MG, Graham SJ, Schweizer TA. Connectomic markers of symptom severity in sport-related concussion: whole-brain analysis of resting-state fMRI. Neuroimage Clin. 2018;18:518–26. https://doi.org/10.1016/j.nicl.2018.02.011.
106. Hellstrøm T, Kaufmann T, Andelic N, Soberg HL, Sigurdardottir S, Helseth E, et al. Predicting outcome 12 months after mild traumatic brain injury in patients admitted to a neurosurgery service. Front Neurol. 2017;8:125. https://doi.org/10.3389/fneur.2017.00125.
107. Yuan W, Wade SL, Quatman-Yates C, Hugentobler JA, Gubanich PJ, Kurowski BG. Structural connectivity related to persistent symptoms after mild TBI in adolescents and response to aerobic training: preliminary investigation. J Head Trauma Rehabil. 2017;32:378–84. https://doi.org/10.1097/HTR.0000000000000318.
108. Johnson B, Gay M, Zhang K, Neuberger T, Horovitz SG, Hallett M, et al. The use of magnetic resonance spectroscopy in the subacute evaluation of athletes recovering from single and multiple mild traumatic brain injury. J Neurotrauma. 2012;29:2297–304. https://doi.org/10.1089/neu.2011.2294.
109. Gardner A, Iverson GL, Stanwell P. A systematic review of proton magnetic resonance spectroscopy findings in sport-related concussion. J Neurotrauma. 2014;31:1–18. https://doi.org/10.1089/neu.2013.3079.
110. MacMaster FP, McLellan Q, Harris AD, Virani S, Barlow KM, Langevin LM, et al. N-acetyl-aspartate in the dorsolateral prefrontal cortex long after concussion in youth. J Head Trauma Rehabil. 2020;35:E127–35. https://doi.org/10.1097/HTR.0000000000000535.
111. Alosco ML, Tripodis Y, Rowland B, Chua AS, Liao H, Martin B, et al. A magnetic resonance spectroscopy investigation in symptomatic former NFL players. Brain Imaging Behav. 2020;14(5):1419–29. https://doi.org/10.1007/s11682-019-00060-4.
112. George EO, Roys S, Sours C, Rosenberg J, Zhuo J, Shanmuganathan K, et al. Longitudinal and prognostic evaluation of mild traumatic brain injury: a 1H-magnetic resonance spectroscopy study. J Neurotrauma. 2014;31:1018–28. https://doi.org/10.1089/neu.2013.3224.
113. Hayes JP, Bigler ED, Verfaellie M. Traumatic brain injury as a disorder of brain connectivity. J Int Neuropsychol Soc. 2016;22:120–37. https://doi.org/10.1017/S1355617715000740.
114. Etkin A, Maron-Katz A, Wu W, Fonzo GA, Huemer J, Vértes PE, et al. Using fmri connectivity to define a treatment-resistant form of post-traumatic stress disorder. Sci Transl Med. 2019;11:eaal3236. https://doi.org/10.1126/scitranslmed.aal3236.
115. Moreno-López L, Manktelow AE, Sahakian BJ, Menon DK, Stamatakis EA. Anything goes? Regulation of the neural processes underlying response inhibition in TBI patients. Eur Neuropsychopharmacol. 2017;27:159–69. https://doi.org/10.1016/j.euroneuro.2016.12.002.
116. Khan MA, Houck DR, Gross AL, Zhang XL, Cearley C, Madsen TM, et al. NYX-2925 is a novel NMDA receptor-specific Spirocyclic-β-lactam that modulates synaptic plasticity processes associated with learning and memory. Int J Neuropsychopharmacol. 2018;21:242–54. https://doi.org/10.1093/ijnp/pyx096.
117. Patel M, Tapan P. The Impact of Mild Traumatic Brain injury on Neuronal Networks and Neurobehavior. Publicly Accessible Penn Dissertations; 2013. p. 788.

Functional Magnetic Resonance Imaging in Sport-Related Concussions

11

Veronik Sicard, Danielle C. Hergert, and Andrew R. Mayer

Introduction

Sport-related concussion (SRC) remains a poorly understood clinical phenomenon, despite the numerous cases in athletics. This can primarily be attributed to the variable and inconsistent definition of concussion (also referred to as mild traumatic brain injury; mTBI), as well as the heterogeneity of the clinical manifestation and prognosis [1, 2]. Spontaneous recovery following a SRC is currently determined by clinical observations and self-reported symptoms rather than objective markers [3]. Findings from standard clinical neuroimaging techniques (computerized tomography [CT] scans; T_1- and T_2-weighted images) are typically negative for the majority of cases [1, 4, 5]. Specifically, two large recent studies of SRC reported positive findings of less than 1% on typical magnetic resonance imaging (MRI) sequences [6, 7].

These null findings on standard neuroimaging initially helped to propagate the view that SRC did not lead to frank neuronal pathology. However, an accumulating body of literature indicates that SRC may result in lingering impairments [for reviews see 8–11], with evidence of neuronal pathology remaining present long after the traditional clinical outcome measures (e.g., balance and cognitive testing)

V. Sicard · D. C. Hergert
The Mind Research Network/Lovelace Biomedical and Environmental Research Institute, Albuquerque, NM, USA

A. R. Mayer (✉)
The Mind Research Network/Lovelace Biomedical and Environmental Research Institute, Albuquerque, NM, USA

Department of Psychiatry and Behavioral Sciences, University of New Mexico, Albuquerque, NM, USA

Department of Neurology, University of New Mexico, Albuquerque, NM, USA

Department of Psychology, University of New Mexico, Albuquerque, NM, USA
e-mail: amayer@mrn.org

have returned to normal [12]. This has resulted in a proliferation of studies that have attempted to define more objective imaging biomarkers of SRC [13, 14]. Given functional MRI's ability to non-invasively perform in vivo measurements during demanding cognitive tasks [15] and to characterize intrinsic neuronal activity [16, 17], dozens of studies have subsequently used this imaging technique to better understand the pathophysiology of concussion.

This chapter first describes the physiological underpinnings of the blood oxygen level-dependent (BOLD) response measured by fMRI and how it can be altered by a concussive insult as well as various analytic considerations. Next, it provides a review of research using evoked fMRI paradigms, functional connectivity (fcMRI), and multimodal imaging studies that included BOLD imaging component to investigate the cognitive and psychological sequelae of SRC. The general benefits and drawbacks of both evoked fMRI and fcMRI studies are then discussed in the context of the SRC literature, including clinical heterogeneity in participant selection criteria, presence of symptoms, variations in scan time post-injury, history of multiple SRC, and sub-concussive head impacts exposure.

fMRI Physiology and Putative Effects of SRC

The ability of fMRI to dynamically measure brain function during higher order cognitive and emotional tasks represents a clear advantage relative to other imaging techniques that are only capable of measuring structural integrity such as susceptibility-weighted imaging (SWI) and diffusion tensor imaging (DTI). Moreover, unlike other functional techniques (e.g., electrophysiological [EEG] and optical imaging), fMRI is capable of probing both superficial cortical and deep gray structures, a powerful advantage given that shear stresses are more likely to accumulate in these regions [18].

The relationship between neurotransmission and resultant hemodynamic activity, referred to as neurovascular coupling, remains an active area of investigation [19]. During intrinsic activity (i.e., at rest, in the absence of evoked activity), the cerebral metabolic rate of glucose (CMR_{glu}), cerebral metabolic rate of oxygen ($CMRO_2$), and cerebral blood flow (CBF) are tightly coupled to maintain homeostasis [20–22]. Following excitatory neuronal transmission, metabolic demands change and energy (glucose) is required to reverse ionic influx that results in depolarization while the excess glutamate needs to be rapidly removed from the synaptic cleft [23–25]. Astrocytes take up excess glutamate, convert it to glutamine, and release vasoactive agents [23], while neurons concurrently release nitric oxide. These events likely contribute to vasodilation and a concomitant increase in CBF. Importantly, there is a decoupling between CBF and oxidative metabolism following neurotransmission, which leads to an excess of oxygenated blood, a decrease in the ratio of deoxyhemoglobin relative to oxyhemoglobin, and a subsequent increase in MR signal due to the differences in magnetic properties between the two forms of hemoglobin [26]. As such, the BOLD response represents an amalgamation of signals derived from the ratio of oxy-to-deoxyhemoglobin, with contributions of CBF, and cerebral blood volume (CBV) [16, 27, 28].

The shape of the BOLD response is also complex, with the canonical hemodynamic response function (HRF) consisting of two primary components: a positive signal change that peaks approximately 4–6 s post-stimulus onset, and a post-stimulus undershoot (PSU) that peaks 6–10 s after the stimulus ends [29, 30]. The positive phase of the BOLD response has been associated with an increase in CBF and a subsequent change in the ratio of oxy-to-deoxyhemoglobin [29]. The biophysiological origins of the PSU remain more controversial. An early model attributed the PSU to temporal delays between when CBF (earlier response) and CBV (delayed response) returned to baseline levels [29, 31]. More recent work suggests that the duration of the PSU extends beyond the CBV return to baseline [32, 33] and may be driven by increased metabolic demands ($CMRO_2$) following neurotransmission [34–36] or post-synaptic inhibitory activity [37].

SRC can affect the different components of the BOLD response through several individual mechanisms as well as combinatory effects. Foremost, the concussive injury can result in alterations in synchronous neuronal activity, causing downstream effects on BOLD activity by changing the amount of glutamate in the synaptic cleft and the energetic needs of cells following neurotransmission [23, 38]. Direct support for this hypothesis comes from reports of neuronal loss in animal models of fluid percussion injury [39] and abnormal cell signaling [40]. Indirect support comes from findings of altered concentrations of glutamate and glutamine in the semi-acute and chronic stages of concussion during magnetic resonance spectroscopy [41–48].

Concussion has also been shown to directly reduce both CBF and metabolism in pediatric and adult athletes, which could affect the BOLD response [49–52]. Metabolic failure following concussion occurs even in the presence of normal perfusion [53], with an initial decoupling between CBF and CMR_{glu}, followed by a generally reduced cerebral metabolism [54]. Animal models suggest that alterations in CBF and CMR_{glu} may be the longest-lasting physiological deficits of concussion [55], with a handful of studies of athletes suggesting that resolution of CBF abnormalities closely mirrors previous reports from preclinical studies [50–52]. However, one study of adolescents with SRC showed increased CBF in the left insula and left dorsal anterior cingulate cortex (ACC) at 2 weeks post-injury relative to controls, with the elevation in the latter persisting up to 6 weeks post-injury. This increase was associated with more persistent post-concussive physical symptoms [56]. Future research investigating CBF following SRC is needed to better understand its role in recovery and vulnerability of the brain to a second concussive impact.

Brain trauma may also directly affect the structural integrity of the microvasculature. Animal models indicate a semi-acute reduction in capillary number and diameter both at the injury site and distally [57–59], with other studies suggesting that experimental TBI results in alterations to the reactivity of microvessel smooth muscle [60]. This latter effect has been confirmed in studies using fMRI and transcranial Doppler ultrasound to measure cerebral vascular reactivity in the acute phase of SRC in collegiate athletes [61–63].

To complement evoked studies of BOLD activity, researchers are increasingly turning to measures of fcMRI to examine neuronal health following SRC using resting-state scans. Connectivity studies are based on intrinsic neuronal fluctuations that synchronously occur over spatially distributed networks in both animals and humans [16, 64]. The majority (60–80%) of the brain's energy resources is expended to maintain homeostasis and intrinsic neuronal activity likely contributes to this heavy metabolic load [65, 66]. These intrinsic fluctuations in neuronal activity tend to alias to low-frequency fluctuations (0.01–0.10 Hz) in the BOLD signal, and therefore can be measured on any MRI scanner with a conventional echo-planar sequence. Several different properties of intrinsic activity can be examined including, but not limited to, static connectivity, dynamic connectivity, regional homogeneity, and the amplitude of low-frequency fluctuations [67]. Previous research indicates changes in baseline metabolism following a concussive injury [54] as well as an abnormal slow-wave electrophysiological activity during passive mental activity [68, 69], providing the biological relevance for fcMRI as a biomarker of concussion.

fcMRI has several advantages over more traditional evoked fMRI studies. Foremost, using a relatively simple task (i.e., passively maintaining fixation), it is possible to probe the neuronal integrity of the multiple sensory, motor, and cognitive networks that exist in the human brain. This can occur without concerns about practice effects or decreased novelty associated with multiple administrations of a task, potentially confounding the results. Specifically, a now seminal study from Smith and colleagues indicated that intrinsic neuronal activity measured from 36 participants was organized into distinct networks that mirror activity evoked across a variety (30,000 archival data sets) of cognitive challenges [70]. Further, fcMRI eliminates the complex requirements for presenting sensory stimuli and monitoring motor responses (e.g., interfacing with a computer, projecting stimuli, special non-ferrous motor response devices), rendering it more feasible for performing clinical scans.

Several limitations need to be considered when analyzing fcMRI data. During resting-state scans, participants are simply asked to either fixate on a visual stimulus or close their eyes for a relatively brief period (~5–10 min). As such, resting state paradigms have been criticized based on the general lack of control over participants' mental activities and the inability to specify what cognitive tasks participants performed in the scanner [71]. Similarly, athletes with SRC do not perform difficult cognitive tasks during resting-state scans, which may be of greater clinical relevance given that patients tend to report more cognitive problems during difficult tasks in everyday life [15, 72, 73]. Another critique of fcMRI studies is that the various analytic approaches (e.g., seed-based analysis vs. independent component analysis vs. graph theory metrics) that are used to parse network activation can result in different findings during data analyses of the same subjects [67]. Finally, noise has a more direct influence on the correlation coefficient in fcMRI relative to evoked signals [74], which can further complicate the interpretation of group-wise results.

Analytic Considerations for fMRI Studies

Several analytic considerations should be taken into account when performing fMRI research in SRC. Foremost, investigators have traditionally used region of interest (ROI) or voxel-wise analyses to compare the BOLD response between concussed and control athletes. However, these analytic methods assume that the heterogeneous initial injury conditions (e.g., a blow to the left temple, a blow to the jaw with rotational acceleration, a force transmitted to the occipital cortex following an indirect impact), result in a homogeneous pattern of gray matter abnormalities that would survive group-wise statistics [75]. Indeed, to survive group-wise statistics, ROI and voxel-wise analyses assume that there is a high degree of spatial overlap in disruptions to BOLD functioning. Although lesions tend to be more common in the diencephalon, midbrain, limbic circuit, and prefrontal cortex [13, 76], the premise of the spatial overlap assumption is likely to be flawed.

Second, despite the known complexity of the hemodynamic response function (HRF), previous studies have typically estimated a single parameter (typically a beta coefficient) by convolving a canonical HRF, such as a gamma variate or a double-gamma variate function, with known experimental conditions (e.g., onset of a particular trial) to derive a predictor function (e.g., regressor). Importantly, this assumes that the different components of the HRF (positive phase and PSU) and their relationship to each other are unaffected by concussion. Animal models suggest that the acute and sub-acute phases of injury are associated with significant disruptions to metabolism and microvasculature, both of which could impact the HRF [57, 77, 78]. Although basic visual stimuli were associated with an increased volume of activation within the visual cortex in individuals with mild-to-severe TBI, there were no differences in the basic shape of the HRF when compared to controls. Others reported an earlier time-to-peak, a positive magnitude shift in the estimated HRF, and a reduced PSU within the visual cortex and medial temporal cortex for semiacute concussed participants relative to healthy controls [79]. Additional fMRI studies modeling the full time course of a deconvolved HRF are needed to explicitly compare the different components of the HRF as well as their individual sensitivity and specificity to provide additional information about underlying neuropathology that is not available with more standard fMRI analyses (Fig. 11.1).

Third, as previously stated, the BOLD signal is temporally sluggish and represents an indirect measure of neuronal activity, resulting from a complex mixture of many underlying physiological processes. As most of these physiological processes may be affected by trauma, it is unfeasible to "isolate" a single biological mechanism that underlies an abnormal BOLD response when fMRI is collected alone [80]. This, along with the heterogeneity of SRC, makes the use of multimodal imaging beneficial to understand biological processes, potential covariates, and changes over time indexed with imaging techniques through the confirmation of multiple sources of information [81]. Indeed, defining recovery based on any single variable (i.e., symptom-free) or a single imaging modality potentially risks a premature

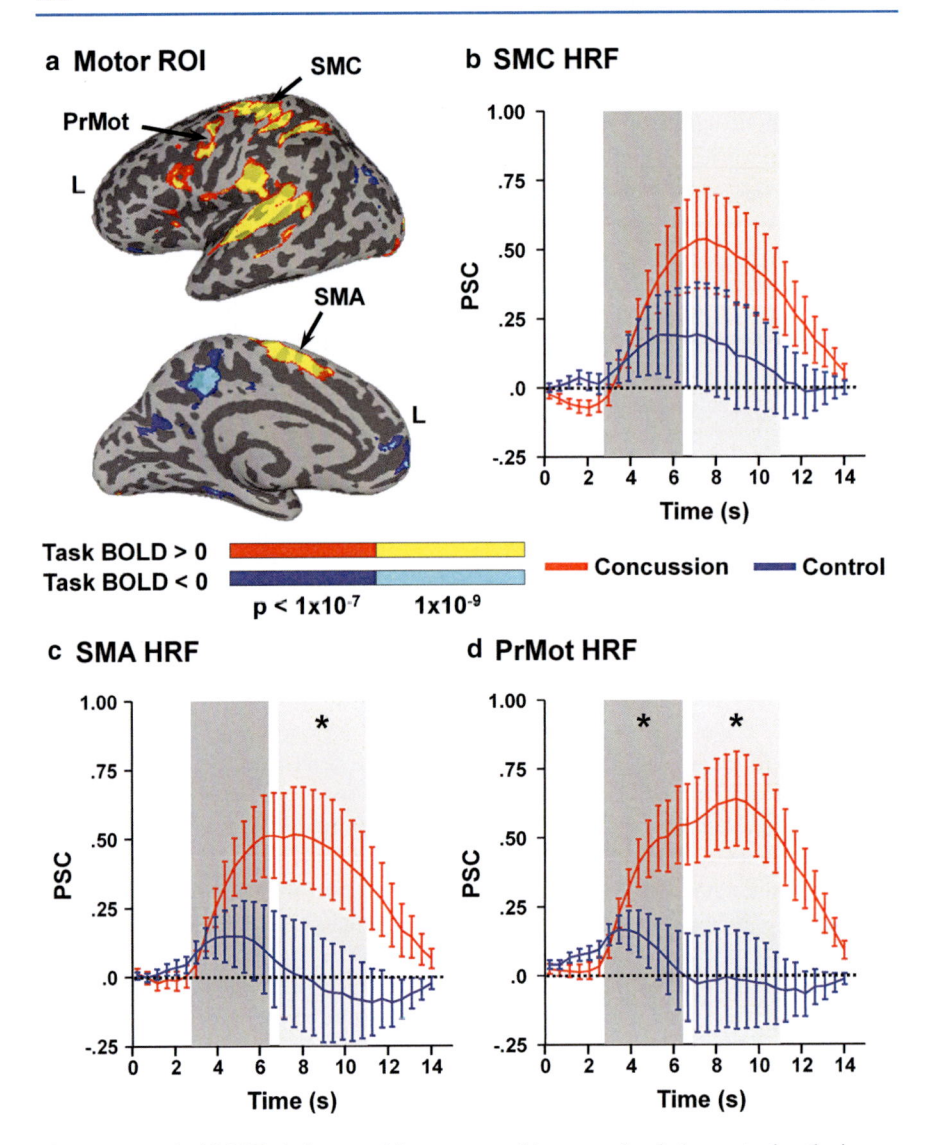

Fig. 11.1 Evoked BOLD during a multisensory cognitive control task demonstrating the importance of examining the entire hemodynamic response function (HRF) for abnormalities. Panel (**a**) depicts a priori regions of interest (ROI) within motor circuitry including the left sensorimotor cortex (SMC), bilateral supplementary motor area (SMA), and left premotor area (PrMot). ROI were derived from a contrast comparing the active trials relative to baseline, collapsing across both concussion and control groups. Inflated views of increased activation relative to baseline are denoted in warm colors for the lateral medial portions of the left (L) hemisphere, whereas decreased activation is denoted in cool colors. Panels (**b**), (**c**), and (**d**) present the percent signal change (PSC) values for the entire BOLD HRF within these ROI. Shaded bars indicate the expected peak (dark gray; 2.76–6.44 s) and inhibitory (light gray; 9.90–11.04 s) phases of the HRF during a stimulus cue presentation, with asterisks denoting significant group differences (concussion group [red line] > control group [blue line]) within a phase. Error bars represent the standard error to the mean. (Data adapted from Mayer et al. [209])

return-to-play decision that may put athletes at risk for worse outcomes, should a repeat, temporally proximate SRC occur.

Fourth, fMRI signals are critically linked to CBF and the dysregulation of autonomic control of neurovascular coupling. Therefore, investigators may calibrate the BOLD signal with arterial spin labeling (ASL) measures of CBF [76, 82–85]. Hypercapnic normalization is another frequently used technique that is achieved through the administration of CO_2, a voluntary breath-hold scan, or more regularized breathing [86, 87]. This method assumes that hypercapnia has a limited effect on neural activity and oxygen metabolism and, thus, primarily measures CBF and/or CVR [88, 89]. Previous results suggest that the hypercapnia method accounts for variability in subject vasculature and physiology differences during task performance, as well as changes in magnetic field strength [63, 90–92]. In recent years, several studies of concussions have observed perturbations in CVR in acute and chronic phases of injury [85, 93–96], providing support for calibrating the BOLD signal. SRC has also been associated with greater reductions in BOLD activity during the early phase of a respiratory challenge task, primarily in frontal and prefrontal areas, whereas no significant effects on resting global CBF were observed [61]. Collectively, these results highlight the importance of examining neurovascular response to physiological stressors after a SRC in conjunction with standard BOLD measurements.

Review of the Current Literature on Functional Imaging and SRC

Review of Evoked fMRI Studies

SRC has been associated with acute and chronic impairments in executive functions/working memory, attention, and memory [8, 97]. fMRI can be useful in examining the integrity of brain regions or networks underlying these cognitive changes. Abnormal brain activation patterns during working memory tasks have been consistently reported in the SRC literature. Seminal studies using the N-back task suggested a complex relationship between cognitive load and functional activation at 1 month post-injury, with hyperactivation observed within the dorsolateral prefrontal cortex (DLPFC) and lateral parietal cortex during moderate load, whereas hypoactivation was observed during low and high loads compared to healthy controls [98, 99]. More recently, a longitudinal study of university athletes has indicated that hyperactivation of the inferior parietal lobe in concussed when compared to the control group persisted 2 months post-injury, despite no differences in neurobehavioral performance [100]. Hypoactivation of different brain regions was also observed in two studies using similar working memory tasks. Specifically, hypoactivation was observed within the DLPFC of athletes with persistent post-concussion symptoms [101], and within the ventral ACC, medial temporal gyri, and the occipital cortex of both recovered and symptomatic athletes [85]. Overall, these studies provide support for changes in neuronal activity of brain regions implicated in working memory following SRC.

Hyperactivation has been reported during other cognitive and motor tasks. Specifically, it has been observed within the DLPFC, parietal cortex, and hippocampus during a virtual reality spatial memory task in recently concussed, yet asymptomatic athletes, relative to non-concussed controls [102]. Similarly, using a sensorimotor coordination and memory task, hyperactivation of frontoparietal regions was observed in recently concussed intercollegiate football players, even in the absence of differences in neurobehavioral performance [103]. Additionally, the increased BOLD response has been documented in several brain regions during oculomotor tasks, ranging from the acute to the chronic phase of SRC, even in the absence of cognitive alterations [104–106]. The degree of hyperactivation may be indicative of a prolonged recovery profile in athletes, particularly when accompanied with sparse and diffuse activation patterns [107], and suggests the presence of compensatory neural mechanisms following SRC [103].

Associations between self-reported symptom intensity and differential activation patterns within several regions, including the working memory and attention networks, have been shown in athletes following SRC [101, 108, 109]. Specifically, symptom intensity in concussed athletes was associated with hyperactivation of frontal and parietal cortical regions within the first week of injury [109]. In contrast, a series of studies from Chen and colleagues found an association between persistent post-concussion symptoms and hypoactivation of prefrontal regions during visual and verbal working memory tasks [101, 108]. They also reported more diffuse activation patterns in the symptomatic athletes relative to controls [101], with activation peaks outside the ROIs [108]. Together, these results indicate that persistent symptoms may be predictors of changes in frontal and parietal brain activation in the chronic phase of injury.

The possible effects of a history of multiple SRC and repetitive sub-concussive impacts on BOLD response are still not well described, with a few published studies yielding variable results. Evidence of hypoactivation of left hemispheric language regions during a verbal learning memory task was observed in former high school athletes with a history of multiple SRC when compared to former athletes who never sustained a concussion [110]. Yet, null results have also been reported in active high school and college athletes with a history of SRC [111, 112]. Thus, more work is needed to fully understand the contribution of multiple concussive injuries on the BOLD response. A single study have examined the effect of head impact exposure to the BOLD response. High school football athletes with embedded sensors in the helmet to tally the number of head hits throughout the season were scanned pre- and post-season. Results indicated that, in the absence of a SRC, athletes with higher numbers of head collision events to the top front of the head, directly above the DLPFC, showed hypoactivation within the DLPFC, accompanied by cognitive impairments on an N-back task [113].

Review of Functional Connectivity Studies

Several fcMRI studies have focused on the default-mode network (DMN), which typically includes medial and lateral parietal, medial prefrontal, and medial and lateral temporal cortices [17]. The DMN is believed to mediate a variety of mental activities such as episodic memory recall and future-oriented thought processes that occur during periods of unconstrained mental activity and therefore is typically associated with deactivation during evoked tasks [114, 115]. SRC studies of the DMN connectivity in the acute and sub-acute phases of injury have shown inconsistent results, with one study showing hyperconnectivity [116], while another study did not find differences between concussed and controls unless participants underwent a physical stress challenge [117]. There is also evidence of changes in resting-state networks from playing a single season of football in children and adolescents [118], with the delta power spectrum of the DMN providing a good classification accuracy between youth athletes in the low and the high head impacts exposure group [119].

Multiple fcMRI studies using whole-brain analysis have documented acute [120], sub-acute [121, 122], and persistent [123–125] differences between concussed athletes and controls following SRC in additional networks outside the DMN, including areas underlying memory, attention, and executive functions. Differences in regional homogeneity (ReHo), a metric of local connectivity, have also been observed at 1 month post-concussion, but not at more acute time points in a large cohort of collegiate athletes relative to healthy contact sports athletes [126]. Similar results were found in a study of network-based statistics and average nodal strength [127]. In contrast, alterations of ReHo in the middle and superior frontal gyri, areas associated with the DMN, have been observed in concussed athletes 24 h post-injury [128]. A recent study indicated acute elevations in ReHo in frontal regions that are typically associated with the DMN, whereas other resting-state metrics, such as average nodal strength, and the relative amplitude of slow oscillations of resting-state fMRI (fractional amplitude of low-frequency fluctuations; fALFF), did not show differences between concussed athletes and controls [67]. Moreover, a history of multiple SRC and exposure to repetitive, yet sub-concussive head impacts from contact sports participation has been associated with fcMRI. For instance, increased connectivity between the areas in frontal cortices, hippocampus, and cingulate cortices was observed in football players with a history of multiple SRC relative to healthy controls without football or concussion history [129].

All of these studies analyzed fcMRI from a static connectivity perspective that computes the average functional coupling among the brain regions across a scan length. More recent studies have used dynamic functional analysis, where the focus is on the dynamic evolution of fcMRI during the entire scan [130, 131]. Such an approach enables the extraction of additional information regarding abnormalities in neural network communication, which may be complementary to findings from static connectivity analyses (Fig. 11.2). This approach was used in two studies of SRC. One study showed that at time of return to play, concussed athletes with both higher symptom intensity and prolonged recovery had altered scale-free dynamics

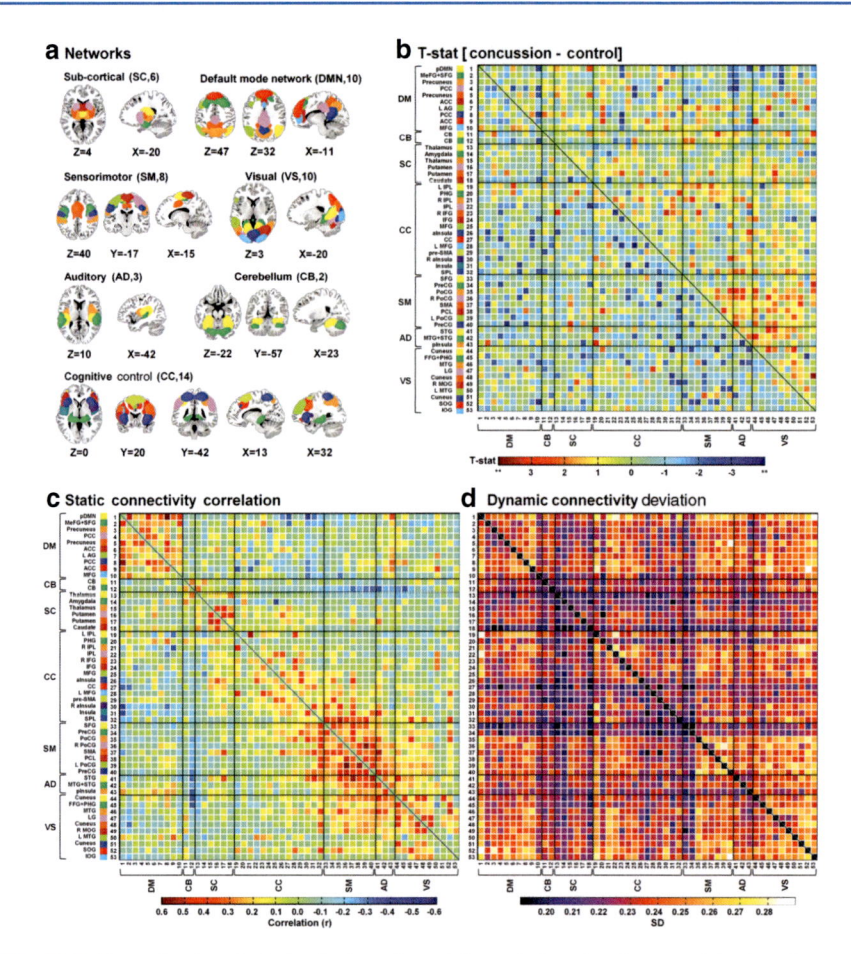

Fig. 11.2 Exemplar data depicting both static and dynamic functional connectivity in cohorts of adult mTBI patients and matched healthy controls. Panel (**a**) depicts the 53 intrinsic connectivity networks (ICN) derived across both mTBI and control participants following group independent component analysis. Individual ICN are clustered into seven overarching networks: subcortical (SC; 6 ICN); default mode network (DMN; 10 ICN); sensorimotor (SM; 8 ICN); visual (VS; 10 ICN); auditory (AD; 3 ICN); cerebellum (CB; 2 ICN); and cognitive control (CC; 14 ICN). Sagittal (X), coronal (Y), and axial (Z) slice locations are presented according to the Montreal Neurological Institute system. The color-coding for each ICN within each of the seven major networks is presented within Panel (**b**), as well as t-statistics representing independent sample comparisons of static (above diagonal) and dynamic (below diagonal) functional connectivity (fcMRI) across the two groups. Individual labels include: L, left; R, right; pDMN, posterior default mode network; MeFG, medial frontal gyrus; SFG, superior frontal gyrus; PCC, posterior cingulate cortex; ACC, anterior cingulate cortex; AG, angular gyrus; MFG, middle frontal gyrus; IPL, inferior parietal lobule; PHG, parahippocampal gyrus; IFG, inferior frontal gyrus; aInsula, anterior insula; CC, cingulate cortex; pre-SMA, pre-supplementary motor area; SPL, superior parietal lobule; PreCG, precentral gyrus; PoCG, postcentral gyrus; SMA, supplementary motor area; PCL, paracentral lobule; STG, superior temporal gyrus; MTG, middle temporal gyrus; pInsula, posterior insula; FFG, fusiform gyrus; LG, lingual gyrus; MOG, middle occipital gyrus; SOG, superior occipital gyrus; IOG, inferior occipital gyrus. ** indicates different upper/lower t-limits (3.7 for static; 3.9 for dynamic). Panel (**c**) presents the pair-wise Pearson correlation values (r), while panel (**d**) presents the standard deviation (SD) of the pair-wise Pearson correlation values across the 126 sliding windows, for concussion (under diagonal) and control groups (above diagonal). (Data adapted from Mayer et al. [210])

relative to control athletes [132]. Further, differences in dwell times for multiple connectivity states were also observed between former athletes with a history of multiple SRC and healthy controls that did not report a SRC [133]. Thus, this dynamic connectivity may provide an additional avenue to study changes related to SRC and additional studies are needed.

In summary, multiple fcMRI metrics have shown sensitivity to SRC, with studies reporting abnormalities in static and dynamic functional connectivity at various time points post-concussion, such as acutely and at time of return to play, with conflicting evidence of prolonged abnormalities that may be explained by the use of different connectivity metrics. Based on these studies, fcMRI appears to be well poised for interrogating connectivity within all major structures and networks of the brain following SRC.

Added Value of Multimodal Imaging

Multimodal MRI studies have indicated concomitant alterations of perfusion, function, chemistry, and brain microstructure at various time points after SRC [134–138]. Recent studies in SRC suggested that group-based differences in BOLD activity may be driven by a mixed effect from vascular and metabolic origins, providing support for the use of multimodal MRI imaging [85, 139]. Specifically, concomitant alterations of DMN connectivity and increased cerebrovascular reactivity (CVR) (Fig. 11.3), a measure of vasculature integrity, have been observed in college athletes a few months post-concussion when compared to healthy controls [139]. Further, a recent study using a working memory paradigm found both reduced BOLD activation and reduced CVR in the ventral ACC and the medial temporal gyri in concussed athletes 4 months post-concussion relative to the control group, supporting the idea that concussion is associated with both vascular and neural dysfunction [85]. The combination of evoked fMRI and event-related potentials (ERPs) can also add valuable information on brain function, as it can afford both high spatial resolution and temporal fidelity. Following a concussion, the decreased BOLD signal has been associated with abnormal ERPs [140, 141], again supporting that alterations in vascular and neuronal response may be simultaneous.

Finally, a series of multimodal studies of SRC by Churchill and colleagues have highlighted the variability among imaging indices that is consistent with the heterogeneous nature of SRC [134, 142, 143], with time-varying changes in diffusion, function, and CBF being observed. Interestingly, the changes were more prominent when the symptoms are most severe, and the recovery was slow [134, 142].

Psychiatric Sequelae of SRC and fMRI

Functional MRI can also help better understand the underlying neural correlates of the development and recovery of psychiatric symptoms in concussed athletes [144]. The relationship between SRC and psychiatric sequelae has been well documented

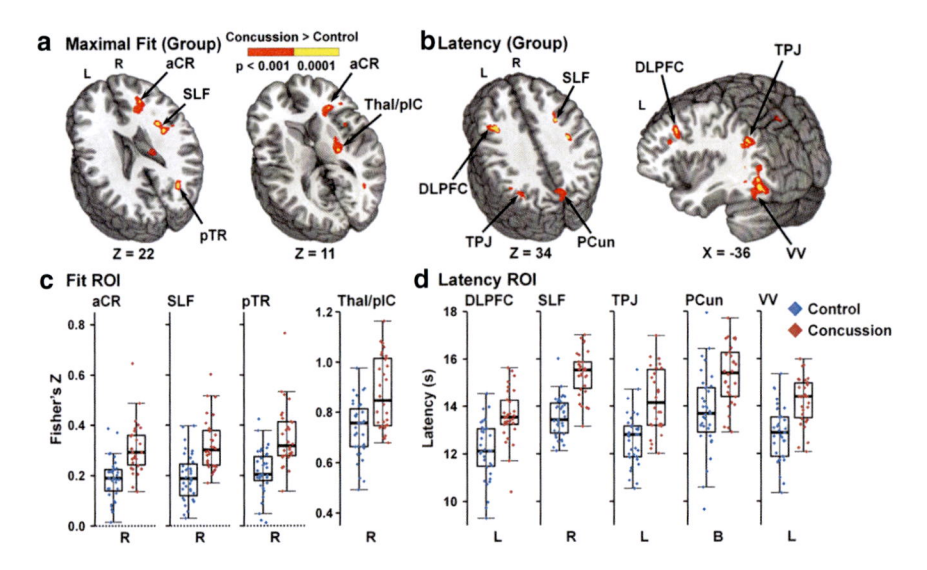

Fig. 11.3 Data depicting the use of BOLD imaging to detect changes in cerebral vascular reactivity (CVR) in a cohort of pediatric concussion patients and controls. Panel (**a**) depicts a main effect of group for increased maximal voxel-wise fit to a subject-specific, variably time-delayed ETCO$_2$ regressor matrix (red: $p < 0.001$; yellow: $p < 0.0001$) for concussed participants relative to healthy controls during a hypercapnia challenge. Displayed regions of interest (ROI) include the right (R) anterior corona radiata (aCR), R superior longitudinal fasciculus (SLF), posterior thalamic radiation (pTR), and R thalamus and posterior internal capsule (Thal/pIC). Similarly, Panel (**b**) depicts a main effect of group for increased latency to maximal voxel-wise fit in the ETCO$_2$ matrix in RBOI that include the left (L) dorsolateral prefrontal cortex (DLPFC), R SLF, L temporoparietal junction (TPJ), bilateral (B) precuneus (PCun), and L ventral visual stream (VV). Coordinates for select axial (Z) and sagittal (X) slices are given according to the Talairach atlas. Panels (**c**) and (**d**) display box and scatter plots of the Fisher's Z (maximal fit; **c**) and latency (**d**) for select ROI region in each group (concussion: red; controls; blue). (Data adapted from Dodd et al. [94])

[128, 145–147], showing elevated symptoms acutely, with partial recovery of psychiatric symptoms within a month of the injury [148, 149]. The potential for long-term psychiatric consequences of SRC remains an important area of study, as a higher incidence of psychiatric symptoms has been shown in retired, professional athletes with a history of SRC compared to those with no reported concussion [150–154]. However, prospective, longitudinal studies are needed to better understand potential moderators and mediators of this relationship.

While premorbid psychopathology and psychosocial changes related to SRC (e.g., loss of position, lack of support from the team) can result in prolonged psychiatric symptoms [2, 144, 145, 155], biologically based disruptions of the emotional processing neural networks can also contribute [148]. Mesocorticolimbic and frontal-subcortical networks and/or their white matter connections may be directly or indirectly affected through shearing forces or inflammation [13, 156]. Additionally, the stress response as a result of SRC engages the sympathetic nervous system and the hypothalamic-pituitary-adrenal (HPA) axis [82, 83, 157–159], resulting in further dysregulation of emotional processing networks [160–162].

fMRI studies of SRC have elucidated brain regions and networks that may be implicated in psychiatric disturbance [128, 148, 163, 164]. Specifically, a longitudinal study showed decreased fcMRI between the DMN and attention regions was observed at 1 day post-injury in collegiate athletes, with improvement at 1 month post-injury above levels in the non-injured, control group, suggesting the presence of compensatory neural response to injury [148]. In the more chronic phase of injury, whole-brain analysis revealed that concussed athletes with depressive symptoms showed less activation of the prefrontal and limbic regions during a working memory task relative to non-depressed concussed athletes and controls [163].

Overall, these fMRI studies have shown that prefrontal regions, limbic regions, and the DMN are some of the most susceptible regions to SRC, areas that are also implicated in increased psychological symptoms [128, 148, 163, 164]. DMN abnormalities have been theorized to be associated with rumination and self-referential thinking, which may link DMN alterations to psychological symptoms [128, 148]. However, causal relationships remain unclear and are likely multifactorial [164].

Overarching Issues in fMRI Research in SRC

As alluded to in the preceding sections, several potential confounds need to be carefully considered when performing and evaluating fMRI studies of SRC. Some common clinical confounds include injury-related pain (orthopedic), fatigue, poor effort, other comorbid medical and psychiatric conditions, and the presence of prescribed medications (e.g., narcotics or sedatives) that may alter neurovascular coupling or complicate the interpretation of BOLD response [165–167]. Some non-specific somatic (e.g., pain and fatigue) or medication confounds can be reduced or eliminated by recruiting orthopedically injured patients as control participants [168–170]. Some psychosocial factors may be specific to athletes [171], thus including healthy athletes as the control group may be a better comparison than community controls. Additionally, it is impossible to disambiguate whether differences in BOLD response result from trauma-induced alterations in neurophysiology, from task-performance differences (e.g., accuracy or reaction time), or a combination of these effects. Interpretation of data from task-based studies is also frequently complicated by learning and/or practice effects, which are minimal during passive rest, providing support for the usage of fcMRI [172–174].

Developing methods for improving the nosology of SRC and understanding of symptom trajectory will be critical for coalescing disparate neuroimaging findings. Currently, there is no single definition or set of diagnostic criteria for SRC [2, 175] or clinical recovery [176]. For example, an athlete who was only dazed following a blow to the head and an athlete who was unconscious for 20 min with a large subdural hematoma can both be classified as having suffered from SRC under current nosology [1, 177]. Additionally, differences between SRC and non-SRC may exist, which can complicate the interpretation of results of studies with mixed samples. While the acute clinical presentation is similar [97, 178], a recent fcMRI study revealed reduced connectivity in the anterior cingulate cortex and posterior cingulate cortex hubs of the DMN in athletes when compared to non-athletes following a concussion [179]. Other groups have observed a decreased fcMRI in athletes that could result from a history of multiple SRC or high exposure to repetitive, subconcussive head impacts [118, 180, 181]. Based on these studies, athletes appear to be a different population because of the inherent risks associated with sports participation.

Furthermore, the nature of SRC itself is heterogeneous, given the variety of clinical features, anatomical location, mechanism of injury, and recovery trajectories [81, 175, 182–184]. Heterogeneity can also arise in SRC as different sports, player positions, and skill levels can be associated with different injury characteristics [175] and, therefore, with potential differences in neuroimaging. For instance, football has been associated with translational forces while boxing has been associated with greater rotational forces which may put boxers at a greater risk for traumatic axonal injuries [175, 185]. Further, a recent study of cognitively unimpaired former collegiate and professional football players suggests that career duration and primary playing position seem to modify the effects of a history of multiple SRC on white matter structure and neural recruitment [186].

fMRI data collection is costly and recruitment of SRC patients who meet strict inclusion criteria (e.g., homogeneous in both injury severity and time since injury with no pre-existing neurological or psychiatric disorders) is challenging. The combination of these factors has resulted in another methodological challenge, namely the utilization of small sample sizes despite the inherently low signal-to-noise ratio of fMRI [38, 187]. Specifically, the majority of fMRI studies following SRC have been reported with sample sizes just at or below commonly accepted recommendations based on statistical power. As a result, these studies may likely be underpowered, suffering from low positive predictive power, and providing poor estimates of the true effect size [187, 188] and potentially contributing to conflicting findings. To combat the problem of small sample sizes, funding agencies have recently developed standard clinical definitions, common data elements, and informational platforms for creating community-wide data-sharing initiatives (e.g., Federal Interagency Traumatic Brain Injury Research; FITBIR). These efforts should accelerate research in this critical area by permitting the pooling of data for meta-analyses, such as recently occurred with the ENIGMA [189] and the NCAA-DoD CARE consortium [67] initiatives.

Finally, while fMRI itself can provide objective information about SRC, fMRI studies may still use self-report measures to establish a diagnosis and gain information on post-concussion symptoms. Importantly, symptom self-report may vary as a function of the sample with SRC populations being associated with the risk of under-reporting neurobehavioral symptoms to return to play faster [190–193], whereas other concussion samples may over-report symptoms [194, 195], especially in the presence of potential financial compensation [196]. Multiple sociological barriers may account for the under-reporting of symptoms ranging from lack of education regarding the seriousness of SRC for parents, players, and coaches, hesitancy to report symptoms that do not result in significant pain, desire not to be removed from play, and stigmatization of concussion as an invisible, non-real injury [190, 193, 197, 198]. The peer pressure to continue to play and not report an injury is particularly important in vulnerable populations such as children who may not comprehend and underestimate the risks involved in continued participation, and in low socioeconomic areas where participation is perceived as a path to future benefit [199–201]. Additional pressures are on the coaching staff who may feel pressured to win and underestimate the risk of returning a player to the field prematurely [202–204].

Conclusion

Sport-related concussion presents diagnostic and prognostic challenges for many reasons, especially because of the heterogeneity of clinical presentation and mechanism of injury. The past two decades were marked by a collective scientific effort to identify and develop biomarkers of SRC, which propelled research using advanced imaging measures. fMRI provides researchers with the ability to non-invasively measure the functional integrity and modulation of neuronal circuitry following SRC at relatively high spatial resolution. Evidence of alterations of brain activation has been observed in the acute, sub-acute, and chronic phases of injury, with the intensity of post-concussion symptoms and the number of remote SRC being associated with more alterations. Further, research shows group differences in both evoked and resting-state activity were observed for concussed athletes who were asymptomatic and declared ready to return to play when compared to controls.

An important feature of SRC is the potential for repeated concussions over the course of an athletic event, a season, or a lifetime. Regardless of the sociological factors, under-reporting of symptoms can lead to premature return-to-play decisions and put players at risk for exacerbated outcomes related to the occurrence of multiple SRC [154, 205–207]. In athletes, the body of literature presented herein suggests that neuronal recovery may lag behind the recovery of behavioral and cognitive symptoms, emphasizing the need for objective biomarkers of when it is truly safe to return to play [12]. Although fMRI studies have provided insights into the brain dysfunctions stemming from SRC, the use of multiple metrics and multimodal imaging will be necessary to fully grasp the multifaceted and time-dependent pattern of neuropathology due to the neurometabolic cascade of concussion [54, 208]. This will be especially true as future studies may attempt to utilize fMRI to aid in the premortem diagnosis of chronic traumatic encephalopathy, a neurodegenerative disorder that has been associated with a history of multiple SRC and high exposure to sub-concussive insults (CTE).

In summary, SRC is associated with a complex, multifaceted, and time-dependent pattern of pathologies due to the neurometabolic cascade of concussion [2, 55]. Although advanced neuroimaging is still in its infancy for detecting pathophysiological markers of trauma, fMRI has helped to reshape our understanding of the neuropathological effects associated with SRC. Given the heterogeneity inherently associated with concussion research [14, 175], well-powered studies with more homogeneous inclusion criteria (time post-injury, injury severity, symptomatic status, history of SRC, sports, and position) are critically needed for truly understanding the underlying pathophysiology and natural recovery course of the injury.

References

1. McCrory P, Meeuwisse W, Dvorak J, Aubry M, Bailes J, Broglio S, Cantu RC, Cassidy D, Echemendia RJ, Castellani RJ, Davis GA, Ellenbogen R, Emery C, Engebretsen L, Feddermann-Demont N, Giza CC, Guskiewicz KM, Herring S, Iverson GL, Johnston KM, Kissick J, Kutcher J, Leddy JJ, Maddocks D, Makdissi M, Manley GT, McCrea M, Meehan WP, Nagahiro S, Patricios J, Putukian M, Schneider KJ, Sills A, Tator CH, Turner M, Vos PE. Consensus statement on concussion in sport-the 5(th) international conference on concussion in sport held in Berlin October 2016. Br J Sports Med. 2017;51(11):838–47.
2. Mayer AR, Quinn DK, Master CL. The spectrum of mild traumatic brain injury: a review. Neurology. 2017;89(6):623–32.
3. Haider MN, Leddy JJ, Pavlesen S, Kluczynski M, Baker JG, Miecznikowski JC, Willer BS. A systematic review of criteria used to define recovery from sport-related concussion in youth athletes. Br J Sports Med. 2018;52(18):1179–90.
4. Harvell BJ, Helmer SD, Ward JG, Ablah E, Grundmeyer R, Haan JM. Head CT guidelines following concussion among the youngest trauma patients: can we limit radiation exposure following traumatic brain injury? Kans J Med. 2018;11(2):1–17.
5. Seabury SA, Gaudette E, Goldman DP, Markowitz AJ, Brooks J, McCrea MA, Okonkwo DO, Manley GT, Adeoye O, Badjatia N, Boase K, Bodien Y, Bullock MR, Chesnut R, Corrigan JD, Crawford K, Diaz-Arrastia R, Dikmen S, Duhaime AC, Ellenbogen R, Feeser VR, Ferguson A, Foreman B, Gardner R, Giacino J, Gonzalez L, Gopinath S, Gullapalli R, Hemphill JC, Hotz G, Jain S, Korley F, Kramer J, Kreitzer N, Levin H, Lindsell C, Machamer J, Madden C, Martin A, McAllister T, Merchant R, Mukherjee P, Nelson L, Noel F, Palacios E, Perl D, Puccio A, Rabinowitz M, Robertson C, Rosand J, Sander A, Satris G, Schnyer D, Sherer M, Stein M, Taylor S, Temkin N, Toga A, Valadka A, Vassar M, Vespa P, Wang K, Yue J, Yuh E, Zafonte R. Assessment of follow-up care after emergency department presentation for mild traumatic brain injury and concussion: results from the TRACK-TBI study. JAMA Netw Open. 2018;1(1):e180210.
6. Klein AP, Tetzlaff JE, Bonis JM, Nelson LD, Mayer AR, Huber DL, Harezlak J, Mathews VP, Ulmer JL, Sinson GP, Nencka AS, Koch KM, Wu Y, Saykin AJ, DiFiori JP, Giza CC, Goldman J, Guskiewicz KM, Mihalik JP, Duma SM, Rowson S, Brooks A, Broglio SP, McAllister T, McCrea MA, Meier TB. Prevalence of potentially clinically significant magnetic resonance imaging findings in athletes with and without sport-related concussion. J Neurotrauma. 2019;36(11):1776–85.
7. Bonow RH, Friedman SD, Perez FA, Ellenbogen RG, Browd SR, Mac Donald CL, Vavilala MS, Rivara FP. Prevalence of abnormal magnetic resonance imaging findings in children with persistent symptoms after pediatric sports-related concussion. J Neurotrauma. 2017;34(19):2706–12.
8. Belanger HG, Spiegel E, Vanderploeg RD. Neuropsychological performance following a history of multiple self-reported concussions: a meta-analysis. J Int Neuropsychol Soc. 2010;16(2):262–7.
9. Moore RD, Kay JJ, Ellemberg D. The long-term outcomes of sport-related concussion in pediatric populations. Int J Psychophysiol. 2018;132(Pt A):14–24.
10. Manley G, Gardner AJ, Schneider KJ, Guskiewicz KM, Bailes J, Cantu RC, Castellani RJ, Turner M, Jordan BD, Randolph C, Dvorak J, Hayden KA, Tator CH, McCrory P, Iverson

GL. A systematic review of potential long-term effects of sport-related concussion. Br J Sports Med. 2017;51(12):969–77.
11. Cunningham J. History of sport-related concussion and long-term clinical cognitive health outcomes in retired athletes: a systematic review. J Athl Train. 2020;55(2):132–58.
12. Joshua K, Erin B, Tracey C, Luke H, Simon K, Leddy John J, Andrew M, Michael MC, Mayumi P, Schneider Kathryn J. What is the physiological time to recovery after concussion? A systematic review. Br J Sports Med. 2017;51(12):935–40.
13. Bigler ED, Maxwell WL. Neuropathology of mild traumatic brain injury: relationship to neuroimaging findings. Brain Imaging Behav. 2012;6(2):108–36.
14. Guenette JP, Shenton ME, Koerte IK. Imaging of concussion in young athletes. Neuroimaging Clin N Am. 2018;28(1):43–53.
15. Narayana S, Charles C, Collins K, Tsao JW, Stanfill AG, Baughman B. Neuroimaging and neuropsychological studies in sports-related concussions in adolescents: current state and future directions. Front Neurol. 2019;10:538.
16. Raichle ME, Mintun MA. Brain work and brain imaging. Annu Rev Neurosci. 2006;29:449–76.
17. Shine JM, Breakspear M. Understanding the brain by default. Trends Neurosci. 2018;41(5):244–7.
18. Zhang L, Yang KH, King AI. A proposed injury threshold for mild traumatic brain injury. J Biomech Eng. 2004;126(2):226–36.
19. Mayer AR, Bellgowan PS, Hanlon FM. Functional magnetic resonance imaging of mild traumatic brain injury. Neurosci Biobehav Rev. 2015;49:8–18.
20. Sokoloff L, Reivich M, Kennedy C, Des Rosiers MH, Patlak CS, Pettigrew KD, Sakurada O, Shinohara M. The [14C]deoxyglucose method for the measurement of local cerebral glucose utilization: theory procedure and normal values in the conscious and anesthetized albino rat. J Neurochem. 1977;28(5):897–916.
21. Murphy K, Birn RM, Bandettini PA. Resting-state fMRI confounds and cleanup. NeuroImage. 2013;80:349–59.
22. Smitha KA, Arun KM, Rajesh PG, Thomas B, Kesavadas C. Resting-state seed-based analysis: an alternative to task-based language fMRI and its laterality index. AJNR Am J Neuroradiol. 2017;38(6):1187–92.
23. Attwell D, Buchan AM, Charpak S, Lauritzen M, Macvicar BA, Newman EA. Glial and neuronal control of brain blood flow. Nature. 2010;468(7321):232–43.
24. Logothetis NK, Wandell BA. Interpreting the BOLD signal. Annu Rev Physiol. 2004;66:735–69.
25. Mangia S, Tkac I, Gruetter R, Van de Moortele PF, Maraviglia B, Ugurbil K. Sustained neuronal activation raises oxidative metabolism to a new steady-state level: evidence from 1H NMR spectroscopy in the human visual cortex. J Cereb Blood Flow Metab. 2007;27(5):1055–63.
26. Fox PT, Raichle ME. Focal physiological uncoupling of cerebral blood flow and oxidative metabolism during somatosensory stimulation in human subjects. Proc Natl Acad Sci USA. 1986;83(4):1140–4.
27. Shen Q, Ren H, Duong TQ. CBF BOLD CBV and CMRO(2) fMRI signal temporal dynamics at 500-msec resolution. J Magn Reson Imaging. 2008;27(3):599–606.
28. Medaglia JD. Functional neuroimaging in traumatic brain injury: from nodes to networks. Front Neurol. 2017;8:407.
29. Buxton RB, Uludag K, Dubowitz DJ, Liu TT. Modeling the hemodynamic response to brain activation. NeuroImage. 2004;23(Suppl 1):S220–33.
30. Cohen M. Parametric analysis of fMRI data using linear systems methods. NeuroImage. 1997;6(2):93–103.
31. Buxton RB, Wong EC, Frank LR. Dynamics of blood flow and oxygenation changes during brain activation: the balloon model. Magn Reson Med. 1998;39(6):855–64.
32. van Zijl PC, Hua J, Lu H. The BOLD post-stimulus undershoot one of the most debated issues in fMRI. NeuroImage. 2012;62(2):1092–102.

33. Liu EY, Haist F, Dubowitz DJ, Buxton RB. Cerebral blood volume changes during the BOLD post-stimulus undershoot measured with a combined normoxia/hyperoxia method. NeuroImage. 2019;185:154–63.
34. Lu H, Golay X, Pekar JJ, van Zijl PC. Sustained poststimulus elevation in cerebral oxygen utilization after vascular recovery. J Cereb Blood Flow Metab. 2004;24(7):764–70.
35. Schroeter ML, Kupka T, Mildner T, Uludag K, von Cramon DY. Investigating the post-stimulus undershoot of the BOLD signal--a simultaneous fMRI and fNIRS study. NeuroImage. 2006;30(2):349–58.
36. van Zijl PC, Hua J, Lu H. The BOLD post-stimulus undershoot one of the most debated issues in fMRI. NeuroImage. 2012;62(2):1092–102.
37. Figley CR, Stroman PW. The role(s) of astrocytes and astrocyte activity in neurometabolism neurovascular coupling and the production of functional neuroimaging signals. Eur J Neurosci. 2011;33(4):577–88.
38. Logothetis NK. What we can do and what we cannot do with fMRI. Nature. 2008;453(7197):869–78.
39. Redell JB, Maynard ME, Underwood EL, Vita SM, Dash PK, Kobori N. Traumatic brain injury and hippocampal neurogenesis: functional implications. Exp Neurol. 2020;331:113372.
40. Dorsett CR, McGuire JL, DePasquale EA, Gardner AE, Floyd CL, McCullumsmith RE. Glutamate neurotransmission in rodent models of traumatic brain injury. J Neurotrauma. 2017;34(2):263–72.
41. Gasparovic C, Yeo R, Mannell M, Ling J, Elgie R, Phillips J, Doezema D, Mayer AR. Neurometabolite concentrations in gray and white matter in mild traumatic brain injury: an 1H-magnetic resonance spectroscopy study. J Neurotrauma. 2009;26(10):1635–43.
42. Henry LC, Tremblay S, Leclerc S, Khiat A, Boulanger Y, Ellemberg D, Lassonde M. Metabolic changes in concussed American football players during the acute and chronic post-injury phases. BMC Neurol. 2011;11:105.
43. Yeo RA, Gasparovic C, Merideth F, Ruhl D, Doezema D, Mayer AR. A longitudinal proton magnetic resonance spectroscopy study of mild traumatic brain injury. J Neurotrauma. 2011;28(1):1–11.
44. Vagnozzi R, Tavazzi B, Signoretti S, Amorini AM, Belli A, Cimatti M, Delfini R, Di Pietro V, Finocchiaro A, Lazzarino G. Temporal window of metabolic brain vulnerability to concussions: mitochondrial-related impairment--part I. Neurosurgery. 2007;61(2):379–88.
45. Vagnozzi R, Signoretti S, Cristofori L, Alessandrini F, Floris R, Isgro E, Ria A, Marziale S, Zoccatelli G, Tavazzi B, Del Bolgia F, Sorge R, Broglio S, McIntosh TK, Lazzarino G. Assessment of metabolic brain damage and recovery following mild traumatic brain injury: a multicentre proton magnetic resonance spectroscopic study in concussed patients. Brain. 2010;133(11):3232–42.
46. McDevitt J, Rubin LH, De Simone FI, Phillips J, Langford D. Association between (GT) n Promoter polymorphism and recovery from concussion: a pilot study. J Neurotrauma. 2020;37(10):1204–10.
47. Gardner AJ, Iverson GL, Wojtowicz M, Levi CR, Kay-Lambkin F, Schofield PW, Zafonte R, Shultz SR, Lin AP, Stanwell P. MR Spectroscopy Findings in Retired Professional Rugby League Players. Int J Sports Med. 2017;38(3):241–52.
48. Alosco ML, Tripodis Y, Rowland B, Chua AS, Liao H, Martin B, Jarnagin J, Chaisson CE, Pasternak O, Karmacharya S, Koerte IK, Cantu RC, Kowall NW, McKee AC, Shenton ME, Greenwald R, McClean M, Stern RA, Lin A. A magnetic resonance spectroscopy investigation in symptomatic former NFL players. Brain Imaging Behav. 2019;14(5):1419–29.
49. Churchill NW, Hutchison MG, Graham SJ, Schweizer TA. Symptom correlates of cerebral blood flow following acute concussion. Neuroimage Clin. 2017;16:234–9.
50. Meier TB, Bellgowan PS, Singh R, Kuplicki R, Polansky M, Mayer AR. Recovery of cerebral blood flow following sports-related concussion. JAMA Neurol. 2015;72(5):530–8.
51. Wang Y, West JD, Bailey JN, Westfall DR, Xiao H, Arnold TW, Kersey PA, Saykin AJ, McDonald BC. Decreased cerebral blood flow in chronic pediatric mild TBI: an MRI perfusion study. Dev Neuropsychol. 2015;40(1):40–4.

52. Wang Y, Nelson Lindsay D, LaRoche Ashley A, Pfaller Adam Y, Nencka Andrew S, Koch Kevin M, McCrea Michael A. Cerebral blood flow alterations in acute sport-related concussion. J Neurotrauma. 2016;33(13):1227–36.
53. Vespa PM, O'Phelan K, McArthur D, Miller C, Eliseo M, Hirt D, Glenn T, Hovda DA. Pericontusional brain tissue exhibits persistent elevation of lactate/pyruvate ratio independent of cerebral perfusion pressure. Crit Care Med. 2007;35(4):1153–60.
54. Barkhoudarian G, Hovda DA, Giza CC. The molecular pathophysiology of concussive brain injury - an update. Phys Med Rehabil Clin N Am. 2016;27(2):373–93.
55. Giza CC, Hovda DA. The new neurometabolic cascade of concussion. Neurosurgery. 2014;75(Suppl 4):S24–33.
56. Stephens JA, Liu P, Lu H, Suskauer SJ. Cerebral blood flow after mild traumatic brain injury: associations between symptoms and post-injury perfusion. J Neurotrauma. 2018;35(2):241–8.
57. Park E, Bell JD, Siddiq IP, Baker AJ. An analysis of regional microvascular loss and recovery following two grades of fluid percussion trauma: a role for hypoxia-inducible factors in traumatic brain injury. J Cereb Blood Flow Metab. 2009;29(3):575–84.
58. Buckley EM, Miller BF, Golinski JM, Sadeghian H, McAllister LM, Vangel M, Ayata C, Meehan WP III, Franceschini MA, Whalen MJ. Decreased microvascular cerebral blood flow assessed by diffuse correlation spectroscopy after repetitive concussions in mice. J Cereb Blood Flow Metab. 2015;35(12):1995–2000.
59. Tagge CA, Fisher AM, Minaeva OV, Gaudreau-Balderrama A, Moncaster JA, Zhang XL, Wojnarowicz MW, Casey N, Lu H, Kokiko-Cochran ON, Saman S, Ericsson M, Onos KD, Veksler R, Senatorov VV Jr, Kondo A, Zhou XZ, Miry O, Vose LR, Gopaul KR, Upreti C, Nowinski CJ, Cantu RC, Alvarez VE, Hildebrandt AM, Franz ES, Konrad J, Hamilton JA, Hua N, Tripodis Y, Anderson AT, Howell GR, Kaufer D, Hall GF, Lu KP, Ransohoff RM, Cleveland RO, Kowall NW, Stein TD, Lamb BT, Huber BR, Moss WC, Friedman A, Stanton PK, AC MK, Goldstein LE. Concussion microvascular injury and early tauopathy in young athletes after impact head injury and an impact concussion mouse model. Brain. 2018;141(2):422–58.
60. Logsdon AF, Lucke-Wold BP, Turner RC, Huber JD, Rosen CL, Simpkins JW. Role of microvascular disruption in brain damage from traumatic brain injury. Compr Physiol. 2015;5(3):1147–60.
61. Churchill NW, Hutchison MG, Graham SJ, Schweizer TA. Evaluating cerebrovascular reactivity during the early symptomatic phase of sport concussion. J Neurotrauma. 2019;36(10):1518–25.
62. Len TK, Neary JP, Asmundson GJ, Goodman DG, Bjornson B, Bhambhani YN. Cerebrovascular reactivity impairment after sport-induced concussion. Med Sci Sports Exerc. 2011;43(12):2241–8.
63. Militana AR, Donahue MJ, Sills AK, Solomon GS, Gregory AJ, Strother MK, Morgan VL. Alterations in default-mode network connectivity may be influenced by cerebrovascular changes within 1 week of sports related concussion in college varsity athletes: a pilot study. Brain Imaging Behav. 2016;10:559–68.
64. Elliott ML, Knodt AR, Cooke M, Kim MJ, Melzer TR, Keenan R, Ireland D, Ramrakha S, Poulton R, Caspi A, Moffitt TE, Hariri AR. General functional connectivity: shared features of resting-state and task fMRI drive reliable and heritable individual differences in functional brain networks. NeuroImage. 2019;189:516–32.
65. Hyder F, Patel AB, Gjedde A, Rothman DL, Behar KL, Shulman RG. Neuronal-glial glucose oxidation and glutamatergic-GABAergic function. J Cereb Blood Flow Metab. 2006;26(7):865–77.
66. Mangia S, Giove F, Tkac I, Logothetis NK, Henry PG, Olman CA, Maraviglia B, Di Salle F, Ugurbil K. Metabolic and hemodynamic events after changes in neuronal activity: current hypotheses theoretical predictions and in vivo NMR experimental findings. J Cereb Blood Flow Metab. 2009;29(3):441–63.
67. Meier TB, Espana LY, Mayer AR, Harezlak J, Nencka AS, Wang Y, Koch KM, Wu YC, Saykin AJ, Giza CC, Goldman J, DiFiori JP, Guskiewicz KM, Mihalik JP, Brooks A, Broglio

SP, McAllister T, McCrea MA. Resting-state fMRI metrics in acute sport-related concussion and their association with clinical recovery: a study from the NCAA-DOD CARE consortium. J Neurotrauma. 2020;37(1):152–62.
68. Huang M, Theilmann RJ, Robb A, Angeles A, Nichols S, Drake A, Dandrea J, Levy M, Holland M, Song T, Ge S, Hwang E, Yoo K, Cui L, Baker DG, Trauner D, Coimbra R, Lee RR. Integrated imaging approach with MEG and DTI to detect mild traumatic brain injury in military and civilian patients. J Neurotrauma. 2009;26(8):1213–26.
69. Huang MX, Nichols S, Robb A, Angeles A, Drake A, Holland M, Asmussen S, D'Andrea J, Chun W, Levy M, Cui L, Song T, Baker DG, Hammer P, McLay R, Theilmann RJ, Coimbra R, Diwakar M, Boyd C, Neff J, Liu TT, Webb-Murphy J, Farinpour R, Cheung C, Harrington DL, Heister D, Lee RR. An automatic MEG low-frequency source imaging approach for detecting injuries in mild and moderate TBI patients with blast and non-blast causes. NeuroImage. 2012;61(4):1067–82.
70. Smith SM, Fox PT, Miller KL, Glahn DC, Fox PM, Mackay CE, Filippini N, Watkins KE, Toro R, Laird AR, Beckmann CF. Correspondence of the brain's functional architecture during activation and rest. Proc Natl Acad Sci U S A. 2009;106(31):13040–5.
71. Chou YH, Sundman M, Whitson HE, Gaur P, Chu ML, Weingarten CP, Madden DJ, Wang L, Kirste I, Joliot M, Diaz MT, Li YJ, Song AW, Chen NK. Maintenance and representation of mind wandering during resting-state fMRI. Sci Rep. 2017;7:40722.
72. Belanger HG, Vanderploeg RD, Curtiss G, Warden DL. Recent neuroimaging techniques in mild traumatic brain injury. J Neuropsychiatry Clin Neurosci. 2007;19(1):5–20.
73. Cook MJ, Gardner AJ, Wojtowicz M, Williams WH, Iverson GL, Stanwell P. Task-related functional magnetic resonance imaging activations in patients with acute and subacute mild traumatic brain injury: a coordinate-based meta-analysis. Neuroimage Clin. 2020;25:102129.
74. Saad ZS, Gotts SJ, Murphy K, Chen G, Jo HJ, Martin A, Cox RW. Trouble at rest: how correlation patterns and group differences become distorted after global signal regression. Brain Connect. 2012;2(1):25–32.
75. Mayer AR, Bedrick EJ, Ling JM, Toulouse T, Dodd A. Methods for identifying subject-specific abnormalities in neuroimaging data. Hum Brain Mapp. 2014;35(11):5457–70.
76. Liau J, Liu TT. Inter-subject variability in hypercapnic normalization of the BOLD fMRI response. NeuroImage. 2009;45(2):420–30.
77. Harris NG, Verley DR, Gutman BA, Thompson PM, Yeh HJ, Brown JA. Disconnection and hyper-connectivity underlie reorganization after TBI: a rodent functional connectomic analysis. Exp Neurol. 2016;277:124–38.
78. Steinman J, Cahill LS, Koletar MM, Stefanovic B, Sled JG. Acute and chronic stage adaptations of vascular architecture and cerebral blood flow in a mouse model of TBI. NeuroImage. 2019;202:116101.
79. Mayer AR, Toulouse T, Klimaj S, Ling J, Pena A, Bellgowan P. Investigating the properties of the hemodynamic response function following mild traumatic brain injury. J Neurotrauma. 2014;31(2):189–97.
80. Shin SS, Bales JW, Edward Dixon C, Hwang M. Structural imaging of mild traumatic brain injury may not be enough: overview of functional and metabolic imaging of mild traumatic brain injury. Brain Imaging Behav. 2017;11(2):591–610.
81. Reid LB, Boyd RN, Cunnington R, Rose SE. Interpreting intervention induced neuroplasticity with fMRI: the case for multimodal imaging strategies. Neural Plast. 2016;2016:2643491.
82. Di Battista AP, Rhind SG, Churchill N, Richards D, Lawrence DW, Hutchison MG. Peripheral blood neuroendocrine hormones are associated with clinical indices of sport-related concussion. Sci Rep. 2019;9(1):18605.
83. Hutchison MG, Mainwaring L, Senthinathan A, Churchill N, Thomas S, Richards D. Psychological and physiological markers of stress in concussed athletes across recovery milestones. J Head Trauma Rehabil. 2017;32(3):E38–48.
84. Stefanovic B, Warnking JM, Pike GB. Hemodynamic and metabolic responses to neuronal inhibition. NeuroImage. 2004;22(2):771–8.

85. Coverdale NS, Fernandez-Ruiz J, Champagne AA, Mark CI, Cook DJ. Co-localized impaired regional cerebrovascular reactivity in chronic concussion is associated with BOLD activation differences during a working memory task. Brain Imaging Behav. 2020;14(6):2438–49.
86. Bandettini PA, Wong EC. A hypercapnia-based normalization method for improved spatial localization of human brain activation with fMRI. NMR Biomed. 1997;10(4–5):197–203.
87. Thomason ME, Glover GH. Controlled inspiration depth reduces variance in breath-holding-induced BOLD signal. NeuroImage. 2008;39(1):206–14.
88. Sicard KM, Duong TQ. Effects of hypoxia hyperoxia and hypercapnia on baseline and stimulus-evoked BOLD CBF and CMRO2 in spontaneously breathing animals. NeuroImage. 2005;25(3):850–8.
89. Zappe AC, Uludag K, Oeltermann A, Ugurbil K, Logothetis NK. The influence of moderate hypercapnia on neural activity in the anesthetized nonhuman primate. Cereb Cortex. 2008;18(11):2666–73.
90. Biswal BB, Kannurpatti SS, Rypma B. Hemodynamic scaling of fMRI-BOLD signal: validation of low-frequency spectral amplitude as a scalability factor. Magn Reson Imaging. 2007;25(10):1358–69.
91. Cohen ER, Rostrup E, Sidaros K, Lund TE, Paulson OB, Ugurbil K, Kim SG. Hypercapnic normalization of BOLD fMRI: comparison across field strengths and pulse sequences. NeuroImage. 2004;23(2):613–24.
92. Thomason ME, Foland LC, Glover GH. Calibration of BOLD fMRI using breath holding reduces group variance during a cognitive task. Hum Brain Mapp. 2007;28(1):59–68.
93. Chan ST, Evans KC, Rosen BR, Song TY, Kwong KK. A case study of magnetic resonance imaging of cerebrovascular reactivity: a powerful imaging marker for mild traumatic brain injury. Brain Inj. 2015;29(3):403–7.
94. Dodd AB, Lu H, Wertz CJ, Ling JM, Shaff NA, Wasserott BC, Meier TB, Park G, Oglesbee SJ, Phillips JP, Campbell RA, Liu P, Mayer AR. Persistent alterations in cerebrovascular reactivity in response to hypercapnia following pediatric mild traumatic brain injury. J Cereb Blood Flow Metab. 2020;40(12):2491–504.
95. Alan MW, Ellis Michael J, Ruth GM, Vincent W, Roshan R, Fisher Joseph A, David M, Jeffrey L, Lawrence R. Brain MRI CO2 stress testing: a pilot study in patients with concussion. PLoS One. 2014;9(7):e102181.
96. Sushmita P, Sorond Farzaneh A, Sydney L, Justin F, Murphy Megan N, Hynan Linda S, Tonia S, Bell Kathleen R. Impaired cerebral vasoreactivity despite symptom resolution in sports-related concussion. J Neurotrauma. 2019;36(16):2385–90.
97. Belanger HG, Vanderploeg RD. The neuropsychological impact of sports-related concussion: a meta-analysis. J Int Neuropsychol Soc. 2005;11(4):345–57.
98. McAllister TW, Saykin AJ, Flashman LA, Sparling MB, Johnson SC, Guerin SJ, Mamourian AC, Weaver JB, Yanofsky N. Brain activation during working memory 1 month after mild traumatic brain injury: a functional MRI study. Neurology. 1999;53(6):1300–8.
99. McAllister TW, Sparling MB, Flashman LA, Guerin SJ, Mamourian AC, Saykin AJ. Differential working memory load effects after mild traumatic brain injury. NeuroImage. 2001;14(5):1004–12.
100. Dettwiler A, Murugavel M, Putukian M, Cubon V, Furtado J, Osherson D. Persistent differences in patterns of brain activation after sports-related concussion: a longitudinal functional magnetic resonance imaging study. J Neurotrauma. 2014;31(2):180–8.
101. Chen JK, Johnston KM, Frey S, Petrides M, Worsley K, Ptito A. Functional abnormalities in symptomatic concussed athletes: an fMRI study. NeuroImage. 2004;22(1):68–82.
102. Slobounov SM, Zhang K, Pennell D, Ray W, Johnson B, Sebastianelli W. Functional abnormalities in normally appearing athletes following mild traumatic brain injury: a functional MRI study. Exp Brain Res. 2010;202(2):341–54.
103. Jantzen KJ, Anderson B, Steinberg FL, Kelso JA. A prospective functional MR imaging study of mild traumatic brain injury in college football players. AJNR Am J Neuroradiol. 2004;25(5):738–45.

104. Clough M, Mutimer S, Wright DK, Tsang A, Costello DM, Gardner AJ, Stanwell P, Mychasiuk R, Sun M, Brady RD, McDonald SJ, Webster KM, Johnstone MR, Semple BD, Agoston DV, White OB, Frayne R, Fielding J, O'Brien TJ, Shultz SR. Oculomotor cognitive control abnormalities in Australian rules football players with a history of concussion. J Neurotrauma. 2018;35(5):730–8.
105. Johnson B, Zhang K, Hallett M, Slobounov S. Functional neuroimaging of acute oculomotor deficits in concussed athletes. Brain Imaging Behav. 2015;9(3):564–73.
106. Johnson B, Hallett M, Slobounov S. Follow-up evaluation of oculomotor performance with fMRI in the subacute phase of concussion. Neurology. 2015;85(13):1163–6.
107. Lovell MR, Pardini JE, Welling J, Collins MW, Bakal J, Lazar N, Roush R, Eddy WF, Becker JT. Functional brain abnormalities are related to clinical recovery and time to return-to-play in athletes. Neurosurgery. 2007;61(2):352–9.
108. Chen JK, Johnston KM, Collie A, McCrory P, Ptito A. A validation of the post concussion symptom scale in the assessment of complex concussion using cognitive testing and functional MRI. J Neurol Neurosurg Psychiatry. 2007;78(11):1231–8.
109. Pardini JE, Pardini DA, Becker JT, Dunfee KL, Eddy WF, Lovell MR, Welling JS. Postconcussive symptoms are associated with compensatory cortical recruitment during a working memory task. Neurosurgery. 2010;67(4):1020–7.
110. Terry DP, Adams TE, Ferrara MS, Miller LS. FMRI hypoactivation during verbal learning and memory in former high school football players with multiple concussions. Arch Clin Neuropsychol. 2015;30(4):341–55.
111. Elbin RJ, Covassin T, Hakun J, Kontos AP, Berger K, Pfeiffer K, Ravizza S. Do brain activation changes persist in athletes with a history of multiple concussions who are asymptomatic? Brain Inj. 2012;26(10):1217–25.
112. Terry DP, Faraco CC, Smith D, Diddams MJ, Puente AN, Miller LS. Lack of long-term fMRI differences after multiple sports-related concussions. Brain Inj. 2012;26(13–14):1684–96.
113. Talavage TM, Nauman E, Breedlove EL, Yoruk U, Dye AE, Morigaki K, Feuer H, Leverenz LJ. Functionally-detected cognitive impairment in high school football players without clinically-diagnosed concussion. J Neurotrauma. 2014;31(4):327–38.
114. Buckner RL, Andrews-Hanna J, Schacter D. The brain's default network: anatomy function and relevance to disease. Ann N Y Acad Sci. 2008;1124:1–38.
115. Xu X, Yuan H, Lei X. Activation and connectivity within the default mode network contribute independently to future-oriented thought. Sci Rep. 2016;6:21001.
116. Newsome MR, Li X, Lin X, Wilde EA, Ott S, Biekman B, Hunter JV, Dash PK, Taylor BA, Levin HS. Functional connectivity Is altered in concussed adolescent athletes despite medical clearance to return to play: a preliminary report. Front Neurol. 2016;7:116.
117. Zhang K, Johnson B, Gay M, Horovitz SG, Hallett M, Sebastianelli W, Slobounov S. Default mode network in concussed individuals in response to the YMCA physical stress test. J Neurotrauma. 2012;29(5):756–65.
118. Murugesan G, Saghafi B, Davenport E, Wagner B, Urban J, Kelley M, Jones D, Powers A, Whitlow C, Stitzel J, Maldjian J, Montillo A. Single season changes in resting state network power and the connectivity between regions: distinguish head impact exposure level in high school and youth football players. Proc SPIE Int Soc Opt Eng. 2018;10575:105750F.
119. Murugesan G, Famili A, Davenport E, Wagner B, Urban J, Kelley M, Jones D, Whitlow C, Stitzel J, Maldjian J, Montillo A. Changes in resting state MRI networks from a single season of football distinguishes controls low and high head impact exposure. Proc IEEE Int Symp Biomed Imaging. 2017;2017:464–7.
120. Churchill NW, Hutchison MG, Graham SJ, Schweizer TA. Connectomic markers of symptom severity in sport-related concussion: whole-brain analysis of resting-state fMRI. Neuroimage Clin. 2018;18:518–26.
121. Slobounov SM, Gay M, Zhang K, Johnson B, Pennell D, Sebastianelli W, Horovitz S, Hallett M. Alteration of brain functional network at rest and in response to YMCA physical stress test in concussed athletes: RsFMRI study. NeuroImage. 2011;55(4):1716–27.

122. Borich M, Babul AN, Yuan PH, Boyd L, Virji-Babul N. Alterations in resting-state brain networks in concussed adolescent athletes. J Neurotrauma. 2015;32(4):265–71.
123. Czerniak SM, Sikoglu EM, Liso Navarro AA, McCafferty J, Eisenstock J, Stevenson JH, King JA, Moore CM. A resting state functional magnetic resonance imaging study of concussion in collegiate athletes. Brain Imaging Behav. 2015;9(2):323–32.
124. Guell X, Arnold Anteraper S, Gardner AJ, Whitfield-Gabrieli S, Kay-Lambkin F, Iverson GL, Gabrieli J, Stanwell P. Functional connectivity changes in retired Rugby league players: a data-driven functional magnetic resonance imaging study. J Neurotrauma. 2020;37(16):1788–96.
125. Churchill N, Hutchison MG, Leung G, Graham S, Schweizer TA. Changes in functional connectivity of the brain associated with a history of sport concussion: a preliminary investigation. Brain Inj. 2017;31(1):39–48.
126. Meier TB, Bellgowan PS, Mayer AR. Longitudinal assessment of local and global functional connectivity following sports-related concussion. Brain Imaging Behav. 2017;11(1):129–40.
127. Kaushal M, Espana LY, Nencka AS, Wang Y, Nelson LD, McCrea MA, Meier TB. Resting-state functional connectivity after concussion is associated with clinical recovery. Hum Brain Mapp. 2019;40(4):1211–20.
128. Meier TB, Espana LY, Mayer AR, Harezlak J, Nencka AS, Wang Y, Koch KM, Wu YC, Saykin AJ, Giza CC, Goldman J, DiFiori JP, Guskiewicz KM, Mihalik JP, Brooks A, Broglio SP, McAllister T, McCrea MA. Resting-state fMRI metrics in acute sport-related concussion and their association with clinical recovery: a study from the NCAA-DOD CARE consortium. J Neurotrauma. 2019;37(1):152–62.
129. Meier TB, Lancaster MA, Mayer AR, Teague TK, Savitz J. Abnormalities in functional connectivity in collegiate football athletes with and without a concussion history: implications and role of neuroactive kynurenine pathway metabolites. J Neurotrauma. 2017;34(4):824–37.
130. Calhoun VD, Miller R, Pearlson G, Adali T. The chronnectome: time-varying connectivity networks as the next frontier in fMRI data discovery. Neuron. 2014;84(2):262–74.
131. Hutchison RM, Womelsdorf T, Allen EA, Bandettini PA, Calhoun VD, Corbetta M, Della Penna S, Duyn JH, Glover GH, Gonzalez-Castillo J, Handwerker DA, Keilholz S, Kiviniemi V, Leopold DA, de Pasquale F, Sporns O, Walter M, Chang C. Dynamic functional connectivity: promise issues and interpretations. NeuroImage. 2013;80:360–78.
132. Churchill NW, Hutchison MG, Graham SJ, Schweizer TA. Scale-free functional brain dynamics during recovery from sport-related concussion. Hum Brain Mapp. 2020;41(10):2567–82.
133. Saurabh S, Sebastien N, Foad T, Charles T, Richard W, David M, Robin G, Brenda C, Carmela TM, Kozloski James R. Multimodal dynamic brain connectivity analysis based on graph signal processing for former athletes with history of multiple concussions. IEEE Trans Signal Inf Process Netw. 2020;6:284–99.
134. Churchill NW, Hutchison MG, Richards D, Leung G, Graham SJ, Schweizer TA. Neuroimaging of sport concussion: persistent alterations in brain structure and function at medical clearance. Sci Rep. 2017;7(1):8297.
135. Zhang K, Johnson B, Pennell D, Ray W, Sebastianelli W, Slobounov S. Are functional deficits in concussed individuals consistent with white matter structural alterations: combined FMRI & DTI study. Exp Brain Res. 2010;204(1):57–70.
136. Manning KY, Schranz A, Bartha R, Dekaban GA, Barreira C, Brown A, Fischer L, Asem K, Doherty TJ, Fraser DD, Holmes J, Menon RS. Multiparametric MRI changes persist beyond recovery in concussed adolescent hockey players. Neurology. 2017;89(21):2157–66.
137. Manning KY, Llera A, Dekaban GA, Bartha R, Barreira C, Brown A, Fischer L, Jevremovic T, Blackney K, Doherty TJ, Fraser DD, Holmes J, Beckmann CF, Menon RS. Linked MRI signatures of the brain's acute and persistent response to concussion in female varsity rugby players. Neuroimage Clin. 2019;21:101627.
138. Shenton ME, Hamoda HM, Schneiderman JS, Bouix S, Pasternak O, Rathi Y, Vu MA, Purohit MP, Helmer K, Koerte I, Lin AP, Westin CF, Kikinis R, Kubicki M, Stern RA, Zafonte R. A review of magnetic resonance imaging and diffusion tensor imaging findings in mild traumatic brain injury. Brain Imaging Behav. 2012;6(2):137–92.

139. Champagne AA, Coverdale NS, Germuska M, Cook DJ. Multi-parametric analysis reveals metabolic and vascular effects driving differences in BOLD-based cerebrovascular reactivity associated with a history of sport concussion. Brain Inj. 2019;33(11):1479–89.
140. Bottari C, Gosselin N, Chen JK, Ptito A. The impact of symptomatic mild traumatic brain injury on complex everyday activities and the link with alterations in cerebral functioning: exploratory case studies. Neuropsychol Rehabil. 2017;27(5):871–90.
141. Gosselin N, Bottari C, Chen JK, Petrides M, Tinawi S, de Guise E, Ptito A. Electrophysiology and functional MRI in post-acute mild traumatic brain injury. J Neurotrauma. 2011;28(3):329–41.
142. Churchill NW, Hutchison MG, Richards D, Leung G, Graham SJ, Schweizer TA. The first week after concussion: blood flow brain function and white matter microstructure. Neuroimage Clin. 2017;14:480–9.
143. Churchill N, Hutchison M, Richards D, Leung G, Graham S, Schweizer TA. Brain structure and function associated with a history of sport concussion: a multi-modal magnetic resonance imaging study. J Neurotrauma. 2017;34(4):765–71.
144. Ptito A, Chen JK, Johnston KM. Contributions of functional magnetic resonance imaging (fMRI) to sport concussion evaluation. NeuroRehabilitation. 2007;22(3):217–27.
145. Yang J, Peek-Asa C, Covassin T, Torner JC. Post-concussion symptoms of depression and anxiety in division I collegiate athletes. Dev Neuropsychol. 2015;40(1):18–23.
146. Tracey C, Elbin RJ, Erica B, Meghan LF, Kontos Anthony P. A review of psychological issues that may be associated with a sport-related concussion in youth and collegiate athletes. Sport Exerc Perform Psychol. 2017;6(3):220.
147. Rice SM, Parker AG, Rosenbaum S, Bailey A, Mawren D, Purcell R. Sport-related concussion and mental health outcomes in elite athletes: a systematic review. Sports Med. 2018;48(2):447–65.
148. McCuddy WT, Espana LY, Nelson LD, Birn RM, Mayer AR, Meier TB. Association of acute depressive symptoms and functional connectivity of emotional processing regions following sport-related concussion. Neuroimage Clin. 2018;19:434–42.
149. Roiger T, Weidauer L, Kern B. A longitudinal pilot study of depressive symptoms in concussed and injured/nonconcussed National Collegiate Athletic Association Division I student-athletes. J Athl Train. 2015;50(3):256–61.
150. Gouttebarge V, Kerkhoffs GMMJ. Sports career-related concussion and mental health symptoms in former elite athletes. Neurochirurgie. 2021;67(3):280–2.
151. Brett BL, Mummareddy N, Kuhn AW, Yengo-Kahn AM, Zuckerman SL. The relationship between prior concussions and depression is modified by somatic symptomatology in retired NFL athletes. J Neuropsychiatry Clin Neurosci. 2019;31(1):17–24.
152. Decq P, Gault N, Blandeau M, Kerdraon T, Berkal M, ElHelou A, Dusfour B, Peyrin JC. Long-term consequences of recurrent sports concussion. Acta Neurochir. 2016;158(2):289–300.
153. Gouttebarge V, Hopley P, Kerkhoffs G, Verhagen E, Viljoen W, Wylleman P, Lambert MI. Symptoms of common mental disorders in professional Rugby: an international observational descriptive study. Int J Sports Med. 2017;38(11):864–70.
154. Guskiewicz KM, Marshall SW, Bailes J, McCrea M, Harding HP Jr, Matthews A, Mihalik JR, Cantu RC. Recurrent concussion and risk of depression in retired professional football players. Med Sci Sports Exerc. 2007;39(6):903–9.
155. Dikmen SS, Bombardier CH, Machamer JE, Fann JR, Temkin NR. Natural history of depression in traumatic brain injury. Arch Phys Med Rehabil. 2004;85(9):1457–64.
156. Blaylock RL, Maroon J. Immunoexcitotoxicity as a central mechanism in chronic traumatic encephalopathy-A unifying hypothesis. Surg Neurol Int. 2011;2:107.
157. Holsboer F, Lauer CJ, Schreiber W, Krieg JC. Altered hypothalamic-pituitary-adrenocortical regulation in healthy subjects at high familial risk for affective disorders. Neuroendocrinology. 1995;62(4):340–7.
158. Urry HL, van Reekum CM, Johnstone T, Kalin NH, Thurow ME, Schaefer HS, Jackson CA, Frye CJ, Greischar LL, Alexander AL, Davidson RJ. Amygdala and ventromedial prefrontal

cortex are inversely coupled during regulation of negative affect and predict the diurnal pattern of cortisol secretion among older adults. J Neurosci. 2006;26(16):4415–25.
159. Watson D, Pennebaker JW. Health complaints stress and distress: exploring the central role of negative affectivity. Psychol Rev. 1989;96(2):234.
160. Erickson K, Drevets W, Schulkin J. Glucocorticoid regulation of diverse cognitive functions in normal and pathological emotional states. Neurosci Biobehav Rev. 2003;27(3):233–46.
161. Johnson EO, Kamilaris TC, Chrousos GP, Gold PW. Mechanisms of stress: a dynamic overview of hormonal and behavioral homeostasis. Neurosci Biobehav Rev. 1992;16(2):115–30.
162. van der Horn HJ, Out ML, de Koning ME, Mayer AR, Spikman JM, Sommer IE, van der Naalt J. An integrated perspective linking physiological and psychological consequences of mild traumatic brain injury. J Neurol. 2020;267(9):2497–506.
163. Chen JK, Johnston KM, Petrides M, Ptito A. Neural substrates of symptoms of depression following concussion in male athletes with persisting postconcussion symptoms. Arch Gen Psychiatry. 2008;65(1):81–9.
164. van der Horn HJ, Liemburg EJ, Aleman A, Spikman JM, van der Naalt J. Brain networks subserving emotion regulation and adaptation after mild traumatic brain injury. J Neurotrauma. 2016;33(1):1–9.
165. Sperling R, Greve D, Dale A, Killiany R, Holmes J, Rosas HD, Cocchiarella A, Firth P, Rosen B, Lake S, Lange N, Routledge C, Albert M. Functional MRI detection of pharmacologically induced memory impairment. Proc Natl Acad Sci U S A. 2002;99(1):455–60.
166. Vollm B, Richardson P, McKie S, Elliott R, Deakin JF, Anderson IM. Serotonergic modulation of neuronal responses to behavioural inhibition and reinforcing stimuli: an fMRI study in healthy volunteers. Eur J Neurosci. 2006;23(2):552–60.
167. Wagner G, Koch K, Schachtzabel C, Sobanski T, Reichenbach JR, Sauer H, Schlosser RG. Differential effects of serotonergic and noradrenergic antidepressants on brain activity during a cognitive control task and neurofunctional prediction of treatment outcome in patients with depression. J Psychiatry Neurosci. 2010;35(4):247.
168. Hutchison M, Mainwaring LM, Comper P, Richards DW, Bisschop SM. Differential emotional responses of varsity athletes to concussion and musculoskeletal injuries. Clin J Sport Med. 2009;19(1):13–9.
169. Hutchison M, Comper P, Mainwaring L, Richards D. The influence of musculoskeletal injury on cognition: implications for concussion research. Am J Sports Med. 2011;39(11):2331–7.
170. Kontos AP, Elbin RJ, Newcomer Appaneal R, Covassin T, Collins MW. A comparison of coping responses among high school and college athletes with concussion orthopedic injuries and healthy controls. Res Sports Med. 2013;21(4):367–79.
171. Asken BM, Sullan MJ, Snyder AR, Houck ZM, Bryant VE, Hizel LP, McLaren ME, Dede DE, Jaffee MS, DeKosky ST, Bauer RM. Factors influencing clinical correlates of chronic traumatic encephalopathy (CTE): a review. Neuropsychol Rev. 2016;26(4):340–63.
172. Chein JM, Schneider W. Neuroimaging studies of practice-related change: fMRI and meta-analytic evidence of a domain-general control network for learning. Brain Res Cogn Brain Res. 2005;25(3):607–23.
173. Telzer EH, McCormick EM, Peters S, Cosme D, Pfeifer JH, van Duijvenvoorde ACK. Methodological considerations for developmental longitudinal fMRI research. Dev Cogn Neurosci. 2018;33:149–60.
174. Weissman DH, Woldorff MG, Hazlett CJ, Mangun GR. Effects of practice on executive control investigated with fMRI. Brain Res Cogn Brain Res. 2002;15(1):47–60.
175. Rosenbaum SB, Lipton ML. Embracing chaos: the scope and importance of clinical and pathological heterogeneity in mTBI. Brain Imaging Behav. 2012;6(2):255–82.
176. Henry LC, Elbin RJ, Collins MW, Marchetti G, Kontos AP. Examining recovery trajectories after sport-related concussion with a multimodal clinical assessment approach. Neurosurgery. 2016;78(2):232–41.
177. Ruff RM, Iverson GL, Barth JT, Bush SS, Broshek DK. Recommendations for diagnosing a mild traumatic brain injury: a National Academy of Neuropsychology education paper. Arch Clin Neuropsychol. 2009;24(1):3–10.

178. Belanger HG, Curtiss G, Demery JA, Lebowitz BK, Vanderploeg RD. Factors moderating neuropsychological outcomes following mild traumatic brain injury: a meta-analysis. J Int Neuropsychol Soc. 2005;11(3):215–27.
179. Johnson B, Dodd A, Mayer AR, Hallett M, Slobounov S. Are there any differential responses to concussive injury in civilian versus athletic populations: a neuroimaging study. Brain Imaging Behav. 2020;14(1):110–7.
180. Monroe DC, Cecchi NJ, Gerges P, Phreaner J, Hicks JW, Small SL. A dose relationship between brain functional connectivity and cumulative head impact exposure in collegiate water polo players. Front Neurol. 2020;11:218.
181. Reynolds BB, Stanton AN, Soldozy S, Goodkin HP, Wintermark M, Druzgal TJ. Investigating the effects of subconcussion on functional connectivity using mass-univariate and multivariate approaches. Brain Imaging Behav. 2018;12(5):1332–45.
182. Kontos AP, Sufrinko A, Sandel N, Emami K, Collins MW. Sport-related concussion clinical profiles: clinical characteristics targeted treatments and preliminary evidence. Curr Sports Med Rep. 2019;18(3):82–92.
183. Lee H, Wintermark M, Gean AD, Ghajar J, Manley GT, Mukherjee P. Focal lesions in acute mild traumatic brain injury and neurocognitive outcome: CT versus 3T MRI. J Neurotrauma. 2008;25(9):1049–56.
184. Shauna K, Hanks Robin A, Casey Joseph E, Millis Scott R. Neuropsychologic and functional outcome after complicated mild traumatic brain injury. Arch Phys Med Rehabil. 2008;89(5):904–11.
185. Viano DC, Casson IR, Pellman EJ, Zhang L, King AI, Yang KH. Concussion in professional football: brain responses by finite element analysis: part 9. Neurosurgery. 2005;57(5):891–916.
186. Clark MD, Varangis EML, Champagne AA, Giovanello KS, Shi F, Kerr ZY, Smith JK, Guskiewicz KM. Effects of career duration concussion history and playing position on white matter microstructure and functional neural recruitment in Former College and Professional Football Athletes. Radiology. 2018;286(3):967–77.
187. Poldrack RA, Baker CI, Durnez J, Gorgolewski KJ, Matthews PM, Munafo MR, Nichols TE, Poline JB, Vul E, Yarkoni T. Scanning the horizon: towards transparent and reproducible neuroimaging research. Nat Rev Neurosci. 2017;18(2):115–26.
188. Desmond JE, Glover GH. Estimating sample size in functional MRI (fMRI) neuroimaging studies: statistical power analyses. J Neurosci Methods. 2002;118(2):115–28.
189. Dennis EL, Baron D, Bartnik-Olson B, Caeyenberghs K, Esopenko C, Hillary FG, Kenney K, Koerte IK, Lin AP, Mayer AR, Mondello S, Olsen A, Thompson PM, Tate DF, Wilde EA. ENIGMA brain injury: framework challenges and opportunities. Hum Brain Mapp. 2020. Online ahead of print.
190. Beidler E, Bretzin AC, Hanock C, Covassin T. Sport-related concussion: knowledge and reporting behaviors among collegiate club-sport athletes. J Athl Train. 2018;53(9):866–72.
191. Booher MA, Wisniewski J, Smith BW, Sigurdsson A. Comparison of reporting systems to determine concussion incidence in NCAA Division I collegiate football. Clin J Sport Med. 2003;13(2):93.
192. Echemendia RJ, Cantu RC. Return to play following sports-related mild traumatic brain injury: the role for neuropsychology. Appl Neuropsychol. 2003;10(1):48–55.
193. Greenwald RM, Chu JJ, Beckwith JG, Crisco JJ. A proposed method to reduce underreporting of brain injury in sports. Clin J Sport Med. 2012;22(2):83–5.
194. Bianchini KJ, Curtis KL, Greve KW. Compensation and malingering in traumatic brain injury: a dose-response relationship? Clin Neuropsychol. 2006;20(4):831–47.
195. Greve KW, Bianchini KJ, Doane BM. Classification accuracy of the test of memory malingering in traumatic brain injury: results of a known-groups analysis. J Clin Exp Neuropsychol. 2006;28(7):1176–90.
196. Donders J, Lefebre N, Goldsworthy R. Patterns of performance and symptom validity test findings after mild traumatic brain injury. Arch Clin Neuropsychol. 2019;36(3):394–402.
197. Craig Debbie I, Lininger Monica R, Wayment Heidi A, Huffman AH. Investigation of strategies to improve concussion reporting in American football. Res Sports Med. 2020;28(2):181–93.

198. Chrisman SP, Quitiquit C, Rivara FP. Qualitative study of barriers to concussive symptom reporting in high school athletics. J Adolesc Health. 2013;52(3):330–5.
199. Broglio SP, Macciocchi SN, Ferrara MS. Sensitivity of the concussion assessment battery. Neurosurgery. 2007;60(6):1050–7.
200. Van Kampen DA, Lovell MR, Pardini JE, Collins MW, Fu FH. The "value added" of neurocognitive testing after sports-related concussion. Am J Sports Med. 2006;34(10):1630–5.
201. Frederic G, Syd JL. The impact of American Tackle Football-related concussion in youth athletes. AJOB Neurosci. 2011;2(4):48–59.
202. Emily K, Bernice G, Matt H, Baugh Christine M, Calzo Jerel P. Concussion under-reporting and pressure from coaches teammates fans and parents. Soc Sci Med. 2015;134:66–75.
203. Delaney JS, Caron JG, Correa JA, Bloom GA. Why professional football players chose not to reveal their concussion symptoms during a practice or game. Clin J Sport Med. 2018;28(1):1–12.
204. Delaney JS, Lamfookon C, Bloom GA, Al-Kashmiri A, Correa JA. Why university athletes choose not to reveal their concussion symptoms during a practice or game. Clin J Sport Med. 2015;25(2):113–25.
205. Guskiewicz KM, Marshall SW, Bailes J, McCrea M, Cantu RC, Randolph C, Jordan BD. Association between recurrent concussion and late-life cognitive impairment in retired professional football players. Neurosurgery. 2005;57(4):719–26.
206. Curry AE, Arbogast KB, Metzger KB, Kessler RS, Breiding MJ, Haarbauer-Krupa J, DePadilla L, Greenspan A, Master CL. Risk of repeat concussion among patients diagnosed at a pediatric care network. J Pediatr. 2019;210:13–9.
207. Scopaz KA, Hatzenbuehler JR. Risk modifiers for concussion and prolonged recovery. Sports Health. 2013;5(6):537–41.
208. Giza CC, Hovda DA. The neurometabolic cascade of concussion. J Athl Train. 2001;36(3):228–35.
209. Mayer AR, Stephenson DD, Wertz CJ, et al. Proactive inhibition deficits with normal perfusion after pediatric mild traumatic brain injury. Human Brain Mapp. 2019;40:5370–81.
210. Mayer AR, Ling JM, Allen EA, et al. Static and dynamic intrinsic connectivity following mild traumatic brain injury. J Neurotrauma. 2015;32(14):1046–55.

Sports-Related Subconcussive Head Trauma

12

Brian D. Johnson

Introduction

Sports-related concussion (SRC) and subconcussive head trauma have received a lot of attention, not only in the scientific and medical communities, but in the public as well. Widespread media coverage and several high-profile cases have brought into question the damaging and long-term effects of sports-related traumatic brain injury (TBI) [1]. Specifically, there has been a broad range of neurodegenerative diseases and processes that include postconcussion syndrome, posttraumatic stress disorder, cognitive impairment, chronic traumatic encephalopathy (CTE), and *dementia pugilistica* that have been linked to repetitive sports-related head injury of any kind [2]. Research exploring the neuropsychological, neurophysiological, and biomechanical effects of SRC has increased dramatically over the past 20 years [3]. Although still in its infancy, research into the effects of subconcussive head trauma and repetitive head impacts has also begun to grow. The increased understanding of the damaging effects from SRC and subconcussive head trauma has led to changes in sport policy. Despite the growing research, there remain knowledge gaps and an incomplete understanding of the short-term and long-term effects of subconcussive head impacts. Continuous exposure to repetitive subconcussive head impacts sustained over a career has been linked to changes in behavior and neurodegenerative diseases [4]. Traumatic brain injury (TBI) is referred to as the "silent epidemic," as many of the physical, cognitive, behavioral, and emotional symptoms go unrecognized [5]. TBI is not only a major health concern in the United States but is also the leading cause of disability worldwide [6].

B. D. Johnson (✉)
Philips Healthcare, Gainesville, FL, USA

Department of Radiology, University of Texas Southwestern Medical Center, Dallas, TX, USA
e-mail: brian.johnson@philips.com

There is growing concern in clinical practice regarding the immediate and long-term effects of multiple and frequent subconcussive blows in athletes participating in full contact sports. These effects, in terms of neurocognitive, behavioral, and underlying neural substrates, have not been sufficiently studied. In particular, concern is growing about the effect of subconcussive impacts on the head and how it may adversely affect cerebral functions [7–9]. Subconcussive blows are below the threshold to cause a concussion [10] and do not elicit any clinically identifiable concussion signs or symptoms [7–9]. Despite not producing any concussion-related signs and symptoms, subconcussive head impacts should not be overlooked. Animal and human studies have shown that even though these subconcussive blows do not result in apparent behavioral alterations, they can cause damage to the central nervous system [2, 11]. Moreover, subconcussive impacts still have the potential to transfer a high degree of linear and rotational acceleration forces to the brain [12]. Alterations in brain gray matter microstructure and neuropsychological deficits have been shown to correlate with the incidence of exposure to subconcussive head impacts during the participation in contact sports [3]. Unlike concussions, subconcussive blows go undiagnosed and are not assessed by medical professionals during a game or practice. Biomechanical research has revealed the staggering numbers of subconcussive head impacts athletes may receive over the course of a season and a career [1, 13]. Furthermore, postmortem studies have identified that repeated subconcussive impacts may have an accumulative effect [10]. It has been hypothesized that these frequent and repetitive subconcussive impacts exacerbate the cognitive aging process by reducing the cognitive reserve at an accelerated rate and lead to altered neuronal biology that may not present itself till later in life [14]. Recent neuroimaging studies have shown that brain injury does not only come from concussive episodes but exposure to subconcussive blows can also cause pathophysiological changes in the brain [15]. Similar to the research focused on concussion and mild traumatic brain injury (mTBI), the current literature on subconcussive head trauma is limited and study results are often mixed [16]. However, deeper investigations into SRC have revealed that subconcussive head trauma is a significant cause of acute and chronic functional and structural changes in the brain [17].

Animal Models of Subconcussive Head Trauma

It has been known since the late nineteenth century that repeated mild blows to the head in animal experiments could be lethal, even though there was no evidence of structural brain damage [18]. Initial animal models investigating the effects of subconcussive insults revealed that following a single subconcussive blow, there were no behavioral and histologic changes, yet repetitive subconcussive head trauma resulted in permanent injury [19]. Fujita et al. [20] reported that repetitive subthreshold head trauma did not cause axonal or vascular changes in the rat. In an early experiment looking at concussion in the rat, it was noted that following subconcussive blows, the animals showed signs of "posttraumatic amnesia" [21]. Additionally, Govons et al. [21] reported that subconcussive blows produced convulsions in some of the rats, elicited altered activity for 24 h, and that the impact caused the animal to be momentarily stunned. Subconcussive head trauma has shown to decrease the polarizability of the cerebrum, although not to the extent of a full concussive blow [22]. Tedeschi [18] reported that repetitive subconcussive blows received over a short duration in a rat model elicited a higher incidence of ill effects. Furthermore, postmortem examination of these rats revealed widespread evidence of neuronal injury, myelin loss, and glial proliferation. Other studies of subconcussive head trauma have reported neuropsychological changes and ionic fluctuations which have been hypothesized to leave the brain more vulnerable to a repeated injury [23]. In another animal study investigating the effects of subconcussive head trauma induced by a mild lateral fluid percussion, Shultz et al. [10] found that such an injury caused acute neuroinflammation, despite any significant axonal injury, or cognitive, emotional, or sensorimotor alterations. Specifically, they documented a short-term increase in microglia, macrophages, and reactive astrogliosis which returned to normal at a 4-week follow-up. Acute neuroinflammation has also been documented in other animal and human studies of TBI. Repetitive mTBI, similar to neuroinflammation, may have cumulative effects leading to neurodegeneration [10] and has been linked to behavioral impairments after TBI [24]. Conversely, it has been thought that neuroinflammation may have a neuroprotective quality [25] and the brain may be better protected following an initial TBI [26]. Complementary to this notion of neuroprotection, it has also been reported that by gradually increasing the amount of brain injury, animals could tolerate trauma that would otherwise kill normal animals. This so-called trauma resistance was attributed to a stabilization of metabolic processes [27] and the idea of preconditioning has been well-documented for cerebral ischemia [28]. Although postmortem studies have identified that repeated subconcussive head trauma may have an accumulative effect and lead to neurodegenerative diseases [10], Slemmer and Weber [28], using a mechanical stretch to simulate mTBI in hippocampal cell cultures, found that when the tissue was preconditioned they observed a significant decrease in S-100B, indicating a positive effect of glial preconditioning. Moreover, Allen et al. [26] reported a rat model of repetitive mTBI preconditioning served to preserve motor function following a severe TBI and also elicited activation of secondary sites in the brain that may aid in recovery. More recently, utilizing an experimental mouse model of subconcussive head trauma, Tagge et al. [29] demonstrated neuropathological changes in the form of axonopathy, disruption of the blood-brain barrier, astrocytosis, and microgliosis. They also reported that the presence of focal phosphorylated tauopathy was detected in the acute phase of injury. These animal studies give evidence that subconcussive blows to the head are enough to cause injury to the brain.

Biomechanical Studies of Subconcussive Head Trauma

Biomechanical studies focusing on subconcussive head trauma have allowed for the quantification of the number of subconcussive impacts athletes are exposed to. These studies have also shown that significant amounts of force are transmitted to deep midbrain and brainstem structures, that does not result in concussion or loss of consciousness [30]. Characterizing repetitive head impacts by biomechanical properties of frequency, linear acceleration, rotational acceleration, jerk, force, impulse, and impact duration, Broglio et al. [31] found that many variables including player position, location of impact, and practice versus game all contribute to the inhomogeneity of subconcussive trauma. Miyashita et al. [32] reported a similar variation in the biomechanical characteristics of repetitive head impacts in collegiate lacrosse players due to player position and session type. Moreover, session type has been identified as an important variable in the frequency of subconcussive exposure on account of the intensity of games, compared to practice demonstrating a higher incidence of these impacts [33, 34]. Adding to the variability of the biomechanical properties of subconcussive head impacts, there are also differences based on the sport being played. Comparing peak accelerations between football, ice-hockey, and soccer, Nauheim et al. [35] reported that peak accelerations in ice-hockey were significantly higher than those in football and substantially higher than those measured in soccer players. Furthermore, biomechanical studies report that forces like momentum and energy transfer associated with heading the soccer ball are far less than those found in football, boxing, hockey, and other full contact sports [36]. With the advent of new technologies, like the Head Impact Telemetry System (HITS) and wearable sensors, tracking the number and quantification of forces at impact has become more feasible. In a recent study, Broglio et al. [12] used the HITS to measure and record head impacts in 95 high school football players over a 4-year period of time. The results of this study highlighted the number of blows to the head an athlete is exposed to over the course of a season as well as the high degree of linear and rotational acceleration forces sustained during these impacts. Probably, the most shocking data to come out of these studies are the sheer quantity of subconcussive impacts endured during the course of a season, let alone an athlete's career. This number can be in the thousands, with one study reporting players sustaining over 1400 subconcussive blows over the course of a single season [37]. Tracking 1208 high school and collegiate football players over the course of a season, Beckwith et al. [38] found that players sustaining a concussion received more impacts and impacts of higher force on days they were diagnosed with a SRC. Consequently, a recent laboratory study of football helmets found that current varsity helmets are less protective to their older leather helmet counterparts when it comes to subconcussive blows [39].

Subconcussive hits do not only occur in collision sports like football, ice-hockey, and rugby. Soccer is a contact sport and chronic traumatic brain injury (CTBI) has been well documented in the literature [40]. During an average game, a soccer player heads the ball 6–12 times, which is estimated to be over 5000 headers for a 15-year career [11, 36]. However, most of the documented cases of concussion in soccer occur due to the players head contacting another player's head, the ground, or the goal post, not from purposeful heading [41]. The repeated subconcussive blows that are incurred from heading the soccer ball account for many clinical symptoms that span the spectrum from headache to brain damage and can also lead to alterations in acute and chronic cognitive functions [11]. It has long been known that heading of the soccer ball could produce "footballer's migraine" [42]. Analyzing the blood levels of nerve growth factor (NGF) and brain-derived neurotrophic factor (BDNF) of 17 male soccer players before and after a bout of heading training, Bamac et al. [43] measured significant changes in both NGF and BDNF concentrations. Measuring blood levels of the neuroprotein S-100B, which is used as a biomarker to indicate brain damage, Mussack et al. [44] reported transient elevations following a dedicated training session of controlled heading in 61 soccer players. The S-100B levels did return to baseline levels 6 h after the heading session. Increases in S-100B concentrations have also been reported from pregame to postgame in football players [45]. Furthermore, biomechanical studies of full-blown concussive episodes have gone to great lengths to quantify and identify a threshold of concussion to no avail [46], as this is very difficult given the fact that each SRC is different [47]. These biomechanical studies illustrate the sheer volume and potential harmful effects from subconcussive head impacts.

Cognitive Assessment of Subconcussive Head Trauma

Exposure to subconcussive impacts that do not result in any clinically identifiable concussion signs or symptoms is a controversial topic, as researchers and clinicians are divided on their true effects. Some research has shown that subconcussive head trauma may have minimal impact on cognitive functions [48], although there is mounting evidence that subconcussive blows have detrimental effects on cognitive and cerebral functions [7, 15]. It has been hypothesized that exposure to repeated and multiple subconcussive blows throughout an athlete's career may compromise cognitive function [49]. It is becoming more apparent that brain injury does not only come from concussive episodes, but that the accumulation of these subconcussive blows may be detrimental [50]. A history of multiple concussions and subconcussive blows has been linked to depression, cognitive deficits, and progressive neuropathologies that include neurofibrillary tangles and deposits of amyloid plaques seen in Alzheimer's disease [51].

A majority of the literature that exists on acute and chronic sports-related subconcussive head trauma has been focused on soccer, as purposeful heading represents a form of repetitive subthreshold mild brain injury [36]. In a preliminary study, it was found that out of 77 retired Norwegian professional soccer players, 50% reported symptoms linked to heading and 75% suffered from disorientation, headache, and nausea [52]. Further studies by Tysvaer et al. used electroencephalograph (EEG) to evaluate professional soccer players. They found that 35% of the participants had abnormal EEGs and 70% displayed some form of neurological impairment [52, 53]. In addition to these findings, neuropsychological testing (Wechsler Adult Intelligence Scale) of the same soccer players revealed significant differences, compared to controls with one-third of participants' scores low enough to suggest evidence of organic brain damage [54]. Matser et al. [55] reported significant deficits in a neuropsychological assessment of amateur soccer players associated with heading. Specifically, they reported impaired performance in memory, planning, and visual perception processing that was exacerbated by the number of previous concussions a player had sustained. Downs and Abwender [56] reported that subjects with a long history of soccer heading demonstrated slower patterns of motor speed and reaction time. Another study looking at purposeful heading by Witol and Webbe [9] revealed that players with the most reported number of headers had the lowest attention, concentration, and IQ scores. Decreased reaction time and reduced speed performing a motor task have been documented, when assessing the effects of concussive and subconcussive head trauma in soccer [49, 56, 57]. Although there is evidence that a long career, which accounts for many instances of heading the soccer ball, can lead to impaired brain function, it is not clear whether or not this increased likelihood is caused by numerous subconcussive blows or from full-blown concussive episodes [41]. Jordan et al. [58] found that there was a correlation between a history of concussion with increased symptoms in the United States national soccer team players and may suggest that full-blown concussions, as compared to repetitive subconcussive impacts, may be the cause of encephalopathic changes. But it seems evident in the literature that a long soccer career, which amounts to a higher frequency of heading and accumulation of subconcussive blows, contributes to impairments in cognitive function [41, 59]. However, in a review by Rutherford et al. [16] on neuropsychological testing and purposeful heading in soccer literature, they raise certain methodological concerns with a majority of the studies. They conclude that there is preliminary evidence that full-blown concussive episodes can have deleterious effects based upon neuropsychological examination, whereas the effects of subconcussive impacts on neuropsychological tests await more supporting evidence. Not all studies on heading in soccer have reported neuropsychological deficits [42]. In a recent study, Kontos and colleagues [60] used computerized testing in the form of Immediate Post-Concussion Assessment and Cognitive Testing (ImPACT) to test 63 adolescent soccer players. All subjects under study had no current (less than 3 months) history of concussion and were placed into one of the three groups based upon the number of documented headers as observed by the researchers over the course of two practices and games. Their results showed no significant differences between the low , moderate-, and high-frequency heading groups on computerized neuropsychological assessment. However, the authors did note that the males showed lower scores on verbal memory, visual memory, and motor processing, compared to female participants. This decreased performance was attributed to differences based upon sex, even though males headed the ball more often than females.

Similar to the studies looking at the chronic effects of repetitive subconcussive head trauma, initial research looking at the acute effects has produced mixed results. Schmitt et al. [41] tested postural control and recorded subjects' self-reported symptoms immediately and at 24 h following a controlled session of intentional soccer ball heading. They found that prior to, immediately following, and at 24 h after the 40-min session of heading, there were no differences in postural control between the heading group and a control kicking group. Despite not finding any significant difference in postural control, there was an increase in concussion-related symptoms reported by the heading group immediately following the session which resolved before the 24-h follow-up. The main complaints were headache, dizziness, and feeling lethargic. This reported finding was similar to that of Tysvaer [61] who found that 10 min following a session of purposeful heading, all subjects reported suffering from a headache. Consistent with these findings, Mangus et al. [62] and Broglio et al. [63] found no significant acute changes in balance following a session of purposeful heading. In a recent study by Rieder and Jansen [64], they took subjects and divided them into three groups to investigate the effects that a bout of acute heading would have on neuropsychological examination. The three groups consisted of subjects exposed to aerobic training and purposeful heading drills, the second group consisted of subjects only doing the aerobic training, and the third group did not exert themselves physically before neuropsychological testing. Neuropsychological testing was performed 1 week prior to training session and immediately after. The results showed no differences between groups and/or any deficits caused by heading drills. However, there was a higher incidence of headache during and after in the heading cohort, which the authors attributed to the most minor form of head trauma, cranial contusion, which is associated with local or diffuse transient headache. However, Putukian et al. [65] did not report any differences in self-reported symptoms and cognitive function in a pilot study after a soccer training session that included heading. Therefore, symptoms from subconcussive blows may be shorter lived and only detectable immediately after insult. Investigating the role of concussion history on the neurocognitive effects of subconcussive impacts using the Automated Neuropsychological Assessment Metrics, Forbes et al. [66] found no significant differences between the experimental and control group of female high school soccer players. Although the number of headers recorded for both groups was almost identical (24.9 and 24.3), it was far less than the incidence of subconcussive blows documented in other contact sports. Several other studies looking at the effects of heading in soccer report no significant changes in neuropsychological testing following exposure to repetitive head impacts [65, 67–69]. Employing the use of a computerized tablet, Zhang et al. [70] devised a variant of common eye tracking research, prosaccade, and antisaccade by having participants point toward a target (Pro-Point) or point to the opposite target (Anti-Point). Eye tracking research has been shown to be more sensitive in picking up cognitive and functional deficits, compared to standard neuropsychological testing [71–73]. In their study, Zhang et al. [70] tested 12 female high school soccer players following practice that included heading of the soccer ball. No difference was seen between the soccer group, compared to sex and age-matched control group on the Pro-Point task. Although the Anti-Point task, like the antisaccade task used in eye tracking studies, showed that subjects in the soccer group who were exposed to heading demonstrated significantly slower response times, compared to the control group. Following head injury, oculomotor deficits are common and impaired eye movements have been documented in concussion and postconcussion syndrome [71]. Although deficits in eye movement have been documented in concussion, little work has been done to study oculomotor function in subconcussive head impacts. Using a cohort of 12 high school football players, Zonner et al. reported oculomotor dysfunction in the form of increased near point of convergence (NPC) during the beginning of the season that was associated with exposure to subconcussive head impacts [74]. This study supported the previous findings of Kawata et al. [75] that also reported increases in NPC, following the completion of a competitive collegiate football season.

In an early study of boxers, Heilbronner and colleagues [76] were the first to demonstrate changes in cognitive function immediately following a fight when compared to a prefight assessment. Specifically, they noted a decline in verbal and incidental memory, and noted that numerous subconcussive blows may be more deleterious than less frequent full-blown concussions, as the number of rounds a boxer fights better predicts the development of encephalopathy, compared to the number of knockouts. In a study by Ravdin et al. [68] investigating the effects of subconcussive blows, boxers were administered neuropsychological examinations before a fight, after the fight, and at a 1-month follow-up session. They noted that at 1-month postfight, neuropsychological performance had increased beyond baseline assessment taken prior to the fight, which was attributed to pre-bout training that included sparring and weight loss. Repetitive subconcussive head trauma has been hypothesized to be the main cause of neurocognitive dysfunction in boxers and that the accumulation of subconcussive blows may lead to cognitive deterioration of brain function [77].

Shuttleworth-Edwards and Radloff [78] investigated the differences between rugby players and athletes involved in noncontact sports and found that rugby players had a poorer performance on visuomotor processing speed. Additionally, they subdivided the rugby players into two groups, based upon the frequency of the positions to be exposed to subconcussive head trauma. This within-group analysis revealed that the group that regularly receives more subconcussive impacts displayed lower scores on the digit symbol substitution visuomotor task. Interestingly enough, it has been reported that despite a five times greater frequency of head injuries, rugby players outperform soccer players in neuropsychological testing [79]. Additionally, Parker et al. [49] found that the subjects exposed to repeated subconcussive blows in football, rugby, and lacrosse showed increased medial–lateral sway in their gaits. In a study by Killam et al. [80] examining athletes with and without a history of concussion and athletes recovering from concussion to a control group without any history of head trauma, researchers concluded that subconcussive head trauma seen in contact sports produces subclinical cognitive impairments. Similarly, Stephens et al. [69] performed neuropsychological testing on adolescent soccer and rugby players. They reported no evidence of neurological dysfunction in both the soccer and rugby players, when compared to their noncontact counterparts. Although no individual had suffered a recent (within the past 3 years) head injury, those with a previous concussion showed poorer performance on attention measures. Looking at several quality-of-life measures including: executive function, anxiety, depression, emotional and behavior dyscontrol, fatigue, and sleep disturbances, Meehan III et al. [81] found no association of previous concussion in athletes aged 40–70 who had participated in collegiate collision sports.

In a recent study by Miller et al. [48], a neuropsychological assessment of collegiate football players via the Standardized Assessment of Concussion (SAC) and the ImPACT was performed at three time intervals: preseason, midseason, and postseason. No subjects under study received a clinically diagnosed concussion, yet they were exposed to numerous subconcussive blows throughout the season. There were no significant decreases in the overall SAC and ImPACT scores reported, yet significant improvements in visual memory and reaction time were noted. Recently, Talavage et al. [15] reported changes in cerebral functions attributed to multiple subconcussive impacts, as evidenced by declines in the visual working memory in high school football players in the absence of clinical signs of concussion. Although it is common for football players to report headaches following practice, it is not yet known whether this is a posttraumatic phenomenon or caused from subconcussive impacts [82]. However, when looking at 282 high school athletes competing in high-contact sports like football and low-contact sports like soccer, Tsushima et al. [83] found significantly worse performance in processing speed and reaction time in the high-contact group, compared to the low-contact group. Jennings et al. [84] found no significant effects of repetitive head impacts on Child-SCAT3 (Sport Concussion Assessment Tool) scores for youth football players. Similarly using ImPACT and SAC neurocognitive tests, Miller et al. [48] reported no significant changes in scores for 58 collegiate football players exposed to subconcussive impacts during preseason, midseason, and postseason testing. While neurocognitive testing is an important part of the return-to-play process, it may not be specific enough to detect the smaller changes in neurocognition that can be caused by subconcussive head impacts.

Neuroimaging of Subconcussive Head Trauma

Few reports in the literature have found any gross structural differences in the brain following concussive or subconcussive head trauma, as evaluated by computed tomography (CT) and standard magnetic resonance imaging (MRI). CT and conventional MRI for the most part are usually found to be normal following concussion, as it is more of a metabolic reaction to trauma than a structural injury [85]. Although, their use can be invaluable in ruling out more serious injuries like skull fractures and hemorrhages. However, one study that looked at boxers longitudinally saw evidence in 13% of the boxers of progressive brain injury, as well as several boxers presenting with cortical atrophy and *cavum septum pellucidum* (Fig. 12.1) [86]. Another CT study evaluating soccer players saw an increase in cerebral atrophy and ventriculomegaly in 27% and 18% of the professional soccer players, respectively [52, 53]. With the advent of newer MRI techniques, there is hope they will have a higher sensitivity and specificity for detecting brain injury caused by subconcussive trauma. These more advanced MRI techniques (Fig. 12.2) like functional magnetic resonance imaging (fMRI), magnetic resonance spectroscopy (MRS), diffusion tensor imaging (DTI), and susceptibility-weighted imaging (SWI) may offer promise in providing some insight into the injured brain, due to concussion and subconcussive head trauma [2]. Experiments utilizing fMRI to study the short-term and long-term effects of subconcussive repetitive head trauma are

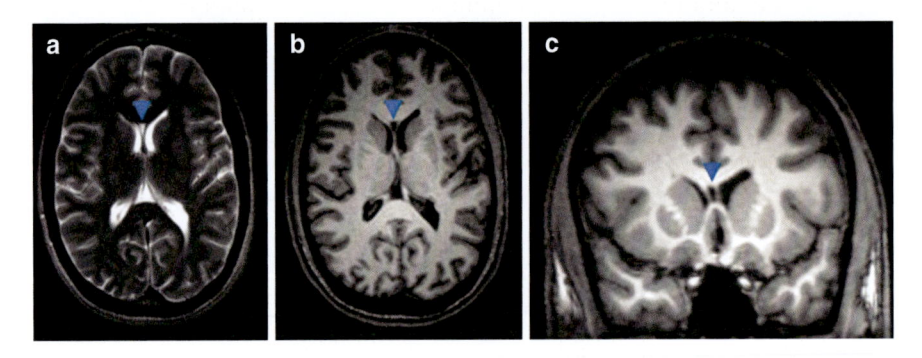

Fig. 12.1 Example of *cavum septum pellucidum* on (**a**) axial T2-weighted, (**b**) axial T1-weighted, and (**c**) coronal T1-weighted MRI

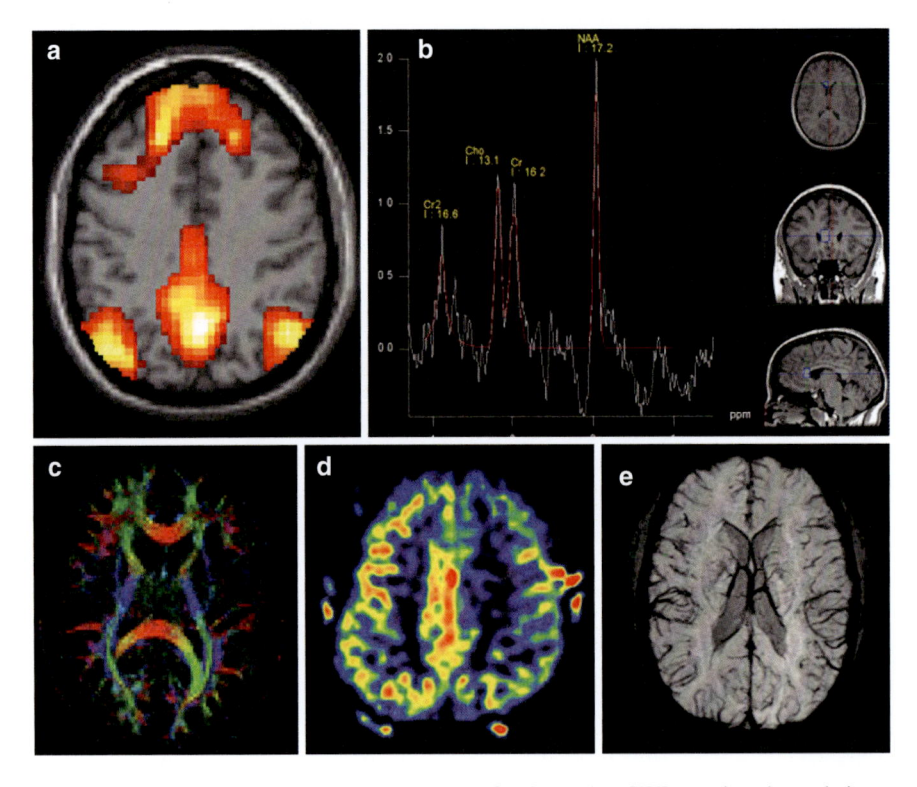

Fig. 12.2 Example of (**a**) fMRI, (**b**) MRS, (**c**) DTI, (**d**) ASL, and (**e**) SWI neuroimaging techniques

growing. Talavage et al. [15] took 11 high school football players and performed an fMRI visual working memory paradigm and baseline neuropsychological testing. They found that the number of collisions was significantly correlated to changes in the subject's fMRI activation. Using resting state functional magnetic resonance imaging (rs-fMRI), Abbas et al. [87] reported functional connectivity differences in the default mode network (DMN) between football players sustaining repetitive head impacts over the course of the season, compared to noncollision athlete controls. Furthermore, differences in functional connectivity were seen between preseason and postseason rs-fMRI scans, indicating the presence of long-term brain changes from these impacts. Looking into the effects of acute exposure to subconcussive head impacts in rugby, Johnson and colleagues [88] reported differences in resting state functional connectivity between pregame and postgame scans (Fig. 12.3). Specifically, they observed increased connectivity from the left supramarginal gyrus to bilateral orbitofrontal cortex and decreased connectivity from the retrosplenial cortex and dorsal posterior cingulate cortex. Furthermore, an analysis based on concussion history revealed that players with a prior history of concussion exhibited only decreased functional connectivity following exposure to subconcussive head trauma, while those with no history showed increased connectivity. Similarly, work by Abbas et al. [87, 89] has shown short-term changes in brain activity following exposure to subconcussive head impacts. These changes observed with fMRI and rs-fMRI show a trend that as the number of subconcussive head impacts increases, there are larger changes in brain activation patterns [90, 91]. Using seed-based connectivity analysis of rs-fMRI, Slobounov et al. [92] revealed changes in functional connectivity to right and left isthmus of the cingulate cortex and left hippocampus in collegiate football players over the course of a single season.

Research using DTI to assess white matter integrity in the brain following exposure to subconcussive head impacts has also increased (Fig. 12.4). Much of the DTI research that has been done to date has focused mainly on measuring changes in DTI metrics from preseason to postseason in males participating in high school and collegiate football. These studies have yielded mixed results in detecting significant changes in fractional anisotropy (FA), mean diffusivity (MD), radial diffusivity (RD), and axial diffusivity (AD). Bazarian et al. [93] took a cohort of nine high school student athletes and performed DTI preseason and postseason at an interval of 3 months apart and, using accelerometers, showed that the subjects sustained between 26 and 399 subconcussive impacts. One subject received a concussion during the season and demonstrated the highest number of voxels in the white matter with significant change in FA and MD from pre- to postseason. The subconcussive group showed the next highest number of voxels with significant FA and MD changes, with most subjects displaying an increase in FA and a decrease in MD. In contrast, Chappell et al. [94] reported an increase in apparent diffusion coefficient (ADC) and a decrease in FA in the deep white matter of 81 professional boxers. They inferred that these abnormalities reported may reflect the cumulative effects of repetitive subconcussive head trauma. Similarly, using DTI, Koerte et al. [95] reported widespread differences in white matter integrity between a small cohort of soccer players with no previous concussive episode, compared to swimmers. Specifically, they observed significantly increased RD in several major white matter tracts including the corpus callosum. Using the Head Impact Telemetry System (HITS™), Davenport et al. [96] monitored 24 male high school football players over the course of a season. In addition, the subjects underwent preseason and postseason assessment via ImPACT and DTI. Correlation analysis revealed a significant

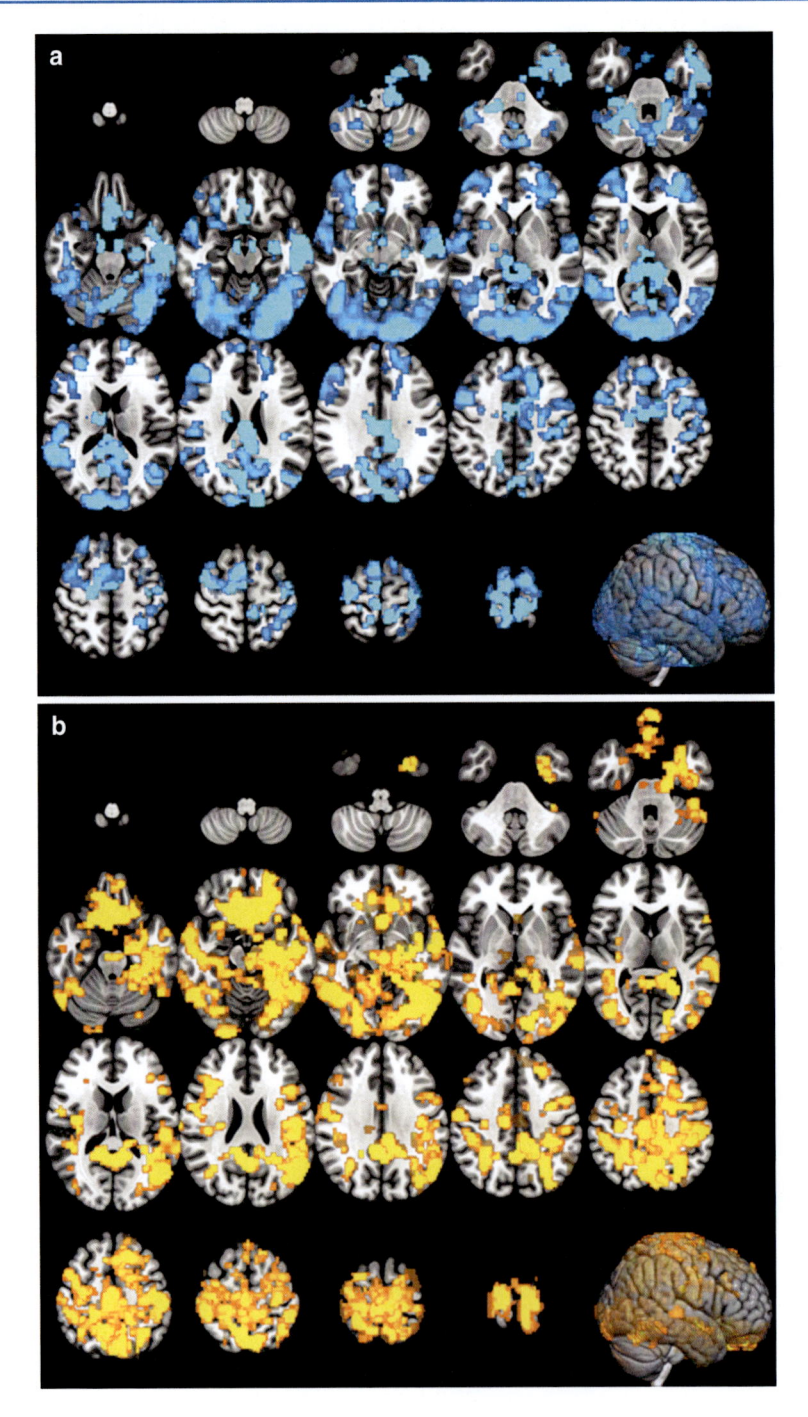

Fig. 12.3 Differences in functional connectivity between rugby players with no history of concussion (**a**) and history of previous concussion (**b**) showing areas of increased functional connectivity (cool colors) and decreased functional connectivity (warm colors). (From Johnson et al. [88])

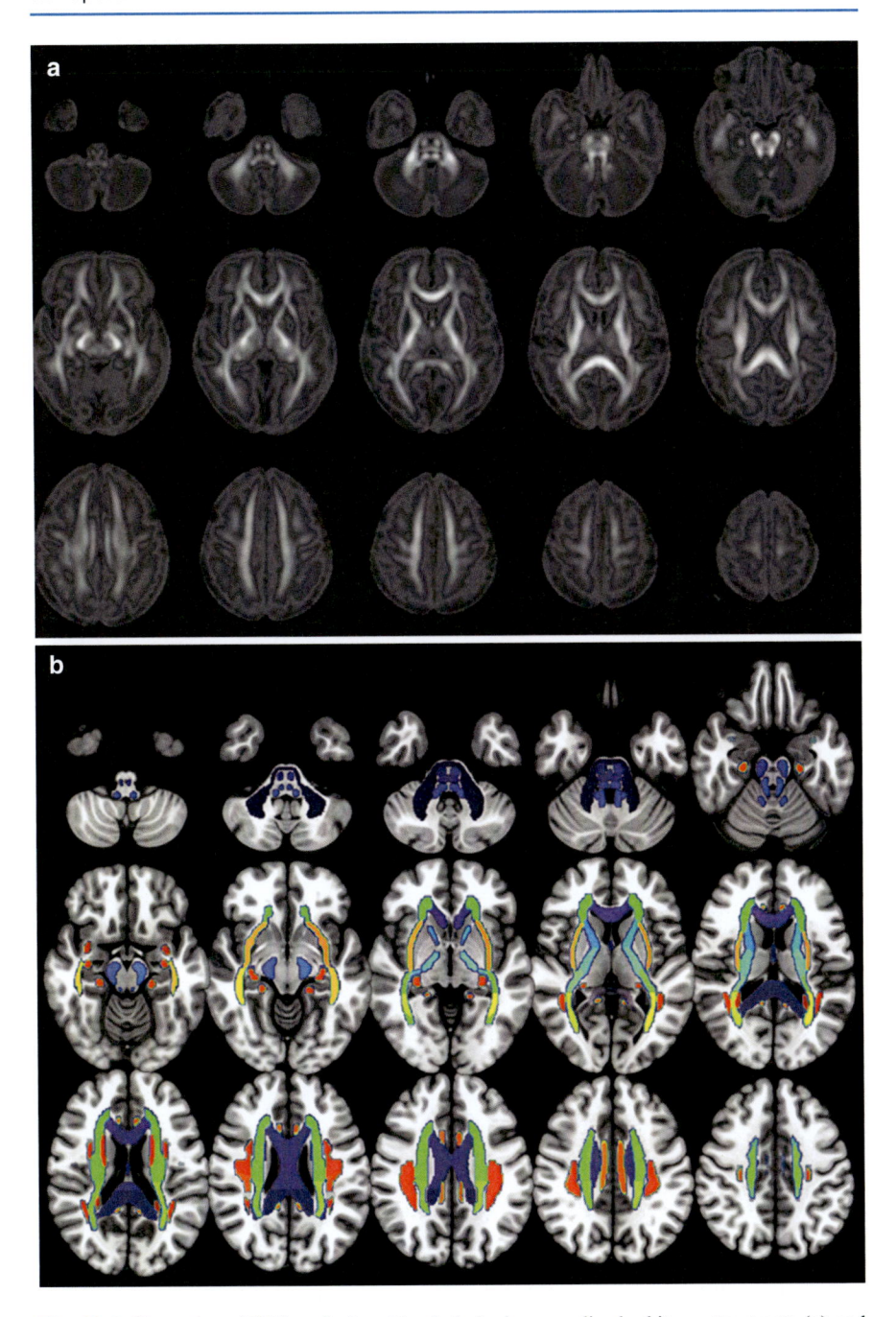

Fig. 12.4 Examples of DTI analysis with whole-brain normalized white matter tracts (**a**) and region of interest white matter tracts (**b**)

linear relationship between changes in fractional anisotropy and the combined components of the risk-weighted cumulative exposure to subconcussive head impacts. Decreases in FA have been reported in the inferior longitudinal fasciculus, forceps minor, forceps major, cingulum, corpus callosum as well as whole-brain white matter [97–101]. Increase in FA have also been observed in the parietal lobe, prefrontal white matter, and whole-brain white matter [99, 102, 103]. This variety of findings is also seen in studies reporting MD, RD, and AD DTI metrics [95, 104–110]. Confounding the literature even more, some studies report no significant differences in DTI metrics [92, 106, 111].

Fewer imaging studies have utilized magnetic resonance spectroscopy (MRS) to investigate neurometabolite changes in the brain following exposure to subconcussive head impacts (Fig. 12.5). Results from these studies also show mixed results. Koerte et al. [112] used MRS to evaluate the long-term effects of repetitive head impacts by scanning 11 retired professional soccer players and reported significant increases in choline (cho) and myo-inositol (mI) which are markers for cell membrane metabolism and glial health. An MRS pilot study of retired professional athletes with a known exposure to concussions and subconcussive head trauma revealed a significant increase in choline (Cho) and glutamate/glutamine (Glx) concentrations [113]. Bari et al. [114] reported significant decreases in Glx metabolites in both male football players and female soccer players. However, Chamard et al. [115] reported no significant changes in neurometabolite concentrations from

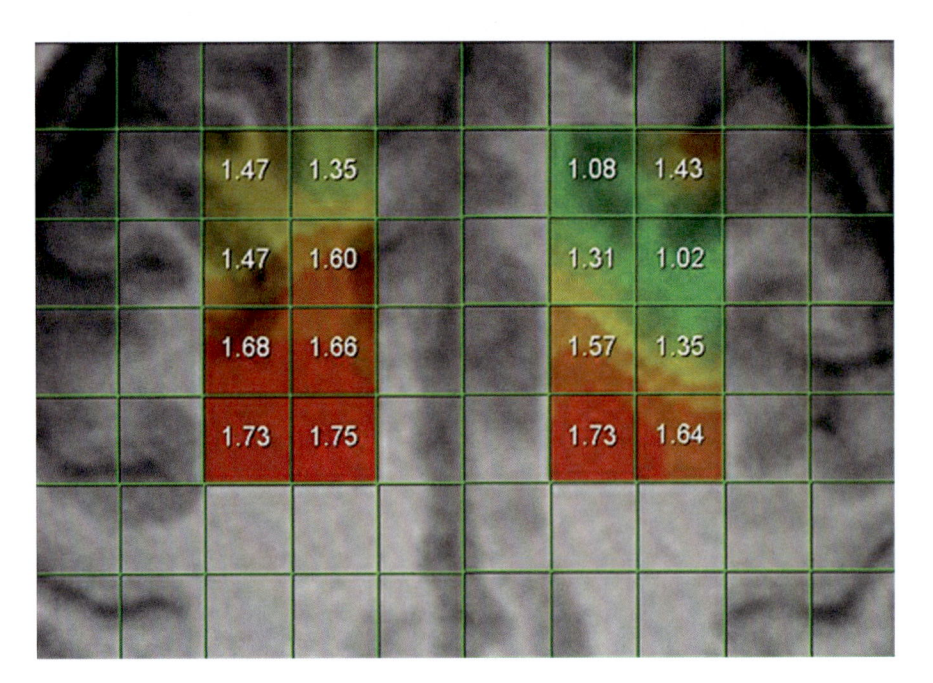

Fig. 12.5 Examples of MRS metabolite maps for NAA/Cho in a concussed athlete showing differences in NAA/Cho homogeneity between the right and left frontal white matter regions

pre- to postseason in male ice-hockey players, but a significant decrease in NAA/Cr in female ice-hockey players. This highlights the importance of gender as an important confound when looking at the SRC and subconcussive literature.

Looking at CTBI in boxers, Bailey and colleagues [116] used transcranial Doppler ultrasound to assess cerebral hemodynamic function. Specifically, the authors looked at dynamic cerebral autoregulation, cerebrovascular reactivity to changes in carbon dioxide (CVR CO_2), and orthostatic tolerance in 12 current professional male boxers, compared to 12 male nonboxers matched for age and physical fitness levels. Results of this study revealed neurocognitive dysfunction and impaired cerebral hemodynamic function, compared to the control group. The CVR CO_2 metric was also correlated with the amount of sparring training the boxers had undergone, not the number of competitive bouts. This study was the first to demonstrate that cerebral hemodynamic function is compromised in CTBI. The authors contributed this hemodynamic and neurocognitive impairment to the mechanical trauma, mostly in the form of subconcussive impacts, experienced from sparring during a career in boxing. Measuring cerebrovascular reactivity in 26 female high school soccer players revealed significant changes in the frontotemporal region of the brain that did not return back to baseline levels till 8 months after the end of the season [117]. Similarly, Champagne et al. documented decreases in cerebral blood flow (CBF) and impaired cerebrovascular reactivity in the DMN [118]. Slobounov et al. [92] utilizing a multimodal imaging approach showed significant increases in global CBF measured by arterial spin labeling (ASL). They also reported that 44% of the players exhibited outlier rates of regional decreases in SWI signal. These changes measured by rs-fMRI, ASL, and SWI were associated with players receiving more high G force impacts. Use of advanced neuroimaging techniques, especially when combined in a multimodal approach, has the potential to characterize the neuropathology of subconcussive head trauma and offer valuable insight into its acute and chronic effects.

Conclusion

Impacts to the head in collision sports are unavoidable, and as serious as concussion is, subconcussive impacts happen much more often. These subconcussive head impacts are now being implicated as a source for the deterioration of cerebral structures and function later in life [12]. Despite being labeled as subconcussive, subthreshold, or subclinical, it is apparent that athletes in contact sports are subjected to an alarming number of these impacts. Contradictory to what the "subconcussive" moniker may imply, subconcussive impacts have shown the ability to cause brain injury [11]. Although the full effect of subconcussive blows on the brain is not known, there is a research focus to understand the immediate and long-term effects they may have [50]. It is important for future research to focus not only on concussive blows, but on varying degrees of head trauma that include subconcussive impacts, as well as time intervals between repetitive sports-related head trauma [2]. Furthermore, empirical evidence suggests that a history of concussion leads to an increased susceptibility to sustain recurrent concussions [119, 120] and further study is needed to explore the effects that subconcussive head trauma may have on those with a history of prior concussion and those without [121]. It appears that like the current SRC literature the research around subconcussive head impacts remains inconsistent with mixed findings. However, it is not hard to believe, despite the overall lack of agreement based on neuropsychological and neuroimaging measures, that subconcussive impacts can cause microstructural and biochemical changes in the brain [37]. Nonetheless, as the research on subconcussive head impacts continues to evolve, so do the policies related to player safety.

References

1. McKee AC, et al. Chronic traumatic encephalopathy in athletes: progressive tauopathy after repetitive head injury. J Neuropathol Exp Neurol. 2009;68(7):709–35.
2. Dashnaw ML, Petraglia AL, Bailes JE. An overview of the basic science of concussion and subconcussion: where we are and where we are going. Neurosurg Focus. 2012;33(6):E5.
3. Mainwaring L, et al. Subconcussive head impacts in sport: a systematic review of the evidence. Int J Psychophysiol. 2018;132:39–54.
4. McKee AC, et al. The spectrum of disease in chronic traumatic encephalopathy. Brain. 2013;136(1):43–64.
5. Langlois JA, Rutland-Brown W, Wald MM. The epidemiology and impact of traumatic brain injury: a brief overview. J Head Trauma Rehabil. 2006;21(5):375–8.
6. Signoretti S, et al. Biochemical and neurochemical sequelae following mild traumatic brain injury: summary of experimental data and clinical implications. Neurosurg Focus. 2010;29(5):E1.
7. Gavett BE, Stern RA, McKee AC. Chronic traumatic encephalopathy: a potential late effect of sport-related concussive and subconcussive head trauma. Clin Sports Med. 2011;30(1):179–88.
8. Martini DN, et al. The chronic effects of concussion on gait. Arch Phys Med Rehabil. 2011;92(4):585–9.
9. Witol AD, Webbe FM. Soccer heading frequency predicts neuropsychological deficits. Arch Clin Neuropsychol. 2003;18(4):397–417.
10. Shultz SR, et al. Sub-concussive brain injury in the Long-Evans rat induces acute neuroinflammation in the absence of behavioral impairments. Behav Brain Res. 2012;229(1):145–52.
11. Bauer JA, et al. Impact forces and neck muscle activity in heading by collegiate female soccer players. J Sports Sci. 2001;19(3):171–9.
12. Broglio SP, et al. Cumulative head impact burden in high school football. J Neurotrauma. 2011;28(10):2069–78.
13. Baugh CM, et al. Chronic traumatic encephalopathy: neurodegeneration following repetitive concussive and subconcussive brain trauma. Brain Imaging Behav. 2012;6(2):244–54.
14. Broglio SP, et al. Cognitive decline and aging: the role of concussive and subconcussive impacts. Exerc Sport Sci Rev. 2012;40(3):138.
15. Talavage TM, et al. Functionally-detected cognitive impairment in high school football players without clinically-diagnosed concussion. J Neurotrauma. 2014;31(4):327–38.
16. Rutherford A, Stephens R, Potter D. The neuropsychology of heading and head trauma in association football (soccer): a review. Neuropsychol Rev. 2003;13(3):153–79.
17. McKee AC, Alosco ML. Assessing subconcussive head impacts in athletes playing contact sports—the eyes have it. JAMA Ophthalmol. 2019;137(3):270–1.

18. Tedeschi C. Cerebral injury by blunt mechanical trauma: special reference to the effects of repeated impacts of minimal intensity; observations on experimental animals. Arch Neurol Psychiatr. 1945;53(5):333–54.
19. Iverson GL, et al. Cumulative effects of concussion in amateur athletes. Brain Inj. 2004;18(5):433–43.
20. Fujita M, Wei EP, Povlishock JT. Intensity-and interval-specific repetitive traumatic brain injury can evoke both axonal and microvascular damage. J Neurotrauma. 2012;29(12):2172–80.
21. Govons S, et al. Brain concussion in the rat. Exp Neurol. 1972;34(1):121–8.
22. Spiegel E, et al. Effect of concussion upon the polarizability of the brain. Am J Physiol. 1946;146(1):12–20.
23. Barkhoudarian G, Hovda DA, Giza CC. The molecular pathophysiology of concussive brain injury. Clin Sports Med. 2011;30(1):33–48.
24. Ramlackhansingh AF, et al. Inflammation after trauma: microglial activation and traumatic brain injury. Ann Neurol. 2011;70(3):374–83.
25. Schmidt OI, et al. Closed head injury—an inflammatory disease? Brain Res Rev. 2005;48(2):388–99.
26. Allen G, Gerami D, Esser M. Conditioning effects of repetitive mild neurotrauma on motor function in an animal model of focal brain injury. Neuroscience. 2000;99(1):93–105.
27. Noble RL, Collip J. A quantitative method for the production of experimental traumatic shock without haemorrhage in unanaesthetized animals. Q J Exp Physiol Cogn Med Sci. 1942;31(3):187–99.
28. Slemmer JE, Weber JT. The extent of damage following repeated injury to cultured hippocampal cells is dependent on the severity of insult and inter-injury interval. Neurobiol Dis. 2005;18(3):421–31.
29. Tagge CA, et al. Concussion, microvascular injury, and early tauopathy in young athletes after impact head injury and an impact concussion mouse model. Brain. 2018;141(2):422–58.
30. Pellman EJ, et al. Concussion in professional football: location and direction of helmet impacts—part 2. Neurosurgery. 2003;53(6):1328–41.
31. Broglio SP, et al. Head impacts during high school football: a biomechanical assessment. J Athl Train. 2009;44(4):342–9.
32. Miyashita T, et al. Frequency and location of head impacts in Division I men's lacrosse players. Athl Train Sports Health Care. 2016;8(5):202–8.
33. Reynolds BB, et al. Practice type effects on head impact in collegiate football. J Neurosurg. 2016;124(2):501–10.
34. Reynolds BB, et al. Quantifying head impacts in collegiate lacrosse. Am J Sports Med. 2016;44(11):2947–56.
35. Naunheim RS, et al. Comparison of impact data in hockey, football, and soccer. J Trauma Acute Care Surg. 2000;48(5):938–41.
36. Spiotta AM, Bartsch AJ, Benzel EC. Heading in soccer: dangerous play? Neurosurgery. 2012;70(1):1–11.
37. Khurana VG, Kaye AH. An overview of concussion in sport. J Clin Neurosci. 2012;19(1):1–11.
38. Beckwith JG, et al. Head impact exposure sustained by football players on days of diagnosed concussion. Med Sci Sports Exerc. 2013;45(4):737.
39. Bartsch A, et al. Impact test comparisons of 20th and 21st century American football helmets. J Neurosurg. 2012;116(1):222–33.
40. Rabadi MH, Jordan BD. The cumulative effect of repetitive concussion in sports. Clin J Sport Med. 2001;11(3):194–8.
41. Schmitt D, et al. Effect of an acute bout of soccer heading on postural control and self-reported concussion symptoms. Int J Sports Med. 2004;25(05):326–31.
42. Kirkendall DT, Jordan SE, Garrett WE. Heading and head injuries in soccer. Sports Med. 2001;31(5):369–86.

43. Bamaç B, et al. Effects of repeatedly heading a soccer ball on serum levels of two neurotrophic factors of brain tissue, BDNF and NGF, in professional soccer players. Biol Sport. 2011;28(3):177.
44. Mussack T, et al. Serum S-100B protein levels in young amateur soccer players after controlled heading and normal exercise. Eur J Med Res. 2003;8(10):457–64.
45. Rogatzki MJ, et al. Biomarkers of brain injury following an American football game: a pilot study. Int J Immunopathol Pharmacol. 2016;29(3):450–7.
46. Duma SM, Rowson S. Past, present, and future of head injury research. Exerc Sport Sci Rev. 2011;39(1):2–3.
47. Cantu RC. Athletic concussion: current understanding as of 2007. Neurosurgery. 2007;60(6):963–4.
48. Miller JR, et al. Comparison of preseason, midseason, and postseason neurocognitive scores in uninjured collegiate football players. Am J Sports Med. 2007;35(8):1284–8.
49. Parker TM, et al. Balance control during gait in athletes and non-athletes following concussion. Med Eng Phys. 2008;30(8):959–67.
50. Spiotta AM, et al. Subconcussive impact in sports: a new era of awareness. World Neurosurg. 2011;75(2):175–8.
51. Packard RC. Chronic post-traumatic headache: associations with mild traumatic brain injury, concussion, and post-concussive disorder. Curr Pain Headache Rep. 2008;12(1):67–73.
52. Tysvaer A, Storli O, Bachen N. Soccer injuries to the brain. A neurologic and electroencephalographic study of former players. Acta Neurol Scand. 1989;80(2):151–6.
53. Sortland O, Tysvaer A. Brain damage in former association football players. Neuroradiology. 1989;31(1):44–8.
54. Tysvaer AT, Løchen EA. Soccer injuries to the brain: a neuropsychologic study of former soccer players. Am J Sports Med. 1991;19(1):56–60.
55. Matser EJ, et al. Neuropsychological impairment in amateur soccer players. JAMA. 1999;282(10):971–3.
56. Downs DS, Abwender D. Neuropsychological impairment in soccer athletes. J Sports Med Phys Fitness. 2002;42(1):103.
57. Bleiberg J, et al. Duration of cognitive impairment after sports concussion. Neurosurgery. 2004;54(5):1073–80.
58. Jordan SE, et al. Acute and chronic brain injury in United States National Team soccer players. Am J Sports Med. 1996;24(2):205–10.
59. Matser J, et al. A dose-response relation of headers and concussions with cognitive impairment in professional soccer players. J Clin Exp Neuropsychol. 2001;23(6):770–4.
60. Kontos AP, et al. Relationship of soccer heading to computerized neurocognitive performance and symptoms among female and male youth soccer players. Brain Inj. 2011;25(12):1234 41.
61. Tysvaer AT. Head and neck injuries in soccer. Sports Med. 1992;14(3):200–13.
62. Mangus BC, Wallmann HW, Ledford M. Soccer: analysis of postural stability in collegiate soccer players before and after an acute bout of heading multiple soccer balls. Sports Biomech. 2004;3(2):209–20.
63. Broglio S, et al. No acute changes in postural control after soccer heading. Br J Sports Med. 2004;38(5):561–7.
64. Rieder C, Jansen P. No neuropsychological consequence in male and female soccer players after a short heading training. Arch Clin Neuropsychol. 2011;26(7):583–91.
65. Putukian M, Echemendia RJ, Mackin S. The acute neuropsychological effects of heading in soccer: a pilot study. Clin J Sport Med. 2000;10(2):104–9.
66. Forbes CR, Glutting JJ, Kaminski TW. Examining neurocognitive function in previously concussed interscholastic female soccer players. Appl Neuropsychol Child. 2016;5(1):14–24.
67. Rutherford A, et al. Do UK university football club players suffer neuropsychological impairment as a consequence of their football (soccer) play? J Clin Exp Neuropsychol. 2009;31(6):664–81.
68. Ravdin LD, et al. Assessment of cognitive recovery following sports related head trauma in boxers. Clin J Sport Med. 2003;13(1):21–7.

69. Stephens R, et al. Neuropsychological consequence of soccer play in adolescent UK school team soccer players. J Neuropsychiatry Clin Neurosci. 2010;22(3):295–303.
70. Zhang MR, et al. Evidence of cognitive dysfunction after soccer playing with ball heading using a novel tablet-based approach. PLoS One. 2013;8(2):e57364.
71. Heitger MH, et al. Eye movement and visuomotor arm movement deficits following mild closed head injury. Brain. 2004;127(3):575–90.
72. Heitger MH, Anderson T, Jones R. Saccade sequences as markers for cerebral dysfunction following mild closed head injury. In: Progress in brain research. Elsevier; 2002. p. 433–48.
73. Capó-Aponte JE, et al. Visual dysfunctions and symptoms during the subacute stage of blast-induced mild traumatic brain injury. Mil Med. 2012;177(7):804–13.
74. Zonner SW, et al. Oculomotor response to cumulative subconcussive head impacts in US high school football players: a pilot longitudinal study. JAMA Ophthalmol. 2019;137(3):265–70.
75. Kawata K, et al. Effect of repetitive sub-concussive head impacts on ocular near point of convergence. Int J Sports Med. 2016;37(05):405–10.
76. Heilbronner RL, Henry GK, Carson-Brewer M. Neuropsychologic test performance in amateur boxers. Am J Sports Med. 1991;19(4):376–80.
77. Jordan BD, et al. Sparring and cognitive function in professional boxers. Phys Sportsmed. 1996;24(5):87–98.
78. Shuttleworth-Rdwards AB, Radloff SE. Compromised visuomotor processing speed in players of Rugby Union from school through to the national adult level. Arch Clin Neuropsychol. 2008;23(5):511–20.
79. Rutherford A, et al. Neuropsychological impairment as a consequence of football (soccer) play and football heading: preliminary analyses and report on university footballers. J Clin Exp Neuropsychol. 2005;27(3):299–319.
80. Killam C, Cautin RL, Santucci AC. Assessing the enduring residual neuropsychological effects of head trauma in college athletes who participate in contact sports. Arch Clin Neuropsychol. 2005;20(5):599–611.
81. Meehan WP III, et al. Division III collision sports are not associated with neurobehavioral quality of life. J Neurotrauma. 2016;33(2):254–9.
82. Terrell TR. Concussion in athletes. South Med J. 2004;97:837–42.
83. Tsushima WT, et al. Are there subconcussive neuropsychological effects in youth sports? An exploratory study of high-and low-contact sports. Appl Neuropsychol Child. 2016;5(2):149–55.
84. Jennings D, et al. Effects of a season of subconcussive contact on child-SCAT3 scores in 8-12 year-old male athletes. Int J Sports Phys Ther. 2015;10(5):667.
85. Lovell M, Collins M, Bradley J. Return to play following sports-related concussion. Clin Sports Med. 2004;23(3):421–41.
86. McCrory P. Sports concussion and the risk of chronic neurological impairment. Clin J Sport Med. 2011;21(1):6–12.
87. Abbas K, et al. Alteration of default mode network in high school football athletes due to repetitive subconcussive mild traumatic brain injury: a resting-state functional magnetic resonance imaging study. Brain Connect. 2015;5(2):91–101.
88. Johnson B, et al. Effects of subconcussive head trauma on the default mode network of the brain. J Neurotrauma. 2014;31(23):1907–13.
89. Abbas K, et al. Effects of repetitive sub-concussive brain injury on the functional connectivity of default mode network in high school football athletes. Dev Neuropsychol. 2015;40(1):51–6.
90. Robinson ME, et al. The role of location of subconcussive head impacts in FMRI brain activation change. Dev Neuropsychol. 2015;40(2):74–9.
91. Shenk TE, et al. FMRI of visual working memory in high school football players. Dev Neuropsychol. 2015;40(2):63–8.
92. Slobounov SM, et al. The effect of repetitive subconcussive collisions on brain integrity in collegiate football players over a single football season: a multi-modal neuroimaging study. Neuroimage Clin. 2017;14:708–18.

93. Bazarian JJ, et al. Subject-specific changes in brain white matter on diffusion tensor imaging after sports-related concussion. Magn Reson Imaging. 2012;30(2):171–80.
94. Chappell MH, et al. Distribution of microstructural damage in the brains of professional boxers: a diffusion MRI study. J Magn Reson Imaging. 2006;24(3):537–42.
95. Koerte IK, et al. White matter integrity in the brains of professional soccer players without a symptomatic concussion. JAMA. 2012;308(18):1859–61.
96. Davenport EM, et al. Abnormal white matter integrity related to head impact exposure in a season of high school varsity football. J Neurotrauma. 2014;31(19):1617–24.
97. Bahrami N, et al. Subconcussive head impact exposure and white matter tract changes over a single season of youth football. Radiology. 2016;281(3):919–26.
98. Bazarian JJ, et al. Persistent, long-term cerebral white matter changes after sports-related repetitive head impacts. PLoS One. 2014;9:e94734.
99. Chun IY, et al. DTI detection of longitudinal WM abnormalities due to accumulated head impacts. Dev Neuropsychol. 2015;40(2):92–7.
100. Kuzminski S, et al. White matter changes related to subconcussive impact frequency during a single season of high school football. Am J Neuroradiol. 2018;39(2):245–51.
101. Sollmann N, et al. Sex differences in white matter alterations following repetitive subconcussive head impacts in collegiate ice hockey players. Neuroimage Clin. 2018;17:642–9.
102. Mayinger MC, et al. White matter alterations in college football players: a longitudinal diffusion tensor imaging study. Brain Imaging Behav. 2018;12(1):44–53.
103. Schranz AL, et al. Reduced brain glutamine in female varsity rugby athletes after concussion and in non-concussed athletes after a season of play. Hum Brain Mapp. 2018;39(4):1489–99.
104. Foss KDB, et al. Relative head impact exposure and brain white matter alterations after a single season of competitive football: a pilot comparison of youth versus high school football. Clin J Sport Med. 2019;29(6):442–50.
105. Marchi N, et al. Consequences of repeated blood-brain barrier disruption in football players. PLoS One. 2013;8(3):e56805.
106. McAllister TW, et al. Effect of head impacts on diffusivity measures in a cohort of collegiate contact sport athletes. Neurology. 2014;82(1):63–9.
107. Myer GD, et al. Analysis of head impact exposure and brain microstructure response in a season-long application of a jugular vein compression collar: a prospective, neuroimaging investigation in American football. Br J Sports Med. 2016;50(20):1276–85.
108. Myer GD, et al. The effects of external jugular compression applied during head impact exposure on longitudinal changes in brain neuroanatomical and neurophysiological biomarkers: a preliminary investigation. Front Neurol. 2016;7:74.
109. Myer GD, et al. Altered brain microstructure in association with repetitive subconcussive head impacts and the potential protective effect of jugular vein compression: a longitudinal study of female soccer athletes. Br J Sports Med. 2019;53(24):1539–51.
110. Yuan W, et al. White matter alterations over the course of two consecutive high-school football seasons and the effect of a jugular compression collar: a preliminary longitudinal diffusion tensor imaging study. Hum Brain Mapp. 2018;39(1):491–508.
111. Lao Y, et al. A T1 and DTI fused 3D corpus callosum analysis in pre-vs. post-season contact sports players. In: 10th International Symposium on Medical Information Processing and Analysis. International Society for Optics and Photonics. 2015.
112. Koerte IK, et al. Altered neurochemistry in former professional soccer players without a history of concussion. J Neurotrauma. 2015;32(17):1287–93.
113. Lin A, et al. Neurochemical changes in athletes with chronic traumatic encephalopathy. Radiological Society of North America; 2010.
114. Bari S, et al. Dependence on subconcussive impacts of brain metabolism in collision sport athletes: an MR spectroscopic study. Brain Imaging Behav. 2019;13(3):735–49.
115. Chamard E, et al. A prospective study of physician-observed concussion during a varsity university hockey season: metabolic changes in ice hockey players. Part 4 of 4. Neurosurg Focus. 2012;33(6):E4.

116. Bailey DM, et al. Impaired cerebral haemodynamic function associated with chronic traumatic brain injury in professional boxers. Clin Sci. 2013;124(3):177–89.
117. Svaldi DO, et al. Cerebrovascular reactivity changes in asymptomatic female athletes attributable to high school soccer participation. Brain Imaging Behav. 2017;11(1):98–112.
118. Champagne AA, et al. Resting CMRO2 fluctuations show persistent network hyperconnectivity following exposure to sub-concussive collisions. Neuroimage Clin. 2019;22:101753.
119. Giza CC, Hovda DA. The neurometabolic cascade of concussion. J Athl Train. 2001;36(3):228.
120. Guskiewicz KM, et al. Cumulative effects associated with recurrent concussion in collegiate football players: the NCAA concussion study. JAMA. 2003;290(19):2549–55.
121. Kaminski TW, Cousino ES, Glutting JJ. Examining the relationship between purposeful heading in soccer and computerized neuropsychological test performance. Res Q Exerc Sport. 2008;79(2):235–44.

Biomarkers for Concussion

13

Linda Papa

Introduction

Path Toward Blood Test for Concussion

Currently, concussion (which is also known as mild traumatic brain injury) is largely a clinical diagnosis based on injury history, neurologic examination, neuropsychological testing, and, at times, neuroimaging. Early and tailored management of athletes following a concussion can provide them with the best opportunity to avoid further injury. Brain-specific biomarkers measured through a simple blood test could complement the clinical evaluation of concussion and potentially guide management decisions [1–5]. The pursuit of these elusive markers has been most intense over the last decade [6–8]. Previously, human trials examined only moderate to severe TBI but are now expanding to include injuries on the milder end of the TBI spectrum, such as concussion, and subconcussive injuries and the effects of head acceleration events.

The degree of brain injury depends on the primary mechanism/magnitude of injury, secondary insults, and the patient's genetic and molecular response. Following the initial injury, cellular responses and neurochemical and metabolic cascades contribute to secondary injury which may evolve over the ensuing hours and days. These secondary insults can be mediated through physiologic events which decrease the supply of oxygen and energy to the brain tissue or through a cascade of cytotoxic events mediated by molecular and cellular processes. The

L. Papa (✉)
Department of Emergency Medicine, Orlando Regional Medical Center, Orlando, FL, USA

University of Central Florida College of Medicine, Orlando, FL, USA

University of Florida College of Medicine, Gainesville, FL, USA

Florida State University College of Medicine, Tallahassee, FL, USA

Department of Neurology and Neurosurgery, McGill University, Montreal, QC, Canada

release of brain injury biomarkers is not a static process. Studying the time course of a biomarker is critical to optimizing timing and clinical use. The time course (or temporal profile) may be affected by source of the sample, lesion type (mass lesion versus diffuse injury) and location, concomitant extracranial injuries (fractures, solid organ injuries), secondary insults, and individual patient physiology. Biomarkers could reflect these secondary insults as well as blood-brain barrier disruption. Complicating the release of biomarkers is the potential for extracranial sources of release after trauma. In cases when the biomarkers are released from tissues other than the brain, caution must be taken when interpreting results. For instance, S100β can be released from soft tissues, cartilage, and bone after trauma and may not accurately reflect brain injury [9, 10]. Furthermore, individual physiology and pre-existing disease states, such as kidney or liver disease, may alter the metabolism or clearance of a given biomarker.

Key features that would make concussion biomarkers clinically useful include the following: (1) a high sensitivity (come from the brain) and specificity (low or undetectable in blood in non-injury states) for brain injury; (2) the ability to stratify patients by severity of injury (concentration of the biomarker should increase with worsening injury); (3) the timely appearance in accessible biological fluid such as serum, saliva, or urine; (4) a well-defined time course; (5) the ability to monitor injury and response to treatment; (6) the ability to predict functional outcome; and (7) be easily measured [8, 11].

To follow is a review of the most widely studied proteomic biomarkers for mild TBI and concussion in humans. Proteomic biomarkers are often represented by their neuroanatomic location in the central nervous system including astroglia (GFAP, S100β) and neuronal cells, with specific areas of the neuron such as the cell body (UCH-L1) and axon (Tau, neurofilament) (Fig. 13.1). Furthermore, a novel group of promising transcriptomic biomarkers called microRNAs will also be discussed.

Proteomic Biomarkers

Glial Fibrillary Acidic Protein (GFAP) and Ubiquitin C-Terminal Hydrolase (UCH-L1)

GFAP and UCH-L1 for Mild-to-Moderate Traumatic Brain Injury

Glial fibrillary acidic protein (GFAP) is a protein found in the astroglial skeleton of both white and gray brain matter and is used as a histological marker for glial cells. Ubiquitin C-terminal hydrolase-L1 (UCH-L1) is a protein in neurons that is involved in the addition and removal of ubiquitin from proteins that are destined for metabolism and is used as a histological marker for neurons [12, 13].

The specificity of GFAP and UCH-L1 for detecting brain injury has been examined in a number of studies. GFAP and UCH-L1 have been shown to distinguish mild and moderate TBI patients from orthopedic controls and motor vehicle crash controls as well as from those TBI patients with negative computed tomography (CT) scans [10, 14, 15]. In these studies, trauma control patients were exposed to

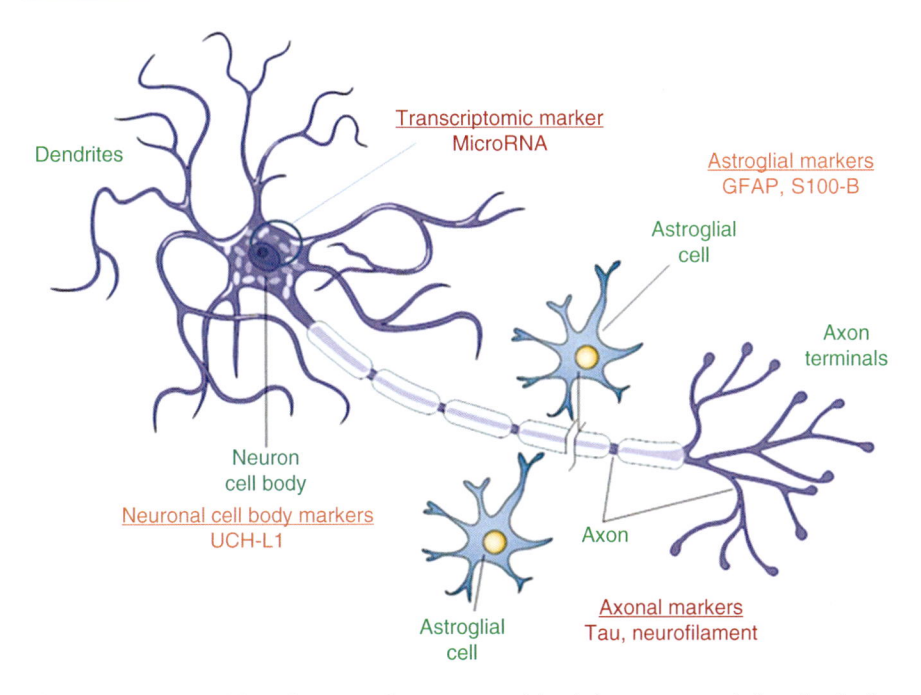

Fig. 13.1 Proteomic biomarkers are often represented by their neuroanatomic location in the central nervous system including astroglia (GFAP, S100β) and neuronal cells, with specific areas of the neuron such as the cell body (UCH-L1) and axon (Tau, neurofilament). A novel group of promising TBI markers include transcriptomic biomarkers called microRNAs

significant trauma including the acceleration-deceleration vectors of motor vehicle collisions and substantial falls. Both GFAP and UCH-L1 showed a graded response to the severity of injury from uninjured to orthopedic trauma, to mild and moderate TBI. However, GFAP appears to be the most brain-specific in the setting of polytrauma with substantial extracranial injuries and fractures [2, 3, 9, 10, 14–16].

The temporal profiles of GFAP and UCH-L1 over a week following a mild traumatic brain injury have been clearly described in a large cohort of emergency department trauma patients. GFAP consistently identified concussion over 7 days. GFAP also detected with good accuracy traumatic intracranial lesions on head computed tomography (CT) and neurosurgical intervention over a week [15]. GFAP was detectible in serum within an hour of concussion and remained elevated for several days after rendering it a promising contender for clinical use for concussion diagnosis within a week of injury [15]. In contrast, UCH-L1 rose rapidly within 30 min of injury and peaked at 8 h after injury and decreased steadily over 48 h with small peaks and toughs over 7 days – making UCH-L1 a very early marker of concussion [15].

Over the last decade, glial fibrillary acidic protein (GFAP) and ubiquitin C-terminal Hydrolase (UCH-L1) have been found in several distinct studies to detect traumatic intracranial CT scan lesions and predict neurosurgical intervention in adults with mild to moderate TBI [10, 14, 15, 17–20]. More recently, these findings have been replicated in children [2, 3, 21, 22]. In early 2018, GFAP and UCH-L1 were FDA approved for clinical use in adult patients with mild to moderate TBI to help determine the need for CT scan within 12 h of injury [23]. The approval was based on the ability to find lesions on a CT scan but was not approved to diagnose a concussion. Moreover, it was not approved for use in children.

GFAP and UCH-L1 for Concussion and Subconcussive Brain Injury

Computed tomography (CT) is the standard imaging modality for assessing damage in TBI during the acute phase of injury. CT scan can detect macroscopic traumatic lesions such as skull fractures, intracranial hematomas, contusions, subarachnoid hemorrhages, and swelling. However, the more subtle injuries associated with mild TBI are often not demonstrated by this imaging modality. This discrepancy is evidenced by the lack of CT abnormalities in patients with cognitive, physical, and behavioral dysfunction following a mild TBI. Therefore, CT does not have sufficient sensitivity to detect damage incurred in mild TBI. This group of TBI patients represents the greatest challenge to accurate diagnosis and outcome prediction. Metting et al. found that patients with axonal injury on MRI, but not CT, had elevated GFAP levels. Similarly, Yue et al. assessed GFAP in mild TBI patients with a negative CT scan and found GFAP was able to detect MRI lesions with an area under the curve of 0.78 despite the CT scan not showing any lesions [24]. UCH-L1 was not examined in either of these studies.

A significantly understudied group in whom biomarkers are rarely examined are individuals who experience head trauma without symptoms of concussion. They are often classified as having "no injury" when, in fact, they may represent milder forms of concussion that do not elicit the typical signs or symptoms associated with concussion. Such injuries have been referred to as subconcussive injuries or head acceleration events. Emerging data have demonstrated that significant alterations in brain function can occur in the absence of clinically obvious symptoms following even a single head trauma [25–27]. The issue of subconcussive trauma has been a particular concern in military personnel [28] and in athletes, as repetitive subconcussive impacts have the potential for long-term deleterious effects [27, 29, 30]. To address this deficiency, a recent study evaluated how GFAP and UCH-L1 behave in subconcussive trauma in a large cohort of children and adult trauma patients presenting to three-level I trauma centers with a Glasgow Coma Scale (GCS) score of 15 and a normal mental status. The biomarkers were measured at 20 distinct time-points in patients with concussive, subconcussive, and non-concussive trauma (Fig. 13.2). Although blood levels of both GFAP and UCH-L1 showed incremental increases from body trauma (lowest levels), to head trauma without concussion (higher levels than body trauma), to concussion (highest levels), GFAP was much better in distinguishing between the groups than UCH-L1. UCH-L1 was expressed at much higher levels than GFAP in those with non-concussive trauma, particularly in children, suggesting that UCH-L1 is either not completely brain-specific or ultrasensitive to subtle impacts [22]. In athletes, UCH-L1 has shown elevations in both concussive

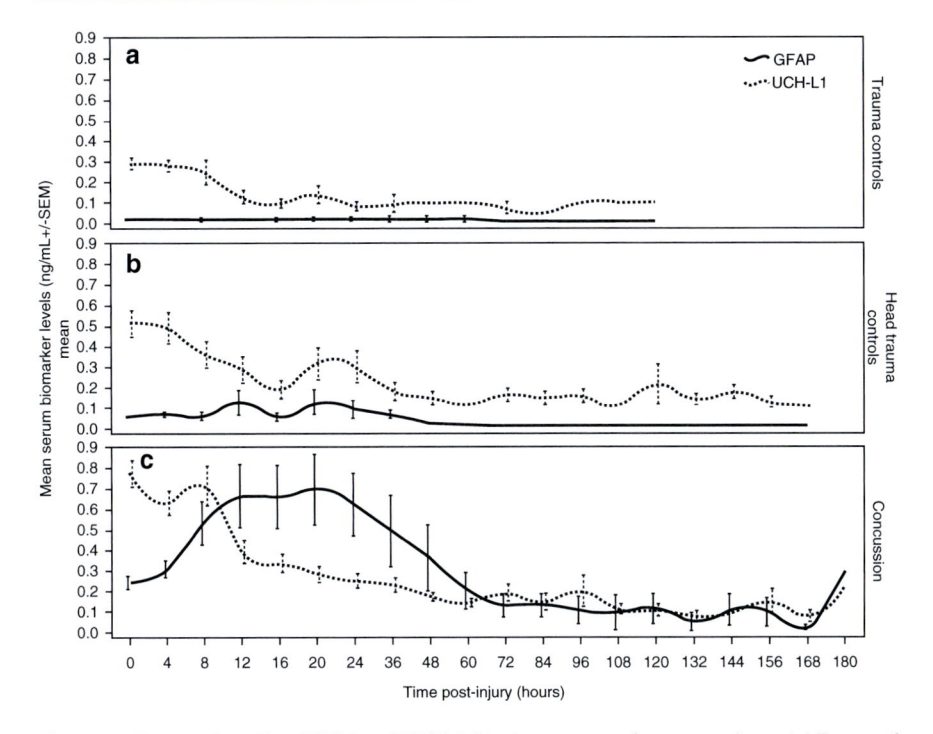

Fig. 13.2 Temporal profile of GFAP and UCH-L1 in three groups of trauma patients. (**a**) Temporal profile of GFAP and UCH-L1 in body trauma control patients. Means with error bars representing SEM. (**b**) Temporal profile of GFAP and UCH-L1 in head trauma control patients. Means with error bars representing SEM. (**c**) Temporal profile of GFAP and UCH-L1 in trauma patients with concussion. Means with error bars representing SEM. GFAP, glialfibrillary acidic protein; UCH-L1, ubiquitin C-terminal hydrolase. (Taken from Papa et al. [22])

[31] and subconcussive trauma [32]. However, these results are not consistent in all studies [33, 34].

Other Potential Proteomic Biofluid Biomarkers of Concussion

A systematic review of biomarkers in sports-related concussion showed that there have been at least eleven different biomarkers assessed in athletes [5]. Besides GFAP and UCH-L1, other potential biomarkers include S100β, neuron-specific enolase, tau, neurofilament, amyloid beta, and brain-derived neurotrophic factor. Some correlate with the number of hits to the head (soccer), acceleration/deceleration forces (jumps, collisions, and falls), post-concussive symptoms, trauma to the body versus the head, and dynamics of injury [5]. Some of these and other novel markers are discussed below.

S100β

S100β is expressed in astrocytes and helps to regulate intracellular levels of calcium. It is considered a marker of astrocyte injury or death. Of note, it can also be found in cells that are not neuronal such as adipocytes, chondrocytes, and melanoma cells and, therefore, it is not brain-specific [35, 36]. Despite this, S100β is one of the most extensively studied biomarkers for TBI [4, 5, 37].

A number of studies have found correlations between elevated serum levels of S100β and CT abnormalities in adults and children [4, 38]. Elevated concentrations of S100β in serum have been associated with increased incidence of post-concussive symptoms, problems with cognition, and traumatic abnormalities on MRI [39–43]. However, there are also a number of studies negating these findings [16, 44–46]. Similarly, several studies have shown that serum S100β increases after concussive [31, 47, 48] and subconcussive brain injury [34, 49, 50]. However, a number of studies have shown a poor association with other prognostic parameters [33, 46, 51]. Peripheral sources of S100β complicate its use as a brain-specific marker, particularly in the setting of polytrauma. S100β has been shown to be elevated in injured patients with peripheral trauma who have had no direct head trauma [2, 10, 52]. Since many of these results have been inconsistently reproduced, the clinical value of S100β in TBI, particularly mild TBI and concussion, is still controversial. Despite these inconsistent findings, S100β has been approved for use by TBI patients in Europe.

Tau Protein

Tau is an intracellular, microtubule-associated protein that is amplified in axons and is involved with assembling axonal microtubule bundles and participating in anterograde axoplasmic transport [53]. Tau lesions are apparently related to axonal disruption such as in trauma or hypoxia [54, 55]. After release, it is proteolytically cleaved at the N- and C-terminals. In a study by Shaw et al., an elevated level of C-Tau was associated with a poor outcome at hospital discharge and with an increased chance of an intracranial injury on head CT [56]. However, these findings were not reproducible when C-Tau was measured in peripheral blood in mild TBI [57]. Two additional studies showed that C-Tau was a poor predictor of CT lesions and a poor predictor of post-concussive syndrome [44, 58]. Similarly, Bulut et al. found total Tau (T-Tau) differentiated patients with intracranial injury from those without intracranial injury [59]. However, they were not able to detect milder injuries.

In 2014, a study of professional hockey players showed that serum T-Tau outperformed S-100B and NSE in detecting concussion at 1 h after injury and that levels were significantly higher in post-concussion samples at all times compared with preseason levels [48]. T-Tau at 1 h after concussion also correlated with the number of days it took for concussion symptoms to resolve. Accordingly, T-Tau remained significantly elevated at 144 h in players with post-concussive symptoms (PCS) lasting more than 6 days versus players with PCS for less than 6 days [48].

Phosphorylated-Tau (P-Tau) is also being examined as a potential biomarker for brain trauma. Following TBI, axonal injury is coupled to Tau hyperphosphorylation, leading to microtubule instability and Tau-mediated neurodegeneration [60]. The

P-tau level has been shown to outperform the T-tau level in distinguishing CT positive from CT negative cases and identifying patients with poor outcome [61]. Moreover, several months after TBI, P-Tau has been shown to be elevated in TBI patients compared to healthy controls. The ratio between P-Tau and T-Tau has shown similar results [61]. High levels of total and phosphorylated Tau have been found in postmortem samples of TBI patients and athletes [62, 63]. Further study is needed to elucidate the role of T-Tau and P-Tau in detecting chronic encephalopathy.

Neurofilaments

Neurofilaments are heteropolymeric components of the neuron cytoskeleton that consist of a 68 kDa light neurofilament subunit (NF-L) backbone with either 160 kDa medium (NF-M) or 200 kDa heavy subunit (NF-H) side-arms [64]. Following TBI, calcium influx into the cell contributes to a cascade of events that activates calcineurin, a calcium-dependent phosphatase that dephosphorylates neurofilament side-arms, presumably contributing to axonal injury [65]. Phosphorylated NF-H has been found to be elevated in the CSF of adults and children with severe TBI [66, 67]. It remains significantly elevated after a few days in children with poor outcome and diffuse axonal injury (DAI) on initial CT scan [67]. Similarly, in a study by Vajtr et al. serum NF-H was much higher in patients with DAI over 10 days after admission with highest levels from day 4 to day 10 [68].

In a cohort of professional hockey players who underwent blood biomarker assessment at 1, 12, 36, and 144 h after concussion and at return-to-play, serum NF-L increased over time and returned to normal at return-to-play. Also, serum NF-L levels were higher in players with prolonged post-concussive symptoms [69]. In a group of amateur boxers, serum NF-L concentrations showed elevations 7–10 days after about and subsequently decreased following 3 months of rest. Levels were also significantly correlated with the number of hits to the head [69]. Moreover, NF-L has been shown to increase in adult soccer players following repetitive subconcussive head impacts compared to baseline levels, however, only after 24 h of the impacts [70]. In contrast, NF-L levels in blood taken at baseline and at 6- and 14-days post-concussion in contact sport athletes showed no differences between any of the pre-post timepoints [71].

Transcriptomic Biomarkers

MicroRNAs as the Next Generation of Biomarkers for Concussion

Initial exploration of TBI biomarkers began using animal models. These models have been helpful in providing histologic and pathophysiologic information on potential biomarkers. As a result, the selection of TBI biomarkers has been based on neuroanatomic location and on mechanisms of injury induced by trauma such as neuroinflammation and ischemia.

A novel set of biomarkers, called microRNAs (miRNA), are now being studied as the next generation of biomarkers for many diseases and disorders such as cancer, cardiovascular, and neurodegenerative diseases [72]. MiRNAs are small (19–28 nucleotides) endogenous RNA molecules that regulate protein synthesis at the post transcriptional level. MiRNAs can be detected in serum and can be an indicator of disease pathology in neuronal cells. MiRNAs are relatively abundant in biofluids such as cerebrospinal fluid, serum, and urine and are relatively stable at variable pH conditions, resistant to repeated freeze thaw and enzymatic degradation. Due to these properties, miRNA has advantages over protein-based markers. The utility of miRNAs as diagnostic markers of mild TBI or concussion has recently been explored [73–77]. In 2016, Bhomia et al. identified specific and sensitive miRNA-based biomarkers for mild and moderate TBI using real-time PCR methodology [74]. Samples from human subjects with mild to severe TBI were compared to trauma and normal controls and identified 10 miRNA signatures miR-151-5p, miR-328, miR-362-3p, miR-486, miR-505*, miR-451, miR-30d, miR-20a, miR-195, and miR-92a. Moreover, Johnson et al. identified 6 salivary miRNAs with overlapping CSF alterations (miR-182-5p, miR-221-3p, miR-26b-5p, miR-320c, miR-29c-3p, and miR-30e-5p) that distinguished children with TBI from healthy controls [75]. In a study by the same group, 52 children with concussion had 5 salivary miRNAs (miR-320c, miR-133a-5p, miR-769-5p, let-7a-3c, and miR-1307-3p) that were associated with prolonged post-concussive symptoms [76].

More recently, studies have been evaluating the role of microRNA in sports-related concussion. In one recent study, microRNA biomarkers measured pre- and post-season in collegiate football players were associated with worsening neurocognitive functioning over the course of a season in those with no concussions [78]. The study found significant elevations in circulating miRNA measured before the athletic season began and prior to any contact practices. All the players had significantly elevated levels compared to non-athlete controls ($p < 0.001$) suggesting residual circulating miRNA biomarkers from prior concussive and subconcussive impacts [78, 79]. Pre-season miRNA levels predicted baseline SAC scores with very good areas under the curve, the highest being miR-195 (0.90), miR-20a (0.89), miR-151-5p (0.86), miR-505* (0.85), and miR-9-3p (0.77). Athletes who demonstrated worsening neurocognitive function from pre- to post-season showed elevations in concentrations of miRNAs over the same period. The miRNAs with the most significant increases over the course of the season were miR-505*, miR-362-3p, miR-30d, miR-92a, and miR-486. Similarly, a study of saliva miRNA levels from 32 rugby players detected 5 miRNAs (miR-27b-3p, miR-142-3p, let-7i, miR-107, and miR-135b-5p) at 48 to 72 h after sports-related concussion that correlated with reaction time on ImPACT testing and predicted concussion better than other protein biomarkers [80].

Conclusion

TBI biomarkers measured through a simple blood test have the potential to provide invaluable information for the management of concussion by facilitating diagnosis and risk stratification; offering timely information about the pathophysiology of injury; monitoring recovery; and furnishing opportunities for drug target identification and surrogate measures for future clinical trials. In light of their timeliness, accuracy, and risk stratification potential, biofluid biomarkers with reliable sensitivity and specificity would be welcomed tools in treating concussion. This is especially so in settings limited by acute care resources such as in rural settings and non-hospital environments such as the playing field, battlefield, and primary care practices.

References

1. Papa L. Potential blood-based biomarkers for concussion. Sports Med Arthrosc Rev. 2016;24:108–15.
2. Papa L, Mittal MK, Ramirez J, et al. In children and youth with mild and moderate traumatic brain injury, glial fibrillary acidic protein out-performs S100beta in detecting traumatic intracranial lesions on computed tomography. J Neurotrauma. 2016;33:58–64.
3. Papa L, Zonfrillo MR, Ramirez J, et al. Performance of glial fibrillary acidic protein in detecting traumatic intracranial lesions on computed tomography in children and youth with mild head trauma. Acad Emerg Med. 2015;22:1274–82.
4. Papa L, Ramia MM, Kelly JM, Burks SS, Pawlowicz A, Berger RP. Systematic review of clinical research on biomarkers for pediatric traumatic brain injury. J Neurotrauma. 2013;30:324–38.
5. Papa L, Ramia MM, Edwards D, Johnson BD, Slobounov SM. Systematic review of clinical studies examining biomarkers of brain injury in athletes after sports-related concussion. J Neurotrauma. 2015;32:661–73.
6. Papa L. Exploring the role of biomarkers for the diagnosis and management of traumatic brain injury patients. In: Man TK, Flores RJ, editors. Poteomics – human diseases and protein functions. 1st ed. In Tech Open Access Publisher; 2012.
7. Papa L, Edwards D, Ramia M. Exploring serum biomarkers for mild traumatic. In: Kobeissy FH, editor. Brain neurotrauma: molecular, neuropsychological, and rehabilitation aspects. Boca Raton: Taylor & Francis Group; 2015.
8. Papa L, Wang KKW. Raising the bar for traumatic brain injury biomarker research: methods make a difference. J Neurotrauma. 2017;34:2187–9.
9. Pelinka LE, Kroepfl A, Leixnering M, Buchinger W, Raabe A, Redl H. GFAP versus S100B in serum after traumatic brain injury: relationship to brain damage and outcome. J Neurotrauma. 2004;21:1553–61.
10. Papa L, Silvestri S, Brophy GM, et al. GFAP out-performs S100beta in detecting traumatic intracranial lesions on computed tomography in trauma patients with mild traumatic brain injury and those with extracranial lesions. J Neurotrauma. 2014;31:1815–22.
11. Papa L, Robinson G, Oli M, et al. Use of biomarkers for diagnosis and management of traumatic brain injury patients. Expert Opin Med Diagn. 2008;2:937–45.
12. Tongaonkar P, Chen L, Lambertson D, Ko B, Madura K. Evidence for an interaction between ubiquitin-conjugating enzymes and the 26S proteasome. Mol Cell Biol. 2000;20:4691–8.
13. Gong B, Leznik E. The role of ubiquitin C-terminal hydrolase L1 in neurodegenerative disorders. Drug News Perspect. 2007;20:365–70.

14. Papa L, Lewis LM, Falk JL, et al. Elevated levels of serum glial fibrillary acidic protein breakdown products in mild and moderate traumatic brain injury are associated with intracranial lesions and neurosurgical intervention. Ann Emerg Med. 2012;59:471–83.
15. Papa L, Brophy GM, Welch RD, et al. Time course and diagnostic accuracy of glial and neuronal blood biomarkers GFAP and UCH-L1 in a large cohort of trauma patients with and without mild traumatic brain injury. JAMA Neurol. 2016;73:551–60.
16. Metting Z, Wilczak N, Rodiger LA, Schaaf JM, van der Naalt J. GFAP and S100B in the acute phase of mild traumatic brain injury. Neurology. 2012;78:1428–33.
17. Papa L, Lewis LM, Silvestri S, et al. Serum levels of ubiquitin C-terminal hydrolase distinguish mild traumatic brain injury from trauma controls and are elevated in mild and moderate traumatic brain injury patients with intracranial lesions and neurosurgical intervention. J Trauma Acute Care Surg. 2012;72:1335–44.
18. Welch RD, Ellis M, Lewis LM, et al. Modeling the kinetics of serum glial fibrillary acidic protein, ubiquitin carboxyl-terminal hydrolase-L1, and S100B concentrations in patients with traumatic brain injury. J Neurotrauma. 2017;34:1957–71.
19. Lewis LM, Schloemann DT, Papa L, et al. Utility of serum biomarkers in the diagnosis and stratification of mild traumatic brain injury. Acad Emerg Med. 2017;24:710–20.
20. Bazarian JJ, Biberthaler P, Welch RD, et al. Serum GFAP and UCH-L1 for prediction of absence of intracranial injuries on head CT (ALERT-TBI): a multicentre observational study. Lancet Neurol. 2018;17:782–9.
21. Papa L, Mittal MK, Ramirez J, et al. Neuronal biomarker ubiquitin C-terminal hydrolase detects traumatic intracranial lesions on computed tomography in children and youth with mild traumatic brain injury. J Neurotrauma. 2017;34:2132–40.
22. Papa L, Zonfrillo MR, Welch RD, et al. Evaluating glial and neuronal blood biomarkers GFAP and UCH-L1 as gradients of brain injury in concussive, subconcussive and non-concussive trauma: a prospective cohort study. BMJ Paediatr Open. 2019;3:e000473.
23. FDA authorizes marketing of first blood test to aid in the evaluation of concussion in adults. US Food & Drug Administration. 2018. Accessed July 2, 2018.
24. Yue JK, Yuh EL, Korley FK, et al. Association between plasma GFAP concentrations and MRI abnormalities in patients with CT-negative traumatic brain injury in the TRACK-TBI cohort: a prospective multicentre study. Lancet Neurol. 2019;18:953–61.
25. Zhou Y, Kierans A, Kenul D, et al. Mild traumatic brain injury: longitudinal regional brain volume changes. Radiology. 2013;267:880–90.
26. Bailes JE, Petraglia AL, Omalu BI, Nauman E, Talavage T. Role of subconcussion in repetitive mild traumatic brain injury. J Neurosurg. 2013;119:1235–45.
27. Bailes JE, Dashnaw ML, Petraglia AL, Turner RC. Cumulative effects of repetitive mild traumatic brain injury. Prog Neurol Surg. 2014;28:50–62.
28. Tate CM, Wang KK, Eonta S, et al. Serum brain biomarker level, neurocognitive performance, and self-reported symptom changes in soldiers repeatedly exposed to low-level blast: a breacher pilot study. J Neurotrauma. 2013;30:1620–30.
29. Gavett BE, Stern RA, McKee AC. Chronic traumatic encephalopathy: a potential late effect of sport-related concussive and subconcussive head trauma. Clin Sports Med. 2011;30:179–88, xi.
30. Huber BR, Alosco ML, Stein TD, McKee AC. Potential long-term consequences of concussive and subconcussive injury. Phys Med Rehabil Clin N Am. 2016;27:503–11.
31. Meier TB, Nelson LD, Huber DL, Bazarian JJ, Hayes RL, McCrea MA. Prospective assessment of acute blood markers of brain injury in sport-related concussion. J Neurotrauma. 2017;34:3134–42.
32. Joseph JR, Swallow JS, Willsey K, et al. Elevated markers of brain injury as a result of clinically asymptomatic high-acceleration head impacts in high-school football athletes. J Neurosurg. 2018:1–7.
33. Asken BM, Bauer RM, DeKosky ST, et al. Concussion BASICS III: serum biomarker changes following sport-related concussion. Neurology. 2018;91:e2133–e43.
34. Puvenna V, Brennan C, Shaw G, et al. Significance of ubiquitin carboxy-terminal hydrolase L1 elevations in athletes after sub-concussive head hits. PLoS One. 2014;9:e96296.

35. Zimmer DB, Cornwall EH, Landar A, Song W. The S100 protein family: history, function, and expression. Brain Res Bull. 1995;37:417–29.
36. Olsson B, Zetterberg H, Hampel H, Blennow K. Biomarker-based dissection of neurodegenerative diseases. Prog Neurobiol. 2011;95:520–34.
37. Schulte S, Podlog LW, Hamson-Utley JJ, Strathmann FG, Struder HK. A systematic review of the biomarker S100B: implications for sport-related concussion management. J Athl Train. 2014;49:830–50.
38. Heidari K, Vafaee A, Rastekenari AM, et al. S100B protein as a screening tool for computed tomography findings after mild traumatic brain injury: systematic review and meta-analysis. Brain Inj. 2015;29:1146–57.
39. Ingebrigtsen T, Romner B. Management of minor head injuries in hospitals in Norway. Acta Neurol Scand. 1997;95:51–5.
40. Waterloo K, Ingebrigtsen T, Romner B. Neuropsychological function in patients with increased serum levels of protein S-100 after minor head injury. Acta Neurochir. 1997;139:26–31; discussion 31–2.
41. Ingebrigtsen T, Romner B. Serial S-100 protein serum measurements related to early magnetic resonance imaging after minor head injury. Case report. J Neurosurg. 1996;85:945–8.
42. Ingebrigtsen T, Waterloo K, Jacobsen EA, Langbakk B, Romner B. Traumatic brain damage in minor head injury: relation of serum S-100 protein measurements to magnetic resonance imaging and neurobehavioral outcome. Neurosurgery. 1999;45:468–75; discussion 75–6.
43. Heidari K, Asadollahi S, Jamshidian M, Abrishamchi SN, Nouroozi M. Prediction of neuropsychological outcome after mild traumatic brain injury using clinical parameters, serum S100B protein and findings on computed tomography. Brain Inj. 2015;29:33–40.
44. Bazarian JJ, Zemlan FP, Mookerjee S, Stigbrand T. Serum S-100B and cleaved-tau are poor predictors of long-term outcome after mild traumatic brain injury. Brain Inj. 2006;20:759–65.
45. Lima DP, Simao Filho C, Abib Sde C, de Figueiredo LF. Quality of life and neuropsychological changes in mild head trauma. Late analysis and correlation with S100B protein and cranial CT scan performed at hospital admission. Injury. 2008;39:604–11.
46. Dorminy M, Hoogeveen A, Tierney RT, Higgins M, McDevitt JK, Kretzschmar J. Effect of soccer heading ball speed on S100B, sideline concussion assessments and head impact kinematics. Brain Inj. 2015;29:1158–64.
47. Kiechle K, Bazarian JJ, Merchant-Borna K, et al. Subject-specific increases in serum S-100B distinguish sports-related concussion from sports-related exertion. PLoS One. 2014;9:e84977.
48. Shahim P, Tegner Y, Wilson DH, et al. Blood biomarkers for brain injury in concussed professional ice hockey players. JAMA Neurol. 2014;71:684–92.
49. Kawata K, Rubin LH, Takahagi M, et al. Subconcussive impact-dependent increase in plasma S100beta levels in collegiate football players. J Neurotrauma. 2017;34:2254–60.
50. Zonner SW, Ejima K, Bevilacqua ZW, et al. Association of increased serum S100B levels with high school football subconcussive head impacts. Front Neurol. 2019;10:327.
51. Babcock L, Byczkowski T, Wade SL, Ho M, Bazarian JJ. Inability of S100B to predict postconcussion syndrome in children who present to the emergency department with mild traumatic brain injury: a brief report. Pediatr Emerg Care. 2013;29:458–61.
52. Pelinka LE, Kroepfl A, Schmidhammer R, et al. Glial fibrillary acidic protein in serum after traumatic brain injury and multiple trauma. J Trauma. 2004;57:1006–12.
53. Teunissen CE, Dijkstra C, Polman C. Biological markers in CSF and blood for axonal degeneration in multiple sclerosis. Lancet Neurol. 2005;4:32–41.
54. Kosik KS, Finch EA. MAP2 and tau segregate into dendritic and axonal domains after the elaboration of morphologically distinct neurites: an immunocytochemical study of cultured rat cerebrum. J Neurosci. 1987;7:3142–53.
55. Higuchi M, Lee VM, Trojanowski JQ. Tau and axonopathy in neurodegenerative disorders. NeuroMolecular Med. 2002;2:131–50.
56. Shaw GJ, Jauch EC, Zemlan FP. Serum cleaved tau protein levels and clinical outcome in adult patients with closed head injury. Ann Emerg Med. 2002;39:254–7.

57. Chatfield DA, Zemlan FP, Day DJ, Menon DK. Discordant temporal patterns of S100beta and cleaved tau protein elevation after head injury: a pilot study. Br J Neurosurg. 2002;16:471–6.
58. Ma M, Lindsell CJ, Rosenberry CM, Shaw GJ, Zemlan FP. Serum cleaved tau does not predict postconcussion syndrome after mild traumatic brain injury. Am J Emerg Med. 2008;26:763–8.
59. Bulut M, Koksal O, Dogan S, et al. Tau protein as a serum marker of brain damage in mild traumatic brain injury: preliminary results. Adv Ther. 2006;23:12–22.
60. Rubenstein R, Chang B, Davies P, Wagner AK, Robertson CS, Wang KK. A novel, ultrasensitive assay for tau: potential for assessing traumatic brain injury in tissues and biofluids. J Neurotrauma. 2015;32:342–52.
61. Rubenstein R, Chang B, Yue JK, et al. Comparing plasma phospho tau, total tau, and phospho tau-total tau ratio as acute and chronic traumatic brain injury biomarkers. JAMA Neurol. 2017;74:1063–72.
62. Puvenna V, Engeler M, Banjara M, et al. Is phosphorylated tau unique to chronic traumatic encephalopathy? Phosphorylated tau in epileptic brain and chronic traumatic encephalopathy. Brain Res. 2016;1630:225–40.
63. Alosco ML, Tripodis Y, Fritts NG, et al. Cerebrospinal fluid tau, Abeta, and sTREM2 in Former National Football League Players: modeling the relationship between repetitive head impacts, microglial activation, and neurodegeneration. Alzheimers Dement. 2018;14:1159–70.
64. Julien JP, Mushynski WE. Neurofilaments in health and disease. Prog Nucleic Acid Res Mol Biol. 1998;61:1–23.
65. Buki A, Povlishock JT. All roads lead to disconnection?--traumatic axonal injury revisited. Acta Neurochir. 2006;148:181–93; discussion 93-4.
66. Siman R, Toraskar N, Dang A, et al. A panel of neuron-enriched proteins as markers for traumatic brain injury in humans. J Neurotrauma. 2009;26:1867–77.
67. Zurek J, Bartlova L, Fedora M. Hyperphosphorylated neurofilament NF-H as a predictor of mortality after brain injury in children. Brain Inj. 2012;25:221–6.
68. Vajtr D, Benada O, Linzer P, et al. Immunohistochemistry and serum values of S-100B, glial fibrillary acidic protein, and hyperphosphorylated neurofilaments in brain injuries. Soud Lek. 2013;57:7–12.
69. Shahim P, Zetterberg H, Tegner Y, Blennow K. Serum neurofilament light as a biomarker for mild traumatic brain injury in contact sports. Neurology. 2017;88:1788–94.
70. Wirsching A, Chen Z, Bevilacqua ZW, Huibregtse ME, Kawata K. Association of acute increase in plasma neurofilament light with repetitive subconcussive head impacts: a pilot randomized control trial. J Neurotrauma. 2019;36:548–53.
71. Wallace C, Zetterberg H, Blennow K, van Donkelaar P. No change in plasma tau and serum neurofilament light concentrations in adolescent athletes following sport-related concussion. PLoS One. 2018;13:e0206466.
72. Jin XF, Wu N, Wang L, Li J. Circulating microRNAs: a novel class of potential biomarkers for diagnosing and prognosing central nervous system diseases. Cell Mol Neurobiol. 2013;33:601–13.
73. Balakathiresan N, Bhomia M, Chandran R, Chavko M, McCarron RM, Maheshwari RK. MicroRNA let-7i is a promising serum biomarker for blast-induced traumatic brain injury. J Neurotrauma. 2012;29:1379–87.
74. Bhomia M, Balakathiresan NS, Wang KK, Papa L, Maheshwari RKA. Panel of serum MiRNA biomarkers for the diagnosis of severe to mild traumatic brain injury in humans. Sci Rep. 2016;6:28148.
75. Hicks SD, Johnson J, Carney MC, et al. Overlapping microRNA expression in saliva and cerebrospinal fluid accurately identifies pediatric traumatic brain injury. J Neurotrauma. 2017;35(1):64–72.
76. Johnson JJ, Loeffert AC, Stokes J, Olympia RP, Bramley H, Hicks SD. Association of salivary microRNA changes with prolonged concussion symptoms. JAMA Pediatr. 2018;172:65–73.
77. Mitra B, Rau TF, Surendran N, et al. Plasma micro-RNA biomarkers for diagnosis and prognosis after traumatic brain injury: a pilot study. J Clin Neurosci. 2017;38:37–42.

78. Papa L, Slobounov SM, Breiter HC, et al. Elevations in microRNA biomarkers in serum are associated with measures of concussion, neurocognitive function, and subconcussive trauma over a single National Collegiate Athletic Association Division I Season in collegiate football players. J Neurotrauma. 2019;36:1343–51.
79. Abbas K, Shenk TE, Poole VN, et al. Alteration of default mode network in high school football athletes due to repetitive subconcussive mild traumatic brain injury: a resting-state functional magnetic resonance imaging study. Brain Connect. 2015;5:91–101.
80. Di Pietro V, Porto E, Ragusa M, et al. Salivary microRNAs: diagnostic markers of mild traumatic brain injury in contact-sport. Front Mol Neurosci. 2018;11:290.

Genetics in Concussion

14

Alexa E. Walter

Concussion and the Role of Genetics

Concussion, or mild traumatic brain injury (mTBI), is a heterogenous brain trauma that is currently challenging to clinically diagnose and treat. mTBI, or sport-related concussion (SRC), is defined as a traumatic brain injury induced by biomechanical forces with common features including (a) a direct blow to the face, head, neck, or body with force transmitted to the head; (b) rapid onset of short-lived impaired neurological function that resolves spontaneously; and (c) a range of clinical symptoms that may or may not involve the loss of consciousness [1]. These injuries are diagnosed by medical providers, typically using the individual's subjective reporting of symptoms as the vast majority of computerized tomography and magnetic resonance imaging findings are negative [2]. The large majority of individuals recover from the injury within 7–10 days [3]; however, there is a growing population (10–20%) whose recovery is more delayed and develops into post-concussion syndrome [4].

Premorbid status has been shown to affect both risk [5] and recovery of SRC [6]. Risk of concussion has been associated with prior concussion history, participation in collision sports for men, participation in soccer for women, being female, age, and previous history of migraine headache (for a review see [5]). More well studied are premorbid characteristics and their role in recovery; however, these findings are very mixed (for a review see [6]).

Due to the heterogeneity of this injury, it has been assumed that genetic variability may play a role in the evolution of injury. The increased susceptibility to injury or different patterns of recovery after an injury has become a recent area of research in this field. The role of genetics has been well documented in Alzheimer's disease [7], Parkinson's disease [8], amyotrophic lateral sclerosis [9], and severe traumatic brain injury [10], but the link to concussion or mTBI is still relatively unknown.

A. E. Walter (✉)
Department of Kinesiology, Pennsylvania State University, University Park, PA, USA

Therefore, this chapter only focuses on the link of genetics to concussion or mTBI, including both the link to the previous history of injury/risk of injury or to an individual's recovery after injury.

Brief Biology of Genetics

Individuals inherently have variation in their DNA, called polymorphisms, due to alterations in the sequence. These polymorphisms are defined as one of two or more variants of a particular DNA sequence. The most common type of polymorphism involves variation at a single base pair, termed single-nucleotide polymorphisms (SNPs) (Fig. 14.1). The majority of polymorphisms do not affect gene function; however, some can change gene expression or function.

SNPs are the simplest form of genetic differences, altering one single nucleotide pair and commonly occur in an individual's DNA (one in every 1000 nucleotides). These SNPs can occur in the exons (coding regions) or introns (non-coding regions) thereby affecting the resulting protein in different ways (Fig. 14.2). While SNPs are

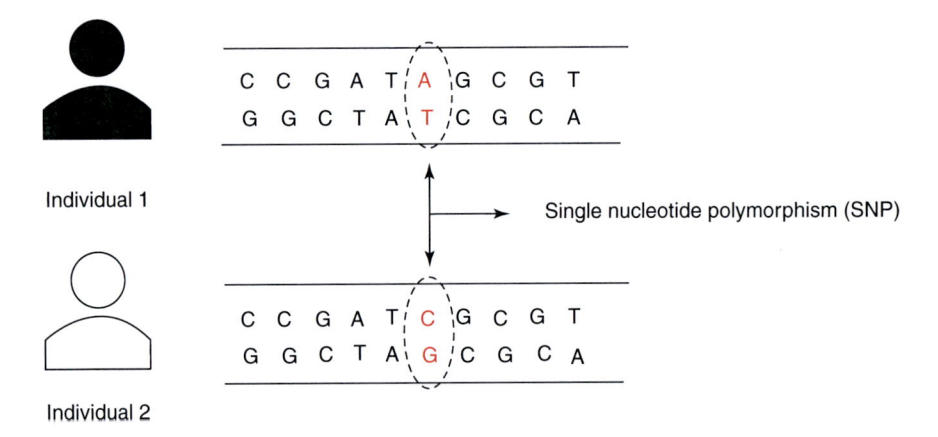

Fig. 14.1 Representation of a single-nucleotide polymorphism

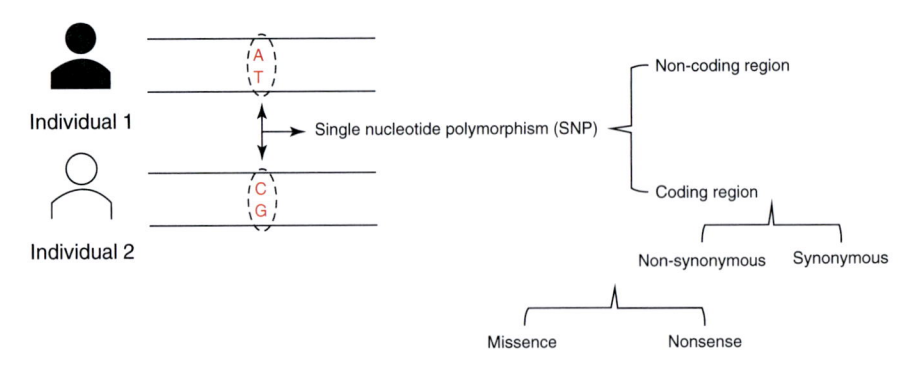

Fig. 14.2 Types of SNPs based on their location on the exon or intron

commonly used when studying genetics, other methods exist as well. Variable number tandem repeats (VNTRs) are short sequences of DNA (20–100 bp) repeated in tandem, while short tandem repeats (STRs) are sequences of DNA, normally 2–7 bp, that are repeated in tandem. Genome-wide association studies (GWAS) study the entire genome and identify all variable SNPs. GWAS is currently the most inclusive way to study genetics.

While all of these methods are feasible experimental techniques, the use of SNP analysis in this field is by far the most common. To our knowledge, no GWAS studies have been done to date on mTBI or concussion, somewhat limiting the potential utility of these findings in the larger context of understanding injury. The following text aims to summarize the current status of the literature involving SNP or VNTR genotypes and their association with concussion or mTBI in both athletic and military populations.

APOE

Apolipoprotein E (*APOE*) is the most studied gene in relation to concussion and mTBI. apoE (the protein) binds to various fats to form a lipoprotein which then packages cholesterol and other fats and carries them through the bloodstream. It is the major apolipoprotein produced in the central nervous system and is synthesized by astrocytes and microglial and during times of stress, neurons [11]. It exists in three isoforms coded by three alleles (ε2, ε3, ε4) [12, 13], and ε4 has been the focus of much neurological research.

In regard to the risk of obtaining a concussion or mTBI, there are mixed findings on the involvement of *APOE*. When examining the role of ε4 (rs7412 and rs429358) in military populations, Dretsch and colleagues ran two studies, one studying 231 soldiers [14] and the other on 438 soldiers [15], and found no link between genotype and previous mTBI history. There are numerous studies examining the link between ε4 and concussion history in college-aged athletes. The majority found no significant link [16–21], while one study (n = 1056) found that the ε4 allele was associated with a reduced risk of concussion [22]. Only one study, however, reported a significant association between a history of concussion and having all of the *APOE* rare alleles [18].

When examining the *APOE* G-219T promoter region (rs405509) in college athletes, Cochrane and colleagues found no relationship to previous concussion history [20]. However, Abrahams and colleagues when studying rugby players found that the TT genotype was associated with reduced concussion susceptibility [19]. Contradictory, Terrell and colleagues demonstrated in 195 college athletes that the TT genotype was associated with a threefold increase in risk for the history of concussion and a fourfold increased odds of concussion with loss of consciousness [17]. Tierney and colleagues also reported an association between the promotor minor allele (T allele) and experiencing more than two previous concussions [18].

Additional work has been done examining the link between the presence of the ε4 allele and recovery after injury. A study examining outcomes in children and adolescents demonstrated a link between ε4 allele and lower GSC scores but no difference in neurocognitive ability or symptom presentation [23]. In studies on college athletes, Cochrane and colleagues ($n = 250$) demonstrated that individuals with the ε4 allele had slower reaction time, as measured by the ImPACT test, compared with non-ε4 carriers. There were no differences in cognitive results with the SNP for *APOE* G-219T promotor [20].

Work by Merritt and colleagues also demonstrated changes in neurocognitive scores with the presence of the ε4 allele. There were no differences when examining mean neurocognitive standardized scores; however, individuals with the ε4 allele had a greater number of impaired scores post-injury and had greater variability in their scores [24]. Furthermore, the same group of researchers showed that the presence of the ε4 allele can affect symptoms presentation post-injury, with those individuals with ε4 allele presenting with a higher severity of symptoms [25, 26].

BDNF

Brain-derived neurotrophic factor (*BDNF*) is involved with neuronal survival through its role in the growth and maturation of neurons [27]. Elevated *BNDF* activity level has the potential to restore neural connectivity and facilitate neuroplastic changes leading to adaptive repair [28]. In particular, the Met allele has been associated with abnormal storage and secretion of *BDNF* [29].

A study on college athletes ($n = 87$) revealed no relationship between *BDNF* and previous history of concussion [21]. Two studies involving military personnel demonstrated that individuals with the Met/Met genotype had an increased lifetime history of concussion ($n = 231$ [14] and $n = 458$ [15]).

DRD

Dopamine receptors (DRD) are G protein-coupled receptors involved with dopamine transmission and therefore are implicated in many processes including motivation, learning and memory, and fine motor control [30]. *DRD2* and *DRD4* are the more commonly studied variants of this gene. *DRD2* encodes the D2 subtype of the dopamine receptor, involved in the inhibition of adenylyl cyclase [31] and *DRD4* encodes the D4 subtype of the dopamine receptor, involved in the inhibition adenylyl cyclase [32]. They have been linked to various neurological and psychiatric concisions, including schizophrenia, Parkinson's disease, impulsivity, and attention-deficit hyperactivity disorder [33].

In a study on 250 college athletes, Cochrane and colleagues found no link between *DRD2* genotype (rs1800497) and concussion history or neurocognitive performance [20]. Similarly, in studies of military personnel, Drestsch and colleagues also found no association between *DRD2* genotype and prior concussions [14, 15].

A study by Abrahams and colleagues examined the role of both *DRD4* (rs1800955) and *DRD2* (rs12364283 and rs1076560) on previous concussion history; 301 rugby athletes from high school (junior) and professional (senior) teams demonstrated that the *DRD4* CC genotype was associated with decreased concussion susceptibility in the junior players. Furthermore, the TT and CT genotypes were associated with lower reward dependence behaviors in both the junior and senior players. The *DRD2* genotypes alone were not related to previous concussion history; however, when the combination of DRD2 alleles (A – C – C) was used they were associated with decreased concussion susceptibility in junior players [19].

COMT

Catechol-O-methyl transferase (*COMT*) is involved with the breakdown of dopamine in the prefrontal cortex [34, 35]. It plays a critical role in cell death, cellular dysfunction, and central nervous system inflammation and seems to be associated with impulsivity [20, 33].

When examining the link to previous concussion history, studies on college athletes revealed no link of genotype (rs4680) to previous concussion history [20, 21]. There was found to be a link to neurocognitive performance with individuals with Val/Val genotype having worse impulse control scores, as measured by ImPACT, as compared to Met-carrying individuals [20].

Interleukins

Interleukin 6 (*IL6*) is a pro-inflammatory cytokine and anti-inflammatory myokine secreted by T cells and macrophages. It is heavily involved in the immune responses as well as involved in encoding a pleiotropic cytokine involved in inflammation and maturation of B cells [36, 37]. The C allele has been associated with lower levels of *IL6* while the G allele is associated with higher levels [10, 38]. It has been implicated in mTBI pathology as it can suppress post-injury neuroinflammation, neuronal injury, and motor coordination deficits [39].

A study on 1056 college athletes demonstrated a significant association between the CC genotype for the IL-6 receptor (rs22281450) and increased concussion risk (3 times greater risk) [22]. There was no association between previous concussions and *IL6* (rs1800796). A study on 87 college athletes using rs1800795 also found no association between genotype and previous concussions [21].

Other work from Mc Fie and colleagues examined the role of *IL1B* (rs16944) and *IL6* (rs1800795) in 163 rugby players. There was no association with previous concussion history for either SNP; however, there was reduced symptom severity in both the rs16944 C allele and the rs1800795 C allele. When a combination of the two SNPs was used, the C-C inferred allele construct demonstrated higher symptom counts and prolonged symptom duration [40].

Tau

Microtubule-associated protein tau (MAPT) is encoded by the *MAPT*, or *TAU*, gene and is involved with tau protein regulation and binding to microtubules [41]. Two SNPs, rs2435211 and rs2435200, were examined in work by Abrahams and colleagues. Studying 303 rugby players from high school (junior) and professional (senior) levels, they found that rs2435200 AA genotype was associated with reduced susceptibility to multiple concussions (66%) and rs2435200 AG genotype was associated with increased susceptibility (134%) in senior players. rs2435211 was not associated with concussion history. The inferred haplotype using both SNPs (T-G) was associated with increased susceptibility for concussion in the senior players [42].

Work in 195 college athletes demonstrated no link between *Tau* Ser53Pro (rs2258689) or *Tau* His47Tyr (rs10445337) and previous concussion history [17]. This was further confirmed in a study of 1056 college athletes where neither *Tau* Ser53Pro nor *Tau* His47Tyr were associated with previous concussion [22].

Single Study Genes Examined

The following genes were only examined in 1 published study to our knowledge and are briefly summarized.

KIAA0319 *KIAA0319* is involved in the regulation of neuronal migration and cell adhesion, especially in the cerebral cortex [43, 44]. Using the SNP rs4504469, a study by Walter and colleagues on 87 college athletes demonstrated a significant association between genotype and previous concussion history. Individuals with the TT genotype had the lowest risk for previous concussion [21].

SLC17A7 The synaptic uptake of glutamate involves vesicular transporters, which are encoded by a subfamily of genes located on chromosome 19 (*SLC17A7*) and chromosomes 11 and 12. A study by Madura and colleagues found that the *SLC17A7* promotor (rs74174284) was not linked to the history of previous injury but was linked with recovery. Individuals with the G allele were 6.33 times more likely to have prolonged recovery rates and perform worse on motor speed tests, as measured by ImPACT, than individuals with the CC phenotype [45].

CACNA1A Calcium voltage-gated channel subunit alpha1 (*CACNA1A*) is involved with altering the configuration of Ca^{2+} pore-forming component and is primarily expressed in neuronal tissue. It is essential for proper neuron communication. A study by McDevitt and colleagues examined 40 athletes and found that individuals with the *CACNA1A* (rs704326) GG genotype had a prolonged recovery. The rs35737760 SNP had no association with the severity of injury [46].

NEFH Neurofilament heavy (*NEFH*) is important for mature axon function and may be involved in forming neuronal filamentous networks. In a study on 96 athletes, McDevitt and colleagues found no association between the rare allele, using rs165602, and history of concussion or symptom recovery [47].

GRINA2A N-methyl-D-aspartate receptor 2A sub-unit (*GRIN2A*) is an NMDA glutamate receptor subunit which has been implicated in influencing the magnitude of neuron dysfunction. A study on 87 athletes using rs3219790 examined the long allele (≥25 repeats) and the short allele (<25 repeats), and found that LL carriers were 6 times more likely to have a longer recovery compared to SS carriers [48].

CASP8 Caspase 8 (*CASP8*) encodes a cysteine-aspartic acid protease and is involved in the execution of cell apoptosis. A study by Mc Fie and colleagues examined rs3834129 in 163 rugby players and found no link between genotype and concussion history or severity [40].

DARC Duffy antigen receptor of chemokines (DARC) encodes a glycosylated membrane protein that is a non-specific receptor for many chemokines and is expressed on Purkinje cells [49, 50]. It has been shown to be upregulated at the BBB [51] and transports inflammatory chemokines across the BBB. In a study on 87 college athletes, using rs2814778, it was found to have no relation to previous concussion history [21].

PARP1 Poly(ADP-ribose) polymerase 1 (*PARP1*) modifies various nuclear proteins by poly ADP-ribosylation. This modification is DNA-dependent and is involved in the regulation of various cellular processes including differentiation, proliferation, tumor transformation, and cell damage and death [52, 53]. In a study on 87 college athletes, using rs3219119, there was no link between genotype and previous concussion history [21].

TPH2 Tryptophan hydroxylase 2 (TPH2) is involved in regulating the production of serotonin and has a role as a trans-synaptic messenger in axonal and dendritic growth [54, 55]. It has been linked to various psychiatric disorders as well as impulsivity and impaired response inhibition [33]. In a study on 87 college athletes, using rs1386483, there was no link between genotype and previous concussion history [21].

NGB Neuroglobin encodes oxygen-binding proteins expressed in the central and peripheral nervous system where it may be involved in facilitating oxygen transfer across the BBB and increase oxygen availability [56, 57]. In 87 college athletes, using rs3783988, there was no link between genotype and previous concussion history [21].

Implications and Future Work

The use of individuals' genetics for health purposes has been a growing area of research and it can be assumed that there is a link between concussion and genetics. However, at this time, the findings are still fairly limited. Studies involving genetics often are aiming to address susceptibility to concussion or risks associated with recovery from injury. While individual studies employ different techniques and gene selection, in combination they reveal some core findings that will be discussed.

Overall, there is limited evidence of a genotype predicting previous concussion history. *NGB, TPH2, PARP1, DARC, CASP8, GRINA2A, NEFH, CACNA1A,* and *SLC17A7* were all examined by single studies and showed no association with the risk of injury. However, *SLC17A7* (G allele), *CACNA1A* (GG phenotype), and *GRINA2A* (long allele, LL) were all associated with longer recoveries after injury. The only gene to predict previous concussion history was *KIAA0319,* with the TT genotype having the lowest risk of previous concussion [21]. In animal models, reduced expression of *KIAA0319* negatively affected the adhesion of neurons to the glial skeleton, impacting neuronal migration [43]. These findings, or lack of findings, should be replicated with further work and could suggest future theoretical frameworks to consider when studying the underlying physiology of injury or the role of genetics in susceptibility to concussion.

More commonly studied genes also revealed limited, and sometimes contradictory, findings in regard to risk of injury. *Tau* genotypes were found to be both not related [17, 22] and related to the susceptibility of injury [19]. *COMT* genotypes were found to be not related to the risk of injury [20, 21] but were related to worse outcomes after injury, specifically in individuals with the Val/Val genotype [20]. *BDNF* genotypes were found to have no association with concussion risk in college athletes [21] but did have an association in military populations. Specifically, individuals with the Met/Met genotype had increased history of concussion [14, 15]. *DRD2* also had no link to concussion risk both in athletic [19, 20] or military populations [14, 15]. *DRD4* was found to have an association with concussion risk with the CC genotype having decreased susceptibility to injury [19]. *IL6* was found to have no association with concussion risk [21, 40] and an increased risk for concussion specifically individuals with the CC genotype [22]. In regards to outcome, the C allele of *IL6* was associated with reduced symptom severity [40].

APOE is the most commonly studied gene in association with concussion risk and recovery. However, most studies show no link between *APOE,* specifically ε4, and concussion risk. Only one study [22] demonstrated that the ε4 allele was associated with a reduced risk of concussion. Use of the promoter region SNP of *APOE* also revealed highly mixed findings: one study shows no association [20], one shows reduced risk [19], and one shows increased risk [17].

Findings on recovery after injury and the association of *APOE* are more in agreement. Typically, the presence of ε4 is associated with worse outcomes after injury, specifically lower GCS scores [23], slower reaction times [20], and greater variability in neurocognitive testing results and more severity of symptoms [24–26].

As with the single study genes, these genes also reveal limited findings in regard to the risk of injury and warrant further exploration. Much larger sample sizes are needed as the sample sizes in the studies included are small for a genetic study (largest $n = 1056$) and this could be contributing to some of the mixed findings demonstrated. Ideally, more comprehensive and rigorous examinations of genotypes should be done instead of focusing on single SNPs. Using GWAS technology would provide a more comprehensive look at genetic susceptibility and the potential interactions that may exist as it is highly unlikely that one individual SNP is a risk factor. Instead, it is more likely that it is an interaction of many, maybe hundreds of, SNPs that is contributing to the high variability in risk of and recovery after injury.

Overall, these studies highlight the beneficial use of genetics as a growing field to consider when understanding injury susceptibility. However, the findings should be interpreted with some caution. Primarily these studies are done on college-aged male, contact sport athletes, and are done in small sample sizes. Additionally, as well as little diversity in sex, there is often little diversity in race. This limits the generalizability of results to other sports teams as well as the general population. Furthermore, the use of an individual's premorbid status as a binary screening tool for participation is currently cautionary. Each of these factors, at this time, should not be used in isolation, but instead should be evaluated to shed light on the observed variability seen and to gain insights into potential physiological consequences of injury.

References

1. McCrory P, Meeuwisse W, Dvořák J, Aubry M, Bailes J, Broglio S, et al. Consensus statement on concussion in sport-the 5th international conference on concussion in sport held in Berlin, October 2016. Br J Sports Med. 2017;51:838–47.
2. Ellis MJ, Leiter J, Hall T, McDonald PJ, Sawyer S, Silver N, et al. Neuroimaging findings in pediatric sports-related concussion. J Neurosurg Pediatr. 2015;16:241–7.
3. Lovell MR, Collins MW, Iverson GL, Johnston KM, Bradley JP. Grade 1 or "ding" concussions in high school athletes. Am J Sports Med. 2004;32:47–54.
4. Graham R, Rivara FP, Ford MA, Spicer CM, Committee on Sports-Related Concussions in Youth; Board on Children, Youth and Families, et al. Treatment and management of prolonged symptoms and post-concussion syndrome [Internet]. In: Sports-related concussions in youth: improving the science, changing the culture. Washington, DC: National Academies Press; 2014. [cited 2020 Jan 20]. Available from: https://www.ncbi.nlm.nih.gov/books/NBK185342/.
5. Scopaz KA, Hatzenbuehler JR. Risk modifiers for concussion and prolonged recovery. Sports Health. 2013;5:537–41.
6. Iverson GL, Gardner AJ, Terry DP, Ponsford JL, Sills AK, Broshek DK, et al. Predictors of clinical recovery from concussion: a systematic review. Br J Sports Med. 2017;51:941–8.
7. Nikolac Perkovic M, Pivac N. Genetic markers of Alzheimer's disease. Adv Exp Med Biol. 2019;1192:27–52.
8. Kim CY, Alcalay RN. Genetic forms of Parkinson's disease. Semin Neurol. 2017;37:135–46.
9. Mejzini R, Flynn LL, Pitout IL, Fletcher S, Wilton SD, Akkari PA. ALS genetics, mechanisms, and therapeutics: where are we now? Front Neurosci. 2019;13:1310. Available from: https://www.ncbi.nlm.nih.gov/pmc/articles/PMC6909825/.
10. Bennett ER, Reuter-Rice K, Laskowitz DT. Genetic influences in traumatic brain injury. In: Laskowitz D, Grant G, editors. Translational research in traumatic brain injury [internet]. Boca

Raton: CRC Press/Taylor and Francis Group; 2016. Available from: http://www.ncbi.nlm.nih.gov/books/NBK326717/.
11. Mahley RW. Central nervous system lipoproteins: ApoE and regulation of cholesterol metabolism. Arterioscler Thromb Vasc Biol. 2016;36:1305–15.
12. Weisgraber KH, Rall SC, Mahley RW. Human E apoprotein heterogeneity. Cysteine-arginine interchanges in the amino acid sequence of the apo-E isoforms. J Biol Chem. 1981;256:9077–83.
13. Bekris LM, Millard SP, Galloway NM, Vuletic S, Albers JJ, Li G, et al. Multiple SNPs within and surrounding the apolipoprotein E gene influence cerebrospinal fluid apolipoprotein E protein levels. J Alzheimers Dis. 2008;13:255–66.
14. Dretsch MN, Williams K, Emmerich T, Crynen G, Ait-Ghezala G, Chaytow H, et al. Brain-derived neurotropic factor polymorphisms, traumatic stress, mild traumatic brain injury, and combat exposure contribute to postdeployment traumatic stress. Brain Behav. 2016;6:e00392. Available from: https://www.ncbi.nlm.nih.gov/pmc/articles/PMC4834940/.
15. Dretsch MN, Silverberg N, Gardner AJ, Panenka WJ, Emmerich T, Crynen G, et al. Genetics and other risk factors for past concussions in active-duty soldiers. J Neurotrauma. 2017;34:869–75.
16. Kristman VL, Tator CH, Kreiger N, Richards D, Mainwaring L, Jaglal S, et al. Does the apolipoprotein epsilon 4 allele predispose varsity athletes to concussion? A prospective cohort study. Clin J Sport Med. 2008;18:322–8.
17. Terrell TR, Bostick RM, Abramson R, Xie D, Barfield W, Cantu R, et al. APOE, APOE promoter, and tau genotypes and risk for concussion in college athletes. Clin J Sport Med. 2008;18:10–7.
18. Tierney RT, Mansell JL, Higgins M, McDevitt JK, Toone N, Gaughan JP, et al. Apolipoprotein E genotype and concussion in college athletes. Clin J Sport Med. 2010;20:464–8.
19. Abrahams S, Mc Fie S, Patricios J, Suter J, Posthumus M, September AV. An association between polymorphisms within the APOE gene and concussion aetiology in rugby union players. J Sci Med Sport. 2018;21(2):117–22.
20. Cochrane GD, Sundman MH, Hall EE, Kostek MC, Patel K, Barnes KP, et al. Genetics influence neurocognitive performance at baseline but not concussion history in collegiate student-athletes. Clin J Sport Med. 2018;28(2):125–9.
21. Walter A, Herrold AA, Gallagher VT, Lee R, Scaramuzzo M, Bream T, et al. KIAA0319 genotype predicts the number of past concussions in a division I football team: a pilot study. J Neurotrauma. 2019;36:1115–24.
22. Terrell TR, Abramson R, Barth JT, Bennett E, Cantu RC, Sloane R, et al. Genetic polymorphisms associated with the risk of concussion in 1056 college athletes: a multicentre prospective cohort study. Br J Sports Med. 2018;52:192–8.
23. Moran LM, Taylor HG, Ganesalingam K, Gastier-Foster JM, Frick J, Bangert B, et al. Apolipoprotein E4 as a predictor of outcomes in pediatric mild traumatic brain injury. J Neurotrauma. 2009;26:1489–95.
24. Merritt VC, Rabinowitz AR, Arnett PA. The influence of the apolipoprotein E (APOE) gene on subacute post-concussion neurocognitive performance in college athletes. Arch Clin Neuropsychol. 2018;33:36–46.
25. Merritt VC, Ukueberuwa DM, Arnett PA. Relationship between the apolipoprotein E gene and headache following sports-related concussion. J Clin Exp Neuropsychol. 2016;38:941–9.
26. Merritt VC, Arnett PA. Apolipoprotein E (APOE) ε4 allele is associated with increased symptom reporting following sports concussion. J Int Neuropsychol Soc. 2016;22:89–94.
27. Yoshii A, Constantine-Paton M. Postsynaptic BDNF-TrkB signaling in synapse maturation, plasticity, and disease. Dev Neurobiol. 2010;70:304–22.
28. Figurov A, Pozzo-Miller LD, Olafsson P, Wang T, Lu B. Regulation of synaptic responses to high-frequency stimulation and LTP by neurotrophins in the hippocampus. Nature. 1996;381:706–9.
29. Egan MF, Kojima M, Callicott JH, Goldberg TE, Kolachana BS, Bertolino A, et al. The BDNF val66met polymorphism affects activity-dependent secretion of BDNF and human memory and hippocampal function. Cell. 2003;112:257–69.

30. Gurevich EV, Gainetdinov RR, Gurevich VV. G protein-coupled receptor kinases as regulators of dopamine receptor functions. Pharmacol Res. 2016;111:1–16.
31. Bunzow JR, Van Tol HH, Grandy DK, Albert P, Salon J, Christie M, et al. Cloning and expression of a rat D2 dopamine receptor cDNA. Nature. 1988;336:783–7.
32. Van Tol HH, Bunzow JR, Guan HC, Sunahara RK, Seeman P, Niznik HB, et al. Cloning of the gene for a human dopamine D4 receptor with high affinity for the antipsychotic clozapine. Nature. 1991;350:610–4.
33. Hehar H, Yeates K, Kolb B, Esser MJ, Mychasiuk R. Impulsivity and concussion in juvenile rats: examining molecular and structural aspects of the frontostriatal pathway. PLoS One. 2015;10:e0139842.
34. Garris PA, Collins LB, Jones SR, Wightman RM. Evoked extracellular dopamine in vivo in the medial prefrontal cortex. J Neurochem. 1993;61:637–47.
35. Chen J, Lipska BK, Halim N, Ma QD, Matsumoto M, Melhem S, et al. Functional analysis of genetic variation in catechol-O-methyltransferase (COMT): effects on mRNA, protein, and enzyme activity in postmortem human brain. Am J Hum Genet. 2004;75:807–21.
36. Yasukawa K, Hirano T, Watanabe Y, Muratani K, Matsuda T, Nakai S, et al. Structure and expression of human B cell stimulatory factor-2 (BSF-2/IL-6) gene. EMBO J. 1987;6:2939–45.
37. Kamimura D, Ishihara K, Hirano T. IL-6 signal transduction and its physiological roles: the signal orchestration model. Rev Physiol Biochem Pharmacol. 2003;149:1–38.
38. Hulkkonen J, Pertovaara M, Antonen J, Pasternack A, Hurme M. Elevated interleukin-6 plasma levels are regulated by the promoter region polymorphism of the IL6 gene in primary Sjögren's syndrome and correlate with the clinical manifestations of the disease. Rheumatology. 2001;40:656–61.
39. Yang SH, Gangidine M, Pritts TA, Goodman MD, Lentsch AB. Interleukin 6 mediates neuroinflammation and motor coordination deficits after mild traumatic brain injury and brief hypoxia in mice. Shock. 2013;40:471–5.
40. Mc Fie S, Abrahams S, Patricios J, Suter J, Posthumus M, September AV. Inflammatory and apoptotic signalling pathways and concussion severity: a genetic association study. J Sports Sci. 2018;36:2226–34.
41. Barbier P, Zejneli O, Martinho M, Lasorsa A, Belle V, Smet-Nocca C, et al. Role of tau as a microtubule-associated protein: structural and functional aspects. Front Aging Neurosci. 2019;11:204.
42. Abrahams S, Mc Fie S, Patricios J, Suter J, September AV, Posthumus M. Toxic TAU: the TAU gene polymorphisms associate with concussion history in rugby union players. J Sci Med Sport. 2019;22:22–8.
43. Paracchini S, Thomas A, Castro S, Lai C, Paramasivam M, Wang Y, et al. The chromosome 6p22 haplotype associated with dyslexia reduces the expression of KIAA0319, a novel gene involved in neuronal migration. Hum Mol Genet. 2006;15:1659–66.
44. Francks C, Paracchini S, Smith SD, Richardson AJ, Scerri TS, Cardon LR, et al. A 77-kilobase region of chromosome 6p22.2 is associated with dyslexia in families from the United Kingdom and from the United States. Am J Hum Genet. 2004;75:1046–58.
45. Madura SA, McDevitt JK, Tierney RT, Mansell JL, Hayes DJ, Gaughan JP, et al. Genetic variation in SLC17A7 promoter associated with response to sport-related concussions. Brain Inj. 2016;30:908–13.
46. McDevitt J. CNS voltage-gated calcium channel gene variation and prolonged recovery following sport-related concussion. Orthop J Sports Med. 2016;4:2325967116S00074. Available from: https://www.ncbi.nlm.nih.gov/pmc/articles/PMC4901914/.
47. McDevitt JK, Tierney RT, Mansell JL, Driban JB, Higgins M, Toone N, et al. Neuronal structural protein polymorphism and concussion in college athletes. Brain Inj. 2011;25:1108–13.
48. McDevitt J, Tierney RT, Phillips J, Gaughan JP, Torg JS, Krynetskiy E. Association between GRIN2A promoter polymorphism and recovery from concussion. Brain Inj. 2015;29:1674–81.
49. Szabo MC, Soo KS, Zlotnik A, Schall TJ. Chemokine class differences in binding to the Duffy antigen-erythrocyte chemokine receptor. J Biol Chem. 1995;270:25348–51.

50. Gardner L, Patterson AM, Ashton BA, Stone MA, Middleton J. The human Duffy antigen binds selected inflammatory but not homeostatic chemokines. Biochem Biophys Res Commun. 2004;321:306–12.
51. Minten C, Alt C, Gentner M, Frei E, Deutsch U, Lyck R, et al. DARC shuttles inflammatory chemokines across the blood-brain barrier during autoimmune central nervous system inflammation. Brain. 2014;137:1454–69.
52. Kraus WL, Hottiger MO. PARP-1 and gene regulation: progress and puzzles. Mol Asp Med. 2013;34:1109–23.
53. Virág L, Robaszkiewicz A, Rodriguez-Vargas JM, Oliver FJ. Poly(ADP-ribose) signaling in cell death. Mol Asp Med. 2013;34:1153–67.
54. Markett S, de Reus MA, Reuter M, Montag C, Weber B, Schoene-Bake J-C, et al. Serotonin and the Brain's Rich Club-Association between molecular genetic variation on the TPH2 gene and the structural connectome. Cereb Cortex. 2017;27:2166–74.
55. Walther DJ, Bader M. A unique central tryptophan hydroxylase isoform. Biochem Pharmacol. 2003;66:1673–80.
56. Dewilde S, Kiger L, Burmester T, Hankeln T, Baudin-Creuza V, Aerts T, et al. Biochemical characterization and ligand binding properties of neuroglobin, a novel member of the globin family. J Biol Chem. 2001;276:38949–55.
57. Sun Y, Jin K, Mao XO, Zhu Y, Greenberg DA. Neuroglobin is up-regulated by and protects neurons from hypoxic-ischemic injury. Proc Natl Acad Sci U S A. 2001;98:15306–11.

Part IV

Sport-Related Concussion in Pediatric Populations

Predicting Postconcussive Symptoms After Mild Traumatic Brain Injury in Children and Adolescents: 2020 Update

15

Keith Owen Yeates

Introduction

Mild traumatic brain injuries (TBI) are a common occurrence in children and adolescents. Annually, as many as 800,000 youth aged 0–17 in the United States are seen in emergency departments for TBI, and the large majority of these injuries are mild in severity [1]. The total number of youth sustaining mild TBI each year is far higher, however; many mild TBI are cared for outside of hospital settings—at least another 800,000 are seen as outpatients [2]—and even more likely never receive any formal medical attention. Indeed, estimates are that 1.1–1.9 million children and adolescents sustain sports-related concussions, a type of mild TBI, each year, with many never coming to medical attention [3].

Systematic reviews suggest that most children recover from mild TBI, at least in terms of clinical presentation, in a matter of weeks [4–6]. However, a substantial body of literature indicates that a small but significant proportion of children with mild TBI experience persistent postconcussive symptoms (PCS), and that persistent PCS occur more often after mild TBI than after injuries not involving the head or among healthy children [7–9]. PCS include a range of somatic (e.g., headache, dizziness), cognitive (e.g., inattention, forgetfulness), and affective (e.g., irritability, disinhibition) symptoms commonly reported after mild TBI, albeit not specific to that condition. Persistent PCS are linked to negative consequences for children's longer-term psychosocial functioning and quality of life [10–13].

A key issue for the purposes of clinical management is how to predict which children with mild TBI will go on to display persistent PCS [14]. This chapter

K. O. Yeates (✉)
Department of Psychology, University of Calgary, Calgary, AB, Canada

Alberta Children's Hospital Research Institute, University of Calgary, Calgary, AB, Canada

Hotchkiss Brain Institute, University of Calgary, Calgary, AB, Canada
e-mail: kyeates@ucalgary.ca

represents an update of an earlier version in the first edition of this book, incorporating research published in the past 7 years. This chapter begins by describing a schematic model for predicting PCS following mild TBI in children and adolescents. It then reviews the existing literature regarding the prediction of PCS, examining both injury-related and non-injury-related factors as possible prognostic indicators. The chapter next summarizes conceptual and methodological issues that arise in research on the prediction of the outcomes of mild TBI and describes recent advances in the development of evidence-based decision rules that help to predict which children are at high risk for poor outcomes after mild TBI. The chapter concludes with suggestions for future research directions.

A Model for PCS

Figure 15.1 portrays a general schematic model for predicting PCS following mild TBI in youth [15]. The model draws on previous theories of children's adaptation to illness, including the Disability-Stress-Coping Model [16] and the Transactional Stress and Coping Model [17], as well as on models of adaptation specific to mild TBI [18, 19]. The model does not reflect the specificity or complexity of more recent systems science analyses of mild TBI [20] but is similar to other recent approaches in providing a broad biopsychosocial framework for understanding recovery [21].

The model presumes that the occurrence of PCS following mild TBI will depend on the combined influences of premorbid child and family factors, the nature of the injury, and post-injury child and family factors. The model also assumes that the influences of these factors can be both direct and indirect. For example, changes in brain structure or function associated with mild TBI may give rise to PCS directly because of the effect of brain impairment on behavior, but they also may result in PCS indirectly by affecting children's cognitive functioning or ability to cope with stress, which in turn mediates an increased risk of PCS.

Importantly, the relationship between various risk factors and PCS is assumed to vary as a function of time since injury [22]. Shortly after an injury, the onset of PCS is more likely to depend on premorbid child and family factors and injury characteristics. The likelihood that PCS will persist over time may depend more on children's

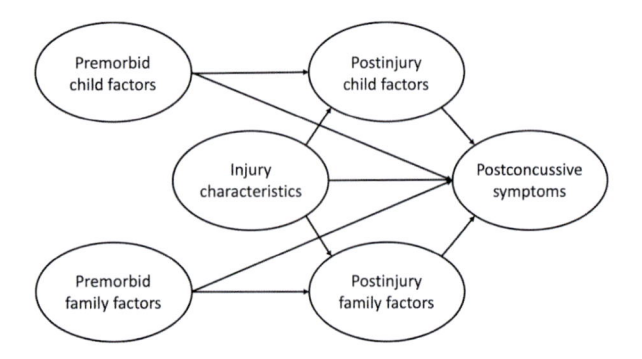

Fig. 15.1 Schematic biopsychosocial model for study of postconcussive symptoms in children with mild traumatic brain injury

and parents' post-injury responses to injury, as well as on the other stressors and resources in their lives. Premorbid factors and injury characteristics may be relevant to both acute and chronic symptoms. However, the influence of post-injury child and parent responses and other stressors and resources may be more pronounced than premorbid factors or injury characteristics for persistent symptoms. In other words, the way in which children and their parents react to the acute disruptions associated with mild TBI is likely to be a significant determinant of the persistence of PCS.

Predictors of PCS

In recent years, research examining the prediction of PCS in children after mild TBI has expanded significantly [14]. The research varies in methodological quality, however, with only a few studies involving prospective recruitment of representative samples of children with mild TBI and appropriate comparison groups who are followed longitudinally. Few studies have examined both injury and non-injury factors as potential predictors of PCS, much less compared their relative contributions at different times post-injury [22]. The following sections provide an overview of existing research about the predictors of PCS.

Injury Factors

A variety of injury factors have been considered as potential predictors of PCS. One is the occurrence of previous concussions or mild TBI. An early study of a national birth cohort suggested that multiple concussions did not result in specific cognitive deficits [23], but subsequent studies of sports concussions found evidence for cumulative effects [24]. Recent studies suggest that the impact of previous concussion may depend on how long it has been since the previous injury and whether the previous injury was associated with a longer time to recovery. Children whose previous concussions occurred more recently, or resulted in symptoms for at least 1 week, demonstrated more protracted symptoms after mild TBI than did children whose previous concussions occurred further in the past or did not result in PCS [25, 26].

Various indices of injury severity have also been studied as potential predictors of PCS. Acute symptom burden is perhaps the most consistent predictor of persistent PCS; some specific symptoms, such as headache/migraine and dizziness, also are predictive. Acute clinical signs that also have been shown to be associated with an increased risk of PCS include loss of consciousness [7, 8, 13, 27, 28], posttraumatic amnesia [28, 29], and balance problems [30]. The presence of intracranial abnormalities on acute neuroimaging has also been associated with increased PCS [8, 13, 27, 31]. Several indirect proxies for injury severity have also been associated with an increased likelihood of PCS, including hospital admission [8, 13, 32], high-speed mechanism of injury—particularly motor vehicle collision [8, 33], referral for CT scanning [34], and the presence of associated injuries not involving the head [8, 29].

Non-injury Factors

Demographic factors such as age and sex are among the non-injury factors most commonly studied as predictors of PCS. The relationship of age to PCS is inconsistent. Several studies have found greater PCS among adolescents than younger children [7, 26, 30], while others have found evidence of more PCS among younger as compared to older children [8]. Differences in results across studies may reflect whether PCS were assessed by self-report or by parent ratings; adolescents tend to report more PCS than younger children, but parents may report more PCS for younger than older children. Few studies have specifically examined whether age moderates the effects of mild TBI on PCS; one showed evidence for larger group differences (mild TBI vs. orthopedic injury) for PCS among younger versus older children [8].

Sex has been a more consistent predictor of PCS, such that girls and their parents typically report more symptoms than boys [8, 26, 30]. However, differences in PCS between children with mild TBI and those with orthopedic injuries do not appear to be more pronounced for girls than boys, suggesting that sex is not a moderator of PCS after mild TBI, but instead that girls and their parents in general may report more symptoms than boys [8, 35].

Pre-injury symptoms are the non-injury factor that consistently accounts for the most variance in PCS [22, 36]. Pre-injury symptoms are typically assessed retrospectively after injury and so may be subject to bias, except in sports concussion research where pre-injury baselines are possible. However, retrospective ratings of pre-injury symptoms tend not to differ for children with mild TBI versus those with orthopedic injuries [22], suggesting that bias is likely minimal if the ratings are obtained shortly after the injury occurs. More generally, pre-injury psychiatric disorders increase the risk of PCS, although attention deficit hyperactivity disorder and learning disabilities specifically are not clearly prognostic [37].

Children's cognitive abilities may also be related to PCS after mild TBI. Although neurocognitive deficits typically resolve within a few weeks after mild TBI when measured using traditional paper-and-pencil tasks [4, 5], computerized testing has the potential to reveal longer lasting deficits in complex processing speed [38]. Neuropsychological testing can be used to identify not only those children who show acute post-injury decrements in their cognitive functioning, but also those who have low cognitive reserve, and both types of children may be at risk for PCS. Cognitive ability has been shown to be a significant moderator of PCS, such that children of lower cognitive ability with mild TBI-associated abnormalities on neuroimaging are especially prone to PCS [39]. More research is needed to determine whether post-acute cognitive deficits on neuropsychological testing are predictive of PCS.

Various aspects of children's psychological functioning also can help account for PCS. Children with mild TBI are at greater risk for PCS relative to children with orthopedic injuries if they rely on avoidance or wishful thinking to cope with their injuries as compared to more problem-focused coping strategies [40]. Children with high levels of psychological resilience also are less likely to demonstrate PCS [41], while those with higher levels of somatization and internalization of symptoms are more likely [42].

A variety of environmental factors may also predict PCS. For instance, family socioeconomic status is negatively correlated with self-reports of PCS [8], and parent psychological distress is positively correlated with PCS [36, 43]. Somewhat surprisingly, children whose families were higher functioning and had more environmental resources were more likely to demonstrate somatic PCS following mild TBI than those from poorer functioning homes with fewer resources [44]. This finding runs counter to previous research among children with severe TBI showing that the effects of TBI are exacerbated in the context of poorer premorbid family functioning [45].

Relative Contributions of Injury Versus Non-injury Factors

Few studies have directly compared injury versus non-injury factors as predictors of PCS. In a large prospective cohort study of children aged 0–18 years [7], family functioning and parent adjustment measured post-acutely did not account for differences in PCS across the first year post-injury as a function of injury status or severity, although the specific contributions of the former variables were not estimated statistically.

Another prospective cohort study examined the prediction of PCS during the first year post-injury in children aged 8–16 years with mild TBI or mild orthopedic injuries [22]. Predictors included demographic variables, premorbid child factors, family factors, and injury factors. Injury factors predicted parent and child ratings of PCS but showed a decreasing contribution over time. Demographic variables consistently predicted symptom ratings across time. Premorbid child factors, especially retrospective ratings of premorbid symptoms, accounted for the most variance in PCS. Family factors, particularly parent adjustment, consistently predicted parent, but not child, ratings of PCS.

In a third prospective cohort study [34], children aged 2–12 years with either mild TBI or minor bodily trauma were followed for 3 months post-injury. Potential predictors of PCS included injury and demographic variables, premorbid child behavior and sleep, and premorbid parental stress. Mild TBI was a stronger predictor of PCS in the first week compared to 1–3 months post-injury. Older age at injury and preexisting learning problems were significant predictors of PCS beyond 1 month post-injury. Family factors, including higher levels of parental stress, higher socioeconomic status, and Anglo-Saxon ethnicity, consistently predicted greater PCS.

Finally, in a recent prospective cohort study [46], children aged 4–15 years with mild TBI, complicated mild TBI, or orthopedic injury were studied across the first year post-injury. Potential predictors included preinjury demographic, child, and family factors. PCS were more common in the two mild TBI groups than in the orthopedic injury group; they also were associated with female sex, adolescence, preinjury symptoms and mood problems, lower family income, poorer family functioning, and lower social support.

Collectively, the findings from these studies suggest that mild TBI predicts increased PCS in the first weeks to months following injury but shows a decreasing contribution over time. In contrast, non-injury factors are more consistently related to PCS and may display an increasingly strong association over time.

Research Issues

Definition of Mild TBI

A variety of methodological shortcomings have characterized previous research on mild TBI [47]. One of the major limitations involves the definition of mild TBI, which has varied substantially across studies, along with associated inclusion/exclusion criteria [26, 48]. Most studies have defined mild TBI based on Glasgow Coma Scale scores ranging from 13 to 15 [49], but they have been inconsistent in applying other criteria, such as presence or duration of loss of consciousness (LOC) or posttraumatic amnesia (PTA) [50]. Some previous studies exclude children whose injuries are accompanied by positive findings on neuroimaging (i.e., complicated mild TBI), while some definitions of mild TBI include such children. Many studies have not clearly defined both the lower and upper limits of severity of mild TBI, which can range from brief alterations in mental status without loss of consciousness to more severe signs and symptoms (e.g., LOC, persistent PTA, seizures). Issues of definition and classification are especially problematic in studies of infants and younger children, for whom traditional measures of injury severity such as the Glasgow Coma Scale may not be valid [51].

A related nosological issue concerns the definition and relationship of concussion versus mild TBI [52, 53]. The terms are often used interchangeably. However, some have argued that they are distinct disorders, with concussion being less severe than mild TBI, while others see them as overlapping but not identical, most often viewing concussion as a subset of mild TBI; yet others have taken an opposing perspective, viewing mild TBI as a subset of all concussion. The lack of a single and specific diagnostic nosology for classifying the different types of mild TBI at different stages post-injury represents a significant barrier to progress in the field.

Outcome Measurement

PCS are typically measured using questionnaires and rating scales, often completed by both children and their parents. Parent–child agreement regarding PCS is significant but modest [54, 55], suggesting that both child and parent's reports should be explored in studies of mild TBI. Only parent ratings may be available for infants and younger children, but the validity of ratings in that age range warrants further investigation. The reporting of PCS may also depend on the format for symptom reporting. For example, in adults, rating scales elicit reports of more symptoms than do open-ended structured interviews [56, 57].

Previous studies have also frequently treated PCS as if they occur along a single dimension. However, research indicates that PCS in children with mild TBI are multidimensional, with clear distinctions between somatic, cognitive, and emotional symptoms [58, 59]. The dimensions of PCS not only can be distinguished psychometrically, but also follow distinct trajectories following mild TBI [8]. They also appear to be distinct from other kinds of symptoms, such as those associated with posttraumatic stress disorder [60, 61].

The definition and measurement of persistent PCS is a key methodological and conceptual issue. Many definitions of persistent PCS are based on a simple count of new or worse symptoms, while other definitions are based on standardized measures of change (e.g., reliable change or normative definitions). A recent study showed that misclassification rates among healthy children were higher for simple versus standardized change definitions [62]. Although inter-method agreement was superior among standardized change algorithms, significant variation existed for identifying children with mild TBI who had "recovered" (i.e., those who did not meet individual criteria for PPCS) across definitions, calling into question the true incidence rate of PPCS. Importantly, the findings raise significant concern about the use of simple change scores for diagnosis of PPCS in clinical settings.

Assessment of Risk Factors

The assessment of risk factors that predict outcomes following mild TBI has been problematic. Most studies have not adequately characterized the severity of children's injuries. Children with mild TBI are often treated as a homogenous group, without regard to whether factors such as LOC or abnormalities on neuroimaging increase the risk of negative outcomes. Advanced neuroimaging techniques, such as susceptibility-weighted and diffusion tensor imaging, may also provide a more sensitive assessment of injury severity in mild TBI [63–66].

Research also needs to incorporate measures of non-injury-related risk factors as possible predictors. In many cases, children with premorbid learning or behavior problems are omitted from studies, although they may be at particular risk for persistent postconcussive symptoms [14]. As noted earlier, a variety of non-injury factors are likely relevant to the prediction of PCS and may moderate its occurrence after mild TBI, including children's premorbid cognitive ability and coping skills [39, 40], demographic factors and socioeconomic status [8, 22], and parent and family functioning [22, 36, 43, 44].

Prediction Versus Moderation

Research on the prediction of PCS often fails to distinguish between predictors and moderators, yet this distinction is critical to understanding whether a particular risk factor is specifically associated with worse outcomes among children with mild TBI versus children in general. A relevant example is the role of sex or gender as a risk factor for PCS. Many existing studies of sex differences lack a comparison group of healthy children or children with injuries not involving the head, and instead simply compare males and females with mild TBI. However, the absence of a comparison group precludes any determination of whether sex actually moderates the effects of mild TBI versus simply accounting for variation in outcomes in a nonspecific fashion, irrespective of mild TBI [35]. Similar concerns can be raised about many studies pertaining to other risk factors. The inclusion of appropriate comparison groups, and testing of statistical interactions between group status and risk factors, is necessary to conclude that any risk factor moderates the likelihood of PCS specifically after mild TBI.

Alternative Explanations

Previous research has rarely considered potential alternative explanations for persistent PCS, such as response validity, pain, and symptom exaggeration. Performance on response validity testing has been shown to account for substantial variance in cognitive test performance among children with mild TBI [67], although it did not account for group differences in PCS in other studies [38, 68]. Pain has not been widely examined, but it is a common consequence of mild TBI and may contribute to poor cognitive test performance and also exacerbate related symptom complaints [69]. Finally, some children or parents may be prone to symptom exaggeration, perhaps because of the lay expectations associated with mild TBI [70]. Research that incorporates indices of symptom exaggeration may help to determine whether reports of PCS after mild TBI are influenced by such expectations.

Timing of Outcome Assessment

Research on mild TBI has often been cross-sectional and focused on relatively short-term outcomes. This problem is compounded in some studies by retrospective recruitment of participants from among clinical referrals or hospital admissions, resulting in significant ascertainment bias. Prospective and longitudinal studies of unselected samples are necessary to examine how the relationship of risk factors to PCS varies post-injury [22, 29].

The timing of assessments is particularly critical in longitudinal studies [71]. Acute post-injury assessments are often desirable, not only to document the immediate effects of mild TBI, but also to obtain retrospective measures of children's premorbid symptoms as soon as possible after the injury and thereby increase the validity of parent recall. The timing of subsequent assessments should be based in part on the expected course of recovery following mild TBI. Given that research suggests that PCS resolve in 2–3 months in most cases of mild TBI [6, 8], more frequent assessment during the first few weeks to months post-injury is warranted. However, longer-term assessments are needed to determine whether PCS result in significant ongoing impairment in children's social or academic functioning.

Prediction of Individual Outcomes

Studies of mild TBI have focused on outcomes at a group level, in part because most common statistical techniques yield results that are based on group averages. Thus, most research on the prediction of PCS is variable-centered and reflects only group trends [72]. In clinical practice, however, we want to know whether mild TBI is likely to be followed by persistent PCS in a particular patient. One way to focus on individual outcomes is to divide children with mild TBI into subgroups based on certain characteristics and then determine if outcomes are different for children in the different subgroups. Parsing a sample of children with mild TBI into those with versus those without LOC or neuroimaging abnormalities exemplifies this approach [8].

A second approach is to identify individuals with a given outcome, such as persistent PCS, and then determine the risk factors linked to this outcome [28]. For instance, analyses of reliable change also can be used to identify individual children who display unusually large increases in PCS compared to pre-injury estimates and to study the risk factors associated with such increases [73]. Figure 15.2 is drawn from a study of reliable change in PCS after mild TBI. The figure shows the proportion of children with mild TBI showing reliable increases in somatic symptoms as a function of loss consciousness or abnormalities on magnetic resonance imaging, as compared to children with orthopedic injuries [13].

Advanced statistical techniques can assist in the prediction of individual outcomes. Growth curve modeling permits the investigation of change at an individual level in relation to multiple risk factors [8]. Mixture modeling can be used to empirically derive latent classes of individuals [74]; for instance, subtypes of children with mild TBI can be identified based on initial clinical presentation or on different symptom trajectories [75]. Figure 15.3 provides an example of this approach; it shows symptom trajectories of PCS in children with mild TBI and orthopedic injuries [27]. In this study, children with mild TBI were more likely than those with orthopedic injuries to demonstrate trajectories involving high acute levels of PCS. Moreover, children with mild TBI whose acute clinical presentation reflected

Fig. 15.2 Probability of reliable change in somatic symptoms as a function of group membership. Children with mild TBI are divided into those (**a**) with and without LOC and (**b**) with and without abnormalities on MRI. (Modified with permission from Yeates et al. [13]. © 2012 by American Medical Association)

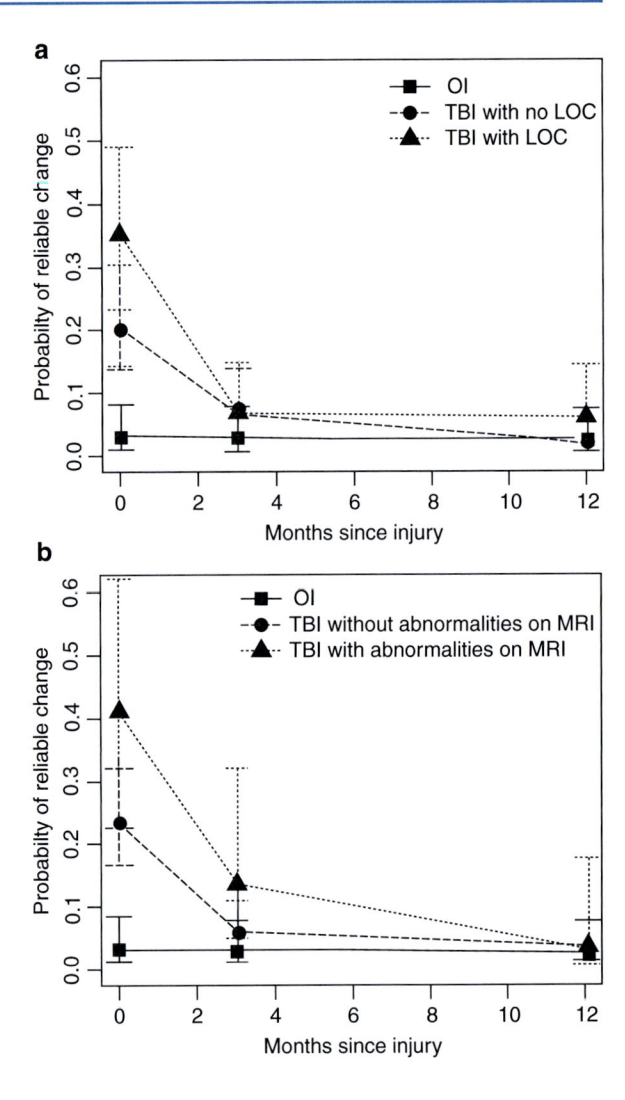

more severe injury were especially likely to demonstrate such trajectories, in contrast to those with mild TBI with less severe acute presentations.

Building Prognostic Models and Decision Rules

In the long run, prognostic models and decision rules are needed so that clinicians can use them to predict which children with mild TBI will demonstrate persistent PCS. To be clinically useful, research on outcome prediction must be methodologically rigorous [76]. Sample sizes need to be relatively large. Predictors should be selected based on previous research and expert opinion. The number of predictors

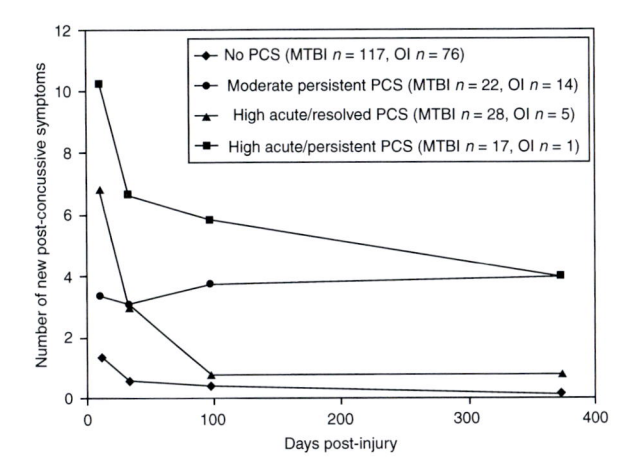

Fig. 15.3 Illustration of developmental trajectory analysis of postconcussive symptoms in children with mild TBI (mTBI) or orthopedic injuries (OI). Four latent groups were identified on the basis of the number of new postconcussive symptoms reported at four occasions post-injury, irrespective of whether participants were in the mTBI or OI group. (Modified with permission from Yeates et al. [27]. © 2009 by American Academy of Pediatrics)

should be kept reasonably small, to avoid overfitting of models. Both outcomes and predictors need to be defined precisely, measured with good reliability, and readily obtainable. Statistical models should use valid approaches to managing missing data and appropriate techniques for the selection of predictors and estimation of prognostic effects. Model performance needs to be assessed in terms of both calibration (i.e., agreement between observed outcome frequencies and predicted probabilities) and discrimination of those with versus without persistent PCS. Models need to be validated, and the results of modeling should be presented in a readily applicable format.

A recent seminal study that incorporated these features sought to derive and validate a clinical risk score for persistent PCS among children presenting to the emergency department (ED) with acute concussion [26]. The study included 3063 children aged 5–17 years who were seen at 9 EDs and were then assessed for PCS at 4 weeks post-injury. The sample was split into derivation and validation cohorts. Statistical modeling was used to develop a 12-point risk score, as shown in Table 15.1, based on the variables of female sex; age of 13 years or older; physician-diagnosed migraine history; prior concussion with symptoms lasting longer than 1 week; symptoms of headache, sensitivity to noise, fatigue; answering questions slowly on clinical exam; and errors on balance testing. The risk score discriminated between children with and without persistent PCS with modest accuracy and performed substantially better than physician prediction alone. The risk score holds significant promise as a tool for improving clinical care of mild TBI.

Table 15.1 Clinical risk score for predicting persistent postconcussive symptoms at 4 weeks post-injury in children presenting to the emergency department

Predictors	Number of risk points for persistent postconcussive symptoms
Age group, years	
5–7	0
8–12	1
13–< 18	2
Sex	
Male	0
Female	2
Prior concussion and symptom duration	
No prior concussion; symptom duration <1 week	0
Prior concussion; symptom duration ≥1 week	1
Physician-diagnosed migraine history	
No	0
Yes	1
Observed answering questions slowly	
No	0
Yes	1
Balance error scoring system tandem stance no. of errors	
0–3	0
≥ 4 or physically unable to undergo testing	1
Headache reported	
No	0
Yes	1
Sensitivity to noise reported	
No	0
Yes	1
Fatigue reported	
No	0
Yes	2

Future Directions

Future research on the prediction of PCS after mild TBI in children must adopt a biopsychosocial approach that acknowledges the contributions of risk factors at multiple levels of analysis—biological, psychological, and environmental. At the biological level, genetic and epigenetic variables may play an important role. The apolipoprotein E gene has not been found to predict PCS after mild TBI in children [77], but many other candidate genes should be examined [78]. Research at the biological level may also yield more sensitive and precise measures of brain injury that predict outcomes. For instance, various fluid biomarkers and advanced neuroimaging techniques are being considered both as indicators of underlying brain injury in mild TBI and possible predictors of PCS [79, 80].

At the psychological level, future research may identify more sensitive measures of the effects of mild TBI on cognitive functioning. Computerized testing has the advantage of being able to assess reaction time, which has been shown to be sensitive to concussion [38]. More research is needed to determine if early post-injury cognitive deficits predict persistent PCS. Research on children's psychological characteristics, such as somatization and psychological resilience, also will be important for understanding the risk of persistent PCS.

Finally, at the environmental level, further research is needed to clarify which aspects of the family and broader social environment are related to the occurrence of PCS following mild TBI in children [22, 44]. The identification of interventions that can reduce the risk of PCS also will be critically important. Clinical trials and comparative effectiveness studies of both pharmacological and non-pharmacological interventions are needed [81].

For future research to have the greatest impact, the methodological issues reviewed earlier need to be addressed. Researchers need to find a common diagnostic nosology with clear criteria, and also a shared definition of persistent PCS. Large prospective studies of children with mild TBI and appropriate comparison groups that assess both injury-related and non-injury-related risk factors are needed to refine existing prognostic models and decision rules for predicting PCS [82]. The use of common data elements will enable harmonization of studies and pooling of data that can be assessed using advanced statistical techniques such as machine learning [83].

A key long-term goal for research on the outcomes of mild TBI is to further develop prognostic models and decision rules to incorporate developmental considerations and allow for individual variability in the importance of different risk factors. Ideally, these advances will enable clinicians to provide parents and children with evidence-based information regarding the effects of mild TBI and to identify those children who are most at risk for demonstrating negative outcomes. Healthcare providers can then target at-risk children and their families for appropriate management [84].

Acknowledgments Portions of this manuscript were published in the first edition of this book. The work was supported by grant R01HD76885 from the National Institutes of Health and grant FDN143304 from the Canadian Institutes of Health Research to the author.

References

1. Centers for Disease Control and Prevention. Surveillance report of traumatic brain injury-related emergency department visits, hospitalizations, and deaths—United States, 2014. Centers for Disease Control and Prevention, U.S. Department of Health and Human Services. 2019.
2. Zogg CK, Haring RS, Xu L, Canner JK, AlSulaim HA, Hashmi ZG, et al. The epidemiology of pediatric head injury treated outside of hospital emergency departments. Epidemiology. 2018;28:269–79.
3. Bryan MA, Rowhani-Rahbar A, Comstock D, Rivara F, on behalf of the Seattle Sports Concussion Research Collaborative. Sports- and recreation-related concussions in US youth. Pediatrics. 2016;138:e20154635.
4. Babikian T, Asarnow R. Neurocognitive outcomes and recovery after pediatric TBI: meta-analytic review of the literature. Neuropsychology. 2009;23:283–96.

5. Carroll LJ, Cassidy JD, Peloso PM, Borg J, von Holst H, et al. Prognosis for mild traumatic brain injury: results of the WHO collaborating centre task force on mild traumatic brain injury. J Rehabil Med. 2004;43(Suppl):84–105.
6. Davis GA, Anderson V, Babl FE, Gioia GA, Giza CC, et al. What is the difference in concussion management in children as compared to adults? A systematic review. Br J Sports Med. 2017;51·949–57.
7. Barlow KM, Crawford S, Stevenson A, Sandhu SS, Belanger F, Dewey D. Epidemiology of postconcussion syndrome in pediatric mild traumatic brain injury. Pediatrics. 2010;126:e374–81.
8. Taylor HG, Dietrich A, Nuss K, Wright M, Rusin J, et al. Post-concussive symptoms in children with mild traumatic brain injury. Neuropsychology. 2010;24:148–59.
9. Yeates KO. Mild traumatic brain injury and postconcussive symptoms in children and adolescents. J Int Neuropsychol Soc. 2010;16:953–60.
10. McKinlay A, Dalrymple-Alford JC, Horwood LJ, Fergusson DM. Long term psychosocial outcomes after mild head injury in early childhood. J Neurol Neurosurg Psychiatry. 2002;73:281–8.
11. Moran LM, Taylor HG, Rusin J, Bangert B, Dietrich A, Nuss KE, Wright M, Minich N, Yeates KO. Quality of life in pediatric mild traumatic brain injury and its relationship to postconcussive symptoms. J Pediatr Psychol. 2012;37:736–44.
12. Novak Z, Aglipay M, Barrowman N, Yeates KO, Beauchamp MH, et al., on behalf of the Pediatric Emergency Research Canada (PERC) 5P Concussion Team. Association of persistent post-concussion symptoms with pediatric quality of life. JAMA Pediatr. 2016;170:e162900.
13. Yeates KO, Kaizar E, Rusin J, Bangert B, Dietrich A, et al. Reliable change in post-concussive symptoms and its functional consequences among children with mild traumatic brain injury. Arch Pediatr Adolesc Med. 2012;166:585–684.
14. Zemek RL, Farion KJ, Sampson M, McGahern C. Prognosticators of persistent symptoms following pediatric concussion: a systematic review. JAMA Pediatr. 2013;167:259–65.
15. Yeates KO, Taylor HG. Neurobehavioral outcomes of mild head injury in children and adolescents. Pediatr Rehabil. 2005;8:5–16.
16. Wallander JL, Varni JW. Adjustment in children with chronic physical disorders: programmatic research on a disability-stress-coping model. In: La Greca AM, Siegal L, Wallander JL, Walker CE, editors. Stress and coping with pediatric conditions. New York: Guilford Press; 1992. p. 279–98.
17. Thompson RJ, Gil KM, Keith BR, Gustafson KE, George LK, Kinney TR. Psychological adjustment of children with sickle cell disease: stability and change over a 10-month period. J Consult Clin Psychol. 1994;62:856–60.
18. Kay T, Newman B, Cavallo M, Ezrachi O, Resnik M. Toward a neuropsychological model of functional disability after mild traumatic brain injury. Neuropsychology. 1992;6:371–84.
19. Wood RL. Understanding the 'miserable minority': a diathesis-stress paradigm for post-concussional syndrome. Brain Inj. 2004;18:1135–53.
20. Kenzie ES, Parks EL, Bigler ED, Wright D, Lim MM, et al. The dynamics of concussion: mapping pathophysiology, persistence, and recovery with causal-loop diagramming. Front Neurol. 2018;9:203.
21. McCrea M, Broshek DK, Barth JT. Sports concussion assessment and management: future research directions. Brain Inj. 2015;29:276–82.
22. McNally KA, Bangert B, Dietrich A, Nuss K, Rusin J, et al. Injury versus non-injury factors as predictors of post-concussive symptoms following mild traumatic brain injury in children. Neuropsychology. 2013;27:1–12.
23. Bijur PE, Haslum M, Golding J. Cognitive outcomes of multiple head injuries in children. J Dev Behav Pediatr. 1996;17:143–8.
24. Collins MW, Lowell MR, Iverson GL, Cantu RC, Maroon JC, Field M. Cumulative effects of concussion in high school athletes. Neurosurgery. 2002;51:1175–81.
25. Eisenberg MA, Andrea J, Meehan W, Mannix R. Time interval between concussions and symptom duration. Pediatrics. 2013;132:1–10.

26. Zemek R, Barrowman N, Freedman SB, Gravel J, Gagnon I, et al., for the Pediatric Emergency Research Canada (PERC) 5P Concussion Team. Clinical risk score for persistent post-concussion symptoms among children with acute concussion presenting to the emergency department. JAMA. 2016;315:1014–25.
27. Yeates KO, Taylor HG, Rusin J, Bangert B, Dietrich A, et al. Longitudinal trajectories of postconcussive symptoms in children with mild traumatic brain injuries and their relationship to acute clinical status. Pediatrics. 2009;123:735–43.
28. McCrea M, Guskiewicz K, Randolph C, Barr WB, Hammeke TA, et al. Incidence, clinical course, and predictors of prolonged recovery time following sports-related concussion in high school and college athletes. J Int Neuropsychol Soc. 2012;18:1–12.
29. Ponsford J, Willmott C, Rothwell A, Cameron P, Ayton G, et al. Cognitive and behavioral outcomes following mild traumatic head injury in children. J Head Trauma Rehabil. 1999;14:360–72.
30. Babcock L, Byczkowski T, Wade SL, Ho M, Mookerjee S, Bazarian JJ. Predicting postconcussion syndrome after mild traumatic brain injury in children and adolescents who present to the emergency department. JAMA Pediatr. 2013;167:156–61.
31. Levin HS, Hanten G, Roberson G, Li X, Ewing-Cobbs L, et al. Prediction of cognitive sequelae based on abnormal computed tomography findings in children following mild traumatic brain injury. J Neurosurg Pediatr. 2008;1:461–70.
32. McKinlay A, Grace RC, Horwood LJ, Fergusson DM, MacFarlane MR. Long-term behavioural outcomes of pre-school mild traumatic brain injury. Child Care Health Dev. 2010;36:22–30.
33. Lumba-Brown A, Tang K, Yeates KO, Zemek R, for the Pediatric Emergency Research Canada 5P Concussion Team. Post-concussion symptom burden in children following motor vehicle collisions. J Am Coll Emerg Physicians Open. 2020;1(5):938–46.
34. Anderson V, Davis GA, Takagi M, Dunne K, Clarke C, et al. Trajectories and predictors of clinician-determined recovery after child concussion. J Neurotrauma. 2020;37:1392–400.
35. Yeates TM, Taylor HG, Bigler ED, Minich NM, Tang K, et al. Sex differences in the outcomes of mild traumatic brain injury in children presenting to the emergency department. J Neurotrauma. 2021; https://doi.org/10.1089/neu.2020.7470.
36. Ollson KA, Lloyd OT, Lebrocque RM, McKinlay L, Anderson VA, Kennardy JA. Predictors of post-concussion symptoms at 6 and 18 months following mild traumatic brain injury. Brain Inj. 2013;27:145–57.
37. Iverson GL, Gardner AJ, Terry DP, Ponsford JL, Sills AK, et al. Predictors of clinical recovery from concussion: a systematic review. Br J Sports Med. 2017;51:941–8.
38. Chadwick L, Roth E, Minich NM, Taylor HG, Bigler ED, et al. Cognitive outcomes in children with mild traumatic brain injury: an examination using the National Institutes of Health Toolbox Cognition Battery. J Neurotrauma. 2021; https://doi.org/10.1089/neu.2020.7513.
39. Fay TB, Yeates KO, Taylor HG, Bangert B, Dietrich A, et al. Cognitive reserve as a moderator of postconcussive symptoms in children with complicated and uncomplicated mild traumatic brain injury. J Int Neuropsychol Soc. 2009;16:94–105.
40. Woodrome SE, Yeates KO, Taylor HG, Rusin J, Bangert B, et al. Coping strategies as a predictor of post-concussive symptoms in children with mild traumatic brain injury versus mild orthopedic injury. J Int Neuropsychol Soc. 2011;17:317–26.
41. Durish CL, Yeates KO, Brooks BL. Psychological resilience as a predictor of symptom severity in adolescents with poor recovery following concussion. J Int Neuropsychol Soc. 2019;25:346–54.
42. Grubenhoff JA, Currie D, Comstock RD, Juarez-Colunga E, Bajaj L, Kirkwood MW. Psychological factors associated with delayed symptom resolution in children with concussion. J Pediatr. 2016;174:27–32.
43. Ganesalingam K, Yeates KO, Ginn MS, Taylor HG, Dietrich A, et al. Family burden and parental distress following mild traumatic brain injury in children and its relationship to postconcussive symptoms. J Pediatr Psychol. 2008;33:621–9.
44. Yeates KO, Taylor HG, Rusin J, Bangert B, Dietrich A, et al. Premorbid child and family functioning as predictors of post-concussive symptoms in children with mild traumatic brain injuries. Int J Dev Neurosci. 2012;30:231–7.

45. Yeates KO, Taylor HG, Drotar D, Wade SL, Klein S, et al. Pre-injury family environment as a determinant of recovery from traumatic brain injuries in school-age children. J Int Neuropsychol Soc. 1997;3:617–30.
46. Ewing-Cobbs L, Cox CS, Clark AE, Holubkov R, Keenan HT. Persistent postconcussion symptoms after injury. Pediatrics. 2018;142:e20180939.
47. Dikmen SS, Levin HS. Methodological issues in the study of mild head injury. J Head Trauma Rehabil. 1993;8:30–7.
48. Williams DH, Levin HS, Eisenberg HM. Mild head injury classification. Neurosurgery. 1990;27:422–8.
49. Teasdale G, Jennett B. Assessment of coma and impaired consciousness: a practical scale. Lancet. 1974;2:81–4.
50. Crowe LM, Hearps S, Anderson V, Broland ML, Phillips N, et al. Investigating the variability in mild traumatic brain injury definitions: a prospective cohort study. Arch Phys Med Rehabil. 2018;99:1360–9.
51. Durham SR, Clancy RR, Leuthardt E, Sun P, Kamerling S, et al. CHOP infant coma scale ('infant face scale'): a novel coma scale for children less than 2 years of age. J Neurotrauma. 2000;17:729–37.
52. Bodin D, Yeates KO, Klamar K. Definition and classification of concussion. In: Apps JN, Walter KD, editors. Pediatric and adolescent concussion: diagnosis, management, and outcome. New York: Springer; 2012. p. 9–20.
53. Mayer AR, Quinn DK, Master CL. The spectrum of mild traumatic brain injury: a review. Neurology. 2017;89:623–321.
54. Gagnon I, Teel E, Gioia G, Aglipay M, Barrowman N, et al. Parent-child agreement on post-concussion symptoms in the acute postinjury period. Pediatrics. 2020;146:e20192317.
55. Hajek CA, Yeates KO, Taylor HG, Bangert B, Dietrich A, et al. Agreement between parents and children on ratings of postconcussive symptoms following mild traumatic brain injury. Child Neuropsychol. 2011;17:17–33.
56. Iverson GL, Brooks BL, Ashton VL, Lange RT. Interview versus questionnaire symptom reporting in people with the postconcussion syndrome. J Head Trauma Rehabil. 2010;25:23–30.
57. Nolin P, Villemure R, Heroux L. Determining long-term symptoms following mild traumatic brain injury: method of interview affects self-report. Brain Inj. 2006;20:1147–54.
58. Ayr LK, Yeates KO, Taylor HG, Browne M. Dimensions of post-concussive symptoms in children with mild traumatic brain injuries. J Int Neuropsychol Soc. 2009;15:19–30.
59. Gioia GA, Schneider JC, Vaughan CG, Isquith PK. Which symptom assessments and approaches are uniquely appropriate for paediatric concussion? Br J Sports Med. 2009;43(Suppl):i13–22.
60. Bryant RA, Harvey AG. Post-concussive symptoms and posttraumatic stress disorder after mild traumatic brain injury. J Nerv Ment Dis. 1999;187:302–5.
61. Hajek CA, Yeates KO, Taylor HG, Bangert B, Dietrich A, et al. Relationships among postconcussive symptoms and symptoms of PTSD in children following mild traumatic brain injury. Brain Inj. 2010;24:100–9.
62. Mayer AR, Stephenson DD, Dodd AB, Robertson-Benta CR, Reddy SP, et al. A comparison of methods for classifying persistent post-concussive symptoms in children. J Neurotrauma. 2020;37(13):1504–11.
63. Ashwal S, Tong KA, Bartnik-Olson B, Holshouser BA. Neuroimaging. In: Kirkwood MW, Yeates KO, editors. Mild traumatic brain injury in children and adolescents: from basic science to clinical management. New York: Guilford Press; 2012. p. 162–95.
64. Beauchamp MH, Ditchfield M, Babl FE, Kean M, Catroppa C, Yeates KO, Anderson V. Detecting traumatic brain lesions in children: CT vs MRI vs susceptibility weighted imaging (SWI). J Neurotrauma. 2011;28:915–27.
65. Chu Z, Wilde EA, Hunter JV, McCauley SR, Bigler ED, et al. Voxel-based analysis of diffusion tensor imaging in mild traumatic brain injury in adolescents. AJNR Am J Neuroradiol. 2010;31:340–6.

66. Ware A, Shukla A, Lebel C, Goodrich-Hunsaker N, Abildskov A, et al. Post-acute white matter microstructure predicts post-acute and chronic post-concussive symptom severity following mild traumatic brain injury in children. Neuroimage Clin. 2020;25:102106.
67. Kirkwood M, Yeates KO, Randolph C, Kirk J. The implications of symptom validity test failure for ability-based test performance in a pediatric sample. Psychol Assess. 2012;24:36–45.
68. Sroufe NS, Fuller DS, West BT, Singal BM, Warschausky SA, Maio RF. Postconcussive symptoms and neurocognitive function after mild traumatic brain injury in children. Pediatrics. 2010;125:e1331–9.
69. Kwan V, Vo M, Noel M, Yeates KO. A scoping review of pain in children following traumatic brain injury: is there more than headache? J Neurotrauma. 2018;35:877–88.
70. Mittenberg W, DiGiulio DV, Perrin S, Bass AE. Symptoms following mild head injury: expectation as aetiology. J Neurol Neurosurg Psychiatry. 1992;55:200–4.
71. Taylor HG, Alden J. Age-related differences in outcome following childhood brain injury: an introduction and overview. J Int Neuropsychol Soc. 1997;3:555–67.
72. Laursen B, Hoff E. Person-centered and variable-centered approaches to longitudinal data. Merrill Palmer Q (Wayne State Univ Press). 2006;52:377–89.
73. McCrea M, Barr WB, Guskiewicz K, Randolph C, Marshall SW, et al. Standard regression-based methods for measuring recovery after sport-related concussion. J Int Neuropsychol Soc. 2005;11:58–69.
74. Nagin DS. Group-based modeling of development. Cambridge, MA: Harvard University Press; 2005.
75. Yeates KO, Tang K, Barrowman N, Freedman SB, Gravel J, et al., for the Pediatric Emergency Research Canada (PERC) Predicting Persistent Postconcussive Problems in Pediatrics (5P) Concussion Team. Derivation and initial validation of clinical phenotypes of children presenting with concussion acutely in the emergency department: latent class analysis of a multicentre, prospective cohort, observational study. J Neurotrauma. 2019;36:1758–67.
76. Mushkudiani NA, Hukkelhoven CWPM, Hernandez AV, Murray GD, Choi SC, et al. A systematic review finds methodological improvements necessary for prognostic models in determining traumatic brain injury outcomes. J Clin Epidemiol. 2008;61:331–43.
77. Moran LM, Taylor HG, Ganesalingam K, Gastier-Foster JM, Frick J, et al. Apolipoprotein E4 as a predictor of outcomes in pediatric mild traumatic brain injury. J Neurotrauma. 2009;26:1489–95.
78. Kurowski BG, Treble-Barna A, Pilipenko V, Wade SL, Yeates KO, et al. Genetic influences on behavioral outcomes after childhood TBI: a novel systems biology-informed approach. Front Genet. 2019;10:481.
79. Mannix R, Levy R, Zemek R, Yeates KO, Arbogast K, et al. Fluid biomarkers of pediatric mild traumatic brain injury: a systematic review. J Neuro-Oncol. 2020;37:2029–44.
80. Mayer AR, Kaushal M, Dodd AB, Hanlon FM, Shaff NA, et al. Advanced biomarkers of pediatric mild traumatic brain injury: progress and perils. Neurosci Biobehav Rev. 2018;94:149–65.
81. Mannix R, Zemek R, Yeates KO, Atabaki S, Badway M, et al. Practice patterns in pharmacological and non-pharmacological therapies for children with mild traumatic brain injury: a survey of 15 Canadian and United States centers. J Neurotrauma. 2019;36:2886–94.
82. Yeates KO, Beauchamp M, Craig W, Doan Q, Zemek R, et al., on behalf of Pediatric Emergency Research Canada. Advancing Concussion Assessment in Pediatrics (A-CAP): a prospective, concurrent cohort, longitudinal study of mild traumatic brain injury in children: study protocol. BMJ Open. 2017;7:e017012.
83. Broglio SP, Kontos AP, Levin H, Schneider K, Wilde EA, et al., on behalf of the Sport-Related Concussion CDE Working Group. The National Institute of Neurological Disorders and Stroke and Department of Defense sport-related concussion common data elements version 1.0 recommendations. J Neurotrauma. 2018;35:2276–783.
84. Kirkwood MW, Yeates KO, Taylor HG, Randolph C, McCrea M, Anderson VA. Management of pediatric mild traumatic brain injury: a neuropsychological review from injury through recovery. Clin Neuropsychol. 2008;22:769–800.

Long-Term Effects of Pediatric Mild Traumatic Brain Injury

16

Rimma Danov

Introduction

While there might be some discrepancy in the reported rates of pediatric brain injury among numerous published studies, younger children tend to have higher rates of brain injury than older children (based on emergency room visits: 0–4-year-old group rate is 1256 per 100,000 versus 15–19-year-old group rate is 757 per 100,000 children) [1]. Sixteen percent of children under 10 years of age sustain at least one traumatic brain injury (TBI) [1] and approximately 80% of these head injuries are mild [2]. According to the National Pediatric Trauma Registry, about 76% of all pediatric brain injuries are mild and only 10% are moderate and 15% are severe [3]. Given these staggering rates, brain injury presents a significant health risk to children, and even the mild form of brain injury may sometimes create significant obstacles in children's lives at home and in school.

The most recent consensus statement regarding concussion, or mild TBI, is that while it may cause neuropathological changes, they are largely associated with functional deficits rather than structural abnormalities, wherein the latter are traditionally detected by neuroimaging [4]. Thus, thousands of children every year sustain mild head injuries and experience various neuropathological changes that greatly affect their academic, behavioral, emotional, and cognitive functioning. While the majority of children with mild TBI recover within the first few weeks or months, a subgroup of these children continues to suffer from persistent cognitive and emotional deficits that compromise their academic performance, social interactions, and emotional stability.

R. Danov (✉)
Private Neuropsychology Clinic, Brooklyn, NY, USA
e-mail: drdanov@neuropsychnyc.com

The actual number of children with mild TBI who are unfortunate to experience long-term functional deficits varies from author to author. Kraus [5] showed that only 10% of children with closed head injury experienced moderate disability. Bruce and Schut [6] concluded that approximately 50% of children continue to experience some form of long-term cognitive deficits post TBI. Other authors have determined that 11% of children in their research sample displayed symptoms 3 months after a mild brain injury and 2.3% of this sample continued to display cognitive and emotional symptoms 1 year later [7]. Thus, while researchers utilize various outcome measures of post-TBI symptoms and focus on different age groups, which likely generates the diversity in rates and severity of functional dysfunction and neuropsychological symptoms, one fact remains clear: a lot of children sustain relatively mild head injuries and appear seemingly well after the first few months post TBI, when pain, scrapes, and bumps disappear, but some of them continue to suffer from disturbing cognitive and emotional symptoms.

Even if only 2–10% of children with a mild brain injury are struggling to learn in school, appropriately interact with peers and adults, and keep up with the increasing social and academic demands, it is important to advance our understanding of a mild TBI in order to help these children. So far, our current knowledge about structural and metabolic changes that occur at different points of time after a mild brain injury point to the need to reassess, intervene, and address the long-term post-TBI deficits at different points of time, in addition to most immediate post-injury care. Such protracted cognitive, emotional, and behavioral difficulties should be addressed as soon as they arise, even if they become pronounced sometime after the injury, so that these children can receive the needed treatment and return to their normal developmental trajectory.

Short-Term Versus Long-Term Post-Concussion Symptoms

Common short-term cognitive symptoms of pediatric brain injury, such as impaired attention, processing speed, visual perception, working memory, motor functioning, emotional lability, and hyperactivity have been observed and documented by numerous studies over the years [8]. It appears that these symptoms may affect virtually all areas of functioning in children. For instance, in addition to having trouble sustaining focus, quickly and accurately processing new information, and retaining new facts, concussed children tend to have fewer friends and experience poor social skills and increased emotional lability [9, 10]. Their family relationships may be compromised as well [11] and their academic performance is likely to decline [11, 12].

Moreover, Wozniak and his group [13] showed that traumatic injury to the white matter in the supracallosal region is specifically related to overt behavioral deficits, such as hyperactivity, aggression, and attention deficit. In this study, while children with mild and moderate brain injury did not differ from controls in general intelligence scores, their sustained focus and behavioral and emotional regulation were impaired when assessed 6–12 months after the brain injury. This finding is very important in the understanding of post-TBI functioning and performance, as it illustrates that, unlike the core intellectual abilities, which remain largely resilient to a mild white matter trauma, regulatory functions and efficiency skills are much more susceptible to impairment. This is a critical aspect of post-TBI life, as regulatory functions and efficiency skills are essential functions that allow one to utilize core intellectual abilities while completing academic tasks, listening to and following daily directions, and navigating social conflicts and relationships.

As our understanding of mild TBI expands, we see that many children may quickly recover from the external head trauma and return to school, but some of them remain irritable, easily angered, hyperactive and fidgety, have difficulty sustaining focus, effectively planning and organizing their activities and study material, adequately capturing and processing new concepts and rules, retaining new facts, and retrieving information they have recently learned. They may also omit or misread social cues and display inappropriate reactions to daily stressors and changes in their environment. As we know, cognitive skills, academic abilities, and emotional stability are closely intertwined in many educational and social activities that children engage in a daily basis. Thus, it is difficult to separate where poor focus and retention problems end and irritability and frustration begin, when a child fails to listen to and follow directions, inhibit impulses, and sustain his focus to solve a math problem and, instead, fidgets and talks in class and disrupts his classmates. As a result, while these children have seemingly recovered from their mild head injury that they might have sustained on a playground or while playing sports, their entire life, including behaviors, relationships, and academic performance, come under assault of residual cognitive deficits and mood changes that cause ongoing disruption and anguish.

Over the past decades, we have learned a lot about the immediate head injury symptoms that children may experience during the first days and weeks post TBI. While immediate symptoms of a mild brain injury in children have been extensively documented, more recent research studies focus on identifying long-term cognitive symptoms, such as memory impairment that persists in some children 2 years post TBI [14]. Barlow and her colleagues [7] investigated mild brain injury in children and showed that 11% of children displayed post-concussion symptoms 3 months after the injury, and 1 year later these symptoms were still seen in 2.3% of injured children. These studies help us develop a better understanding of how and why some children's recovery patterns differ from the majority of their peers, who have also sustained a mild TBI, and how persistent post-injury symptoms alter their normal developmental trajectory.

We can glean answers to these questions from the unique developmental processes that take place in a growing child's brain. Children's brain differs significantly from the adult brain and it is not just by virtue of being less mature or less capable. There are multiple developmental processes that are constantly changing the matrix of a child's brain, making it more or less sensitive to various brain insults, treatment efforts, and environmental changes and stressors. Some of those developmental factors include ongoing myelination, sensitivity to oxidative stress, higher water content, open sutures, and brain plasticity [15, 16]. In fact, it is believed that maturation of white matter continues until approximately 30 years of age, as summarized by Maxwell in 2012. Since the brain development is such a fluid process, any insult to the growing brain at any specific time would technically produce a different outcome because the brain was at a different state of the development, with certain developmental goals already accomplished and certain developmental goals still at various stages of completion.

Over the past two decades, several authors have suggested that the damage caused by a traumatic injury to a developing brain can interfere with such processes as neuronal myelination and frontal lobe maturation [17, 18]. Indeed, during childhood and adolescence, a child's brain is constantly undergoing a major construction of complex cortical networks, making it possible for a child to utilize self-regulation of emotions and behavior, sustain focus on lengthy assignments, organize his belongings and activities, and reflect on, compare, and associate various concepts. It is a complex, multidimensional scaffolding process that would be suspended and/or interrupted if some aspects of it are damaged and cannot, at least for some period of time, play their role in advancing the higher order skills and supporting the associated cerebral functions. Levin [19] specifically questioned whether diffuse injury, which often occurs in mild brain injury cases, disrupts the development of networks that support higher order cognitive functions in childhood.

Thus, if a mild cerebral insult produces diffuse injury, it may not be always detected by the traditional neuroimaging studies [4]. Yet, it still sets off a disruption of the ongoing myelination and maturation of white matter in a child's brain. How long can this disruption last for before it generates long-lasting effect on the cognitive, academic, and emotional maturity of a child? If some skill development is suspended for some time after the mild TBI, how does it affect the development of associated skills and how long does it take for the specific skill expansion, or evolution, to catch up with its original developmental goal?

Cognitive Impairment and Structural Abnormalities

In the past decades, numerous research findings have provided a tremendous help in understanding the short-term and long-term effects of a focal brain damage on cognitive functioning. For example, studies that used neuropsychological measures of cognitive abilities and MRI results have determined that extrafrontal and temporal lesion volume predicted memory deficits as late as 1 year after brain injury [20]. Also, Power and colleagues [21] concluded that combined frontal and extrafrontal lesions predicted attention deficits 5 years after TBI, while the severity of individual frontal lesions were not predictive of attentional function. Furthermore, other researchers have determined that the uncinate fasciculus area of the brain is sensitive to executive dysfunction in children [22].

However, if a mild TBI produces mainly diffuse white matter injury, which is not always detected by the traditional MRI scans, how can we illuminate the disruption of a complex web of constantly evolving cortical networks and its protracted effect over time on child's functioning at home and in school? Such interruption in the maturation of white matter of a child's brain may not only delay the advancement of the existing skills but also delay the acquisition of more complex abilities. Indeed, in a growing child's brain that undergoes rapid restructuring and layering of cognitive and emotional skills, a delay in maturation of lower-level abilities may significantly disrupt the scaffolding of higher-level abilities. While this hypothesis is not entirely new, recent studies investigating mild TBI have offered more support as they have found persistent cognitive impairments, as measured by neuropsychological tests, correlated with metabolic disruptions and structural impairments in the brain.

It has been noted that conventional MRI can measure small lesions or hemorrhages and MRI findings correlate with neuropsychological and psychiatric outcome, but MRI may also underestimate diffuse axonal injury that is frequently seen in mild TBI [13]. While traditional MRI studies are not always able to detect structural impairment in mild brain injury cases [4], newer neuroimaging techniques, like diffusion tensor imaging (DTI), offer a more precise method of measuring postconcussion changes that occur in the while matter and contribute to persistent postconcussion symptoms and functional impairment months after the mild TBI.

DTI studies measure the integrity of the white matter fibers via diffusion of water molecules [23]. If some axons are damaged and myelin sheath has diminished, the inter-axonal water volume increases. Therefore, DTI can detect injured axons and destroyed myelin even in mild TBI by measuring the integrity of white matter fibers; such axonal injury was observed months after the brain injury [13]. This is a relatively new advancement in the detection of neuronal injury over the traditional MRI scan, which is not able to "see" such minor brain damage. In addition to being able to detect minor, yet important changes in white matter shortly after the brain injury, DTI can detect long-term axonal injuries. For example, Bendlin and colleagues [24] described long-term impairments of white matter, as seen in DTI studies 1 year after the injury. Her group detected specific axonal injury via fractional anisotropy and mean diffusivity reduction that was much greater than normal white matter changes expected in age-matched peers.

Thus, DTI technique allows us to detect some structural abnormalities in concussed individuals that were not visible on traditional neuroimaging studies, but those abnormalities remained for months or more post TBI. While these structural abnormalities might be minor, they are not inconsequential and do contribute to significant functional impairment that disturbs a brain injured child's ability to complete schoolwork, learn new information, develop new skills, and effectively interact with and adapt to his environment. In the recent years, such functional dysfunction, which is traditionally measured by neuropsychological tests, was found to correlate with structural abnormalities, as detected by DTI, further supporting the idea that even mild brain injury may produce long-term cognitive functional impairments in some individuals.

For example, Wozniak and colleagues [13] showed that decreased cortical white matter fractional anisotropy, as measured by DTI, is associated with impaired neurocognitive test scores, mainly with executive functioning and motor speed neuropsychological measures (tests and rating scales) 6–12 months after the injury. This study has shown that children with mild and moderate brain injury had lower fractional anisotropy in three white matter regions—inferior frontal, superior frontal, and supracallosal regions. When DTI study results were compared to neuropsychological test results, fractional anisotropy in frontal and supracallosal regions correlated with neuropsychological test scores on measures of executive functioning, while fractional anisotropy in supracallosal region correlated with test scores measuring motor speed, and supracallosal fractional anisotropy correlated with behavioral ratings. This group concluded that greater impairment of white matter in the frontal lobe were associated with functional deficits, as reflected in low scores on specific neuropsychological measures (the Tower of London and the reports and ratings of daily behaviors on the Behavior Rating Inventory of Executive Function), which measure executive functions such as planning, impulse control, sustained focus, self-monitoring, and other aspects of executive, or frontal lobe, functions. Thus, while the detected axonal damage was minimal, children with mild and moderate brain injury in this study demonstrated measurable cognitive and behavioral deficits. Such findings of objective neuropsychological tools, in combination with advanced technology, further solidify the notion that diffuse axonal injury can cause persistent disruption in a child's daily functioning. Knowing this, we can help children and their families effectively cope with and remediate multiple changes in cognition, academics, and behavior.

Treble and research group [25] detected a significant structural abnormality of the corpus collosum via brain MRI DTI imaging in children with severe, moderate, and complicated mild TBI. This study also determined the connection of this structural damage to a long-term working memory impairment, especially visual spatial working memory. Specifically, this study confirmed a correlation between decreased functional anisotropy (FA) values and higher radial diffusivity in callosal subregions connecting anterior and posterior parietal cortical regions and deficient verbal working memory, while such abnormality involving callosal subregions connecting anterior and posterior parietal as well as temporal cortical regions correlated with visuospatial working memory deficits.

Cognitive Impairment and Metabolic Abnormalities

Further support for the notion of post-concussion functional disruption comes from research studies that focused on metabolic abnormalities secondary to TBI. Different neurochemical concentrations reflect different neuropathological processes that occur at different stages of life and post-injury period. Some of these metabolic changes, which have been detected from infancy to later childhood, up to 16 years of age, are involved in the normal course of development and contribute to the development of various cognitive and emotional abilities [26].

Recent studies have shown that post-traumatic metabolic changes may signal the presence of axonal injury that is not always easily identified. For example, lower NAA concentration may reflect neuronal and axonal damage, which is consistent with diffuse axonal injury but not seen on traditional MRI studies [27]. Researchers have also detected specific changes in *N*-acetyl aspartate (NAA) and choline (Cho) levels in mild and severe pediatric TBI cases, with Cho levels decreasing in the first year after the brain injury; in severe TBI cases, decreased Cho levels may reflect neuronal death and cerebral atrophy [28, 29]. Cholines, such as glycerolphosphocholine and phosphocholine, are markers of a cell membrane synthesis and repair, while NAA is a marker of neuronal and axonal functioning. Thus, any post-traumatic changes in the brain cell metabolic concentrations signal the disruption of the cell integrity and functioning. Interestingly, NAA concentration changes post TBI are associated not only with axonal loss due to various trauma mechanisms, but also with milder forms of axonal injury, such as axonal swelling, stretching, and myelin damage.

The influence of metabolic changes in the growing child brain on everyday functioning is undeniable. As brain injury triggers a chain reaction of certain metabolic changes in a child's brain, it disrupts the normal ratio of metabolic concentrations that is necessary for optimal functioning in school and at home. Specifically, Chertkoff Walz and his colleagues [28] have determined that higher metabolic concentration is associated with better academic skills and social competence. They also showed positive correlation between Cho levels and spatial, spelling, and pragmatic language abilities.

Thus, a growing body of research leads us to believe that even mild brain injury may cause an ongoing disruption in the normative developmental changes in the brain metabolism, which, in turn, compromises the integrity of child's neuropsychological functioning, as reflected in cognitive difficulties, declining academic performance, and social-emotional problems that disrupt the lives of some children after a mild TBI.

Post-Concussion Recovery and Assessment Challenges

Recovery from mild brain injury is also laced with peculiarities that are specific to a growing child's brain. Several researchers have concluded that some aspects of a child's brain, such as plasticity and functional reorganization, are helpful in recovery from a focal brain injury but not from a diffuse brain injury [19, 30, 31]. White matter at different stages of development may respond differently to the traumatic process and if some higher-level skills, such as social comprehension, sustained and divided attention, impulse inhibition, or complex reasoning, did not have a chance to develop before the onset of TBI, concussed children may experience slowed maturation of these skills in the following months. In fact, Gerrard-Morris and colleagues [32] showed that deficits in pragmatic language emerged some 12 months after the brain injury, while Anderson and colleagues [33] showed that memory problems did not emerge in young children until 1 year after the brain injury. These long-term effects may be different for children in different age groups, but it is important to know that if some children are just too young to demonstrate full-fledged abilities involving social communication (pragmatic language) or certain aspects of memory, their cognitive impairment and social deficits may not be acknowledged, measured, and remediated following their mild brain injury.

Levin and Hanten [34] have pointed out a well-accepted fact that the executive system in children is undergoing such significant and rapid changes that it greatly complicates the study of the effects of brain injury on pediatric executive system. As a result, children who sustained a brain injury, including frontal lobe injury specifically, at a younger age, when organization, impulse control, self-regulation, and other frontal lobe functions are not developed and matured yet, may not demonstrate executive system deficits until much later in life. Thus, we may not appreciate the extent of the brain injury until after the child has recovered from all external and overt physical and cognitive symptoms.

Moreover, the age of onset of TBI and the severity of injury are not the only variables affecting the outcome of pediatric TBI, as different brain functions may suffer different long-term post-concussion effects. One study investigated the variability in dysexecutive symptom expression in children post TBI, specifically looking at focal versus diffuse brain injury and the extent of frontal lobe involvement and the effect of pre-injury functioning [35]. This research group determined that children who sustain a concussion at a younger age are more vulnerable to executive skill impairment and long-term deficits. In fact, when concussed children were assessed 2 years post injury, 14–50% of them performed below grade level in math. Other authors have also showed that the development of arithmetic skills is most vulnerable to the effects of TBI, while word recognition was relatively unchanged [36]. Their finding is not surprising, as math is an academic achievement ability that builds upon such cognitive skills such as sustained focus, sequencing, planning, spatial reasoning, planning, and organization—the same cognitive abilities that are often impaired by a concussion.

In addition, it was determined that attentional control and literacy mature by approximately 8 years of age, while goal setting and arithmetic skills mature by approximately 12 years [35]. Thus, if some children sustain a brain injury before 8 or 12 years of age, they may experience protracted post-TBI deficits, including the delay in maturation of attention control, literacy, goal setting, and arithmetic skills, which were not so obvious shortly after their brain injury.

Now, when a student scores low on a math test, experiences difficulty in reasoning and developing a multistep plan for a science project, has trouble sustaining focus on lengthy standardized tests, falls under the peer pressure to engage in maladaptive behaviors, or displays poor judgment in friendship choices, teachers and parents do not immediately connect these academic and behavioral problems with a concussion that took place last summer or during a winter break. Thus, concussed children may end up following a dwindling road of poor academic performance and conflicts with peers and adults, while their caretakers and educators are not recognizing these problems as long-term symptoms of a mild brain injury and may mistakenly attribute some failures to adolescent attempts to establish independence and a rebellion against authority. Therefore, they do not proactively monitor concussed children for possible academic and cognitive problems in order to address them at the earliest point of time and in their mildest form, which is easier to remediate.

School work is the major responsibility of a child, and it requires a child to utilize all of his cognitive and socio-emotional resources. Academic activities depend on the executive skills, as students are required to reason and apply appropriate rules and formulas, sustain focus for prolonged period of time, organize their assignments, plan their study and test preparation activities, extract essential elements from a reading material, compare and contrast facts, and perform many other executive functions. Social interactions also heavily depend on executive skills, as children are required to monitor their environment and behavior, regulate their emotional reactions and behavioral actions in accordance with social norms, inhibit impulses to act and talk when necessary, etc. In fact, researchers are actively studying the effects of the executive system on the adolescents' educational performance, and Arnett and her group [37] specifically noted that teenagers' emotional and behavioral regulation directly affected their grades in school after a concussion. This finding also confirms the understanding that some skills, such as executive functions, are not heavily used until older childhood, which leaves younger children with TBI with a potential protracted TBI-related deficit in their ability to manage time, plan and sustain focus on complex assignments, retrieve and utilize the stored social knowledge in various social situations, prioritize activities, inhibit impulse for immediate gratification, and regulate negative emotions and urges. These are all very important abilities that allow children to establish and maintain appropriate and rewarding relationships with peers and adults, behave and regulate their mood and attention so that they can learn in class, and adapt and apply their new knowledge and skills to ever-changing life circumstances. While younger children who seemingly recover from a TBI do not experience much demand on their executive system, adolescents naturally experience a heavy executive system demand and TBI survivors undergo even more challenging adjustments in self-regulation than their peers.

Thus, if some protracted post-TBI deficits do not come to the surface until months later, children who sustained a mild brain injury during their summer vacation may be viewed as fully recovered when they start their new academic year in September. It is possible that we do not consider a concussion as a precipitating factor when some children start experiencing pragmatic language deficits, aggression, hyperactivity, frequent conflicts, and social interaction problems months after their concussion, as at that point their brain injury incident is so far removed that parents and teachers may believe that these problems are not related to a brain injury. Of course, a thorough neuropsychological assessment is required in such cases to rule out developmental disorders that also involve pragmatic language deficits and social interaction problems, such as Asperger's disorder and pervasive developmental disorder. Neuropsychological assessment and academic achievement testing are also needed to rule out specific pre-TBI learning disabilities involving math, reading, and writing in children who display declining academic performance post TBI. In essence, neuropsychological evaluation becomes an essential tool in bringing all these different pieces of a puzzle together in order to sort out preexisting conditions, protracted post-TBI symptoms, and normally developing brain functions. It is a complicated task, but certainly worth attempting for the sake of a happier and satisfying life for the child.

Neuropsychologists who specialize in the assessment of children and developmental disorders possess a unique expertise to evaluate functional integrity of child's brain immediately after the brain injury and at a later time, when some children might be experiencing long-term effects of a brain injury that prevent them from adequately adapting to changing academic, cognitive, and social demands of their peer group and the environment. Hence, the timeline for monitoring concussed children should include a visit at least 12 months post brain injury. Subsequent neuropsychological assessments can be performed at 24 months post TBI mark if prior evaluation detected any lingering cognitive, emotional, or behavioral deficits. If no such deficits were detected at 24 months mark post-brain injury, concussed children can be discharged from a neuropsychological care. Additional follow up is suggested if they display any newfound difficulties in social, emotional, academic, or general cognitive functioning, such as difficulty reading social cues, negotiating conflicts, inhibiting impulses at age-appropriate level, or developing higher order reasoning, academic, and comprehension skills.

The necessity of the follow up neuropsychological evaluation is highlighted by the findings of a meta-analysis conducted by Babikian and Asarnow [38] that showed children with moderate and severe TBI not only showed cognitive deficits months after the injury but demonstrated even greater difference from non-injured peers 2 years later. Specifically, their analysis of multiple studies using neuropsychological tests to measure cognitive abilities revealed what was already known to neuropsychologists—many children with moderate and severe TBI experience deficits in processing speed, attention, visual perception, and memory functions during the first 5 months post injury. However, while some of these cognitive functions improve within the first 2 years, select cognitive deficits, such as immediate and delayed verbal memory, executive functioning, processing speed, and attention, fell even farther behind their age norm as seen on neuropsychological testing 2 years post TBI. Moreover, 2 years after the injury, children with moderate and severe TBI scored lower on the IQ test than their non-injured peers. Scores on tests of working memory, visual perception, and visual memory were similar among injured and non-injured children, suggesting that visual memory and visual perception skills appear to be the most resilient in children. While working memory test scores were also included in this group, clinical experience indicates that working memory can also be very susceptible to long-term effects of TBI due to the involvement of attention and concentration functions. In fact, research studies point to a much greater role of working memory in the completion of a wide range of daily and academic tasks, similarly to the well-known role of the executive functioning, and the prevalence of a long-term working memory deficit, especially visual spatial working memory, in children with severe, moderate, and complicated mild TBI [25].

Neuropsychological measures provide objective, structured symptom assessment and ecologically valid functional description of executive (i.e., organization, emotional regulation, self-monitoring of performance and behavior, social judgment, goal-directed behavior, problem solving, abstraction, impulse control), memory, motor, language, attention, speed, information processing, emotional, and behavioral abilities relative to child's age norm, which are critical in post-injury return to school, home life, sports, and social settings. The wealth of objective data gathered during the neuropsychological assessment allows neuropsychologists to track the developmental trajectory of cognitive and behavioral skills, a foundation for a more targeted, individualized treatment, and intervention plan before cognitive, academic, and behavioral problems have worsened and higher-order cognitive skills have failed to develop. Such comprehensive, objective assessments are critical when tracking the recovery of cognitive skills as well as persistent cognitive deficits, as neuropsychological tests determine how far child's cognitive abilities fall from the age norm and if certain cognitive skills are not developing at the expected pace compared to non-injured peers. Such objective measurements take much of the guesswork out of the decision loop and provide hard evidence of whether cognitive deficits are actually present or not when a child continues to complain of headaches, dizziness, emotional lability, and sleep disturbance that complicate the picture by intertwining with cognition. The work of Wade and her group [39] highlights the effect of psychotherapy targeting specific executive deficit in problem solving on the reduction of depressed and anxious mood and somatic complaints in adolescents who suffered mild to severe TBI. Their study clearly indicated that detecting an executive deficit through a neuropsychological instrument and improving it via non-medicinal problem-solving psychotherapy helped adolescents resolve and adapt to common life problems and stressors that triggered psychiatric, emotional, and neurological complaints.

Furthermore, neuropsychologists are in the unique position of determining whether the observed cognitive and psychological difficulties are due to the post-concussion syndrome or preexisting learning disabilities, developmental delays, behavioral disorders, or mood disorders. After all, it is the neuropsychological assessment that can distinguish if the child's failure to remember new information in class is due to preexisting attention deficit, post-TBI acquired memory encoding or retention deficit, or TBI-related mood disorder or insomnia that diminished motivation and mental stamina to study. Neuropsychologists can also distinguish if the recent moodiness, avoidance of academic demand, confrontations with teachers, and involvement in destructive peer groups are the result of hormonal changes and the strive for independence and new identity, or the outcome of executive dysfunction in adolescents who are believed to have recovered from a TBI 3 years ago. Knowing the correct etiology of observed difficulties can lead to a timely choice of the most effective treatment modality such as cognitive rehabilitation and retraining, behavioral therapy, or psychostimulant medication. Professional guidance based on neuropsychological objective test findings has always been welcomed by teachers, parents, neurologists, speech and occupational therapists, psychotherapists, and other specialists who are involved in child's care, as neuropsychological test results carefully measure the trajectory of emotional regulation, executive, reasoning, and other cognitive and neuropsychological skills over time in order to detect child's response to treatment modalities and support the need for specialized educational and vocational services or guardianship.

Conclusion

The wealth of the existing research knowledge, supported by the ever-developing technology that helps us to detect even minor effects of brain injury, allows more precise investigation of concussion diagnosis and short-term and long-term symptomatology. It also prompts us to consider recovery patterns and the developmental level of child's individual skill sets, which may or may not have matured at the time of the injury. We know now that brain injury may impede the development of any cognitive or emotional abilities while they are at their "budding" stage and that impairment becomes more apparent at a later time, when a child fails to acquire, mature, and demonstrate more advanced skills.

Some children who sustained a concussion return to classrooms and appear to have fully recovered, yet may still experience cognitive, emotional, and behavioral problems at a later time because those particular skills were not required or utilized at the age when they sustained a concussion; hence, their impairment was not "visible." However, as the social and academic demands increase with time, some children who sustained a mild brain injury may fail to adapt to the changing environment because they did not fully develop and acquire higher-order skills that support a steady learning curve and make a successful adaptation possible. This hypothesis resonates with findings that showed that behavioral and emotional problems, including impulsivity, aggressive behaviors, and frequent mood changes, increase with time after the TBI, while physical and cognitive complaints decrease [40].

Of course, the long-term effects of concussion on children's brain development are dependent on many factors, including age at the time of concussion; pre-concussion level of cognitive, behavioral, and emotional development; and resources available to help them recover and catch up on developmental milestones. Since such a multitude of variables are involved, research studies may produce varying results based on the different characteristics of pediatric samples and measurement tools involved. We do not have a precise matrix of all these factors yet, but future pediatric concussion research may help us construct a concussion evaluation and recovery model that would include protracted effects of a mild TBI and, hence, allow us to identify the child's trajectory of recovery from a concussion and the future development of specific cognitive, emotional, and behavioral skills.

The treatment of such long-term effects of concussions would depend on the type and severity of their symptoms and would need to be tailored to individual characteristics of these children and their environment. While frequent repetitive neuropsychological testing would not be necessary, occasional neuropsychological assessments of concussed children produce important information about their overall cognitive, emotional, and behavioral development, including their adjustment to changing peer environment and academic demands. Thus, useful guidelines can be generated for concussed children's parents, teachers, school psychologists, and caretakers as to which cognitive, emotional, or behavioral weaknesses exist in a child's neuropsychological profile and how to reduce them (e.g., specialized educational services and accommodations, social skills and communication skills group therapy to improve reasoning, pragmatic language and social interactions, and cognitive rehabilitation and retraining).

Children who are unfortunate to experience long-term effects of a mild brain injury could be identified before their post-concussion symptoms have seriously interfered with their academic performance and peer relationships and limited their future educational and career advancement. Adopting more proactive approach to identifying such weaknesses in children with mild TBI should certainly yield better functioning and happier children who can truly state that they have survived a brain injury and successfully developed their cognitive, emotional, and behavioral skills up to par with their age-matched peers.

References

1. Faul M, Xu L, Wald M, Coronado V. Traumatic brain injury in the United States: emergency department visits, hospitalizations and deaths. Atlanta: U.S. Department of Health and Human Services, Centers for Disease Control and Prevention, National Center for Injury Prevention and Control; 2010.
2. Wortzel HS, Granacher RP. Mild traumatic brain injury update: forensic neuropsychiatric implications. J Am Acad Psychiatry Law. 2015;43:499–505.
3. Lescohier I, DiScala C. Blunt trauma in children: causes and outcomes of head versus extracranial injury. Pediatrics. 1993;91:721–5.
4. McCrory P, Meeuwisse WH, Aubry M, Cantu B, Dvorák J, Echemendia RJ, et al. Consensus statement on concussion in sport: the 4th international conference on concussion in sport held in Zurich, November 2012. Br J Sports Med. 2013;47:250–8.
5. Kraus JF. Epidemiological features of brain injury in children: occurrence, children at risk, causes and manner of injury, severity, and outcomes. Trauma Head Inj Child. New York: Oxford University Press; 1995. p. 22–39.
6. Bruce, DA, Schut L. Concussion and contusion following pediatric head trauma. In: McLaurin RL (Ed.), Pediatric neurosurgery: Surgery of the developing system. New York: Grune and Stratton. 1982;301–8.
7. Barlow KM, Crawford S, Stevenson A, Sandhu SS, Belanger F, Dewey D. Epidemiology of post-concussion syndrome in pediatric mild traumatic brain injury. Pediatrics. 2010;126:e374–81.
8. Matz PG. Classification, diagnosis, and management of mild traumatic brain injury: a major problem presenting in a minor way. Semin Neurosurg. 2003;14:125–30.
9. Prigatano GP, Gupta S. Friends after traumatic brain injury in children. J Head Trauma Rehabil. 2006;21:505–13.
10. Janusz JA, Kirkwood MW, Yeates KO, Taylor HG. Social problem-solving skills in children with traumatic brain injury: long-term outcomes and prediction of social competence. Child Neuropsychol. 2002;8:179–94.
11. Hawley CA. Reported problems and their resolution following mild, moderate and severe traumatic brain injury amongst children and adolescents in the UK. Brain Inj. 2003;17:105–29.
12. Hooper SR, Alexander J, Moore D, Sasser HC, Laurent S, King J, et al. Caregiver reports of common symptoms in children following a traumatic brain injury. NeuroRehabilitation. 2004;19:175–89.
13. Wozniak JR, Krach L, Ward E, Mueller BA, Muetzel R, Schnoebelen S, et al. Neurocognitive and neuroimaging correlates of pediatric traumatic brain injury: a diffusion tensor imaging (DTI) study. Arch Clin Neuropsychol. 2007;22:555–68.
14. Levin HS, Hanten G, Zhang L, Swank PR, Ewing-Cobbs L, Dennis M, et al. Changes in working memory after traumatic brain injury in children. Neuropsychology. 2004;18:240–7.

15. Bauer R, Fritz H. Pathophysiology of traumatic injury in the developing brain: an introduction and short update. Exp Toxicol Pathol. 2004;56:65–73.
16. Bigler ED, Maxwell WL. Neuropathology of mild traumatic brain injury: relationship to neuroimaging findings. Brain Imaging Behav. 2012;6:108–36.
17. Ewing-Cobbs L, Prasad MR, Swank P, Kramer L, Cox CS, Fletcher JM, et al. Arrested development and disrupted callosal microstructure following pediatric traumatic brain injury: relation to neurobehavioral outcomes. NeuroImage. 2008;42:1305–15.
18. Thatcher RW. Maturation of the human frontal lobes: physiological evidence for staging. Dev Neuropsychol. 1991;7:397–419.
19. Levin HS. Neuroplasticity following non-penetrating traumatic brain injury. Brain Inj. 2003;17:665–74.
20. Salorio CF, Slomine BS, Grados MA, Vasa RA, Christensen JR, Gerring JP. Neuroanatomic correlates of CVLT-C performance following pediatric traumatic brain injury. J Int Neuropsychol Soc. 2005;11:686–96.
21. Power T, Catroppa C, Coleman L, Ditchfield M, Anderson V. Do lesion site and severity predict deficits in attentional control after preschool traumatic brain injury (TBI)? Brain Inj. 2007;21:279–92.
22. Johnson CP, Juranek J, Kramer LA, Prasad MR, Swank PR, Ewing-Cobbs L. Predicting behavioral deficits in pediatric traumatic brain injury through uncinate fasciculus integrity. J Int Neuropsychol Soc. 2011;17:663–73.
23. Basser PJ, Jones DK. Diffusion-tensor MRI: theory, experimental design and data analysis - a technical review. NMR Biomed. 2002;15:456–67.
24. Bendlin BB, Ries ML, Lazar M, Alexander AL, Dempsey RJ, Rowley HA, et al. Longitudinal changes in patients with traumatic brain injury assessed with diffusion-tensor and volumetric imaging. NeuroImage. 2008;42:503–14.
25. Treble A, Hasan KM, Iftikhar A, Stuebing KK, Kramer LA, Cox CS, et al. Working memory and corpus callosum microstructural integrity after pediatric traumatic brain injury: a diffusion tensor tractography study. J Neurotrauma. 2013;30:1609–19.
26. van der Knaap MS, van der Grond J, van Rijen PC, Faber JA, Valk J, Willemse K. Age-dependent changes in localized proton and phosphorus MR spectroscopy of the brain. Radiology. 1990;176:509–15.
27. Holshouser BA, Tong KA, Ashwal S. Proton MR spectroscopic imaging depicts diffuse axonal injury in children with traumatic brain injury. AJNR Am J Neuroradiol. 2005;26:1276–85.
28. Walz NC, Cecil KM, Wade SL, Michaud LJ. Late proton magnetic resonance spectroscopy following traumatic brain injury during early childhood: relationship with neurobehavioral outcomes. J Neurotrauma. 2008;25:94–103.
29. Parry L, Shores A, Rae C, Kemp A, Waugh M-C, Chaseling R, et al. An investigation of neuronal integrity in severe paediatric traumatic brain injury. Child Neuropsychol. 2004;10:248–61.
30. Anderson VA, Morse SA, Catroppa C, Haritou F, Rosenfeld JV. Thirty month outcome from early childhood head injury: a prospective analysis of neurobehavioural recovery. Brain J Neurol. 2004;127:2608–20.
31. Suskauer SJ, Huisman TAGM. Neuroimaging in pediatric traumatic brain injury: current and future predictors of functional outcome. Dev Disabil Res Rev. 2009;15:117–23.
32. Gerrard-Morris A, Taylor HG, Yeates KO, Walz NC, Stancin T, Minich N, et al. Cognitive development after traumatic brain injury in young children. J Int Neuropsychol Soc. 2010;16:157–68.
33. Anderson VA, Catroppa C, Rosenfeld J, Haritou F, Morse SA. Recovery of memory function following traumatic brain injury in pre-school children. Brain Inj. 2000;14:679–92.
34. Levin HS, Hanten G. Executive functions after traumatic brain injury in children. Pediatr Neurol. 2005;33:79–93.
35. Anderson V, Catroppa C. Recovery of executive skills following paediatric traumatic brain injury (TBI): a 2 year follow-up. Brain Inj. 2005;19:459–70.

36. Ewing-Cobbs L, Fletcher JM, Levin HS, Iovino I, Miner ME. Academic achievement and academic placement following traumatic brain injury in children and adolescents: a two-year longitudinal study. J Clin Exp Neuropsychol. 1998;20:769–81.
37. Arnett AB, Peterson RL, Kirkwood MW, Taylor HG, Stancin T, Brown TM, et al. Behavioral and cognitive predictors of educational outcomes in pediatric traumatic brain injury. J Int Neuropsychol Soc. 2013;19:881–9.
38. Babikian T, Asarnow R. Neurocognitive outcomes and recovery after pediatric TBI: meta-analytic review of the literature. Neuropsychology. 2009;23:283–96.
39. Wade SL, Taylor HG, Cassedy A, Zhang N, Kirkwood MW, Brown TM, et al. Long-term behavioral outcomes after a randomized, clinical trial of counselor-assisted problem solving for adolescents with complicated mild-to-severe traumatic brain injury. J Neurotrauma. 2015;32:967–75.
40. Yeates KO, Taylor HG, Barry CT, Drotar D, Wade SL, Stancin T. Neurobehavioral symptoms in childhood closed-head injuries: changes in prevalence and correlates during the first year postinjury. J Pediatr Psychol. 2001;26:79–91.

Multimodal Approaches to Preventing Asymptomatic Repetitive Head Injury in Adolescent Athletes

17

Thomas M. Talavage, Eric A. Nauman, and Taylor A. Lee

Introduction

In 2010, Talavage et al. demonstrated that a high percentage of athletes participating in contact sports, in this case American football, exhibited dramatic changes in neurophysiology without presenting discernable symptoms. Since then, the effects of these repetitive head acceleration events (rHAEs)—rapid head movements associated with direct blows to the head as well as whiplash motions resulting from impacts to the body—have been clarified using a range of neuroimaging techniques including functional magnetic resonance imaging (FMRI), diffusion tensor imaging (DTI), magnetic resonance spectroscopy (MRS), and susceptibility weighted imaging (SWI). These injuries have generally been categorized using the label "subconcussive" injuries, but this is a misnomer, related to conflation of the *diagnosis* of "concussion," as determined by the presentation of particular symptoms, with the underlying pathophysiology. Rather, the injuries induced by exposure to rHAE are merely "asymptomatic," consistent in the lack of external dysfunction with the presence of clear physiological abnormalities, like as in early stages of multiple neurodegenerative disorders (e.g., Alzheimer's disease, Parkinson's disease, and

---

T. M. Talavage (✉)
Department of Biomedical Engineering, University of Cincinnati, Cincinnati, OH, USA
e-mail: talavatm@ucmail.uc.edu

E. A. Nauman
School of Mechanical Engineering, Purdue University, West Lafayette, IN, USA

Weldon School of Biomedical Engineering, Purdue University, West Lafayette, IN, USA

Department of Basic Medical Sciences, Purdue University, West Lafayette, IN, USA

T. A. Lee
School of Mechanical Engineering, Purdue University, West Lafayette, IN, USA

Huntington's disease) in which substantial alteration in brain structure and health can occur prior to the onset of symptoms.

This distinction between *subconcussive* and *asymptomatic* events is critical because researchers have for many years been trying to quantify the particular type of head impact that "causes" a concussion. Every attempt to ascertain the magnitude of this elusive hit has been unproductive given the underlying assumption that a singular event has occurred. Rather, the majority of concussions are influenced by the prior history of head impacts, certainly over the season in question and possibly from previous seasons (e.g., [1, 2]). More importantly, erroneous focus on "the hit" that causes a concussion has produced confusion in the larger community. A number of studies have attempted to generate injury risk curves associated with the magnitude of experienced rHAEs [3–5], or to define a threshold above which diagnosis of a concussion is deemed likely [6–9]. However, such efforts are critically flawed, as they both ignore the underlying pathophysiology brought about by asymptomatic injuries, and generally have failed to model *all* experienced rHAEs, focusing only on those events which led to the diagnosis of a concussion. As in any detection problem, a reliance on only the true positives leads to limited statistical power and fails to yield effective decision criteria.

Within the context of separating the pathophysiology from the symptomatology, a critical clinical challenge is to retain an emphasis on detection of concussion—a clear sign that brain injury *has* occurred—while also recognizing that the *lack* of observation of the symptoms associated with a concussion does not equate to a brain being healthy (see Fig. 17.1).

Acknowledgment of this key fact—that the symptoms and pathophysiology are related, but not equivalent [10]—represents a first step toward understanding and preventing longer-term consequences of rHAE-related brain injuries. While the alterations observed in such cases have been found to be consistent in location (e.g., white matter injures in the corpus callosum or other central tracts) and nature (e.g., decoupling of cerebrovascular reactivity; and alterations in neurotransmitter production or consumption) with those injuries observed to be present when an athlete exhibits symptoms that lead to the clinical diagnosis of a "concussion" (c.g., loss of balance, impaired vision, slurred speech, and inability to control crying), there does not yet exist evidence directly linking particular elements of pathophysiology to symptomatology.

When we consider athletics, and particularly youth athletics, we must weigh the additional factor of the developing brain in our examination of the relationship between pathophysiology and symptomatology. The past several decades emphasizing early or on-field detection/diagnosis of a concussion has led to confusion regarding what is and is not a fundamentally injurious activity, as well as to what is and is not of concern from a neurological perspective. Within the adolescent population, there is an inherent desire to be conservative, and as such, one viewpoint is that no collision-based activities are acceptable, as even the most subtle of rHAEs have been found to produce persistent (if not necessarily permanent) changes in brain structure and function. The counter, perhaps nihilistic, viewpoint is that there is

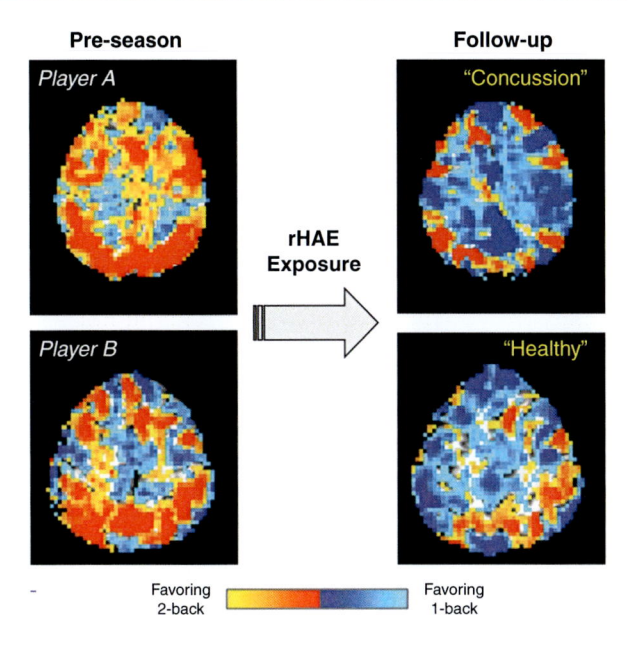

Fig. 17.1 Comparison of task-based functional MRI (FMRI) activation patterns during a working memory task, using pre-participation measures within each subject as a self-control to document the presence of pathophysiologic changes in brain function for both (*top*) symptomatic and (*bottom*) asymptomatic brain injury. The follow-up session for Player A (*top right*) was conducted shortly after completion of a high school football season, within 24 hours of diagnosis of a concussion related to a failed dive. The follow-up session for Player B (*bottom right*) was conducted during a high school football season, within 24 hours of a game that ended a week in which the athlete was exposed to over 200 rHAEs of at least 10 g (assessed using HITS™). Observe that, for both athletes, the broad extent of activation favoring the harder ("2-back") working memory task was greatly reduced following rHAE exposure, with many regions now exhibiting greater activation during the easier ("1-back") task. Note that task performance was not altered at follow-up, relative to the pre-season assessment

nothing that can be done to prevent any such injury so long as youth are likely to engage in activities that involve head collisions. As a result, we tend to be presented with the false choice that one may either participate in these activities and accept (or have accepted on their behalf) whatever risks exist, or that such activities (and their multi-billion-dollar economies) must be eliminated.

In reality, the path laid before the medical community is quite simple—gain a greater understanding of how pathophysiological changes are causally linked to exposure to rHAEs while moderated or mediated by genetic and lifestyle factors, and then develop preventative methodologies (including equipment) and corrective approaches (including potential pharmaceutical treatments) such that the risk of long-term neurological dysfunction is minimized for the vast majority of participating individuals.

Consequently, we seek to explore how asymptomatic injury to the brain is produced by exposure to rHAE, and how subsequent measurable changes in brain health and function may guide future efforts at intervention, both to encourage the recovery and repair from such injury and to prevent such injury from occurring in the first place.

Evidence for Pathophysiology in the Absence of Symptomatology

Given that, by definition, asymptomatic injuries do not produce readily identifiable symptoms, athletes may continue to participate in contact sports after development of an underlying pathophysiological change. Over the past decade, several groups of investigators have examined whether exposure to rHAEs results in changes to brain health. To effectively quantify these changes, it is typically necessary to follow a structural health monitoring paradigm [11, 12]. This paradigm employs a series of steps, including (1) baseline quantitative assessments that may include cognitive testing and neuroimaging; (2) season-spanning recording of rHAE frequency, type, and severity using accelerometers or similar sensors; (3) focused analysis on athletes diagnosed with concussions during the season; and (4) re-evaluation of all athletes at the end of the season. To date, studies using this approach [13–17] have been conducted primarily (but not exclusively) in tackle football athletes, including those participating at the youth, high school, and college levels.

In the initial application of this paradigm, the authors initially reported that approximately half of the high school football athletes studied exhibited extensive within-season alterations in FMRI activation during a visual working memory task [14, 18]. These alterations were best explained by the number of rHAE exposures in the preceding week. After the season, this task-based activation generally trended toward pre-participation levels, suggesting that at least some of the neurophysiological changes were transient. A simultaneous effort implemented by Bazarian and colleagues [13] revealed comparable trends in MRI measures of white matter health.

Subsequent work has demonstrated a general propensity for accumulation of pathophysiological changes throughout the competition season—that is, over the duration of time when athletes are regularly exposed to rHAEs. These studies have further demonstrated that many of the changes in brain function and structure, observed in up to 70% of the studied athletes [12], may be explained using measures of rHAEs—for example, counts and magnitudes [14, 15, 17, 19–28].

Ongoing work is elucidating the time course of the process of brain health alteration and recovery. Alterations in FMRI activations appear to arise as a short-term (within several weeks) consequence of exposure to rHAEs [14], or to be associated with an abrupt increase or decrease in the level of weekly exposure [29, 30]. While some recovery in task-based FMRI activation appears to be possible during a season [12], continued accumulation of rHAEs seems more likely to lead to continued accrual of impairment [31]. These observations imply that some local neuronal "rewiring" may be able to resolve networking inefficiencies, thereby precluding observation of classical symptoms even though the brain is not truly healthy. Other changes in brain health, such as decreased cerebrovascular reactivity [28, 32, 33], alterations in brain chemistry [26, 34], and changes in white matter health [13, 17, 20, 24, 35–38], hint at a gradual buildup of changes over the course of the entire season, with the potential for prolonged alterations that may effectively be persistent if athletes continue to participate in collision-based activities year-round—for example, soccer athletes who participate in club competition in the off-season [33, 39], or football athletes who compete in other collision-based sports (e.g., wrestling, ice hockey, and lacrosse) over the winter and spring (e.g., [34]).

These functionally observed asymptomatic changes may have more profound short-term effects than previously believed. Resting-state functional connectivity has been found to yield robust patterns of connectivity—"fingerprints"—that are unique and reproducible for each individual [40, 41], yet organized into relatively consistent networks across a population (e.g., [42]). These patterns of connectivity have been documented to be appreciably altered in patient populations with neurodegenerative disorders, such as Alzheimer's disease (e.g., [43]), Parkinson's disease (e.g., [44, 45]), and Huntington's disease (e.g., [46–48]). As such, we know that changes in the underlying structure of the brain can be reflected at the network level. Recent work in high school football athletes has documented that even the robust "fingerprint" that is unique to each individual may be altered following prolonged exposure to rHAEs, such that individuals come precariously close to no longer being "themselves" (Fig. 17.2 [49]). It is plausible that this approach toward, but not crossing of, the boundary with a domain in which an individual is no longer unique underpins why most accumulated injuries are classified as "asymptomatic." Further, given that the potential appears to exist for prolonged exposure to rHAEs to fundamentally alter "who" we are, the early detection of asymptomatic injury is even more important.

The asymptomatic pathophysiology and functional alterations noted above suggest that, at least within the competition season, the natural healing processes are unable to overcome the rate at which such injuries accrue. All of the discussed alterations have been found to arise *within* a single season of participation in collision sport competition, and a substantial, but incomplete, recovery within 12–15 weeks of the cessation of rHAE exposure (e.g., [30, 31]). However, while it is good that recovery occurs, there is concern that these asymptomatic injuries might persist more than a few weeks or months beyond the cessation of participation, particularly in sports for which activities have taken on an almost year-round nature (e.g., soccer), or in athletes who participate in multiple collision sports over the course of the calendar year (e.g., football followed by wrestling and/or lacrosse).

As players continue to participate year after year in collision sports, it is logical to be concerned that persistent presence of pathophysiology will lead to permanent alterations in some aspects of brain health. White matter evaluation using DTI has demonstrated troubling differences in football players from season to season with observations of increased fractional anisotropy (FA) and decreased mean diffusivity

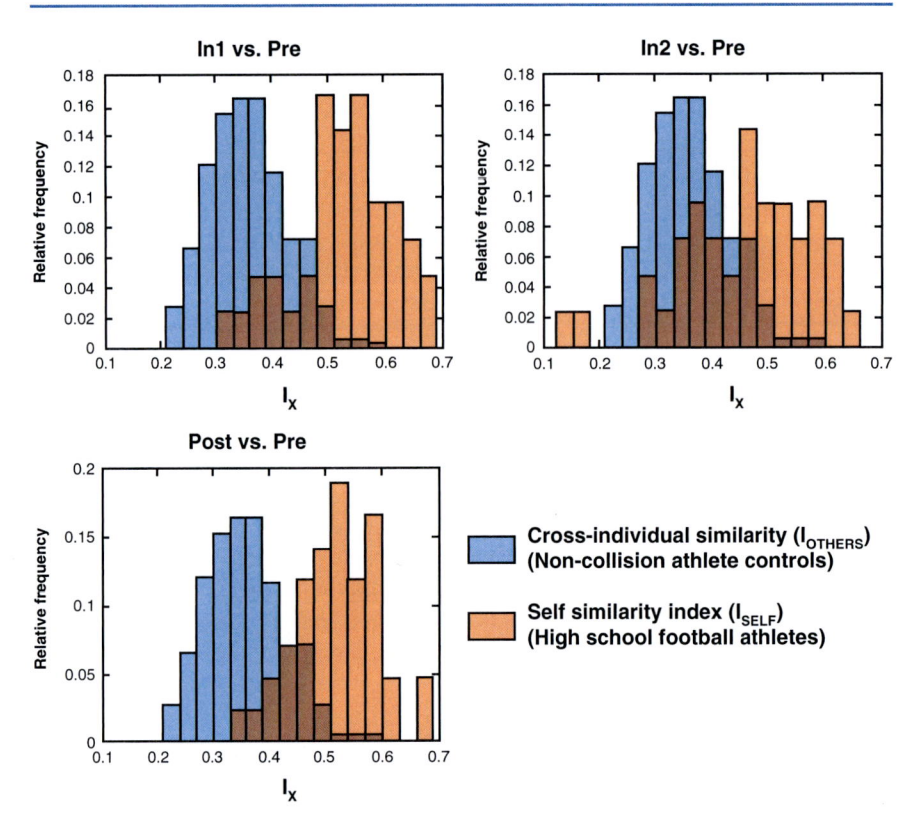

Fig. 17.2 Comparison of functional connectome self-similarity (e.g., Finn et al. [40]; Amico and Goni [41]) in football athletes with cross-individual similarity in non-collision sport athlete controls effected for football athlete assessments during (In1 and In2) and after (Post) a season of high school football. Note that the distribution of self-similarity of football athletes at In2 with themselves at Pre (*middle*) shifts appreciably toward the distribution of cross-individual similarity distribution observed across a corpus of high school non-collision sport athlete controls. This shift suggests that, following extensive exposure to rHAEs, football athlete functional connectomes are changed to the point that many athletes exhibit connectivity as disparate from their (presumed) healthy state at Pre as if they were, in fact, a different individual. (Image based on Bari et al. [49])

(MD), which is typically associated with swelling or inflammation [50]. Evidence for such chronic shifts in brain health exist from metabolomic studies, for which collegiate football athletes assessed prior to the onset of collision activities exhibit highly atypical levels of a range of compounds (e.g., [51]). Such alterations in brain physiology are not entirely without behavioral evidence, as studies using virtual reality-based assessment of balance and motor coordination suggest impairment in some athletes even before the beginning of a season [52]. Note that these deviation measures do, in fact, represent impairments, even though such athletes would be more likely expected to evidence *better* than normal performance.

Therefore, the pathophysiology being observed in adolescent athletes is damage, and it has a meaningful risk of becoming persistent (chronic), should the healing processes remain overwhelmed by the continued accrual of injury.

Contributing Factors to Asymptomatic Injury

We now seek to explore additional factors that contribute to asymptomatic injury. We have documented, above, the evidence arguing for the accrual of asymptomatic injury based on the observation of both pathophysiologic changes in brain structure and function, as well as evidence of behavioral alterations not typically assessed in a clinical setting—that is, the pathophysiology is not truly without symptomatology; rather, the symptomatology of "concussion" is inadequate. The most immediate culprit—rHAE exposure—has been well explored, and while an appreciable (often 20–25%) portion of the variance associated with pathophysiologic changes may be explained by monitoring rHAEs, it is clear that the present acquisition technology and the associated data are insufficient for detection of injury, and likely insufficient to be effective guides for fully effective development of protective technologies and interventions. It is plausible that the variation in athlete height, weight, skill level, chosen protective equipment, and other clinical variables may be categorized through large-scale studies. However, the potential remains for meaningful predisposition of an individual to susceptibility to rHAE-related pathophysiology from the athlete's sex, genome, and other inalterable biological sources. We will here first consider those factors that are inherent and may be important to factor into decisions related to play or return to play (e.g., if they affect recovery), and then move on to factors which may be more likely to be mutable within the context of a sport (e.g., equipment and training).

Genetics

A role for genetics in the incidence and progression of neurodegeneration has previously been established in Alzheimer's disease and Parkinson's disease, among others (e.g., [53, 54]), making it reasonable to suspect a genetic susceptibility in concussion. Early work in this area focused on variation in the apolipoprotein E (*APOE*) gene (e.g., [55–58]) which affects clearance of beta amyloid and mediates the transport of cholesterols in the brain [59]. APOE variants have been related to more severe symptoms and slower recovery after traumatic brain injury [55, 58, 60–64] and may predispose athletes in contact sports to concussion [57, 65].

In addition to APOE variants, other genes are likely to contribute to susceptibility or resistance to brain injury. Several genes critical for normal brain function such as brain-derived neurotrophic factor (BDNF) and the serotonin transporter gene 5-HTT have been suggested to influence the repair and recovery processes after mild traumatic brain injury [66–68] but additional work is needed to elucidate these relationships. A more recent study used a candidate gene approach to demonstrate that the KIAA0319 genotype was statistically correlated with the number of diagnosed concussions in a cohort of contact sport athletes [69]. Interestingly, KIAA0319 variants have been shown to affect the manner in which the neurons adhere to the glial cytoskeleton, potentially altering the way that the cells respond to mechanical impacts [69, 70]. Weaker trends were demonstrated for BDNF, COMT, TPH2, and DARC. These data suggest that the brain's response to rHAEs may be affected by a number of different pathways (plaque clearance, chemical transport, cell-matrix interactions, etc.) and it is unlikely that a single gene will dominate the overall pathophysiology. These results do suggest that there may be individuals with a combination of genetic variants who are predisposed to respond to rHAEs in a negative way. Identifying this population would require a longitudinal study that goes beyond the diagnosis of concussion. To be fruitful, it requires an assay of these genes, with concomitant measurements of brain health via imaging and cognitive assessments, rHAE exposure, age, and sex to elucidate the relevant co-factors.

Sex

Although most studies have focused on male athletes, it is also important to study female athletes to determine the degree to which they are at risk for concussion and neurological changes due to rHAEs. Understanding how rHAEs might differentially affect males and females will provide insight into appropriate rules changes, recommended training techniques, and more accurate diagnostic and rehabilitation practices for each group.

There is ample evidence for differences between males and females regarding concussion, with it seeming appropriate to extend the implications of these findings to risk of asymptomatic injury. Within the domain of diagnosed concussions, high school female athletes are more than twice as likely as male athletes in comparable sports (e.g., soccer, basketball, baseball/softball, cross country, swimming, and track and field) to sustain a concussion [71]. Psychophysical testing following concussion diagnosis reveals that females exhibit slower reaction times relative to baseline than do their male counterparts [72]. Further, females appear not only to be more adversely affected by concussions but they are also more likely to report symptoms, perhaps contributing to their observed higher concussion rates [71, 72].

Psychophysical testing subsequent to soccer heading suggests that sex-related effects can be observed in asymptomatic athletes. As an example, let us consider two evaluations of how reaction times have changed with rHAE exposure for high school-aged soccer players. Zhang et al. [73] found that the reaction time on an anti-point task (stimulus in one direction, select the option in the opposite direction) was loosely related to the number of headers and strongly related to the time dedicated to the sport per week and years of experience for high school female soccer players. In a comparable manner, heading-based rHAE exposure was only found to decrease the speed at which high school-aged male soccer players improved their reaction times over repeated testing [74]. One hypothesis is that the males—likely having stronger neck structures, and greater overall mass with which to absorb incident energy—may simply be less affected by each heading event, but should rHAE exposure be severe enough, they might ultimately mirror the female athletes in exhibiting poorer reaction times.

Neuroimaging studies of athletes dealing with probable asymptomatic injury support the idea that females are differentially at risk for brain injury. While female soccer athletes tend to accrue many fewer head impacts than do their male football counterparts, observed changes in females for cerebrovascular reactivity and brain chemistry are usually no less prevalent, albeit often of lesser magnitude [12, 26, 33]. Measures of brain structure in asymptomatic athletes participating in a common sport have also revealed differences as a function of sex that are unlikely to be caused only by differences in mechanical loading (i.e., extent of rHAE exposure). Female and male collegiate hockey players were evaluated using DTI before and after a season of play, with female athletes exhibiting significant diffusivity differences while males exhibited none [75]. Similarly, female soccer athletes were found to be more sensitive to heading than men, exhibiting lower FA values that were correlated with such exposures than were their male counterparts [76]. As a general rule, these sex-specific observations of pathophysiology are attributed to group differences in the response to the milieu of rHAE severity, frequency, origin (e.g., heading the ball vs. collisions with the ground), as well as physiological or hormonal differences.

Physical Activity/Sport

Differences across physical activities, including sports, will also affect an athlete's exposure to rHAEs, and therefore risk of developing neurological pathophysiology. Football and girls' soccer typically have the highest rates of concussion, so to characterize the rHAEs sustained by these athletes may shed light on how injury accrues, possibly leading to diagnosed concussion [77–79]. While football and female soccer athletes exhibit rHAEs having a similar average peak translational acceleration (PTA), football players sustain more rHAEs over the course of the season, and female soccer players experience a higher average peak angular acceleration (PAA) [80]. The difference in rHAE frequency is likely due to differences in game play and the role that head impacts play within the sports (i.e., football players likely experience a collision on each play, whereas soccer players do not head at every opportunity). It is postulated that the difference in PAA is a consequence of protective equipment—a helmet may reduce linear energy transmission to the head, but the resulting increased radius provides a larger moment arm by which angular acceleration may be induced. While confounded by the linkage of sex and sport, neuroimaging findings suggestive of differential changes in brain chemistry [26] and cerebrovascular reactivity [28, 33] are not inconsistent with the expected differences in rHAE exposure. Further, these studies have documented a common threshold for rHAE exposure (50 g), above which changes in brain health were more likely to be observed in asymptomatic athletes, whether male or female [26, 28].

Competition/Skill Level

One last environmental factor to be addressed here is how the level of play of athletes may affect the frequency and severity of rHAEs. However, it must be noted that, for youth athletes, it is difficult to decouple competition level from age. To this end, let us focus on a comparison of women's soccer at the high school and collegiate levels, given that the size differences between these competitors are lesser than would exist if we contrast early adolescents against older individuals. Within this sport, we do know that the increase in competition level results in a greater exposure to rHAEs, both on a per-game and cumulative basis [39]. These differences most likely arise from the increase in average strength and skill level for college athletes. These increases are found to be amplified in games relative to practices [39, 81], and exhibit appreciable dependence on the position played [81]. Elevated rHAE exposure (both number and magnitude) at the collegiate level would be expected to produce greater risk of asymptomatic injury, and also to be reflected in greater diagnosed concussions. The latter is documented in the literature, both for games relative to practice and the collegiate level relative to high school [77].

Prevention of Asymptomatic Injury

Having now addressed the pathophysiology underlying asymptomatic brain injury and how a range of biological and environmental factors might contribute to or mitigate its accumulation, we may now begin to explore how we might intervene. Because treating an existing brain injury is both exceedingly difficult and has proven to yield mixed results, prevention of injury is the preferred intervention strategy. There are many avenues that one could follow to reduce injuries including the development of improved protective equipment, improved training, exposure monitoring, rule changes, and non-invasive quantitative clinical assessments—all of which fall within the framework of structural health monitoring, which has been used effectively by the airline and automotive industries.

A Framework for Evaluation—Structural Health Monitoring

Structural health monitoring evolved from the case of the De Havilland Comet, the first commercial jet airline. Catastrophic in-flight failures of these planes during the early 1950s led engineers to perform an intensive analysis of fatigue failures, ultimately determined to originate at the corners of square windows and propagate throughout the fuselage of the plane. Every decompression-compression cycle caused small cracks to extend in much the same way that each rHAE increases the magnitude and extent of neurophysiological changes in the brain. In the airline industry, methods for non-destructive evaluation were developed that remain in use today, including acoustic emissions, liquid penetrant testing, eddy current testing of welds, infrared and thermal measurement systems, holography, and vibration analysis. Engineers have further extended structural health monitoring of structural materials by integrating methods originally developed for medical applications such as radiography and computed tomography, ultrasound, and MRI. When these techniques are combined with flight logs and statistical analysis, a true structural health monitoring process can be achieved, and the risks of catastrophic failures in any material decrease substantially.

Utilizing a structural health monitoring model to improve overall brain health can be both effective and economical. If symptomatic TBI can be interpreted as a system failure, then prospective monitoring and predictive modeling of the internal damage can be used to determine when an individual should be clinically evaluated or removed from practice or competition entirely. It should be noted that one of the most important aspects of the prospective monitoring is ensuring that it is quantitative. This requires the acquisition of multiple pre-participation assessments for each individual because there is simply too much variability between individuals to use population averages. To date, this process has demonstrated that male and female collision sport athletes experience asymptomatic brain injuries that alter their neurophysiology at considerably higher rates than the incidence rates for diagnosed concussions. Interestingly, the rates are similar to those found by Baugh et al. [82] using post-season surveys to assess the level of undiagnosed concussions over the course of a season of collegiate football. Thus, this approach to the tracking of accumulated injury and natural repair processes can be used to identify techniques for assessment of brain health (e.g., virtual reality assessments, cognitive testing, and blood biomarkers) that may be cheaper or more effective than present approaches (e.g., expensive MRIs), allowing for streamlining of the care of athletes exposed to rHAEs.

Ultimately, structural health monitoring model provides the necessary framework to evaluate benefits of potential interventions intended to protect athletes from brain injury. Conducting such monitoring in controlled studies can allow for documentation of the nature and extent of benefits from novel interventions such as new training techniques and rule changes, and new designs for protective equipment (both passive and active). Before discussing these two key interventional mechanisms, we must begin by considering how we are to monitor the external events (i.e., rHAEs) that will affect our structure of interest (i.e., the brain).

Intervention—Exposure Monitoring

We must recognize that a fundamental aspect of structural health monitoring as applied to the prevention of TBI is the measurement of rHAE exposure. Moreover, any alterations we might effect to protect athletes will expressly be intended to reduce either the number of or the incident energy associated with the experienced rHAEs. In an ideal world, we would prefer directly to measure the incident energy or its suitable proxy, the force experienced by the recipient of an impact or whiplash movement. Note that this incident force appears to be the more critical component, given that the acceleration profile of experienced rHAEs appears to be relatively independent of the sport being played, and may be relatively independent of the sex of the athlete [80]. This remarkable uniformity of experienced accelerations suggests that differences in historical rates of diagnosed concussions are a consequence of the energy being transmitted through the skull of the athlete, a quantity more directly related to the incident force. However, given that the computation of the incident force requires appreciable instrumentation, we are left with the unfortunate reality that, for the vast majority of sports and age groups, measurement of the incident accelerations is the practical objective. With sufficiently large studies, profiles of experienced rHAEs may be combined with individual physical characteristics to produce sex- (and possibly sport-) specific modeling of the energy transmitted through the skull.

At present, accurate measurement of accelerations associated with rHAEs is a distinct challenge, both from the perspective of implementation and quality of data. Initial efforts at rHAE monitoring focused on the use of sensors embedded in protective equipment (e.g., the helmet). Such systems provided appreciable ease of use, but, due to their not being affixed to the skull, were frequently imprecise [83]. The next generation of devices that were released to the market were intended to be affixed to the head of the athlete, paving the way for conducting larger-scale longitudinal studies in non-helmeted sports. However, while these devices provided improvements in precision, they largely suffered from inaccurate kinematic modeling that made them highly susceptible to errors in estimation of angular acceleration [84]. Further, the need to attach them to the skin—a surface that does not lend itself to strong, yet temporary, adhesion—often led to low reliability in hot or humid conditions and may have contributed to additional inaccuracy [85]. It should also be noted that the need to affix, possibly reattach, and subsequently collect and clean such sensors on a daily basis greatly increases the demand for personnel beyond that which is practical for most youth teams. Simultaneous with the development of these smaller, skin-based devices, work has been ongoing for the development of mouthguard-based sensing, which offers an ideal linkage to the skull and its encased brain, providing one of the most practical measurements of experienced accelerations. Note that many racing sports use ear canal-based sensors, which could offer greater accuracy, but such devices could also reduce hearing acuity—at a minimum increasing the hearing threshold—while also being more prone to displacement in the case of head impacts. Thus, it is likely that future work will emphasize mouthguard-based sensing, as these approaches offer appreciable ease of use as the athlete can be granted control of the dual sensing and protective device, and such protective equipment can readily be made unique to a given athlete, providing appreciable information for kinematic modeling.

Practical measurements of the accelerations associated with rHAEs, combined with personalized kinematic modeling (see below), will allow a complete structural health monitoring approach to be implemented in athletes, permitting both characterization of injury and documentation of reductions in said injury from the interventional approaches described above. Such an approach will also permit identification of thresholds or protective needs for each athlete—providing an ideal case in which every athlete may participate in sport while also minimizing their short- and long-term risks of neurological injury.

Intervention—Training and Rules Changes

Various recommendations have been made to increase the safety of contact sports, related to *how* an athlete participates. It is of interest to find evidence-based interventions that can be easily implemented while maintaining the competitive nature and spectator appeal of the game. Football has been the primary focus of these efforts due to the number of direct, forceful head impacts sustained by these athletes. However, ice hockey and soccer have also sought legislative changes—primarily at the youth level—that might reduce the exposure of participating athletes to rHAEs.

One means to reduce injury has been to change the rules of play to eliminate specific activities that are associated with concussions or other clinically diagnosed head injuries. Ice hockey has sought to reduce the risk of injury at the youth level through the prohibition of body checking [86]. Similarly, soccer in the United States has prohibited the heading of the ball prior to the age of 12 [87]. While an argument is frequently made that not performing or developing these skills in lower levels of play will preclude learning of proper technique, an assessment in ice hockey of the effects on concussions at higher levels of play did not find any deleterious effects of the delayed introduction of body checking [86, 88].

Within football, several recommendations have been made to prevent concussion or to reduce exposure to rHAEs. One recommendation has been that linemen should only start in an "up" (or two-point) stance [89]. This proposal has been documented (see Fig. 17.3) in practice to reduce exposure to rHAEs [90]. Additional football rule change proposals have included minor alterations kickoffs, often thought to be the most dangerous play in football, particularly with regard to concussions. As

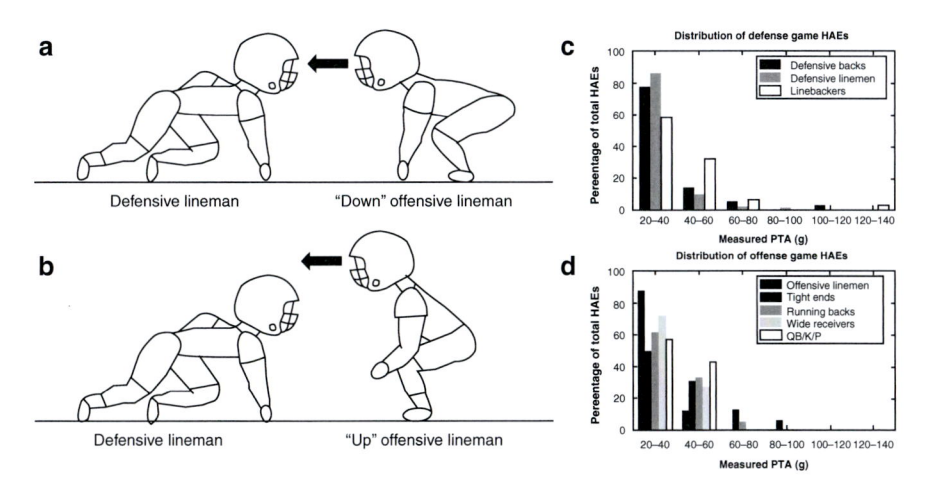

Fig. 17.3 Schematic of the (**a**) "down" (e.g., 3- and 4- point) and (**b**) "up" (e.g., 2-points) starting stances for offensive linemen and distribution of rHAEs by PTA in the game for the (**c**) defense and (**d**) offense [90]. In (**a**) and (**b**), the defensive linemen is on the left and offensive lineman on the right. In (**b**) the offensive linemen in the "up" stance has their head and hands higher than in (**a**) a "down" stance. This could allow the offensive linemen to get their hands in front of them faster to avoid getting hit in the head and keep their head out of the way of an oncoming defensive lineman

with the stance change, implementation of relatively simple changes to the kickoff—moving the kickoff form the 35-yard line to the 40-yard line and the touchback line from the 25-yard line to the 20-yard line—was found to reduce the concussion rate from 10.93 (per 1000 plays) to 2.04 [91].

General changes to training techniques or even simply to the style of play associated with a football team may also reduce the number of rHAEs sustained by players during a season. Implementation in practices of helmetless tackling drills resulted in 26–33% fewer game rHAEs (per athletic exposure) as assessed at various times in a season [92]. Alteration of a team's offensive scheme to be more pass oriented than run oriented has also previously been documented to reduce the number of rHAEs [93]; however, such scheme-level changes are unlikely to be widely implementable, as offensive plans are heavily influenced by coaching philosophy, player talent and skill levels, opponent, and game situation.

Intervention—Protection

Historically, the most appealing solution to reducing head injuries (and, for our purposes, rHAE exposure) has been the use of helmets or other protective equipment. Devices which will absorb or deflect incident energy away from the head, and which to do not inherently force an alteration to the means by which the sport is played, are most desirable. To date, the primary means to affect changes in rHAE exposure have been through helmets, noting that some sports (e.g., soccer and rugby) do not allow for such protection in the absence of a fundamental change to the nature of play.

Since the early twentieth century, helmets have evolved from tooled leather caps to more complex structures with polymer shells, steel, or titanium facemasks, and numerous types of padding inserts [94]. The National Operating Committee on Standards for Athletic Equipment (NOCSAE) produced its first helmet testing standard in 1973, which decreased the rate of head impact-related fatalities [95]. In addition to the certification of existing helmets, their drop tower-based testing protocol (Fig. 17.4a) has been used to evaluate the effects of facemasks [96], after market add-on devices [97], helmet reconditioning [98], and gross differences between helmets from different sports [99]. Interestingly, the most substantive effects were observed between football and lacrosse helmets with football helmets ameliorating impacts to a much greater degree than lacrosse helmets [99]. Unfortunately, the inability to quantify the input force during the drop tower impacts limited its use in designing helmets for specific sports and levels of play.

More recent studies have focused on the use of a Hybrid III headform to obtain more biofidelic data (e.g., [100–104]), especially those associated with sport-specific impacts. Building on these efforts, recent work has integrated a modal hammer with the Hybrid III headform, making it possible to quantify both the input impacts and output accelerations (Fig. 17.4b). These data can be used to help delineate design features that promote energy absorption, an analysis that has been applied to helmets for football [105] and lacrosse [106]. Extending this technology to incorporate a finer-grained frequency analysis (Fig 17.4c) offers further

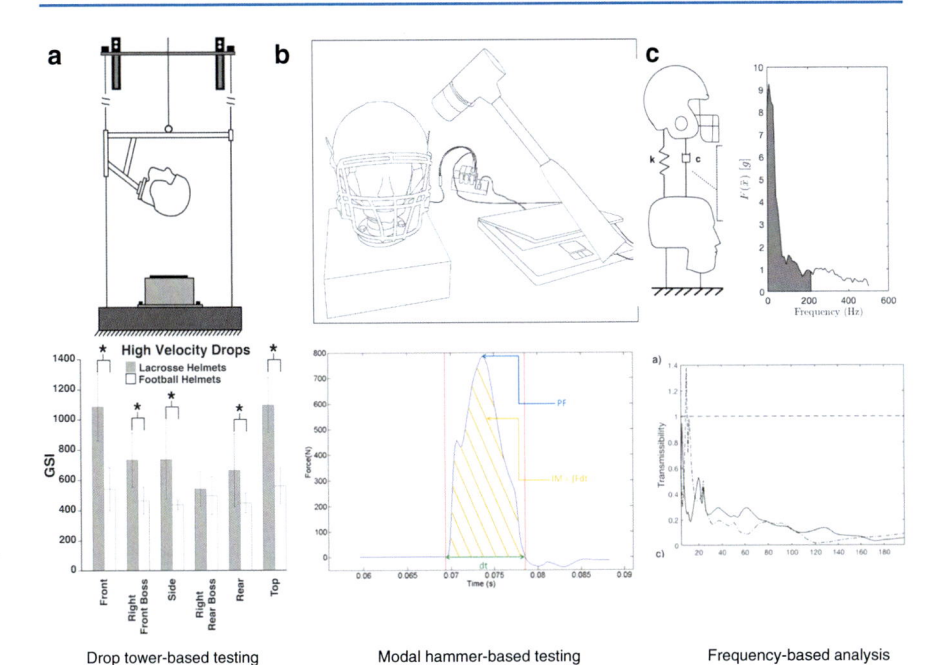

Fig. 17.4 Depiction of methods that have been used to characterize the protective aspects of helmets used in sports such as football or lacrosse. (**a**) The National Operating Committee on Standards for Athletic Equipment initially advocated for use of a drop tower to evaluate the energy absorption of helmets. This test has been superseded by use of a pneumatic ram, allowing for greater ability to quantify accelerations associated with impacts other than to the crown of the helmet. (**b**) Location-specific energy absorption can be better quantified using a modal hammer which allows for quantification of both the input forces and output accelerations [109]. (**c**) Frequency domain analysis of the energy input to, and subsequently transmitted by, a helmet provides a finer-grained quantification of energy absorption, identifying bandwidths in which particular constructions may be more effective at reducing the transmission of incident energy to the head and brain [107]

refinement to the analysis of mechanical load transmission [107]. Continued improvements to helmet testing protocols will undoubtedly offer additional data, but it should be noted that a more fruitful approach would incorporate helmet type into the structural health monitoring framework and use clinical data, especially neuroimaging, to evaluate their efficacy.

Given that many sports (e.g., rugby or soccer) have rules and gameplay that do not lend themselves to the use of helmets or other relatively rigid protective headwear, other approaches to protection have been explored over the past several decades. Such efforts have ranged from cushioned headbands purported to reduce the incident energy from heading the ball or colliding with other athletes to a jugular compression collar that is intended to increase intracranial pressure and reduce relative motion of brain tissue within the skull.

The addition of external padding, whether worn over a helmet [97] or directly on the skull, has proven to reduce accelerations experienced by athletes, but not at a level that is likely to meaningfully alter pathophysiologic changes, given that the reduction (typically fewer than 5 g) is quite small relative to the approximately 50 g thresholds observed (via neuroimaging) to best predict brain alterations [26–28].

One alternative protective measure that has been studied using a structural health monitoring approach—with evidence of some benefit—is the use of jugular compression. Several pilot studies have documented reductions in the alterations of functional activation and white matter structure observed in asymptomatic high school athletes using these devices relative to those who do not [16, 38, 50, 108]. Further, additional preliminary evidence for a protective effect has been derived from pilot study of blast exposure [109]. While it is unclear if measures such as this carry any as-yet unforeseen risks [110], it does indicate that means to prevent asymptomatic injury need not necessarily be of a shield-like nature.

Future Work—Personalization of Injury Prevention and Treatment

The approaches to prevention and intervention outlined above provide good starting points, but all largely involve mechanisms that are intended to limit or prevent rHAE exposure for *all* athletes, even though we have documented above that there are additional factors that may affect the risk for a given *individual* athlete. This point raises the question whether it may be possible to personalize the approach to injury mitigation or prevention, thereby reducing the level of rules or instructional changes required to permit more athletes to participate in more sports, more safely. Such future work may be built on wedding neuroimaging data to improved finite-element (FE) modeling and simulation approaches, allowing each individual rHAE experienced by an athlete to be modeled and combined with ever-improving models of the natural repair processes to predict the level of risk for prolonged accumulation/presence of pathophysiology.

Creating individual FE models from structural neuroimaging data allows for accurate separation of tissues, head sizing and measurements, and implementation of age- or development-specific material properties and physiology. When combined with a player's specific rHAE history (collected by sensors worn during play), the FE model can illuminate specific locations within the brain at which an individual may experience high stress and strain. These locations can be correlated with neuroimaging data to illuminate how stress and strain fields are related to microscale changes in the brain (i.e., changes in metabolite concentration, white matter integrity, and blood flow). Validation of this type of approach has previously been piloted (e.g., [111, 112]), but limitations in telemetry and the detail level of the underlying FE models preclude the widespread adoption of this approach on an individual-athlete basis.

The FE models can be expanded to also incorporate the musculature and muscle activation profiles of an individual's neck. In such a case, the model inputs could be expanded to include characteristics of rHAEs (e.g., force, location, and angle) with acceleration recordings from sensors to better understand the stabilizing contribution of neck muscles. Such data could lead to personalized preventative care strategies for each player to limit the neurological changes by creating player-specific plans to reduce or remove rHAEs while still allowing them to participate in the season. For example, characterization of the role in dissipation of energy from blows to the head played by the coupling of the head to the body could provide feedback allowing each player to focus on improvement of technique or increasing neck strength, whichever might prove more efficient in protection from injury during contact.

In the long run, development of individualized modeling and simulation coupled with a large-scale study incorporating structural health-monitoring approaches could provide not only validation for efforts to characterize the *individualized* pathophysiology of asymptomatic injury (and the genetic susceptibility thereto) but also serve as the basis for evaluating whether particular interventions are efficacious at this individual level. Such a large-scale study would also be expected to permit identification of those characteristics and participation measures most relevant to accumulation of injury, likely reducing the long-term cost and invasiveness of the screening and monitoring necessary to track and fairly predict the risk of accrual of both short- and long-term pathophysiology that might eventually transition from asymptomatic to symptomatic.

References

1. Beckwith JG, Greenwald RM, Chu JJ, Crisco JJ, Rowson S, Duma SM, et al. Timing of concussion diagnosis is related to head impact exposure prior to injury. Med Sci Sports Exerc. 2013;45:747–54.
2. Broglio SP, Lapointe A, O'Connor KL, McCrea M. Head impact density: a model to explain the elusive concussion threshold. J Neurotrauma. 2017;34:2675–83.
3. Funk JR, Rowson S, Daniel RW, Duma SM. Validation of concussion risk curves for collegiate football players derived from HITS data. Ann Biomed Eng. 2012;40:79–89.
4. Rowson S, Duma SM. Development of the STAR evaluation system for football helmets: integrating player head impact exposure and risk of concussion. Ann Biomed Eng. 2011;39:2130–40.
5. Rowson S, Duma SM. Brain injury prediction: assessing the combined probability of concussion using linear and rotational head acceleration. Ann Biomed Eng. 2013;41:873–82.
6. Guskiewicz KM, Mihalik JP, Shankar V, Marshall SW, Crowell DH, Oliaro SM, et al. Measurement of head impacts in collegiate football players: relationship between head impact biomechanics and acute clinical outcome after concussion. Neurosurgery. 2007;61:1244–52; discussion 1252–1253.
7. Broglio SP, Surma T, Ashton-Miller JA. High school and collegiate football athlete concussions: a biomechanical review. Ann Biomed Eng. 2012;40:37–46.
8. Hoshizaki TB, Post A, Kendall M, Cournoyer J, Rousseau P, Gilchrist MD, et al. The development of a threshold curve for the understanding of concussion in sport. Trauma. SAGE Publications;. 2017;19:196–206.
9. Pellman EJ, Viano DC, Tucker AM, Casson IR, Waeckerle JF. Concussion in professional football: reconstruction of game impacts and injuries. Neurosurgery. 2003;53:799–814.
10. Guskiewicz KM, Mihalik JP. Biomechanics of sport concussion: quest for the elusive injury threshold. Exerc Sport Sci Rev. 2011;39:4–11.
11. Talavage T. Medical imaging to recharacterize concussion for improved diagnosis in asymptomatic athletes. Natl Acad Eng [Internet]. 2016;46. Available from: https://nae.

edu/152059/Medical-Imaging-to-Recharacterize-Concussion-for-Improved-Diagnosis-in-Asymptomatic-Athletes

12. Talavage TM, Nauman EA, Leverenz LJ. The role of medical imaging in the recharacterization of mild traumatic brain injury using youth sorts as a laboratory. Front Neurol [Internet]. 2016 [cited 2017 Feb 13];6. Available from: http://www.ncbi.nlm.nih.gov/pmc/articles/PMC4717183/
13. Bazarian JJ, Zhu T, Zhong J, Janigro D, Rozen E, Roberts A, et al. Persistent, long-term cerebral white matter changes after sports-related repetitive head impacts. PLoS One. 2014;9:e94734.
14. Talavage TM, Nauman EA, Breedlove EL, Yoruk U, Dye AE, Morigaki KE, et al. Functionally-detected cognitive impairment in high school football players without clinically-diagnosed concussion. J Neurotrauma. 2014;31:327–38.
15. Slobounov SM, Walter A, Breiter HC, Zhu DC, Bai X, Bream T, et al. The effect of repetitive subconcussive collisions on brain integrity in collegiate football players over a single football season: a multi-modal neuroimaging study. Neuroimage Clin. 2017;14:708–18.
16. Myer GD, Yuan W, Barber Foss KD, Thomas S, Smith D, Leach J, et al. Analysis of head impact exposure and brain microstructure response in a season-long application of a jugular vein compression collar: a prospective, neuroimaging investigation in American football. Br J Sports Med. 2016;50:1276–85.
17. Bahrami N, Sharma D, Rosenthal S, Davenport EM, Urban JE, Wagner B, et al. Subconcussive head impact exposure and white matter tract changes over a single season of youth football. Radiology. 2016;281:919–26.
18. Epstein D. Big hits dominate the debate, but small ones are as traumatic [Internet]. Sports Illustrated Vault | SI.com. 2010 [cited 2020 Dec 23]. Available from: https://vault.si.com/vault/2010/11/01/the-damage-done
19. Breedlove EL, Robinson M, Talavage TM, Morigaki KE, Yoruk U, O'Keefe K, et al. Biomechanical correlates of symptomatic and asymptomatic neurophysiological impairment in high school football. J Biomech. 2012;45:1265–72.
20. Davenport EM, Whitlow CT, Urban JE, Espeland MA, Jung Y, Rosenbaum DA, et al. Abnormal white matter integrity related to head impact exposure in a season of high school varsity football. J Neurotrauma. 2014;31:1617–24.
21. Nauman EA, Breedlove KM, Breedlove EL, Talavage TM, Robinson ME, Leverenz LJ. Post-season neurophysiological deficits assessed by ImPACT and fMRI in athletes competing in American Football. Dev Neuropsychol. 2015;40:85–91.
22. Poole VN, Breedlove EL, Shenk TE, Abbas K, Robinson ME, Leverenz LJ, et al. Subconcussive hit characteristics predict deviant brain metabolism in football athletes. Dev Neuropsychol. 2015;40:12–7.
23. Robinson ME, Shenk TE, Breedlove EL, Leverenz LJ, Nauman EA, Talavage TM. The role of location of subconcussive head impacts in fMRI brain activation change. Dev Neuropsychol. Routledge;. 2015;40:74–9.
24. Davenport EM, Apkarian K, Whitlow CT, Urban JE, Jensen JH, Szuch E, et al. Abnormalities in diffusional kurtosis metrics related to head impact exposure in a season of high school varsity football. J Neurotrauma. 2016;33:2133–46.
25. Merchant-Borna K, Asselin P, Narayan D, Abar B, Jones CMC, Bazarian JJ. Novel method of weighting cumulative helmet impacts improves correlation with brain white matter changes after one football season of sub-concussive head blows. Ann Biomed Eng. 2016;44:3679–92.
26. Bari S, Svaldi DO, Jang I, Shenk TE, Poole VN, Lee T, et al. Dependence on subconcussive impacts of brain metabolism in collision sport athletes: an MR spectroscopic study. Brain Imaging Behav. 2018;
27. Jang I, Chun IY, Brosch JR, Bari S, Zou Y, Cummiskey BR, et al. Every hit matters: white matter diffusivity changes in high school football athletes are correlated with repetitive head acceleration event exposure. NeuroImage Clin. 2019;24:101930.

28. Svaldi DO, Joshi C, EC MC, Music JP, Hannemann R, Leverenz LJ, et al. Accumulation of high magnitude acceleration events predicts cerebrovascular reactivity changes in female high school soccer athletes. Brain Imaging Behav. 2018;
29. Johnson B, Neuberger T, Gay M, Hallett M, Slobounov S. Effects of subconcussive head trauma on the default mode network of the brain. J Neurotrauma. 2014;31:1907–13.
30. Abbas K, Shenk TE, Poole VN, Breedlove EL, Leverenz LJ, Nauman EA, et al. Alteration of default mode network in high school football athletes due to repetitive subconcussive mild traumatic brain injury: a resting-state functional magnetic resonance imaging study. Brain Connect. 2015;5:91–101.
31. Shenk TE, Robinson ME, Svaldi DO, Abbas K, Breedlove KM, Leverenz LJ, et al. FMRI of visual working memory in high school football players. Dev Neuropsychol. 2015;40:63–8.
32. Svaldi DO, Joshi C, Robinson ME, Shenk TE, Abbas K, Nauman EA, et al. Cerebrovascular reactivity alterations in asymptomatic high school football players. Dev Neuropsychol. Routledge;. 2015;40:80–4.
33. Svaldi DO, McCuen EC, Joshi C, Robinson ME, Nho Y, Hannemann R, et al. Cerebrovascular reactivity changes in asymptomatic female athletes attributable to high school soccer participation. Brain Imaging Behav. 2017;11:98–112.
34. Poole VN, Abbas K, Shenk TE, Breedlove EL, Breedlove KM, Robinson ME, et al. MR spectroscopic evidence of brain injury in the non-diagnosed collision sport athlete. Dev Neuropsychol. 2014;39:459–73.
35. Lipton ML, Kim N, Zimmerman ME, Kim M, Stewart WF, Branch CA, et al. Soccer heading is associated with white matter microstructural and cognitive abnormalities. Radiology. 2013;268:850–7.
36. Schranz AL, Manning KY, Dekaban GA, Fischer L, Jevremovic T, Blackney K, et al. Reduced brain glutamine in female varsity rugby athletes after concussion and in non-concussed athletes after a season of play. Hum Brain Mapp. 2018;39:1489–99.
37. Schneider DK, Galloway R, Bazarian JJ, Diekfuss JA, Dudley J, Leach JL, et al. Diffusion tensor imaging in athletes sustaining repetitive head impacts: a systematic review of prospective studies. J Neurotrauma. 2019;36:2831–49.
38. Myer GD, Barber Foss K, Thomas S, Galloway R, DiCesare CA, Dudley J, et al. Altered brain microstructure in association with repetitive subconcussive head impacts and the potential protective effect of jugular vein compression: a longitudinal study of female soccer athletes. Br J Sports Med. 2018;
39. McCuen E, Svaldi D, Breedlove K, Kraz N, Cummiskey B, Breedlove EL, et al. Collegiate women's soccer players suffer greater cumulative head impacts than their high school counterparts. J Biomech. 2015;48:3720–3.
40. Finn ES, Shen X, Scheinost D, Rosenberg MD, Huang J, Chun MM, et al. Functional connectome fingerprinting: identifying individuals using patterns of brain connectivity. Nat Neurosci. 2015;18:1664–71.
41. Amico E, Goñi J. The quest for identifiability in human functional connectomes. Sci Rep [Internet]. 2018 [cited 2020 Dec 22];8. Available from: https://www.ncbi.nlm.nih.gov/pmc/articles/PMC5973945/
42. Yeo BTT, Krienen FM, Sepulcre J, Sabuncu MR, Lashkari D, Hollinshead M, et al. The organization of the human cerebral cortex estimated by intrinsic functional connectivity. J Neurophysiol. 2011;106:1125–65.
43. Contreras JA, Avena-Koenigsberger A, Risacher SL, West JD, Tallman E, McDonald BC, et al. Resting state network modularity along the prodromal late onset Alzheimer's disease continuum. Neuroimage Clin [Internet]. 2019 [cited 2020 Dec 22];22. Available from: https://www.ncbi.nlm.nih.gov/pmc/articles/PMC6357852/.
44. Wu T, Wang L, Chen Y, Zhao C, Li K, Chan P. Changes of functional connectivity of the motor network in the resting state in Parkinson's disease. Neurosci Lett. 2009;460:6–10.
45. Hacker CD, Perlmutter JS, Criswell SR, Ances BM, Snyder AZ. Resting state functional connectivity of the striatum in Parkinson's disease. Brain. 2012;135:3699–711.

46. Thiruvady DR, Georgiou-Karistianis N, Egan GF, Ray S, Sritharan A, Farrow M, et al. Functional connectivity of the prefrontal cortex in Huntington's disease. J Neurol Neurosurg Psychiatry. 2007;78:127–33.
47. Wolf RC, Sambataro F, Vasic N, Schönfeldt-Lecuona C, Ecker D, Landwehrmeyer B. Aberrant connectivity of lateral prefrontal networks in presymptomatic Huntington's disease. Exp Neurol. 2008;213:137–44.
48. Werner CJ, Dogan I, Saß C, Mirzazade S, Schiefer J, Shah NJ, et al. Altered resting-state connectivity in Huntington's disease: resting-state connectivity in HD. Hum Brain Mapp. 2014;35:2582–93.
49. Bari S, Vike N, Nauman E, Talavage T. Brain fingerprint analysis using resting state fMRI in asymptomatic high-school football athletes. *The 26th Annual Meeting of the Organization for Human Brain Mapping*, 23 June–3 July, 2020;1193.
50. Yuan W, Foss KDB, Thomas S, DiCesare CA, Dudley JA, Kitchen K, et al. White matter alterations over the course of two consecutive high-school football seasons and the effect of a jugular compression collar: a preliminary longitudinal diffusion tensor imaging study. Hum Brain Mapp. 2018;39:491–508.
51. Papa L, Slobounov S, Breiter H, Walter A, Bream T, Seidenberg P, et al. Elevations in microRNA biomarkers in serum are associated with measures of concussion, neurocognitive function and subconcussive trauma over a single NCAA division I season in collegiate football players. J Neurotrauma. 2019;36:1343–51.
52. Chen Y, Herrold AA, Martinovich Z, Bari S, Vike NL, Blood AJ, et al. Brain Perfusion Mediates the Relationship Between miRNA Levels and Postural Control. Cerebral Cortex Communications [Internet]. 2020 [cited 2020 Dec 23];1. Available from: https://doi.org/10.1093/texcom/tgaa078.
53. Wexler NS. Venezuelan kindreds reveal that genetic and environmental factors modulate Huntington's disease age of onset. Proc Natl Acad Sci U S A. 2004;101:3498–503.
54. Moss DJH, Pardiñas AF, Langbehn D, Lo K, Leavitt BR, Roos R, et al. Identification of genetic variants associated with Huntington's disease progression: a genome-wide association study. Lancet Neurol. 2017;16:701–11.
55. Smith C, Graham DI, Murray LS, Stewart J, Nicoll JAR. Association of APOE e4 and cerebrovascular pathology in traumatic brain injury. J Neurol Neurosurg Psychiatry. 2006;77:363–6.
56. Kristman VL, Tator CH, Kreiger N, Richards D, Mainwaring L, Jaglal S, et al. Does the apolipoprotein epsilon 4 allele predispose varsity athletes to concussion? A prospective cohort study. Clin J Sport Med. 2008;18:322–8.
57. Terrell TR, Bostick RM, Abramson R, Xie D, Barfield W, Cantu R, et al. APOE, APOE promoter, and Tau genotypes and risk for concussion in college athletes. Clin J Sport Med. 2008;18:10–7.
58. Zhou W, Xu D, Peng X, Zhang Q, Jia J, Crutcher KA. Meta-analysis of APOE4 allele and outcome after traumatic brain injury. J Neurotr. Mary Ann Liebert, Inc., Publishers;. 2008;25:279–90.
59. Bu G. Apolipoprotein E and its receptors in Alzheimer's disease: pathways, pathogenesis and therapy. Nat Rev Neurosci. 2009;10:333–44.
60. Sun X, Jiang Y. Genetic susceptibility to traumatic brain injury and apolipoprotein E gene. Chinese J Traumatol (English Edition). 2008;11:247–52.
61. Crawford F, Wood M, Ferguson S, Mathura V, Gupta P, Humphrey J, et al. Apolipoprotein E-genotype dependent hippocampal and cortical responses to traumatic brain injury. Neuroscience. 2009;159:1349–62.
62. Moran LM, Taylor HG, Ganesalingam K, Gastier-Foster JM, Frick J, Bangert B, et al. Apolipoprotein E4 as a predictor of outcomes in pediatric mild traumatic brain injury. J Neurotrauma. 2009;26:1489–95.
63. Noé E, Ferri J, Colomer C, Moliner B, Chirivella J. APOE genotype and verbal memory recovery during and after emergence from post-traumatic amnesia. Brain Inj. 2010;24:886–92.

64. Ponsford J, McLaren A, Schönberger M, Burke R, Rudzki D, Olver J, et al. The association between apolipoprotein E and traumatic brain injury severity and functional outcome in a rehabilitation sample. J Neurotrauma. 2011;28:1683–92.
65. Tierney RT, Mansell JL, Higgins M, McDevitt JK, Toone N, Gaughan JP, et al. Apolipoprotein E genotype and concussion in college athletes. Clin J Sport Med. 2010;20:464–8.
66. McAllister TW. Polymorphisms in genes modulating the dopamine system: do they influence outcome and response to medication after traumatic brain injury? J Head Trauma Rehabil. 2009;24:65–8.
67. Dretsch MN, Silverberg N, Gardner AJ, Panenka WJ, Emmerich T, Crynen G, et al. Genetics and other risk factors for past concussions in active-duty soldiers. J Neurotrauma. 2017;34:869–75.
68. Panenka WJ, Gardner AJ, Dretsch MN, Crynen GC, Crawford FC, Iverson GL. Systematic review of genetic risk factors for sustaining a mild traumatic brain injury. J Neurotrauma. 2017;34:2093–9.
69. Walter A, Herrold AA, Gallagher VT, Lee R, Scaramuzzo M, Bream T, et al. KIAA0319 genotype predicts the number of past concussions in a division I football team: a pilot study. J Neurotrauma. 2019;36:1115–24.
70. Paracchini S, Thomas A, Castro S, Lai C, Paramasivam M, Wang Y, et al. The chromosome 6p22 haplotype associated with dyslexia reduces the expression of KIAA0319, a novel gene involved in neuronal migration. Hum Mol Genet. 2006;15:1659–66.
71. Kerr ZY, Chandran A, Nedimyer AK, Arakkal A, Pierpoint LA, Zuckerman SL. Concussion Incidence and Trends in 20 High School Sports. Pediatrics [Internet]. American Academy of Pediatrics; 2019 [cited 2020 Dec 22];144. Available from: http://pediatrics.aappublications.org/content/144/5/e20192180.
72. Broshek DK, Kaushik T, Freeman JR, Erlanger D, Webbe F, Barth JT. Sex differences in outcome following sports-related concussion. J Neurosurg. 2005;102:856–63.
73. Zhang MR, Red SD, Lin AH, Patel SS, Sereno AB. Evidence of cognitive dysfunction after soccer playing with ball heading using a novel tablet-based approach. PLoS One. 2013;8:e57364.
74. Koerte IK, Nichols E, Tripodis Y, Schultz V, Lehner S, Igbinoba R, et al. Impaired cognitive performance in youth athletes exposed to repetitive head impacts. J Neurotrauma. 2017;34:2389–95.
75. Sollmann N, Echlin PS, Schultz V, Viher PV, Lyall AE, Tripodis Y, et al. Sex differences in white matter alterations following repetitive subconcussive head impacts in collegiate ice hockey players. Neuroimage Clin. 2018;17:642–9.
76. Rubin TG, Catenaccio E, Fleysher R, Hunter LE, Lubin N, Stewart WF, et al. MRI-defined white matter microstructural alteration associated with soccer heading is more extensive in women than men. Radiology. 2018;289:478–86.
77. Gessel LM, Fields SK, Collins CL, Dick RW, Comstock RD. Concussions among United States high school and collegiate athletes. J Athl Train. 2007;42:495–503.
78. Lincoln AE, Caswell SV, Almquist JL, Dunn RE, Norris JB, Hinton RY. Trends in concussion incidence in high school sports: a prospective 11-year study. Am J Sports Med. SAGE Publications Inc STM;. 2011;39:958–63.
79. Marar M, McIlvain NM, Fields SK, Comstock RD. Epidemiology of concussions among United States high school athletes in 20 sports. Am J Sports Med. 2012;40:747–55.
80. Lee T, Lycke R, Auger J, Music J, Dziekan M, Newman S, et al. Head acceleration event metrics in youth contact sports more dependent on sport than level of play. Proc Inst Mech Eng H. IMECHE;. 2020;0954411920970812
81. Press JN, Rowson S. Quantifying head impact exposure in collegiate women's soccer. Clin J Sport Med. 2017;27:104–10.
82. Baugh CM, Kiernan PT, Kroshus E, Daneshvar DH, Montenigro PH, McKee AC, et al. Frequency of head-impact-related outcomes by position in NCAA division I collegiate football players. J Neurotrauma. 2015;32:314–26.

83. Jadischke R, Viano DC, Dau N, King AI, McCarthy J. On the accuracy of the Head Impact Telemetry (HIT) System used in football helmets. J Biomech. 2013;46:2310–5.
84. Cummiskey B, Schiffmiller D, Talavage TM, Leverenz L, Meyer JJ, Adams D, et al. Reliability and accuracy of helmet-mounted and head-mounted devices used to measure head accelerations. Proceedings of the Institution of Mechanical Engineers, Part P. J Sports Eng Technol. SAGE Publications;. 2017;231:144–53.
85. Wu LC, Nangia V, Bui K, Hammoor B, Kurt M, Hernandez F, et al. In vivo evaluation of wearable head impact sensors. Ann Biomed Eng. 2016;44:1234–45.
86. Emery CA, Black AM. Are rule changes the low-hanging fruit for concussion prevention in youth sport? JAMA Pediatr. 2019;173:309.
87. Yang YT, Baugh CM. US youth soccer concussion policy. JAMA Pediatr. 2016;170:413–4.
88. Emery C, Kang J, Shrier I, Goulet C, Hagel B, Benson B, et al. Risk of injury associated with bodychecking experience among youth hockey players. CMAJ. 2011;183:1249–56.
89. Auerbach PS, Waggoner WH II. It's time to change the rules. JAMA. 2016;316:1260–1.
90. Lee TA, Lycke RJ, Lee PJ, Cudal CM, Torolski KJ, Bucherl SE, et al. Distribution of Head Acceleration Events Varies by Position and Play Type in North American Football. Clinical Journal of Sport Medicine [Internet]. 2020 [cited 2020 Dec 22]; Publish Ahead of Print. Available from: http://journals.lww.com/cjsportsmed/Abstract/9000/Distribution_of_Head_Acceleration_Events_Varies_by.98992.aspx.
91. Wiebe DJ, D'Alonzo BA, Harris R, Putukian M, Campbell-McGovern C. Association between the experimental kickoff rule and concussion rates in ivy league football. JAMA. 2018;320:2035–6.
92. Swartz EE, Myers JL, Cook SB, Guskiewicz KM, Ferrara MS, Cantu RC, et al. A helmetless-tackling intervention in American football for decreasing head impact exposure: a randomized controlled trial. J Sci Med Sport. 2019;22:1102–7.
93. Martini D, Eckner J, Kutcher J, Broglio S. Subconcussive head impact biomechanics: comparing differing offensive schemes. Med Sci Sports Exerc. 2013;45:755–61.
94. Newman JA. Modern sports helmets: their history, science, and art. Schiffer Pub; 2007.
95. Mueller FO. Catastrophic head injuries in high school and collegiate sports. J Athl Train. 2001;36:312–5.
96. Breedlove KM, Breedlove EL, Bowman TG, Arruda EM, Nauman EA. The effect of football helmet facemasks on impact behavior during linear drop tests. J Biomech. 2018;79:227–31.
97. Breedlove KM, Breedlove E, Nauman E, Bowman TG, Lininger MR. The ability of an aftermarket helmet add-on device to reduce impact-force accelerations during drop tests. J Athl Train (Allen Press). 2017;52:802–8.
98. Bowman TG, Breedlove KM, Breedlove EL, Dodge TM, Nauman EA. Impact attenuation properties of new and used lacrosse helmets. J Biomech. 2015;48:3782–7.
99. Breedlove KM, Breedlove EL, Bowman TG, Nauman EA. Impact attenuation capabilities of football and lacrosse helmets. J Biomech. 2016;49:2838–44.
100. Coulson N, Foreman S, Hoshizaki T. Translational and rotational accelerations generated during reconstructed ice hockey impacts on a hybrid III head form. J ASTM Int. West Conshohocken, PA: ASTM International;. 2009;6:1–8.
101. Rousseau P, Hoshizaki T. The influence of deflection and neck compliance on the impact dynamics of a Hybrid III headform. Proceedings of The Institution of Mechanical Engineers, Part P. J Sports Eng Technol. 2009;223:89–97.
102. Walsh ES, Rousseau P, Hoshizaki TB. The influence of impact location and angle on the dynamic impact response of a Hybrid III headform. Sports Eng. 2020;13:135–43.
103. Oeur RA, Gilchrist MD, Hoshizaki TB. Interaction of impact parameters for simulated falls in sport using three different sized Hybrid III headforms. Int J Crashworthiness. Taylor & Francis;. 2019;24:326–35.
104. Oeur RA, Gilchrist MD, Hoshizaki TB. Parametric study of impact parameters on peak head acceleration and strain for collision impacts in sport. Int J Crashworthiness. Taylor & Francis;. 2019;0:1–10.

105. Cummiskey B, Sankaran GN, McIver KG, Shyu D, Markel J, Talavage TM, et al. Quantitative evaluation of impact attenuation by football helmets using a modal impulse hammer. Proceedings of the Institution of Mechanical Engineers, Part P. J Sports Eng Technol. SAGE Publications;. 2019;233:301–11.
106. McIver KG, Sankaran GN, Lee P, Bucherl S, Leiva N, Talavage TM, et al. Impact attenuation of male and female lacrosse helmets using a modal impulse hammer. J Biomech. 2019;95:109313.
107. Leiva-Molano N, Rolley R, Lee T, McIver K, Sankaran G, Meyer J, et al. Evaluation of impulse attenuation by football helmets in the frequency domain. J Biomech Eng. 2020;
108. Myer GD, Yuan W, Barber Foss KD, Smith D, Altaye M, Reches A, et al. The Effects of External Jugular Compression Applied during Head Impact Exposure on Longitudinal Changes in Brain Neuroanatomical and Neurophysiological Biomarkers: A Preliminary Investigation. Front Neurol [Internet]. 2016 [cited 2020 Dec 22];7. Available from: https://www.ncbi.nlm.nih.gov/pmc/articles/PMC4893920/
109. Yuan W, Barber Foss KD, Dudley J, Thomas S, Galloway R, DiCesare C, et al. Impact of low-level blast exposure on brain function after a one-day tactile training and the ameliorating effect of a jugular vein compression neck collar device. J Neurotrauma. 2019;36:721–34.
110. Experts say Panthers shouldn't rush Luke Kuechly back on the field [Internet]. ESPN.com. 2017 [cited 2020 Dec 22]. Available from: https://www.espn.com/blog/nfcsouth/post/_/id/69463/experts-say-panthers-shouldnt-rush-luke-kuechly-back-on-the-field
111. Ji S, Ghadyani H, Bolander RP, Beckwith JG, Ford JC, Mcallister TW, et al. Parametric comparisons of intracranial mechanical responses from three validated finite element models of the human head. Ann Biomed Eng. 2014;42:11–24.
112. Ji S, Zhao W. A pre-computed brain response atlas for instantaneous strain estimation in contact sports. Ann Biomed Eng. 2015;43:1877–95.

Part V

Clinical Management and Rehabilitation of Concussions

Management of Collegiate Sport-Related Concussions

18

Allyssa K. Memmini, Vinodh Balendran, Steven E. Pachman, and Steven P. Broglio

Introduction

Sport-related concussion (SRC), otherwise known as mild traumatic brain injury, is a cerebral neurological disruption induced by traumatic biomechanical forces [1] resulting in acute clinical symptoms. When accounting for both reported and unreported SRC, prevalence of concussion falls between 1.6 and 3.8 million injuries per year [2].

To optimize the student-athlete's (SA) health and well-being, the healthcare provider must rapidly recognize, remove, and evaluate any SA with a suspected SRC. There are several position statements to guide clinicians depending on their healthcare licensure and place of employment. For example, athletic trainers (ATs) would be held to the standards set forth by the National Athletic Trainers' Association (NATA) [3] and the International Concussion in Sport Group [4]. Physicians, on the other hand, would not be held to the standard of the NATA, but would need to comply with the American Medical Society for Sports Medicine (AMSSM) statement [5]. Either healthcare professional practicing within the National Collegiate Athletics Association (NCAA) may be required to follow the guidelines outlined by the NCAA [6]. While it would be impossible to review every position statement (>20 since 2001), this chapter compares and contrasts four key guidelines regarding their clinical recommendations for SRC identification and management: NCAA, NATA, Concussion in Sport Group, and AMSSM.

A. K. Memmini (✉) · V. Balendran · S. P. Broglio
Michigan Concussion Center, University of Michigan, Ann Arbor, MI, USA
e-mail: amemmini@umich.edu; vinodhb@umich.edu; broglio@umich.edu

S. E. Pachman
Montgomery McCracken Walker & Rhoads LLP, Philadelphia, PA, USA
e-mail: spachman@mmwr.com

Concussion Education and Baseline Assessment

NCAA

Institutions within the NCAA are required to provide educational materials to SAs, coaches, ATs, athletics directors, and team physicians every year, with signed acknowledgment that these individuals have read and understood institution's specific SRC management protocol.

Prior to participation in collegiate athletics, SAs undergo a single, preparticipation SRC assessment including, but not limited to: SRC/brain injury history, symptom inventory (total number and severity), and neurocognitive and balance assessments. Following testing, the team physician must clear the SA to participate in sport [7].

NATA

Current guidelines encourage ATs to collaborate with administrators to ensure parents, coaches, and SAs are educated on SRC prevention, mechanisms of injury, recognition, referral, short- and long-term effects, and overall ramifications of improper management [8]. The AT is responsible for all relevant governing bodies' SRC policies, such as at the school, state, and athletic conference levels.

In addition to SAs participating in collision sports undergoing baseline assessments before the start of the competitive season [9, 10], so should adolescent SAs with SRC history and those with comorbid conditions. If resources are readily available, schools should aim to test all SAs on an annual basis [11]. The baseline assessment should consist of a comprehensive medical history questionnaire, physical and neurological evaluations, as well as motor control and neurocognitive assessments [9]. All baseline examinations should be reviewed for intentional suboptimal performance to reduce the risk of SAs from returning to sport prematurely. Baseline evaluations should be administered to small groups in quiet, secluded areas of the athletic training room or clinic.

Concussion in Sport Group

Although baseline assessments provide healthcare providers the opportunity to educate their patients on SRCs, the 2016 consensus group agreed that, although useful, baseline assessments are not necessary to interpret postinjury scores. In addition, inevitable extraneous variables may also influence the interpretations of the postinjury assessment (game vs. clinic setting, postexercise, etc.). If a clinician elects to test SAs, the postinjury environment should replicate the baseline test.

AMSSM

The preparticipation exam (PPE) documents a SA's medical history prior to clearance for sport activity from a healthcare provider. The PPE should capture comorbid conditions such as attention deficit or learning disorders, motion sickness, mood disorders, or family history of migraines. Consistent with other guidelines, the baseline evaluation should include a symptom checklist, balance assessment, and cognitive evaluation as the core components of the initial baseline evaluation. Despite several organizations that recommend baseline assessments prior to the start of sport participation [4, 6], AMSSM indicates baseline testing has been proven to not be as necessary as initially thought, and in some cases is no longer an accepted standard of care in collegiate athletics [6].

Summary

Although differences exist between organizations, the sports medicine staff is encouraged to educate administrators, coaches, and other associated staff about the risks of SRC in collegiate athletics. The NCAA requires educational materials to be provided for SAs and coaches prior to athletic participation, with a signed acknowledgment. In addition, annual baseline assessments may or may not be required for collegiate SAs depending on the requirements established within the institution's SRC management policy. Although baseline assessments are not necessary to interpret postinjury scores, they can be helpful in certain situations.

Injury Identification

Sideline Assessment

NCAA
All SAs experiencing SRC-related signs or symptoms must be immediately removed from participation. Following removal, they must be evaluated by the AT or team physician trained in diagnosis and management of SRCs. The healthcare provider must evaluate the SA using serial clinical evaluations including symptom count and severity, as well as cognitive and balance assessments. Unless a SRC can be ruled out, the SA is required to remain out of sport until the next calendar day.

NATA
Under the suspicion of SRC, the SA must be immediately removed from participation and undergo a multistep evaluation, with the clinical examination consisting of a thorough medical history, general observations, neurologic screening, and assessing mental status, motor control, and balance [12]. If the assessment is conducted solely by an AT, results pertaining to diagnosis should be interpreted conservatively, especially if a physician is not readily available on-site. Once a SRC diagnosis has been

confirmed, the SA must be removed from sport and is not permitted to return to sport unless cleared by a physician, no sooner than the next day.

Concussion in Sport Group
SRC is noted to be an evolving injury during the acute phase with no single diagnostic tool, necessitating the use of an assessment battery. If a SA is suspected of sustaining a SRC, they must be immediately removed from participation and evaluated by a licensed healthcare professional. No SA should be permitted to return to activity, and, therefore, must be serially monitored. The clinician should always err on the side of caution and manage the SA conservatively.

The sideline assessment should consist of a brief neuropsychological evaluation to determine level of cognitive function using attention or memory tasks. Such assessments include the fifth-edition Sport Concussion Assessment Tool (SCAT-5), which is comprised of a symptom list, Glasgow Coma Score, Maddock's Questions, the Standardized Assessment of Concussion (SAC), and a motor control evaluation [13, 14]. This brief assessment should be used as a rapid evaluation tool on the sideline and should not replace a more comprehensive evaluation. Only appropriately trained clinicians can make the injury diagnosis or clear a SA to return to sport on the same day of the suspected injury.

Finally, although the SCAT-5 can be useful during acute injury assessment, it does not appropriately track recovery, with utility decreasing 3–5 days postinjury [5]. Instead, symptom checklists have demonstrated clinical value in assessing recovery trajectories.

AMSSM
Due to an ostensible lack of validated diagnostic tools, confounding comorbidities, and reliance on self-reported symptom surveys, the clinical diagnosis should be made based upon medical history in conjunction with a comprehensive physical examination.

SAs must be immediately removed from participation due to the following circumstances: seizures, loss of consciousness, tonic posturing, gross motor impairments, amnesia, or disorientation. When video of the impact is available, any signs of motor incoordination, postural instability, or vacant look on the SA warrant immediate removal for evaluation [15]. If removed from activity for a suspected SRC, the SA is not permitted to return until at least the next calendar day [16].

The initial assessment includes an injury history from the SA or witnesses, during which the clinician may be able to determine impairments in cognitive processing in conversation with the SA. Depending on the relationship between the SA and the healthcare provider, subtle changes in the SA's personality or performance metrics may be observable, further suggesting a SRC. To confirm diagnosis, there should be a clear mechanism of injury relating to direct or indirect forces to the head and/or body resulting in characteristic signs/symptoms, and neuropsychological assessment if available. Following the history, a multimodal process for diagnosing SRC is recommended so as to increase evaluation specificity and sensitivity [17]. In parallel with the Concussion in Sport Group, the AMSSM recommends the SCAT-5 [18] to appropriately evaluate a suspected SRC. Clinicians should be aware that SAs may not recognize common signs/symptoms associated with SRC, or be fully forthcoming in reporting so as to minimize time loss from athletic participation. Additional components of comprehensive assessment include evaluating neurocognitive, vestibular and/or ocular function, and gait. For example, the vestibulo-ocular motor screening (VOMS) assesses the SA's vestibular ocular reflex, vestibular motion sensitivity, convergence, and saccadic testing [19]. The King-Devick (KD) test assesses saccadic eye movement by asking SAs to quickly read numbers aloud, and whereas simple reaction time may be assessed via weighted-stick drop [20].

It is also important for clinicians to consider conditions which may be of another etiology but may have become unmasked due to the concussive event. These pathologies include migraine/headache disorder, mood disorders, cervicogenic pain, and peripheral vestibular conditions.

Summary

Any SA who appears stunned, dazed, or confused, reports any SRC symptoms, or if there is video evidence suggesting a head injury has occurred must be immediately removed from activity. Those displaying signs of more severe injury (Table 18.1) should seek additional medical care. If a SRC is suspected, they must undergo a comprehensive evaluation in an athletic training room or clinic setting. The evaluation should include a thorough clinical history and exam, supported by an evaluation of neurocognitive status, motor control, and symptoms. In no case should a SA be returned on the same day as the suspected SRC, unless cleared by an appropriate healthcare professional.

Table 18.1 Observable red flags that warrant emergency medical transportation[a]

Neck pain or tenderness
Diplopia
Weakness/tingling/burning into arms or legs
Severe or increasing headache
Seizure or convulsions
Loss of consciousness
Deteriorating mental status
Emesis
Increasingly agitated, restless, or combative

[a]Table has been modified based on the Sport Concussion Assessment Tool (SCAT-5) [18]

Injury Management

NCAA

Passive management of SRC may in fact be detrimental for the SA's recovery. Recent studies suggest prolonged rest may lead to adverse effects including low self-esteem, physical deconditioning, and social isolation from teammates [3, 21, 22]. It is the responsibility of the healthcare provider to be aware of the signs and symptoms associated with an emotional response associated with SRC [3, 21]. Other conditions that may stem from SRC include postconcussion syndrome, sleep dysfunction, headache disorders, or migraines [22].

Currently, there are no empirical data to indubitably outline optimal rehabilitation of concussed SAs. Some clinicians have instead based treatment protocols on clinical profiles such as vestibular symptoms, general fatigue, mood disorders, oculomotor impairments, cognitive dysfunction, or cervicogenic disorder [23]. In patients reporting primarily vestibular symptoms, common rehabilitation includes proprioceptive exercises, assessing the vestibular ocular reflex, and dynamic gait or postural control activities [24]. Patients who report oculomotor-related symptoms are often treated using vision therapies to target convergence and accommodative insufficiencies, ocular misalignments, and impaired eye tracking movements. Clinicians should use these guidelines as a framework and adapt as needed depending on the patient population.

NATA

Management of concussed SAs should be based on the individual's unique needs. Common treatment goals include cessation of symptomology, reestablishment of neurocognitive performance, and restoration of motor control function. In order to avoid an increase in symptoms, current recommendations include limited cognitive and physical activity during the acute recovery period (24–48 hours). It is critical that the SA is not completely withheld from all activities, as isolation from social endeavors may increase SRC symptoms unrelated to the head injury [25].

After symptom cessation, objective assessments should be repeated and compared to baseline values. Caution is warranted in solely using self-reported symptom surveys to determine whether a SA is ready to begin the next stage of return to activity, thus clinicians should opt to use measures of neurocognitive function and motor control in conjunction with symptom severity measures. The decision to begin the return-to-play protocol is appropriate when the SA no longer reports symptoms and performs at baseline scores for neurocognitive and motor control tasks.

During the symptom resolution period, the AT must maintain communication with the team physician regarding the SA's progression, especially if the recovery trajectory is beyond a 14- to 21-day time frame. Although not ideal, some research suggests if baseline measures are not readily available, physicians and ATs may opt to use normative data as a comparison [10]; however, more conservative management strategies are warranted using this method.

Concussion in Sport Group

Current consensus statements recommend that SAs rest until they become asymptomatic. Although rest may minimize brain energy demands after SRC, there is currently insufficient evidence to support the claim that complete rest is beneficial in recovery. As such, SAs are encouraged to engage in light cognitive and physical activity while remaining below their symptom-exacerbation thresholds following the initial acute phase (24–48 hours). They should not engage in vigorous physical activity until cleared by a medical professional to begin the stepwise return-to-sport protocol.

At the time of the consensus meeting, the literature had not readily investigated early interventions, as most individuals recover within 10–14 days. SRCs often present as clusters of symptoms, some concurrent with disruption to the vestibular system or injury to the cervical spine. For those with ongoing symptoms, interventions include targeting psychological, vestibular, and cervical symptoms. In addition, researchers have suggested that active rehabilitation in a controlled environment using subsymptom thresholds during submaximal exercise may further facilitate recovery.

AMSSM

During the acute recovery phase, SAs are oftentimes prescribed mental and physical rest despite insufficient evidence supporting its efficacy [26]. Clinicians should use caution when prescribing rest, as isolation and prolonged rest may lead to increased recovery timelines [27]. Previous recommendations such as "staying in a dark room" and "cocoon therapy" are no longer recommended due to the detrimental effects demonstrated in animal models [4]. Standard guidelines support rest for the first 24–48 hours postinjury, with gradual increase in activity without exacerbating symptoms.

After the acute phase, preliminary evidence suggests subsymptom threshold activity may improve recovery and is safe for acutely concussed individuals as long as they are under the direct supervision of a healthcare provider [28]. From a physiological standpoint, exercise has been proven to increase autonomic function and, thus, promote cerebral blood flow regulation [29]. Other benefits of exercise include neurotrophic factor gene upregulation and general improvements in sleep and mood [30]. Although there are benefits to implementing exercise during the initial stages of recovery, exercise alone does not replace the graduated return-to-sport protocol.

Recovery trajectories among SAs are often influenced on the number and severity of acute symptoms [31], such as subacute headache and depression. As based on current research, those with attention deficit/hyperactivity or other learning disabilities are not at heightened risk for prolonged recovery [31]. Some studies suggest a difference in recovery timelines based on sex, with women reporting longer periods of symptoms [31]. A final predictor of increased symptom burden has been recently suggested in adolescent SAs who present with a lower symptom-limited heart rate threshold during graduated exercise testing (treadmill and biking) within 1 week of injury.

Although various SAs may experience symptom relief with early interventions, others may suffer from persistent symptoms beyond typical recovery trajectories. Clinicians should be aware that prolonged symptoms may not be attributed directly from the SRC, and instead may be a comorbid condition affected by their overall recovery. Recent studies have developed individualized treatment programs for postconcussive symptoms (PPCS), which include oculomotor, sleep, psychological, vestibular, autonomic nervous system, and cervicogenic targeted [32]. To target SAs with PPCS, activities of daily living and aerobic exercise that do not increase symptom severity may be helpful. For example, the Buffalo Concussion Exercise Treatment Protocol is a subsymptom threshold program which has been shown to reduce persistent symptom burden in concussed SAs compared to controls [33].

Furthermore, those with prolonged headache-related symptoms should be evaluated for cervicogenic disorders or cervical dysfunction [32]. Therapists with expertise in vestibular therapy may opt to use "exposure-recovery" therapy in those suffering from prolonged balance impairments [24]. Clinicians must also consider cognitive rehabilitation completed at the symptom subthreshold level, and discussions surrounding the SA's sleep hygiene [34] should be discussed during the first few rehabilitation sessions. If the SA reports symptoms related to comorbid mood disorders, a clinician may choose a multidisciplinary approach using cognitive behavioral therapy to best approach the case [35]. In sum, treating SRCs is a continually evolving process depending on the individual needs of the SA.

Summary

Managing SRCs ultimately depends on the patient's clinical profile. Each document emphasizes "active" rehabilitation by limiting physical and cognitive rest during the early phase of the recovery process, with subsymptom-exacerbation levels thereafter until the formal return-to-play protocol begins. Previous protocols implementing "cocoon therapy" are no longer standard clinical care, and in fact may delay the recovery by endorsing social isolation. In cases where symptom recovery does not follow a typical time course, rehabilitation strategies should focus on specific needs including, but not limited to, cervicogenic or headache disorder, vestibular symptoms, and/or sleep disorders.

Return to Learn

NCAA

Despite growing literature regarding SRC management plans, return-to-learn (RTL) guidelines are explicitly based on expert consensus and, thus, must be implemented for the SAs' specific needs. As such, the RTL protocol should incorporate a multidisciplinary team including team physicians, ATs, coaches, academic representatives, and administrators, as well as the institutions' disability services to best assist each SA as they return to the classroom. According to current research, SAs are more likely to successfully return to the classroom when they are immersed in an environment with a proactive SRC management team with a well-integrated protocol.

It is recommended that SAs do not return to the classroom on the same day of injury. Current recommendations suggest that the SA should remain in their home or residence hall until they can tolerate light cognitive activity, with an incremental return to the classroom. Consistent with normal symptom recovery, SAs may fully RTL within 2 weeks following injury without requiring substantial curriculum, testing modifications, or necessity of creating an Individualized Education Plan (IEP) or 504 Plan.

If symptoms persist beyond 2 weeks, it is the responsibility of the multidisciplinary team to enforce specified academic accommodations such as extended time for assignments or examinations, as well as adjusting their class schedule if necessary. Several institutions offer temporary accommodations for those who have short-term impairments (less than 6 months) and are typically accessible through the department of services for students with disabilities.

If symptomology is prolonged for longer than 6 months, clinicians should consider further neuropsychological testing to determine the magnitude of cognitive impairment, as well as identify any underlying psychological disorders which may be influencing the recovery trajectory. Long-term accommodations, such as an IEP, may be pursued with the assistance of a disability officer.

Successful RTL implementation incorporates several components. Importantly, a case manager, as defined by the multidisciplinary team, is critical in navigating the logistics of academic and athletic profiles of the SA. The medical staff should also consider comorbid psychological conditions that may impact recovery trends such as depression, anxiety, and attention deficit disorder. Finally, SAs should be introduced to campus resources as soon as possible to ensure they are provided appropriate accommodations, such as learning specialists, academic counselors, and services for students with disabilities. Within the office of student disabilities, administrators are responsible for verifying each SA's impairment and ensuring they are adequately supported as they return to the classroom.

NATA

The current NATA position statement does not provide guidance for RTL following SRC. It is recommended that future versions of this statement include appropriate RTL management strategies for the AT and multidisciplinary team.

Concussion in Sport Group

Schools are encouraged to develop a SRC policy for administrators, teachers, SAs, and parents that includes the potential need for academic accommodations. Depending on the needs of the SA, temporary absence from school and assistance with incremental RTL may be necessary. Prior to clearance for return to sport, SAs must completely return to classroom activities without exacerbation of symptoms.

Graduated RTL strategies (Table 18.2) begin by reintroducing daily activities at home without increasing symptoms. Typical activities include reading a book, texting, and computer usage, starting with 5-minute increments and building up the time as tolerated. Next, SAs should be reintroduced to classwork beyond the classroom, such as homework, reading, or other types of cognitive activity in order to increase their cognitive load tolerance. SAs may be able to complete a partial, half, or full day of school with increased breaks throughout the day. The last step in the progression includes gradually returning to a full day of school and catching up on missed work.

AMSSM

Immediately following a SRC, school personnel should be notified to begin monitoring and implementing an individualized RTL protocol [36]. A school health professional, administrator, school nurse, AT, or counselor must be defined as the SA's

Table 18.2 Return-to-school progression[a]

Stage	Aim	Activity	Goal
1	Daily activities at home that do not increase child's symptoms	Reading, texting, and typing (start with 5- to 15-minute increments and gradually increase time)	Gradual return to activities of daily living
2	Classroom activities	Homework and other cognitive activities	Increase tolerance in cognitive load
3	Part-time return to school	Reintroduction to schoolwork and intermittent breaks through the day	Adjust to academic activities
4	Full return to school	Progress to full school days	Full return to academics; make up any missed work

[a]Table has been modified based on the Concussion in Sport Group position statement [4]

point person in order to monitor their recovery, academics, and facilitate effective communication with the medical staff. If a SA requires additional accommodations, teachers are encouraged to develop a plan for missed coursework or exams. Guidance counselors may be needed in order to adjust class schedules to modify attendance, and schools must be prepared to manage both acute and chronic recovery patterns of concussed SAs (Table 18.3). The SAs must completely return to classroom activities without increase in symptomology prior to clearance for return to sport.

Summary

An efficacious RTL protocol consists of a multidisciplinary team including academic staff, physicians, school counselors, coaches, and sports medicine staff. It is imperative that institutions have RTL protocols in place for SAs who sustain a SRC to ensure they receive the appropriate academic accommodations that facilitate their academic goals. Current guidelines suggest starting the RTL progression with activities of daily living, slowly building back up into classroom activities such as homework and reading assignments (Table 18.3) Once the SA is comfortable with school-related activities, they may be able to tolerate attending class part-time. Depending on the length of recovery, it may be beneficial to adjust the SA's schedule, alter the curriculum, encourage permanent testing modifications, or create an IEP. Communication among the multidisciplinary staff is critical to the success of returning a SA back to the classroom setting.

Table 18.3 Recommendations for academic accommodations[a]

Classroom adjustments	School environment adjustments
Periodic breaks throughout the school day	Permit use of headphones to reduce noise sensitivity
Reduce coursework and homework	Limit use of electronic screens including computers, tablets, etc.
Arrange for additional time to complete assignments/projects	Allow the student to leave prior to the end of class to avoid congested hallways
Provide a peer note taker or the teacher's notes	Permit use of sunglasses to reduce light sensitivity
Extra time during quizzes/examinations	Avoid areas of high volume: cafeteria, pep assemblies, lunch room, etc.
Avoid physical activity	
Allow testing in a separate, distraction-free space	
Delay tests or major project deadlines until the students' symptoms no longer affect their work	

[a]Table has been modified based on the AMSSM position statement [5]

Return to Sport Participation

NCAA

No SA removed from sport participation under the suspicion of SRC can be returned within the same calendar day without clearance from a qualified clinician. Once a SRC is diagnosed and symptoms, cognitive, and balance measurements return to preinjury levels, the return to sport participation (RTP) protocol may be initiated under the supervision of a physician or physician designee [37]. The RTP protocol steadily increases exercise intensity, progressing from light aerobic exercise to sport-specific activity, noncontact sports drills, and unrestricted training and sport participation (Table 18.4). Daily progression is based on the SAs' self-reported symptoms before and after activity, with regression to the previous step should symptoms return. Depending on the patient's clinical profile, the RTP protocol may be affected by other comorbidities, with modifications as needed. Prior to full return to sport activity, medical clearance is warranted by the team physician.

NATA

The NATA recommendations for return to sport are similar to the NCAA. Concussed SAs should not begin the RTP progression until SRC symptoms are no longer reported and performance is at or above preinjury baseline measures. The RTP stages are identical to the NCAA, separated by approximately 24 hours [1]. If a SA experiences an increase in symptoms or demonstrates cognitive decline, activity should stop immediately and the SA should return to the previous stage 24 hours later [38]. A typical time frame to be withheld from competition to complete the RTP protocol is approximately 7 days; however, this depends on the individual

Table 18.4 Return-to-sport progression[a]

Stage[b]	Description	Activity
1	Symptom-limited activities of daily living	No physical activity; reintroduction of activities of daily living (walking, etc.)
2	Light aerobic activity	<70% age-predicted maximal heart rate (stationary biking and controlled activities to stress cardiac output)
3	Sport-specific activity	Running, skating, and sport-specific activities without the risk of head impacts
4	Noncontact drills	Training activities with others, progression of resistance training, increased coordination, and thinking
5	Unrestricted practice	Return to normal training activities
6	Full return to sport[c]	Medical clearance from physician/physician designee

[a]Table based on Concussion in Sport Group guidelines [4] supported by the NATA [3] and AMSSM [5] position statements
[b]Stages should be separated by a minimum of 1 calendar day [1]
[c]Written clearance from a healthcare provider may be necessary prior to full return to sport depending on the state laws and regulations [4]

patient. If the patient presents with comorbidities that may affect the recovery trajectory, the AT may lengthen the progression sequence or prolong certain stages. Likewise, SAs experiencing deconditioning due to prolonged removal from activity may require additional aerobic conditioning prior to their full return to sport. Only the physician may shorten the sequence if it is appropriate for the SA.

Concussion in Sport Group

Starting in 2001, the Concussion in Sport Group established, and has continued to support, the use of a graded RTP protocol [39]. Following injury (> 48 hours), SAs are recommended to engage in physical and cognitive rest with symptom-based physical activity progressions via the RTP protocol. Each stage of the protocol is separated by 24 hours, advancing from activities of daily living through unrestricted return to play over approximately 1 week (Table 18.4). SAs reporting symptoms at any stage of the protocol must wait 24 hours to resume activity and regress to the previous stage. Additional interpersonal factors may also influence recovery, making it possible for RTP to extend beyond a typical 1-week time frame.

AMSSM

The RTP progression follows international recommendations with a stepwise increase in physical activity toward sport-specific exercises without exacerbation of symptoms. Prior to the initiation of the RTP protocol, SAs must report as asymptomatic.

The progression is subject to individualization as based upon the SA's age, previous SRCs, and whether the healthcare professional can provide complete supervision during the RTP progression. In addition to physical conditioning at the time of RTP, the SA should also demonstrate psychological readiness prior to unrestricted athletic activity.

Summary

The RTP protocol endorsed by Concussion in Sport Group is consistently endorsed by the organizations evaluated here. The stepwise progression gradually increases the physical demands necessary to be competitive in sports. The gradual progression begins with activities of daily living and progresses through various aerobic activities, noncontact drills, and unrestricted practice before clearance for full return to athletic activity, with 24 hours in-between each phase. If the SA reports any increases in symptoms, they must immediately stop activity and begin at the previous stage 24 hours later. Depending on the individual, a clinician may choose a more conservative approach to the RTP program in order to build their aerobic endurance and confidence during sport-specific activity.

Documentation and Legal Aspects

Today's reality is that following a catastrophic head injury in the sports' context, the first question becomes who—*other* than the injured SA—is responsible for that catastrophic outcome. That question quickly becomes who must ultimately pay the injured SA, or the surviving parents in a death case, to compensate the victim or victim's family for that injury.

Complicating matters is the undefined moving target that is the standard of care concerning the management of SRC. The fact that the "experts" have competing views on the appropriate standard muddies the waters further. On the issue of preseason baseline testing, for example, experts remain divided on whether such testing is required to meet the standard of care, with some arguing that the use of such testing may actually result in exposing the SA to *greater* risk of injury. With this backdrop of confusion, and thus no well-defined standard to hold defendants to, plaintiffs' lawyers have been feasting in this new area of law.

Depending on the facts, defending the conduct at issue can be especially challenging. In some actions, the jury will have to grapple with a complicated medical or scientific theory regarding the cause of the player's injury; in others, the player may be so severely injured that juror sympathy might outweigh a more objective assessment of the facts. In such cases, jurors who are on the proverbial fence regarding whether a defendant met the applicable standard of care may simply return a verdict for the plaintiff so as to avoid having to confront other, likely harder, issues.

Because certain matters are so unpredictable, potential defendants must control what they *can* control. This begins first and foremost with following to the letter any and all applicable SRC policies, procedures, and protocols.

On a more practical issue, a common allegation against healthcare providers, in particular, in SRC cases is "failure to properly document" since, for years now, the recommended approach has been that "all pertinent information" surrounding head injuries be documented. Indeed, the expression "if it's not written, it didn't happen" is a common one that can be dangerous to a defendant in a lawsuit.

The question, thus, sometimes becomes whether certain information is "pertinent." For example, during a player's return-to-play period following a head injury, the injured player generally performs graduated exertional exercises in an AT's presence. But how much detail in the AT's documentation is required to meet the standard of care?

Many would argue—certainly, plaintiffs' lawyers would—that it is insufficient for an AT to record simply that the injured player "performed exertional maneuvers." Questions at the trial of an AT might be raised as to the specifics of the exertional testing—for example, the dates on which the testing was performed, the witnesses to the testing, and the actual maneuvers performed. Even though the AT may have a recollection of the testing performed and the accompanying details, and be willing to testify to the specifics, the absence of such detail in an actual injury record may call into question whether the AT is recalling the specifics accurately. Indeed, trials generally occur years after the alleged conduct.

Because plaintiffs' lawyers will make all efforts to discredit the defendant's testimony, the more detailed the documentation, the more likely a jury will find the defendant to be a credible witness. Thus, ideally, the documentation of all pertinent information surrounding a head injury also should include any details, including the specific testing and maneuvers performed (jumping jacks, knee bends, etc.), dates, times, and specific locations of testing, and the questions asked of the SA during testing and the SA's responses. Simply put, the more detailed the documentation, the better able a defendant may be to defend a lawsuit for an alleged breach of the standard of care.

As SRC lawsuits become even more common, it is crucial for potential defendants to protect themselves as discussed above for the good of their institutions and the safety and health of the SAs. Along these lines, strict adherence to all applicable SRC policies, procedures, and protocols, as well as accurate, complete, and legible documentation is imperative.

Conclusion

Management of SRCs in collegiate athletics continues to pose as a complex practice for healthcare providers. Clinicians are encouraged, if not required, to educate their SAs and coaches and other personnel about common signs/symptoms, as well as the consequences of continuing to participate in sport with a SRC. In some instances, clinicians may need to conduct a baseline evaluation for use in the postinjury assessment, diagnosis, and management process. Tools such as the SCAT-5 offer a standardized approach to injury care and often fulfill professional requirements. Regardless of what tools are used, the clinical examination remains the gold standard for SRC diagnosis. Since symptoms may evolve over time, SAs should not return on the same day as a suspected SRC unless the injury can be ruled out by an appropriate healthcare professional. When appropriate, the graded RTP protocol is now the standard of care for returning a concussed SA back to play, with a complete return to the classroom occurring before unrestricted return to sport participation.

References

1. McCrory P, Meeuwisse WH, Aubry M, Cantu RC, Dvořák J, Echemendia RJ, et al. Consensus statement on concussion in sport: the 4th international conference on concussion in sport, Zurich, November 2012. J Athl Train. 2013;48(4):554–75.
2. Langlois JA, Rutland-Brown W, Wald MM. The epidemiology and impact of traumatic brain injury: a brief overview. J Head Trauma Rehabil. 2006;21(5):375–8.
3. Broglio SP, Cantu RC, Gioia GA, Guskiewicz KM, Kutcher J, Palm M, et al. National athletic trainers' association position statement: management of sport concussion. J Athl Train. 2014;49(2):245–65.
4. McCrory P, Meeuwisse W, Dvorak J, Aubry M, Bailes J, Broglio S, et al. Consensus statement on concussion in sport—the 5th international conference on concussion in sport held in Berlin, October 2016. Br J Sports Med. 2017;51(11):838–47.

5. Harmon KG, Clugston JR, Dec K, Hainline B, Herring S, Kane SF, et al. American medical society for sports medicine position statement on concussion in sport. Br J Sports Med. 2019;53(4):213–25.
6. National Collegiate Athletic Association (NCAA). Interassociation consensus: diagnosis and management of sport-related concussion best practices. Indianapolis, IN; 2016.
7. Parsons JE. 2014-15 NCAA sports medicine handbook. National Collegiate Athletic Association; 2014.
8. McLeod TCV, Schwartz C, Bay RC. Sport-related concussion misunderstandings among youth coaches. Clin J Sport Med. 2007;17(2):140–2.
9. Guskiewicz KM, Bruce SL, Cantu RC, Ferrara MS, Kelly JP, McCrea M, et al. National athletic trainers' association position statement: management of sport-related concussion. J Athl Train. 2004;39(3):280.
10. Schmidt JD, Register-Mihalik JK, Mihalik JP, Kerr ZY, Guskiewicz KM. Identifying impairments after concussion: normative data versus individualized baselines. Med Sci Sports Exerc. 2012;44(9):1621–8.
11. Yakovlev P, Lecours A. The myelogenetic cycles of regional maturation of the brain. In: Regional development of the brain in early life; 1967. p. 3–70.
12. Broglio SP, Guskiewicz KM. Concussion in sports: the sideline assessment. Sports Health. 2009;1(5):361–9.
13. Maddocks DL, Dicker GD, Saling MM. The assessment of orientation following concussion in athletes. Clin J Sport Med. 1995;5(1):32–5.
14. McCrea M, Randolph C, Kelly J. Standardized assessment of concussion (SAC): manual for administration, scoring and interpretation. CNS: Waukesha, WI; 2000.
15. Tucker R, Raftery M, Fuller GW, Hester B, Kemp S, Cross MJ. A video analysis of head injuries satisfying the criteria for a head injury assessment in professional rugby union: a prospective cohort study. Br J Sports Med. 2017;51(15):1147–51.
16. Patricios J, Fuller GW, Ellenbogen R, Herring S, Kutcher JS, Loosemore M, et al. What are the critical elements of sideline screening that can be used to establish the diagnosis of concussion? A systematic review. Br J Sports Med. 2017;51(11):888–94.
17. Broglio SP, Katz BP, Zhao S, McCrea M, McAllister T, Investigators CC. Test-retest reliability and interpretation of common concussion assessment tools: findings from the NCAA-DoD CARE consortium. Sports Med. 2018;48(5):1255–68.
18. Echemendia RJ, Meeuwisse W, McCrory P, Davis GA, Putukian M, Leddy J, et al. The sport concussion assessment tool 5th edition (SCAT-5): background and rationale. Br J Sports Med. 2017;51(11):848–50.
19. Leong DF, Balcer LJ, Galetta SL, Evans G, Gimre M, Watt D. The king–devick test for sideline concussion screening in collegiate football. J Opt. 2015;8(2):131–9.
20. Eckner JT, Kutcher JS, Broglio SP, Richardson JK. Effect of sport-related concussion on clinically measured simple reaction time. Br J Sports Med. 2014;48(2):112–8.
21. Putukian M. How being injured affects mental health. In: Mind, body and sport: Understanding and supporting student-athlete mental wellness; 2014. p. 61–4.
22. Kontos AP, Covassin T, Elbin R, Parker T. Depression and neurocognitive performance after concussion among male and female high school and collegiate athletes. Arch Phys Med Rehabil. 2012;93(10):1751–6.
23. Collins MW, Kontos AP, Reynolds E, Murawski CD, Fu FH. A comprehensive, targeted approach to the clinical care of athletes following sport-related concussion. Knee Surg Sports Traumatol Arthrosc. 2014;22(2):235–46.
24. Schneider KJ, Meeuwisse WH, Nettel-Aguirre A, Barlow K, Boyd L, Kang J, et al. Cervicovestibular rehabilitation in sport-related concussion: a randomised controlled trial. Br J Sports Med. 2014;48(17):1294–8.
25. Silverberg ND, Iverson GL. Is rest after concussion "the best medicine?": recommendations for activity resumption following concussion in athletes, civilians, and military service members. J Head Trauma Rehabil. 2013;28(4):250–9.

26. Schneider KJ, Leddy JJ, Guskiewicz KM, Seifert T, McCrea M, Silverberg ND, et al. Rest and treatment/rehabilitation following sport-related concussion: a systematic review. Br J Sports Med. 2017;51(12):930–4.
27. Thomas DG, Apps JN, Hoffmann RG, McCrea M, Hammeke T. Benefits of strict rest after acute concussion: a randomized controlled trial. Pediatrics. 2015;135(2):213–23.
28. Leddy JJ, Haider MN, Hinds AL, Darling S, Willer BS. A preliminary study of the effect of early aerobic exercise treatment for sport-related concussion in males. Clin J Sport Med. 2019;29(5):353–60.
29. Caplan B, Bogner J, Brenner L, Clausen M, Pendergast DR, Willer B, et al. Cerebral blood flow during treadmill exercise is a marker of physiological postconcussion syndrome in female athletes. J Head Trauma Rehabil. 2016;31(3):215–24.
30. Erickson KI, Voss MW, Prakash RS, Basak C, Szabo A, Chaddock L, et al. Exercise training increases size of hippocampus and improves memory. Proc Natl Acad Sci. 2011;108(7):3017–22.
31. Iverson GL, Gardner AJ, Terry DP, Ponsford JL, Sills AK, Broshek DK, et al. Predictors of clinical recovery from concussion: a systematic review. Br J Sports Med. 2017;51(12):941–8.
32. Makdissi M, Schneider KJ, Feddermann-Demont N, Guskiewicz KM, Hinds S, Leddy JJ, et al. Approach to investigation and treatment of persistent symptoms following sport-related concussion: a systematic review. Br J Sports Med. 2017;51(12):958–68.
33. Leddy JJ, Haider MN, Ellis M, Willer BS. Exercise is medicine for concussion. Curr Sports Med Rep. 2018;17(8):262–70.
34. Hoffman NL, Weber ML, Broglio SP, McCrea M, McAllister TW, Schmidt JD. Influence of postconcussion sleep duration on concussion recovery in collegiate athletes. Clin J Sport Med. 2017;
35. McCarty CA, Zatzick D, Stein E, Wang J, Hilt R, Rivara FP. Collaborative care for adolescents with persistent postconcussive symptoms: a randomized trial. Pediatrics. 2016;138(4):e20160459.
36. McAvoy K, Eagan-Johnson B, Halstead M. Return to learn: transitioning to school and through ascending levels of academic support for students following a concussion. NeuroRehabilitation. 2018;42(3):325–30.
37. Makdissi M, Davis G, Jordan B, Patricios J, Purcell L, Putukian M. Revisiting the modifiers: how should the evaluation and management of acute concussions differ in specific groups? Br J Sports Med. 2013;47(5):314–20.
38. McGrath N, Dinn WM, Collins MW, Lovell MR, Elbin R, Kontos AP. Post-exertion neurocognitive test failure among student-athletes following concussion. Brain Inj. 2013;27(1):103–13.
39. Aubry M, Cantu R, Dvorak J, Graf-Baumann T, Johnston K, Kelly J, et al. Summary and agreement statement of the first international conference on concussion in sport, Vienna 2001. Br J Sports Med. 2002;36(1):6–7.

The Role of the Quantitative EEG (QEEG) in the Assessment and Treatment of the Brain Injured Individual

19

Kirtley E. Thornton

QEEG Background

The QEEG (Fig. 19.1) collects digital EEG information from 19 locations based upon the historical standard 10–20 system, which examines the brain from a mathematically determined spatial viewpoint to ensure a thorough coverage of the brain.

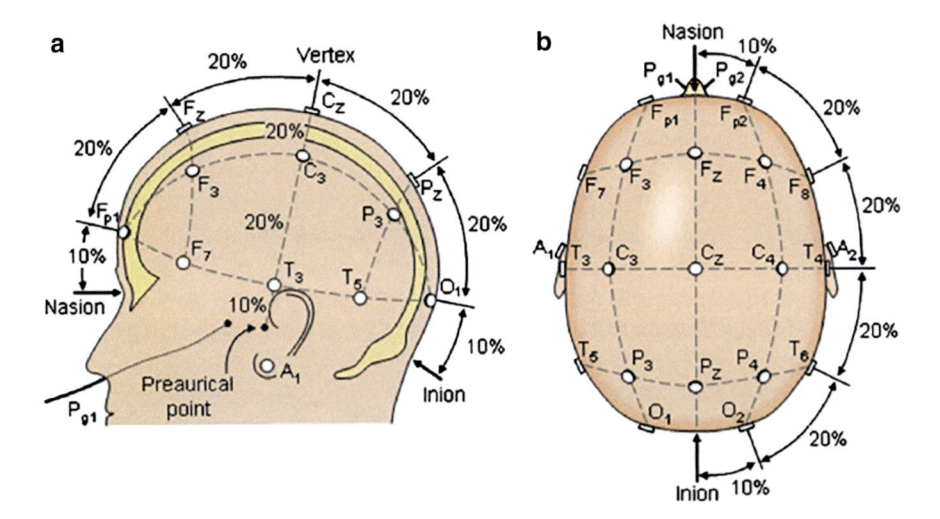

Fig. 19.1 A representation of the 10–20 system. (**a**) represents the lateral view. (**b**) represents the axial view

---

K. E. Thornton (✉)
The Neuroscience Center, Charlotte, NC, USA
e-mail: ket@chp-neurotherapy.com; http://neuroeducation.co

© Springer Nature Switzerland AG 2021
S. M. Slobounov, W. J. Sebastianelli (eds.), *Concussions in Athletics*,
https://doi.org/10.1007/978-3-030-75564-5_19

Quantitative EEG (QEEG) Measures

Activation/Arousal Measures: While there are other measures employed in the QEEG (e.g., peak frequency and peak amplitudes), this chapter reports on only those variables which are critically involved in the brain injured subjects and other presented clinical situations.

RP: Relative magnitude/microvolt or relative power: the relative magnitude of a band defined as the absolute microvolt of the particular band divided by the total microvolt generated at a particular location across all bands.

C: Coherence or spectral correlation coefficients (SCC): the average similarity between the waveforms of a particular band in two locations over the epoch (1 second). The SCC variable is conceptualized as the strength or number of connections between two locations and is a correlation of the magnitudes across a period of time (epoch).

P: Phase: the time lag between two locations of a particular band as defined by how soon after the beginning of an epoch a particular waveform at location #1 is matched in location #2.

The frequencies employed in EEG analysis are delta (0.5–4 Hz), theta (4–8 Hz), alpha (8–13 Hz), beta1 (13–32 Hz), and beta2 (32–64 Hz).

Head Injury Discriminant Approaches

Multiple publications have addressed the issue of discriminating traumatic brain injury (TBI) subjects from normal individuals using statistical approaches [1–12].

There are two reports which have provided impressive and useful discriminant results. Thatcher et al. [1] was able to obtain a discriminant accuracy rate of 90% with mild-to-moderate TBI using eyes-closed QEEG data. Of note was the increased frontal theta coherence, decreased frontal beta phase, increased beta coherence, and reduced posterior alpha relative power. Three independent cross validations within the original research resulted in accuracy rates of 84%, 93%, and 90%. Additional testing using the Thatcher discriminant function [1] in a military setting was correctly able to identify 88% of the soldiers with a blast injury history and 75% with no blast injury history [5].

Work by Barr and colleagues [6] examined EEG recordings immediately post-concussion, at 8 days after, and at 45 days after injury. Using a brain injury algorithm, abnormal features of EEG were detected at the time of injury (and that persisted over time) and contributed most to the discriminant analysis. Some of these features include slow wave increase in relative power, alpha1 and alpha2 decrease in relative power, power asymmetries in theta, and abnormalities in measures of connectivity. The resulting discriminant analysis produced a cutoff score of 65 at which there was a 95% probability of TBI.

Leon-Carrion et al. [13] also did work on the discriminant ability of QEEG in brain injury. They reported the discriminant ability of QEEG to accurately classify brain injury (in the chronic phase; mean 22 months postinjury) in 100% ($N = 48$) and obtained a 75% correct classification in an "external-cross-validation sample" of 33. Coherence measures were the most frequent variables in the function, employing the frequency range 1–30 Hz, similar to the Thatcher research.

Research by Thornton [7–9] has focused on the EEG gamma frequency band. Specifically, they focused on the altered spectral correlation coefficients ((SCC; based upon the Lexicor algorithms) and phase values in the beta2 (gamma; 32–64 Hertz) range) when comparing the TBI group to controls during eyes-closed and different cognitive activation tasks. Results from all three of these studies did not indicate any deficits in the relative power of delta, theta, or alpha. The TBI group did show lower beta2 coherence (SCC) values when compared to controls.

Moreover, Thornton and Carmody [11] and Thornton [10] investigated the use of frontal activity as well as coherence (SCC) and phase relations within the frontal lobe to distinguish between TBI and normal controls (NC) participants. Using frontal coherence and phase relationships, they obtained a 97.5–100% accuracy rate in the discrimination analysis when reanalyzing the data, employing a different approach using five tasks, adding all coherence and phase 32–64 Hz relationships, and adding frontal relative power of 32–64 Hz [10]. This approach resulted in a 100% correct discrimination but decreased to 99% accuracy following the analysis of three cases post publication. Figure 19.2 presents a comparison of the studies which engaged in a discriminant analysis.

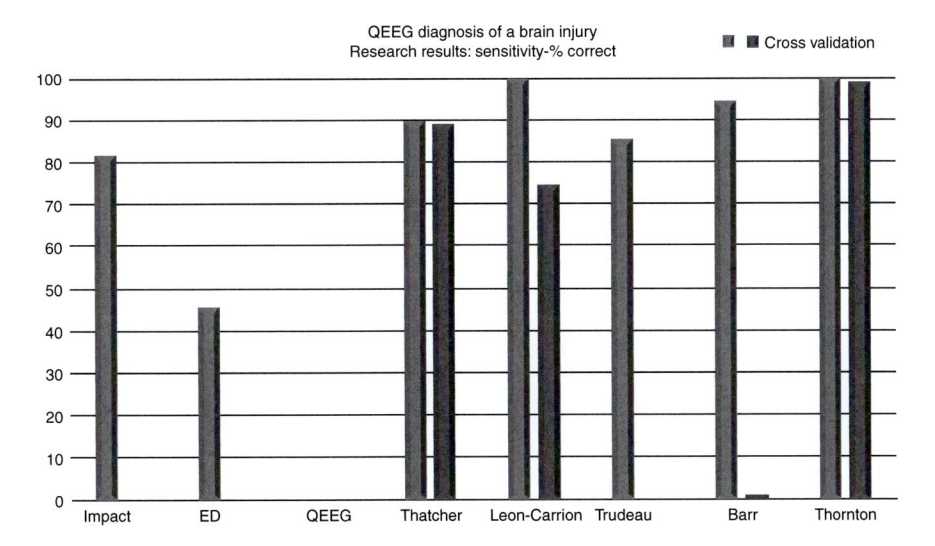

Fig. 19.2 A summary of the discrimination studies. *Impact = Impact Software; ED: Emergency Dept.* The second column represents the cross-validation results for the specific author: Thatcher, et al. [1]; Leon-Carrion et al. [13]; Trudeau et al. [5]; Barr et al. [6]; and Thornton [10]

Methods

The data presented below are based on 88 TBI participants and 109 normal control participants with a mean age of 37 years and 51.7% being female. The time between the date of the head injury and evaluation ranged from 12 days to 30 years. There was also a children group of participants with 49 normal control children (mean age 10.6 years) and 45 children (mean age 10.6 years) who could be classified as having a learning disability (LD). The child sample had 63 males and 31 females. The subjects' identity was protected, and the data were collected in accordance with the Declaration of Helsinki.

Participants underwent a cognitive QEEG evaluation which consisted of an eyes-closed condition (300 seconds), auditory attention task (200 seconds), visual attention task (200 seconds), four auditory memory tasks (200 seconds), one reading task (100 seconds), in addition to a problem-solving (Raven's matrices) task. The auditory attention task consisted of the participant listening to the sound of a pen tapping on a table while their eyes were closed and raising their right index finger when they heard the sound. The visual attention task required the participant to look at a page of upside-down Spanish text. The participant was asked to raise their right index finger when a laser light was flashed on the text. The auditory memory tasks required the participant to listen to four individually administered stories with their eyes closed, quietly recall the story, and then repeat the story back to the examiner. The reading task required the subject to read a story presented on a laminated sheet for 100 seconds, quietly recall the story while their eyes are closed, and then recall the story to the examiner. During all of these tasks, QEEG data were collected. The data for the eyes-closed condition and four cognitive activation tasks (auditory and visual attention, listening, and reading) were employed for the discriminant analysis.

Results

Discriminant Analysis

Figure 19.3 presents the results which indicated the normative reference group ($p < 0.05$) for the SCC and the phase values. The blackened circle is the origin of a metaphorical flashlight which is sending out a beam to three other locations. The

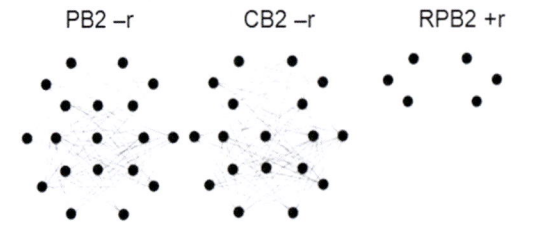

CB2 = Coherence (SCC) Beta2; PB2 = Phase Beta2; RPB2 = Relative Power Beta2.

Fig. 19.3 Discriminant variables used

flashlight locations were chosen according to the number of significant relations emanating from that location. In deciding if whether the source of a connection between two locations (A and B) is A or B, the location with the higher number of other significant relations was determined to be the source. Figure 19.3 presents summary figures of all the significant relations (coherence and phase) as well as the frontal RPB2 locations. The effect is broad and diffusely located and is not primarily focused on the frontal locations, contrary to some opinions. The average standard deviation (*SD*) difference between the normal control and TBI group for the SCC variable was 0.47 and 0.44 for the phase variables ($p < 0.05$). The frontal relative power values of beta2 indicated a similar average *SD* value difference of 0.47 between the TBI and normal group.

Classification Matrices

To determine if the discriminant algorithm could accurately indicate a misclassification, 5 TBI subjects and 5 normal subjects were misclassified for all the tasks. The discriminant analysis was then recalculated to determine if the inaccurate classification was identified. Ten different subjects were selected for each task for a total of 50 misclassifications. The discriminant reanalysis was 100% correct in the identification of all the misclassifications.

Table 19.1 presents the resultant discriminant analysis for the five tasks. As can be seen from this table, the discriminant analysis was 100% effective in

Table 19.1 Classification matrices

		TBI	Normal
Eyes closed			
	Correct	$P = 0.56$	$P = 0.44$
TBI	100	102	0
Normal	100	0	81
Total	100	102	81
Auditory attention		TBI	Normal
	Correct	$P = 0.51$	$P = 0.49$
TBI	100	90	0
Normal	100	0	86
Total	100	90	86
Visual attention		TBI	Normal
	Correct	$P = 0.52$	$P = 0.48$
TBI	100	87	0
Normal	100	0	81
Total	100	87	81
Auditory memory		TBI	Normal
	Correct	$P = 0.45$	$P = 0.55$
TBI	100	88	0
Normal	100	0	109
Total	100	88	109
Reading memory		TBI	Normal
	Correct	$P = 0.46$	$P = 0.54$
TBI	100	75	0
Normal	100	0	87
Total	100	75	87

distinguishing between the TBI and normal participants. The variables employed were the SCC and phase values in the 32–64 Hz range and the RPB2 values for the six frontal locations indicated in Fig. 19.3.

Cognitive and EEG Characteristics of the TBI Population

The critical variables were coherence and phase beta2 and frontal relative power of beta2. There was a nonsignificant correlation between time since accident and the frontal relative power of beta2. There were also nonsignificant correlations between time since accident and left hemisphere coherence beta2 (0.07), left hemisphere phase beta2 (0.15), right hemisphere coherence beta2 (−0.16), and right hemisphere phase beta2 (−0.19). These results indicate the critical discriminating variables do not seem to be improving over time. There also was a pattern of decreasing coherence beta1 (13–32 Hz) over time since accident (Fig. 19.4).

The TBI group's auditory memory score (mean = 37, SD = 18.4)) across the four stories was significantly lower (t = −9.53) than the normative reference group score (mean = 70.5, SD = 28.3; p = 0.000000). There was a nonsignificant correlation between time since injury and auditory memory scores (0.17). The TBI group's reading memory score (mean = 23.3, SD = 18.8) was significantly lower (t = −4.83) than the normative group score (mean = 40, SD = 25.6; p = 0.000003). Thus suggesting a TBI subject's memory does not improve with time.

Gender and Sex Effects: Females More Affected by TBI

Differential sensitivity of the female brain to TBI has been the subject of a number of recent reports, generally supportive of the notion that the female brain has more negative effects post injury [14]. To determine if there is a correlate with this greater sensitivity using QEEG data, the coherence and phase beta2 values were examined between male and female subjects (Fig. 19.5). There were no significant differences in the auditory memory performances of the two groups (male mean = 43, female mean = 55). Figure 19.5 shows that the male TBI brain had higher values on the critical phase and coherence variables, thus indicating that the female brain had lower values and was more negatively affected by TBI. When the relative power of frontal beta2 was examined, there were no sex differences in TBI groups.

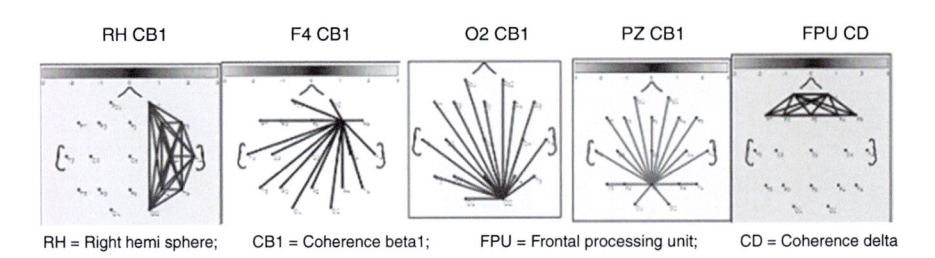

RH = Right hemi sphere;   CB1 = Coherence beta1;   FPU = Frontal processing unit;   CD = Coherence delta

Fig. 19.4 Variables which decrease with greater time since injury

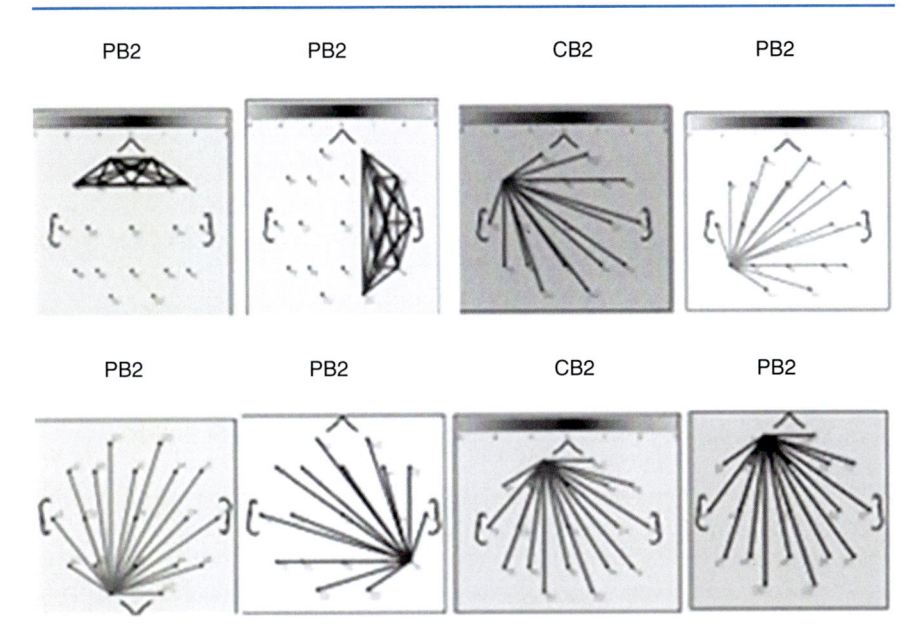

Fig. 19.5 Differences between male and female brains on coherence and phase beta2 (32–64 Hz) values. Note that males are higher than females

When the normal control sample was examined for the phase and coherence differences, there were no significant differences between male and female brain functions. Examining frontal relative power values, the females were significantly higher at all locations ($p < 0.05$) except Fp2. Thus, the normal control sample females were not inherently lower than males on these critical coherence and phase variables. The higher frontal relative power beta2 in the normal female group is not evident in the female TBI group, a finding not easily explained.

The Issue of Determining if Problems Are a Preexisting Learning Disability

A potential diagnostic problem would be the presence of a preexisting learning problem, which could show a similar EEG pattern to a TBI. A preliminary investigation of this problem was undertaken by the author with the clinical data available. Two problems were initially evident:

1. Lack of a sufficient number of adults with learning disability (LD) to compare to the adult TBI group.
2. The presence of a strong developmental pattern showing increases in almost all coherence and phase relations. This developmental pattern would negate the use of comparing the values of children to normal adults or TBI adults, as the child's numbers would be lower strictly due to development patterns.

Thus, the only viable method to assess this diagnostic question would be to compare children with LD to a normal child control group and determine if the LD child patterns deviant from the normative reference group, which theoretically would be similar to the adult TBI patterns from a corresponding adult normative reference group. This is based on the reasonable assumption that a child's TBI pattern would be the same as an adult's TBI pattern. If the LD problem is manifested in lower coherence and phase beta2 values, then there would be a diagnostic problem of differentiating a TBI from a LD.

Figure 19.6 presents the results of this analysis for a group of 49 normal children and 45 children who pursued EEG biofeedback treatment for cognitive / learning problems. They had not undergone a psychoeducational evaluation by the author due to the desire to avoid additional fees to the client. However, they pursued treatment based upon the parents understanding that their child was not performing adequately in the school setting.

Discriminant analysis revealed 25 significant differences involving phase relations and 10 involving coherence relationships. There were 8 variables involving delta, 9 involving theta, 14 involving alpha, 2 involving beta1, and 1 involving beta2. There were 9 phase theta variables and 10 phase alpha variables which were more than the other variables (PD = 3, CD = 5, CT = 0, CA = 5, PB1 = 1, PB2 = 1). Thus, it appears that the learning disability problem electrophysiology resides in the phase theta and phase alpha relations. It also appears that the LD child does not demonstrate a deficit in coherence and phase beta2. The conclusion can be reached that the discriminant is not picking up a previous LD pattern, a clinically useful finding.

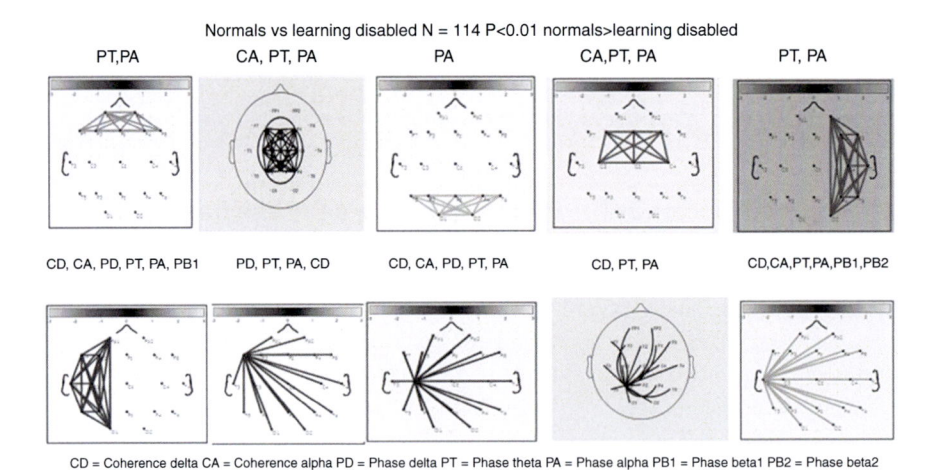

Fig. 19.6 Results for normal control children and cognitive/learning disability children. Figures represent the electrophysiological differences between normal and the learning disabled child

Discussion

Theoretical Considerations

The interventions were based upon the coordinated allocation of resource model of brain functioning. The model states that specific cognitive skills relay upon use of specific QEEG variables to function maximally (albeit overlapping in certain situations). The model employs the flashlight metaphor (a specific location sends out a "beam" to all other locations within a specific frequency) across different cognitive tasks. It also employs a processing unit concept that areas of the brain (frontal, posterior, etc.) have a specific role in cognitive functioning. The interventions were based upon a deficit model as lower values of critical variables are (compared to normative values) critical variables to address in the rehabilitation intervention.

Rehabilitation of the Brain Injured Subjects

In addition to the diagnostic issues, the QEEG has shown to be useful in the rehabilitation of cognitive functioning after TBI. The author reviewed his clinical files from the last 5 years and examined the QEEG data addressing relative power and coherence changes and memory (auditory and reading) improvements in the TBI patients who he had (Table 19.2). For the TBI group, the focus of the interventions

Table 19.2 Participant's characteristics

Group	N	Male	Female	Avg. age	Hand	Raven's avg	*T	*A	*B1	*B2	Avg. # ss
Normal	12	6	6	28.8	R = 11, L = 1	15.4	0	0	1	0	49
TBI	15	9	6	31.1	R = 15	10.6	1	2	2	2	48.3
Adult SLD	17	11	6	23.4	R = 15, L = 2	23.2	0	4	0	0	38.4
Child SLD	15	12	3	10.4	R = 14, L = 1	11.29	0	3	1	0	45.4
Total	59	38	21	23.4	R = 55, L = 4	15.1	1	9	4	2	45.3

Note. An asterisk indicates participants whose relative power values averaged across nine cognitive tasks were greater than 1 SD above the normative values and indicated frequency. Some participants were above the cutoff on two frequencies. *Avg. age* average age calculated within and across groups, *Hand* handedness, *R* right handed, *L* left handed, *Avg.* average Raven's score (participant is administered up to 11 difficult Raven's matrices problems and allowed 400–500 s to provide answers. Scoring employed the following method: 4 points if correct on first guess, 3 points if correct on second guess, 2 points if correct on third guess, and 1 point if correct on fourth guess. The measure is generally considered a measure of nonverbal intelligence); *D* delta, *T* theta, *A* alpha, *B1* beta1, *B2* beta2, *Avg. # ss* estimate of average no. of sessions; and # is an underestimate of actual number as sessions that addressed specific issues (other than CA, CB1, CB2, and posterior relative power values) were not included in the analysis, *TBI* traumatic brain injury, *SLD* specific learning disability

was on the phase and coherence problems. Table 19.3 presents the cognitive changes for the TBI patients as a result of the intervention. A weighted average of the auditory memory improvements across these three studies indicated an average SD improvement of 2.31. Table 19.4 presents the changes on the reading memory scores and comparisons to the reference group. On average, the treated group was performing 0.90 SD and 52% above the normative reference group.

Table 19.3 Raw score/percentage/standard deviation improvement values in auditory memory

Group	Pre-Tx [a] M (SD)[a]	Post-Tx [b] M (SD)[b]	p Level M Diff	ES*	95% CI CI ES*	Avg. # sess[c] Sess[c]	% Changed[d] Change[d]	Norm value /SD[e] (Sample size)[e]	Vs. Norm[f] diff./% diff[f]
TBI (N = 36)	11.7 (7.7)	24 (5.8)	<0.001	1.75	.88, 2.62	1.93	105%	15.7 (5.12)	1.52 (53%)

Note. Asterisks indicates Hedge's unbiased estimate of effect size, with confidence intervals effect size. If values are above 0, then results are significant. *Tx* treatment, *ES* effect size, *CI* confidence interval, *sess* session, *SD* standard deviation
[a] Initial average auditory memory value (immediate and delayed recall score) and standard deviation value (SD) of group
[b] Posttreatment average auditory memory value and SD value of group
[c] Average no. of evaluations employed to obtain posttreatment memory scores
[d] The % change from preevaluation values, that is, (post-pre)/pre
[e] The average memory score of the control group (SD value)
[f] The SD of the posttreatment memory score compared to the normative database values as well as the % difference from the normative values

Table 19.4 Raw score/percentage/standard deviation improvement values in reading memory

Group	Pre-Tx M (SD)[a]	Post-Tx M (SD)[b]	p level M Diff	ES*	CI 95% CI ES*	Avg. Sess[c]	% Change[d]	Norm value (SD) (Sample size)[e]	Vs. norm SD diff./% diff[f]
TBI (N=13)	2.23 (1.38)	5.41 (1.9)	<0.001	1.85	0.94, 2.77	1.69	143%	3.61, (1.5)	1.06/50 %

Note. Asterisks indicate Hedge's unbiased estimate of effect size (1981 and 1985), with confidence intervals effect size. If values are above 0, then results are significant. *Tx* treatment, *ES* effect size, *CI* confidence interval, *TBI* =traumatic brain injury, *sess* session, *SD* standard deviation
[a] Reading memory (immediate and delayed score combined) and SD scores of the original evaluation per 10 s of reading (i.e., participant reads for 100 s; if has a recall score of 10, then the 10-s reading memory value is 1)
[b] Mean and SD of posttreatment reading scores for 10 seconds of reading
[c] The average # of sessions employed to obtain posttreatment reading scores
[d] The % change value (i.e., (post-pre)=pre)
[e] The normative values and SD for adults
[f] The SD difference of the posttreatment measure compared to the normative database as well as the percentage difference

Possible Placebo Effects

It has been a criticism of the EEG biofeedback field that the effects are a result of a placebo effect. This argument has been made by Thibault and Raz [15] who state, "in light of the comparable benefits of veritable-versus-sham feedback, conflicts of interest, and a weak theoretical underpinning, advocating for EEG-nf poses a conundrum...Sparse evidence supports the idea that humans can reliably modulate EEG-nf signals" (p.684). This issue was directly addressed in the Thornton [16] article and has been rebuked for six main reasons including discussions of placebo effects, biochemical effects, specifically neurotransmitters, and empirical evidence (see article for details on all points). The use of the QEEG in TBI assessment/classification and rehabilitation has sound research support. The effectiveness of EEG biofeedback can be understood, not as a placebo effect, but as consistent with a long history on the effectiveness of operant conditioning.

Conclusion

The clinical value of the QEEG in the TBI arena has been documented in this chapter as: (1) highly effective in discriminating between a TBI subject and a normal individual; (2) has shown the specificity in distinguishing between a learning disabled and a normal control (in pediatric cases); (3) has highlighted an important difference in the male and female brain; and (4) has been shown to be efficient in addressing the cognitive problems in patients suffering from a TBI. With the lack of sound diagnostic and treatment options in the management of mTBI, QEEG offers itself as another potential methodology. Its high accuracy of diagnoses (at times 100%) and its utility in cognitive rehabilitation could be useful to clinicians dealing with individuals post mTBI.

References

1. Thatcher RW, Walker RA, Gerson I, Geisler FH. EEG discriminant analyses of mild head trauma. Electroencephalogr Clin Neurophysiol. 1989;73:94–106.
2. Thatcher RW, Biver C, McAlaster R, Salazar A. Biophysical linkage between MRI and EEG coherence in closed head injury. NeuroImage. 1998;8:307–26.
3. Hughes JR, John ER. Conventional and quantitative electroencephalography in psychiatry. J Neuropsychiatry Clin Neurosci. 1999;11:190–208.
4. Tebano MT, Cameroni M, Gallozzi G, Loizzo A, Palazzino G, Pezzini G, et al. EEG spectral analysis after minor head injury in man. Electroencephalogr Clin Neurophysiol. 1988;70:185–9.
5. Trudeau DL, Anderson J, Hansen LM, Shagalov DN, Schmoller J, Nugent S, et al. Findings of mild traumatic brain injury in combat veterans with PTSD and a history of blast concussion. J Neuropsychiatry Clin Neurosci. 1998;10:308–13.

6. Barr WB, Prichep LS, Chabot R, Powell MR, McCrea M. Measuring brain electrical activity to track recovery from sport-related concussion. Brain Inj. Taylor & Francis;. 2012;26:58–66.
7. Thornton KE. The FIG functional integrative QEEG technique and the functional structure of memory functioning in normals and head injured subjects. J Neurother [Internet]. 1996 [cited 2020 Dec 29];2. Available from: http://www.isnr-jnt.org/article/view/17254
8. THORNTON KE. Exploratory investigation into mild brain injury and discriminant analysis with high frequency bands (32–64 Hz). Brain Inj. Taylor & Francis;. 1999;13:477–88.
9. Thornton K. Improvement/rehabilitation of memory functioning with neurotherapy/QEEG biofeedback. J Head Trauma Rehabil. 2000;15:1285–96.
10. Thornton KE. A QEEG activation methodology that obtained 100% accuracy in the discrimination of traumatic brain injured from normal and does the learning disabled show the brain injury pattern? Neuro Regulat. 2014;1:209.
11. Thornton KE, Carmody DP. Traumatic brain injury rehabilitation: QEEG biofeedback treatment protocols. Appl Psychophysiol Biofeedback. 2009;34:59–68.
12. Thornton KE, Carmody DP. Eyes-closed and activation QEEG databases in predicting cognitive effectiveness and the inefficiency hypothesis. J Neurother [Internet]. [cited 2020 Dec 29];13. Available from: http://www.isnr-jnt.org/article/view/16654
13. Leon-Carrion J, Martin-Rodriguez JF, Damas-Lopez J, Martin JMBY, Dominguez-Morales MDR. A QEEG index of level of functional dependence for people sustaining acquired brain injury: the Seville Independence Index (SINDI). Brain Inj. 2008;22:61–74.
14. Munivenkatappa A, Agrawal A, Shukla DP, Kumaraswamy D, Devi BI. Traumatic brain injury: does gender influence outcomes? Int J Crit Illn Inj Sci. 2016;6:70–3.
15. Thibault RT, Raz A. The psychology of neurofeedback: clinical intervention even if applied placebo. Am Psychol. 2017;72:679–88.
16. Thornton KE. Perspectives on placebo: the psychology of neurofeedback. Neuro Regulat. 2018;5:137.

Treatment of Sports-Related Concussion

Michael Gay

Introduction

Sports-related concussion (SRC) or mild traumatic brain injury (mTBI) remains a significant healthcare concern for athletes of all ages. Clinicians and researchers are learning more details about the short- and long-term consequences of trauma to the brain. In 2012, the National Collegiate Athletic Association (NCAA) & the Department of Defense launched the largest study to date on concussion entitled the CARE Consortium. This research effort has yielded several studies advancing our knowledge across a spectrum of brain science in sports-related concussion.

The complexities of the pathophysiologic sequelae in the brain, combined with the clinical manifestation of behavioral signs and symptoms, are what can make the treatment of concussion challenging. Combine the difficulties in diagnosing and treating an athlete recovering from concussion with the pressure surrounding sports culture in America and you create a potentially dangerous environment for the concussed athlete. Moreover, there is an urgency to develop targeted treatments for young athletes as we are beginning to understand the correlations that exist between age of onset for sports-related head impacts and likelihood of repeat trauma [1]. Recent research into high school sports injury rates has revealed an alarming increase in the number of diagnosed concussions each year [2]. These young brains are in their formative years of neurological development and the long-term consequences from brain injury are significant.

In addition, there are tens of thousands of military personnel from multiple battle fronts overseas who have suffered traumatic brain injury and are in need of

M. Gay (✉)
Center for Sports Concussion Research and Services, Department of Kinesiology, Pennsylvania State University, University Park, PA, USA

Department of Intercollegiate Athletics, Penn State Center for Sports Concussion Research and Services, Penn State University, University Park, PA, USA
e-mail: mrg201@psu.edu

treatment and long-term care. This societal increase in brain injury rates has focused the research community's efforts into further understanding tenants of the brain's pathophysiological response to injury as well as short- and long-term clinical manifestations. However, researching effective treatments for mild traumatic brain injury meets with several challenges in forming evidence-based treatment approaches to improve patient outcomes and overall health [3]. Most treatment approaches remain grounded in the clinical domain of "functional recovery" while biomarkers of physiological recovery have not been made clinically meaningful. This intersection between functional and physiological recovery continues to demand our attention in order to maximize our outcomes and reduce the lifelong burden placed on quality of life following concussion.

Definition of Concussion

Reviewing the literature surrounding the treatment for concussion or mild traumatic brain injury (mTBI) requires that we examine the definition and events surrounding concussive injury. There is disparity among researchers on the issue of a unified definition of the term "concussion." The current accepted definition of concussion was re-tasked by the Concussion in Sport Group (CISG) during the first International Conference on Concussion in Sport in Vienna 2001 and has remained unchanged in subsequent examinations by the CISG. This group was comprised of researchers and clinicians from the fields of neuropsychology, sports medical physicians, neurologists, and neurosurgeons among other allied health professionals. These experts were highly involved in research as well as with the diagnosis, treatment, and management of sports-related concussion in patients. The CISG definition is as follows [4]:

"Concussion is defined as a complex pathophysiological process affecting the brain, induced by traumatic biomechanical forces. Several common features that incorporate clinical, pathological, and biomechanical injury constructs that may be used in defining the nature of a concussive head injury include the following:

1. Concussion may be caused by a direct blow to the head, face, neck, or elsewhere on the body with an 'impulsive' force transmitted to the head.
2. Concussion typically results in the rapid onset of short-lived impairment of neurological function that resolves spontaneously.
3. Concussion may result in neuropathological changes, but the acute clinical symptoms largely reflect a functional disturbance rather than structural injury.
4. Concussion results in a graded set of clinical syndromes that may or may not involve loss of consciousness. Resolution of the clinical and cognitive symptoms typically follows a sequential course.
5. Concussion is typically associated with grossly normal structural neuroimaging studies."

Although some medical experts and researchers vary in their approach to the term, in the research literature and in clinical terminology, sports-related concussion is often considered interchangeable with mild traumatic brain injury. In contrast to the CISG- based definition of concussion in 1993, the American Congress of Rehabilitative Medicine defined mTBI as a traumatically induced physiological disruption of brain function, as manifested by focal neurologic deficit(s) that may or may not be transient [5]. This contrasting definition is inclusive, in that mild traumatic brain injury involves some level of both functional and structural disruption to normal brain tissue that may or may not be permanent. The scope of this debate is beyond the intention of this chapter but considering the lack of a true clinical or research-based distinction between concussion and mild traumatic brain injury, the terms will be used interchangeably throughout the text of this chapter.

New Classification of Post-Concussion Syndrome

Athletes who suffer from sports-related concussion experience a variety of clinical symptoms caused by damage and neurologic dysfunction at the cellular level in the brain. Many of these individuals experience a recovery from clinical symptoms within 7–10 days post injury. However, several athletes recovering from sports-related concussion have clinical symptoms lasting 3 months or longer [6]. Formally, a diagnosis of post-concussion syndrome (PCS) is based on clinical symptoms defined by the *Diagnostic and Statistics Manual – Fourth Edition (DSM-IV)* as (1) cognitive deficits in attention or memory and (2) at least 3 or more of the following symptoms: fatigue, sleep disturbance, headache, dizziness, irritability, affective disturbance, apathy, or personality change [7]. In the updated *Diagnostic and Statistics Manual – Fifth Edition (DSM-V),* post-concussion syndrome is now diagnosed as neurocognitive disorder (NCD) of either major or minor classification due to the extent of traumatic brain injury. The specific DSM-5 criteria for neurocognitive disorder (NCD) due to traumatic brain injury are as follows [8]:

I. The criteria are met for major or mild neurocognitive disorder (decline in cognitive ability: memory, concentration, processing speed).
II. There is evidence of a traumatic brain injury – that is, an impact to the head or other mechanisms of rapid movement or displacement of the brain within the skull, with one or more of the following:
   - Loss of consciousness
   - Posttraumatic amnesia
   - Disorientation and confusion
   - Neurological signs (e.g., neuroimaging demonstrating injury; a new onset of seizures; a marked worsening of a preexisting seizure disorder; visual field cuts; anosmia; hemiparesis).
III. The neurocognitive disorder presents immediately after the occurrence of the traumatic brain injury or immediately after recovery of consciousness and persists past the acute post-injury period.

Biomechanics of Concussion

Acute concussion or mTBI is characterized by the disruption of neuronal homeostasis through physical forces transferred to the neuron through direct or indirect mechanical forces. The biomechanics of mTBI are important to understand when looking at the associated physiological damage that is created. These damaging forces include acceleration/deceleration, compression, and distraction or shear forces. Each of these forces creates a different signature within the brain and can have slight differing affects across the relatively isomeric characteristic of brain tissue. Each of these forces should be explored and defined, both singularly and in combination, as concussive injury to the brain. Rarely is brain trauma isotopic in nature (i.e., just stretch or just compression).

The acceleration force injury occurs when the head is fixed and is accelerated rapidly by an external force of an object colliding into it. These acceleration forces drive the inner cranium to collide with a fixed brain within the cranial cavity. In athletics, an example of an acceleration injury would be like the forces absorbed through punches being taken by a boxer or when a football player is "blindsided" by an opposing athlete and the head becomes violently accelerated. In contrast, the deceleration force is created when the head is already in motion and it is rapidly decelerated by a fixed object. A player's head coming into contact with the playing surface or with a fixed object on the playing field like a goal post would be an example of a deceleration force.

Acceleration and deceleration forces of a linear nature produce contusion-type injuries to the brain due to the absorption of compressive forces. A contusion located on the same side relative to the location of the applied external force is labeled a "coup"-type injury. A contusion received by the brain on a side opposite the side of the acceleration/deceleration forces is commonly referred to as a counter coup injury. The degree and depth of penetration for linear forces are modified by its intensity [9]. Mild acceleration/deceleration forces affect namely superficial layers in the brain. In addition, moderate-to-severe compressive forces can affect deeper structures within the brain. Thus, cell viability, structural, and functional disturbance of neurons can involve both cortical (superficial) and subcortical (deep) structures in the brain.

In addition to the damaging nature of linear acceleration/deceleration compressive forces, angular acceleration/deceleration stretches, or shear forces can generate significant trauma in the brain and are often considered more damaging [10]. These may be considered more damaging as the viscoelastic and gelatinous properties of the brain, with its subsequent high-water content, are highly resistant to compression and less resistant to distraction or shear tensile forces. These acceleration/deceleration forces contribute to the destructive distraction and shear forces or "stretch" on the white and gray matter of the brain. In addition, regardless of etiology, focal injury has a tendency to accumulate at the site of a transition in density as in the transition zones of gray matter (neuronal cell bodies) to white matter (neuronal axons), as well as along areas where vessels penetrate the gelatinous matrix of the brain [11]. Angular acceleration/deceleration shear forces can create stretch injuries to the white matter or axons [12, 13].

Neurophysiologic Cascade of Injury

Seminal papers on the pathophysiology of concussion have been developed which have been foundational to our understanding of the traumatic sequelae resulting from the adverse biomechanical forces absorbed in the brain [14–16]. Researchers exploring treatment strategies base their interventions on the ensuing cascade of cellular events within the injured tissue in order to influence adverse effects downstream and ultimately limit the amount of damage to the brain. A brief overview of the different pathophysiological effects of concussion will be helpful as we describe the different treatment strategies outlined in this chapter and give context to the intervention.

Metabolic Dysregulation

Of the most damaging forces, stretch and shear strain forces applied to the neuronal cell body and axon, can cause significant membrane disruption with a cascade of neurometabolic events [17]. Disrupted membranes and altered membrane potentials result in a massive efflux of intracellular excitatory amino acids (EAA) and potassium (K^+) [18]. Additionally, mechanically induced depolarization contributes to the release of EAA-like glutamate. Once glutamate is released and subsequently bound, more intracellular K^+ is released compounding the distressed environment [19]. To restore intracellular homeostasis, the Na^+/K^+ ATP-dependent pumps work in excess [17]. This excess function demands increased amounts of ATP. However, the immediate ATP stores become quickly depleted, as normal oxidative metabolism of ATP is diminished and less effective glycolysis begins. This depletion of ATP available for the cell has been linked to mitochondrial dysregulation in the cell after mTBI [20].

Metabolic dysregulation mediated by compromised mitochondrial function also leads to a decreased glucose metabolic rate and depressed oxidative metabolism [21, 22]. This was primarily due to mitochondrial dysfunction and decreased respiration that is well documented in the literature after concussive injury to the neuron [22, 23]. DiPietro et al. developed a broader theory that the proteins associated with ATP-dependent processes within the cell and associated with the mitochondrial electron transport chain were downregulated at the time of injury as a form of "hibernation" state. It is theorized that this hibernation and hypometabolic state may be neuroprotective in nature and spare the cell from secondary metabolic cell death [24]. However, a prolonged state of metabolic dysregulation and hypometabolism may contribute to the deleterious long-lasting clinical features of minor/major neurocognitive disorder (NCD) often experienced in patients with prolonged symptoms [25].

Oxidative Damage and Apoptosis

The unregulated release of EAA contributes to an increased cellular concentration of Calcium. Increased amounts of intracellular Ca^{++} have direct and indirect consequences in the cell. A direct consequence of the cytosolic presence of Ca^{++} is the altered membrane potentials across the mitochondrial membrane [26]. Moreover, if not corrected, the increasing presence of Ca^{++} within the cell and within the mitochondria can stimulate the release of apoptic precursor proteins (Caspase 3). The indirect consequence of Ca^{++} accumulation in the cell is on the ATP-dependent voltage-gated Ca^{++} channels. This becomes another ATP-dependent process in the cell which requires energy. In the axon, Ca^{++}-mediated activation of catabolic enzymes will affect the cytoarchitecture in the effected microtubule, causing compaction [27]. In addition, Ca^{++}-mediated release of phospholipases works to disrupt cellular membranes of both the neuron and mitochondria, as they both have phospholipid bilayers regulating and protecting intracellular processes. Indirectly, glutamate induces neuronal cell death via stimulation of the N-methyl-D-aspartate (NMDA) receptor site. Through this action, extracellular Ca^{++} continues to enter the cell and activates Ca^{++}-dependent nitric oxide synthase, resulting in excessive nitric oxide formation. Production of free radicals combined with mitochondrial dysfunction, and the resultant upregulation of apoptic pre-cursor signaling proteins, can ultimately contribute to cell death [21, 25, 28, 29].

Among cells which remain viable, there has been some evidence of differential recovery of function between the soma (cell body) and axons of the groups of neurons exposed to injury [30]. The cell body has the density in organelles with the capability of earlier restoration of cell body homeostasis. This is in stark contrast to the axon, which has microtubule structures that are more vulnerable to the stretch and shear forces seen in mTBI. Through the stretch biomechanical forces absorbed, intracellular Ca^{++} stores are released, resulting in increased intra-axonal concentrations [31]. Dysregulation of resting membrane potentials across the axonal cellular membrane contributes to sustained heightened Ca^{++} concentrations, which contribute to secondary axonotomy in some stretched axons [31, 32]. This acute and sustained increase in Ca^{++} concentration leads to a cleaving of neurofilament side arms (leading to compaction) and microtubule disassembly [33]. The healing rates for axonal or white matter tracks can take days, months, or years according to diffuse tensor imaging research and delays in FA value recovery [30].

Inflammation

Neuroinflammation plays a role in neuronal cell death and regeneration and can be activated in mild TBI or concussion [34, 35]. Physical disruption of cellular membranes, unregulated excitotoxicity, altered cerebrovascular response, and mitochondrial dysfunction all contribute to the neurochemical milieu surrounding affected tissues and can contribute to neuronal injury and cell death. Neuroinflammation is characterized by activation of glia, microglia, and astrocytes releasing proinflammatory mediators within the brain. These mediators subsequently recruit immune cells. Activation of the complement cascade and upregulation in the production of proinflammatory cytokines and chemokines define the neuronal inflammatory response and neuronal regenerative response in the brain [36]. This generalized response in the brain contributes to both cellular death and regeneration in the recovering brain tissue. Upregulation of proinflammatory cytokines like tumor necrosis factor-alpha (TNF-α) and a subgroup of interleukins (IL-1, IL-6, IL-18) can facilitate the inflammatory response through activation of local microglial cells, as well as stimulating the expression of various endothelial cellular adhesion molecules (CAM) [37–41]. Cellular adhesion molecules are then responsible for local infiltration of neutrophils, leukocytes, and other inflammatory cells [42]. These neuroinflammatory changes occur in a dose response from repeated subconcussive blows and/or singular mild brain traumatic brain injury [43]. Moreover, these "subconcussive" exposures can trigger the same acute neuroinflammatory response, in the absence of measured behavioral changes, but are shown to increase infiltration of activated microglia/macrophages as part of the inflammatory response [43]. Neuroinflammation as described is a physiological process following concussive injury that can contribute to the cumulative and neurodegenerative effects stemming from repeated "subconcussive" and mild concussive injuries.

Cerebrovascular Response

In addition to the other cellular responses to injury, cerebral blood flow can also be compromised from mild traumatic brain injury [44–46]. Cerebral blood flow can remain compromised in the acute and chronic stages of recovery from mild traumatic brain injury [14, 47–52]. This is possible through uncoupling of the autonomic nervous system's ability to regulate heart rate based on vascular feedback loops from the sympathetic and parasympathetic nervous system [53, 54]. Local release of cytokines leads to perturbations in local perfusion rates within vascular beds surrounding lesion sites [55]. Moreover, these cytokines associated with neuroinflammation are strongly correlated to acute and chronic changes in cerebral blood flow [56]. Alterations in cerebral blood flow can last longer than 1 week in patients recovering from mTBI and can be significantly altered in patients suffering from chronic post-concussion syndrome [57, 58]. It has even been suggested that measurements of cerebral blood flow may act as a biomarker of recovery in athletes recovering from mild traumatic brain injury due the strong connection with neuroinflammation.

Ultimately, correction of these cellular dysfunctions lies in the brain's ability to restore adequate blood flow to the site of injury; restore/preserve cellular membranes; restore/preserve mitochondrial function; increase substrate availability; and limit the inflammatory response to cellular injury. As the brain restores homeostasis, the normal physiologic function of largely intact neuronal cells can remain disrupted.

Chronic Traumatic Encephalopathies

One area of increased attention over the past decade has been the "downstream" effects of repeated head impacts or traumas. These effects have both pathological and clinical features which, in some cases, can be fatal. These disease-states are the result of diffusely distributed neurofibrillary tangles (NFTs) composed of hyperphosphorylated tau protein, the presence of which ultimately disrupts neuronal function in the brain. It has been well established that brain injury, like what is experienced in sports-related concussion, is an environmental risk factor for acute and chronic tauopathy like what is seen in early onset dementia and Alzheimer's Disease [59]. One we hear about most often today is chronic traumatic encephalopathy or CTE. This pathology had been previously explored in the psychiatric literature and identified as "punch drunk" syndrome [60]. Its neuropathological features had been published recently and inform our current accepted features of the disease [61]. Furthering this association of repeated brain trauma and tauopathy was a landmark discovery of hyperphosphorylated tau with specific perivascular distribution reported by Dr. Bennet Omalu in the brain of a deceased football player [62]. Dr. Omalu reported these pathologies found in the brains of professional football players from the NFL who also demonstrated noted behavioral pathologies causing mental illness and ultimately leading to their untimely deaths. Today, CTE has a tissue presentation that is recognized as a distinct neurodegenerative disease neuropathologically defined by perivascular accumulation of abnormally phosphorylated tau protein at the depths of cortical sulci [63]. CTE, like many other taupathies, is attributed to traumatic brain injury stemming from subclinical to clinical head impacts [64].

The underlying mechanisms which ultimately lead to these disease states represent targets for therapeutic intervention which is currently ongoing. Proposed treatment strategies for sports-related concussion or mTBI and its physiological phenomena should attempt to address some of the deleterious pathophysiologic effects outlined above. Some attempts have been made to synthesize the literature to assess clinical *and* physiological features of injury and time course of healing to inform future directions in research on recovery from sports-related concussion [65]. At present, these serial biologic datapoints are not readily available and meaningful to clinicians. Therefore, this chapter provides a summary of the interventions currently being researched around mTBI using available definitions of functional recovery with some biological insight using imaging and animal models of mTBI to help inform the process.

Common Treatment Intervention Strategies

Review of the literature on treatment strategies being researched for sports-related concussion focuses on a few primary areas. Current treatment interventions receiving significant attention in the research include rest, exercise, physical therapy interventions, and psychiatric/psychological interventions. We will examine the research surrounding each of these areas of rest, exercise, physical therapy, and psychiatric/psychological interventions.

Rest for Concussion

The long-standing recommendation of physical and cognitive rest has remained intact since the very first and subsequent concussion in sport group formed and provided concussion management guidelines [66–70]. Most recently, there has been a paradigm shift to introduce exercise or activity at an earlier stage of recovery following an initial period of rest [70]. The prescription of rest has been studied more closely by a few RCTs examining the recommendation and its effects [71, 72]. However, the major difficulties in validating this treatment recommendation across the body of research are largely due to the heterogeneity of research constructs. Attempts are being made to synthesize the information in a meaningful way so that clinicians can make evidence-based decisions for the use of rest and exercise in their treatment and management of athletes recovering from concussion [73, 74]. Prescriptions for *rest* studied in the literature are inconsistently assigned and result in varied timing of rest (i.e., acute vs. sub-acute); duration of rest; definition of rest; type of rest (cognitive vs physical); objective pre- and post-rest measures of "recovery" from concussion. The most glaring omission is the complete absence of neurophysiological biomarkers to assess tissue-based recovery in our patient population. We will attempt to summarize the *different* studies looking at *different* prescriptions of rest following concussion, demonstrating either a benefit, no benefit, or delayed "healing."

The research describing benefits of cognitive and/or physical rest are reported in the literature across decades of study [75–79]. In line with these findings are studies that describe patient prognosis when exposed to early cognitive stress. Dr. Gioia et al. found that school-aged students reported an increase in concussion-related symptoms when they were immediately returned to school [80]. In a prospective cohort study, early cognitive rest was supported by Dr. Brown and colleagues [81]. Brown et al. determined that increased cognitive activity was associated with longer recovery from concussion and therefore supported the idea of early cognitive rest. In addition, a recent study by clinicians at a concussion treatment clinic found that a 7-day period of rest prescribed during *any* phase of recovery post concussion significantly improved cognitive testing measures and symptom reports across high school- and college-aged athletes [78]. Even more, Gibson et al. found no association with early cognitive rest to the duration of symptoms in athletes evaluated and enrolled in a sport concussion clinic [82]. As a result, it is still recommended that adolescents recovering from sports-related concussion have a *brief period*, typically 24–48 hours, of cognitive rest designed to reduce cognitive burden on the brain in order to support recovery and full return to academics [83–87].

Early Activity or Exercise for Concussion

As noted in an earlier section, concussion happens when traumatic forces cause a cascade of physiological effects on the brain. As such, the clinician and guiding physician treating athletes recovering from concussion should employ strategies that look to counteract these damaging physiological effects. In a broad sense, one such strategy has emerged over the past decade: activity or exercise. The health benefits of early movement and exercise following concussion have been reported in the research for decades [88]. Chronic exercise is noted to improve overall function in the brain and specifically clinical outcomes from a wide range of mental illness [89], brain disease [90, 91], cognitive function [92], and trauma [93]. Exercise and acclimation to environmental stresses enhance several neuroprotective mechanisms in the brain [94] and subsequently make the brain more resilient to disease and injury [95, 96]. As such, the prescription of exercise for athletes in their recovery from sports-related concussion is a practical application of the large body of literature for the improvement of patient outcomes in concussion.

In contrast to the previous section, a growing body of research has found no direct benefit from a prescription of rest or *prolonged* rest [88, 97–99]. Moreover, in a recent meta-analysis of RCTs for rest & aerobic exercise, researchers found that protocols that included a normal rest period contributed to longer recovery times and higher symptoms scores on PCSS [100]. Examining the effects of early activity, one study by emergency room physicians assigned patients to either 5 days or 1–2 days of rest followed by a gradual return to activity. The clinician researchers found that rest for 5 days vs. 1–2 days resulted in a larger number of reported symptoms by patients [101]. Confirming this finding, Howell et al. found that athletes who engaged in aerobic activity within the first week post-concussive injury reported lower symptoms severity than their non-exercising peers [102]. Wilson and colleagues also found that children and adolescents recovering from concussion who engaged in early activity report fewer and milder post-concussion symptoms and recovered sooner than their peers who were prescribed relative rest [103]. Translational research using animal models of concussion shows that immediate activity following brain injury upregulated genetic transcription factors supporting healing as well as improved behavioral activity scores in mice [104]. Combined, these findings of benefits *and* non-benefits lead us to the conclusion that this area of initial care using rest needs further investigation to fully understand what clinicians should be prescribing for their athletes recovering from concussion.

As with most areas of promise in the treatment of brain injury, its application remains limited to the objective measures of functional injury resolution. Clinicians still lack the ability to assess physiologic recovery and tissue recovery objectively through readily accessible and relevant biomarkers. So, we will examine the effect that exercise has on the recovering brain through that lens. From the animal and human imagining and physiological research, we can examine how exercise improves overall brain physiology and function in the specific areas effected by sports-related concussive injury.

Neurophysiologic Adaptation to Exercise

Neurovascular Response to Exercise in Concussion

Additionally, it is well known that the vasculature in the brain changes with exercise [105]. Exercise is capable of new vascular formation in the cerebral cortex [106] and strengthening cerebrovascular reactivity [107]. These changes due to exercise positively affect the brain and help to mitigate the strength of negative vascular responses post injury as sports-related concussion causes acute and chronic cerebrovascular reactivity and hypoperfusion [57].

It has been demonstrated that exercise as a treatment modality can restore normal perfusion in the brain to areas previously effected [57]. Exercise has been proven to improve and promote cerebrovascular circulation through reperfusion and angiogenesis in the brain. During exercise, the brain becomes "flush" with heavily oxygenated blood. While humans exercise, the brain is challenged with providing the musculoskeletal system and body organs with an adequate amount of blood to meet the increased metabolic demands. In addition, the body must maintain adequate arterial blood pressures across the entire system. Compared to the dramatic increases across the periphery and organs, the increase in cerebral blood flow is only mild (<30% increase in CBF) up to ~60% Max VO2 [108, 109].

Research looking at patients with chronic post-concussion syndrome has shown differences in cerebrovascular blood flow compared to normal controls in pediatric and adult populations [48, 57, 58, 110]. Consequently, when exercise is prescribed for athletes recovering from concussion, researchers have found restoration of CBF and improved tolerance to exercise [57, 111].

Neuroplasticity, Neurogenesis, and Exercise

Exercise, in particular aerobic exercise, has a long line of research demonstrating its benefit on the improvement in neurogenesis, cognitive function, and plasticity [112–116]. The processes that support these functions also promote healing as the brain recovers from trauma. Exercise enhances the production and release of several factors in the brain and from the periphery, including substances like BDNF, IL-1, VEGF, and lactate, all of which have been indicated in neuroprotective cascades in the brain. Briefly, brain-derived neurotrophic growth factor (BDNF) is believed to be a major factor in hippocampal function, neuronal cell survival, synaptic plasticity, neurogenesis, and mitochondrial biogenesis [117, 118]. Insulin-like growth factor 1 (IGF-1) is a neurotrophic hormone taken up by the brain after exercise. IGF-1 interacts through many complex pathways to promote amyloid β production and the stabilization or preservation of synaptic plasticity in recovery from brain injury [119]. Moreover, studies of exercise following brain injury demonstrated early uptake of IGF-1, which reduced overall brain lesion size [120]. Vascular endothelial growth factor (VEGF) is a cytokine responsible for the restoration/promotion of new blood vessels and long-term potentiation in the brain. Exercise upregulates the production of VEGF in the brain which subsequently works counter to the localized compromised regional cerebral blood flow seen in mTBI through angiogenesis [121]. Finally, lactate is a by-product when pyruvate is broken down by muscle during moderate activity. When its produced at a faster rate that it can be processed, lactate concentrations remain elevated in the blood. This increase in blood lactate is utilized across the body and is also taken up in the brain to support various functions during exercise [122]. Lactate is also used as an energy substrate for neurons recovering from TBI [123]. In addition, lactate is also closely linked with increased VEGF production by binding to lactate receptors in the brain [121].

Mental Illness, Concussion, and Exercise

Over the past decades, exercise has long been prescribed to improve outcomes from patients with mental illness across a spectrum of disorders [124–135]. Trauma-enhanced mental illness is a serious growing public health crisis where adolescent and adult athletes sustaining concussion have an increased susceptibility [136–139]. Moreover, many parents of adolescent patients recovering from concussion are not fully aware that they need diligence in identifying mental health-related symptoms following concussion [140]. Population- based research tells us that school-aged adolescents sustaining a concussion have an increased risk of poor mental health outcomes that includes increased or persistent depression symptoms including attempted suicide [141–144]. This is also supported in research on adults suffering multiple concussions that demonstrate an increase in impulsivity and aggression [145] and symptoms of mental illness like anxiety and depression [146, 147]. The prescription of exercise for the subgroup of concussion with mental illness has demonstrated promising findings.

Exercise, Heat Acclimation, and Neuroprotection

As regular exercisers, athletes have developed many physiologically adaptive responses to stress. One of those areas of stress comes from the environment. Research in the area of heat stress and acclimation during exercise has yielded insights into proposed mechanisms of neuroprotection and neurophysiological adaptation. The brain's adaptations to heat stress may indirectly influence how the brain responds to the added condition of trauma. Known adaptations to heat stress in the areas of vascular response and, more specifically, the upregulation of heat shock proteins are discussed in this section.

As discussed in the previous section, exercise up to 60% VO2 increases global CBF by as much as 30% above which point CBF is maintained or reduced, despite the continued cerebral metabolic demands that often are enhanced during exercise. The introduction of heat stress during moderate-to-heavy exercise enhances the uncoupling between metabolic demands and a subsequent reduction in CBF [148]. In addition, the cerebrovascular demand across the brain is regionally modified in an attempt for the brain to address location-specific activation, which may be compromised in the heat. It has been demonstrated in the literature that anterior hemispheric CBF may be compromised or reduced during exercise in the heat [149]. Therefore, under hyperthermic conditions, this "pre-existing" increased metabolic demand and lowered regional blood flow may in some way contribute to worse outcomes, although it has not been directly assessed in animal models of hyperthermia and concussion [150]. This remains a hypothetical framework that has not been investigated fully.

Animal models and human case studies of heat stress and trauma have given us insight into the underpinnings of worse physiological and clinical outcomes following mild-to-moderate TBI [150, 151]. The brain's ability to preserve brain function and mitigate the stress of heat may be largely modulated by the expression of a group of stabilizing proteins called heat shock proteins. Research in the area of neurophysiological acclimatization to heat has focused on the expression of these heat shock proteins and their role in stabilizing intercellular processes during times of stress and heat induction. These proteins contribute to the local intra- and extracellular environment both directly through stabilization of cellular proteins and indirectly through the up- or downregulation of cytokines responsible for apoptosis, tau protein toxicity, and amyloid plaque formation. This cellular response to heat stress is seen across many tissue and cell types. There are some sub-families of heat shock proteins present in the brain which can provide neuroprotective effects. However, to date, there are no published studies that examine the effects of these sub-groups of heat shock proteins and their effect on mechanically induced neurotrauma (i.e., concussion).

We can however describe the peri- and posttraumatic hyperthermic environment under which these heat shock proteins may play a role. Some sub-families of heat shock proteins and their subsequent functions are described. Heat shock transcription factor-1 (HSF-1) is a precursor for heat shock protein-1 (HSP-1). Its primary role serves in the stabilization of endoplasmic reticulum function and the downregulation of certain proapoptic cytokines [152, 153]. It also supports mitochondrial and cellular function through the preservation of intracellular protein folding within the endoplasmic reticulum. In general, this would assist neurons in the restoration of cellular homeostasis if these proteins and mechanisms are active during mechanically induced neurotrauma.

Heat Shock Protein-27 (HSP-27) is a protein which can have neuroprotective effects against tau protein toxicity. In mTBI, early mechanisms following trauma result in hyperphosphorylated tau. This overexpression of these specific proteins forms neurofibrillary (NF) tangles, which disrupt normal cell function in the brain and can lead to early onset dementia, Alzheimer's, and ultimately, cellular apoptosis. HSP-27, along with other proteins expressed in the astrocyte, has a neuroprotective effect on tau phosphorylation [154]. This decreased expression of tau has the potential to protect against the long-term formation of NF tangles as a result from trauma.

Finally, heat shock protein-70 (HSP-70) has been reported in the research to have a potentially therapeutic effect for patients with Alzheimer's disease (AD). The presence of amyloid plaques in the brain is a result of the overexpression of β-amyloid peptides through beta-amyloid precursor protein phosphorylation. Like the production of NF tangles, β-amyloid plaque deposits disrupt the normal cellular function of neurons and astrocytes in the brains of patients diagnosed with Alzheimer's disease. Both NF tangle and amyloid plaque formation have been the target for research aimed at treating AD. Hoshino et al. focused on the expression of HSP-70 in transgenic mice. Mice with an increased expression of HSP-70 were able to decrease the production of β-APP through decreased expression of β-amyloid-degrading enzymes and TGF-β1, which is a cytokine that stimulates phagocytosis of β-APP [155]. TBI also stimulates the production of β-amyloid plaques. In a sense, an active expression of HSP-70 through heat acclimation training may have a potential benefit in the long-term formation of these damaging plaques.

Heat shock proteins along with other proteins and cellular components can potentially play an important role in the preservation of homeostasis to the injured neuron. It certainly appears that heat shock proteins have a neuroprotective effect as it relates to both the short- and long-term consequences of neuronal stress under controlled conditions. Research in this area using animal models of injury may provide a clearer picture of the functional role these proteins play in preservation of neurons as result of trauma under hyperthermic conditions. These claims of hyperthermia-induced physiological changes have not been substantiated in the research and are therefore a hypothetical framework of neuroprotection in mTBI.

Psychological Treatment of Concussion

Increasing attention has been given to mental health disparities occurring secondary to sports-related brain injury. It is widely accepted that psychological treatment techniques like psychoeducation, cognitive behavioral therapy (CBT), and mindfulness-based treatment techniques are an effective treatment option to improve executive function, reduce PCSS scores, improve quality of life, and reduce symptoms of depression and anxiety in mTBI patients [156, 157]. This section reviews the research surrounding these psychological treatment strategies and their efficacy.

Psychoeducation

There is some evidence to support the use of early psychoeducation about expected post-concussive symptoms and recovery from concussion. Several studies providing early reassurance regarding expected recovery, guidance about managing symptoms, and guidance in resuming pre-injury roles in the acute phase of injury found a significant effect of reported symptoms 3 months later [158]. Minderhoud and colleagues provided patients with a manual on the nature and recovery of symptoms seen in PCS and found significantly reduced reports of PCSS 6 months post injury [159]. In two different studies where patients were issued a manual or pamphlet specifying what symptoms to expect and how to manage symptoms and stress, the patients claimed that the information helped, or they reported fewer symptoms [158, 159]. This trend of reduced symptom reporting has shown up in several other studies involving early psychoeducation as well. This would indicate that early psychoeducation does not prevent the development of symptoms, but rather facilitates better coping strategies and symptom management. This is exactly what Wade and colleagues concluded in their study [160]. They provided patients with an informational sheet about potential symptoms and additional clinical support as needed, but found no objective difference in symptom severity at 6 months post injury. They did, however, find significant improvement in daily functioning and activity [160]. In 2002, Ponsford and colleagues provided patients with a pamphlet on potential symptoms and coping strategies [161]. They found almost identical results to those of Wade with no significant improvements on neuropsychological assessments, but significantly fewer symptoms reported by the treatment group when compared to controls [161]. This is not to say that early education does not have a place in treatment of concussion. It has long been established that patients' appraisal of recovery can have a strong effect on their rate of recovery and overall perceived quality of life. Furthermore, it has been shown that stress can exacerbate concussion symptoms and slow recovery; therefore, early education may be beneficial simply by helping to foster management of symptoms and stress [162]. The inclusion of early education practices in managing patients recovering from concussion is indicated to manage injury-related stress.

Cognitive Behavioral Therapy

Cognitive behavioral therapy (CBT) takes the results of early education and improved symptom coping and management and attempts to apply them to individuals suffering from PCS. Cognitive behavioral therapy targets individuals' maladaptive beliefs, emotions, and cognitive processes [163]. In PCS populations, CBT seeks to improve the emotional appraisal of symptoms, coping, and stress management following injury. In a meta-analysis of RCTs, there were positive effects of cognitive behavioral therapy on sub-acute depression and anxiety scores [157]. In studies of individuals with head injuries, subjects often underestimate the frequency and severity of PCS-like symptoms pre-injury. Comparatively, healthy controls were better able to predict or anticipate potential symptoms of PCS. This difference in perception and expectation of injury can lead to cognitive bias and result in focusing on and exacerbation of symptoms. It has also been found that negative causal attributions and expectation predict persistent symptoms 3 months post injury [163]. Whittaker, Kemp, and House found that patients who expected serious negative consequences were more likely to have persistent symptoms [164]. They also found that severity of injury and symptoms did not better predict persistent symptoms than negative expectations [164]. In pediatric populations, CBT has been used to treat those with prolonged recovery trajectories and improve their ability to cope with and reduce PCS symptoms burden, reduce sleep disturbance, and improve mental health symptom reports [165–168].

Although there are limited studies on maladaptive behaviors and coping in concussed individuals, some studies of more severe TBI have shown that poor coping and maladaptive behaviors such as self-blame and symptom focusing have been associated with worse outcome. It is believed that maladaptive behaviors and perceptions may contribute to the maintenance of PCS and PCS-like symptoms.

Mindfulness-Based Stress Reduction

Mindfulness-based stress reduction (MSBR) is another psychological treatment that focuses on the management of negative thoughts, emotions, and behaviors. It involves mind-body-focused practices such as yoga and meditation that are intended to make one more aware of their internal state and resources. A review of the research on mindfulness techniques shows improvement in function of various structures in the brain and improved functional connectivity across the default mode network (DMN) [169]. Mindfulness-based stress reduction, like other psychological intervention platforms, aims to combat the effects of stress, anxiety, and depression that sometimes accompany mTBI post-injury symptom cluster.

Earlier this decade, research using MSBR in mild-to-moderate TBI patients had produced inconclusive results with regard to objective improvements. One study using a mindfulness-based stress reduction intervention on TBI patients produced no real treatment effect [170]. McMillan and colleagues found no significant effects on objective or subjective measures of cognition, mood, or symptom reporting in a cohort of TBI patients [170].

In a more recent growing body of research, many clinicians are reporting positive interventions from mindfulness-based treatment. In two studies from Bedard and colleagues, they used MBSR interventions at a frequency of one session per week for 8 weeks and demonstrated statistically significant improvements in depression symptoms, reduced pain intensity, and increased energy levels [171, 172]. However, like most of the mindfulness research, it should be noted that Bedard had a small sample size and the MBSR intervention was used as a supplement to another group-based treatment plan; therefore, its result cannot solely be attributed MBSR intervention.

In another small cohort of military mTBI patients, researchers used mindfulness-based classes that met weekly to treat a group of servicemen who reported lingering cognitive effects of concussion 1 year post injury [173]. Treatment using MBSR resulted in fewer reports of cognitive symptoms and lower symptoms associated with PTSD. In a pilot study of MSBR in treating post-concussion syndrome, patients were led by neuropsychological experts trained in MSBR for a 2-hour session once a week for 10 weeks [174]. The study found significant changes in perceived quality of life and self-efficacy, but no significant improvements in symptoms [174]. Similarly, in a study of patients recovering from mild-to-moderate TBI, researchers looked at measures of chronic stress, PCSS, and depressive symptom reports [175]. They reported MSBR reduced chronic stress reports as well as PCSS and depressive symptom scores compared to the active control group. Additionally, Polich and colleagues studied focused attention meditation and a form of mobile neurofeedback in mild-to-moderate TBI patients and discovered an overall reduction in symptom report and anxiety/depression inventory scores [176]. These positive trends are also demonstrated among pediatric mTBI cohorts using MSBR treatment techniques [177].

It would appear that MSBR helps patients to cope with reported symptoms and improve overall mental health recovery following brain injury. Mindfulness-based therapy may be used in conjunction with a treatment plan that provides objective scoring measures that assess mental health status following mild traumatic brain injury.

Conclusion

While great efforts have been made to advance the treatment options for individuals suffering from a concussion or mTBI, there is still no standard of care. This is partly due to the individualized approach many clinicians take, tailoring to the needs of the specific individual. As the knowledge of the physiology of concussion continues to grow, this will further help to develop treatment plans that are scientifically backed and can be tailored to an individual post injury. While rest, exercise and physical activity, and psychological approaches were discussed at length here, various technologies, supplements, and other therapies are being explored for their potential utility in individuals suffering from concussion. Many of these are in the preliminary stages of research and more work is needed to determine their effectiveness to be able to offer individuals suffering from concussion valid, effective, and individually tailored treatment options.

References

1. Schmidt JD, Rizzone K, Hoffman NL, et al. Age at first concussion influences the number of subsequent concussions. Pediatr Neurol. 2018;81:19–24.
2. Lincoln A, Caswell S, Almquist J, Dunn R, Norris J, Hinton R. Trends in concussion incidence in high school sports: a prospective 11-year study. Am J Sports Med. 2011;30(10):958–63.
3. Burke MJ, Fralick M, Nejatbakhsh N, Tartaglia MC, Tator CH. In search of evidence-based treatment for concussion: characteristics of current clinical trials. Brain Inj. 2015;29(3):300–5.
4. McCrory P, Johnston K, Meeuwisse W, Aubry M, Cantu R, Dvorak J, et al. Summary and agreement statement of the 2nd international conference on concussion in sport, Prague 2004. Br J Sports Med. 2005;39:196–204.
5. American Congress of Rehabilitation Medicine. Mild Traumatic Brain Injury Committee, Definition of mild traumatic brain injury. J Head Trauma Rehabil. 1993;8(3):86–7.
6. Willer B, Leddy J. Management of concussion and post-concussion syndrome. Curr Treat Options Neurol. 2006;8(5):415–26.
7. American Psychiatric Association. *Diagnostic and Statistical Manual of Mental Disorders*. Washington, DC, USA: American Psychiatric Association; 1994.

8. American Psychiatric Association. Diagnostic and Statistical Manual of Mental Disorders: DSM-5. Washington, DC, USA: American Psychiatric Association; 2013.
9. Ommaya AK, Gennarelli TA. Cerebral concussion and traumatic unconsciousness. Correlation of experimental and clinical observations of blunt head injuries. Brain. 1974;97(4):633–54.
10. Holbourn A. Mechanics of head injuries. Lancet. 1943;242(6267):438–41.
11. Bigler ED, Maxwell WL. Neuropathology of mild traumatic brain injury: relationship to neuroimaging findings. Brain Imaging Behav. 2012;6(2):108–36.
12. Strich S. Shearing of nerve fibers as a cause of brain damage due to head injury. Lancet II. 1961:443–8.
13. Povlishock J, Becket D, Cheng C, Vaughan G. Axonal change in minor head injury. J Neuropathol Exp Neurol. 1983;42:225–42.
14. Denny-Brown D, Russell W. Experimental cerebral concussion. Brain. 1941;64(2–3):93–164.
15. Giza CC, Hovda DA. The neurometabolic cascade of concussion. J Athl Train. 2001;36(3):228–35.
16. Signoretti S, Vagnozzi R, Tavazzi B, Lazzarino G. Biochemical and neurochemical sequelae following mild traumatic brain injury: summary of experimental data and clinical implications. Neurosurg Focus. 2010;29(5):E1:1–12.
17. Barkhoudarian G, Hovda D, Giza C. The molecular pathophysiology of concussive brain injury. Clin Sports Med. 2010;30:33–48.
18. Farkas O, Lifshitz J, Povlishock JT. Mechanoporation induced by diffuse traumatic brain injury: an irreversible or reversible response to injury? J Neurosci. 2006;26(12):3130–40.
19. Katayama Y, Becker DP, Tamura T, Hovda DA. Massive increases in extracellular potassium and the indiscriminate release of glutamate following concussive brain injury. J Neurosurg. 1990;73:889–900.
20. Gilmer L, Roberts K, Joy K, Sullivan P, Scheff S. Early mitochondrial dysfunction after cortical contusion injury. J Neurotrauma. 2009;26:1271–80.
21. Hovda D, Yoshino A, Kawamata T, Katayama Y, Becker D. Diffuse prolonged depression of cerebral oxidative metabolism following concussive brain injury in the rat: a cytochrome oxidase histochemistry study. Brain Res. 1991;567:1–10.
22. Vagnozzi R, Marmarou A, Tavazzi B, Signoretti S, Di Pietro D, et al. Changes of cerebral energy metabolism and lipid peroxidation in rats leading to mitochondrial dysfunction after diffuse brain injury. J Neurotrauma. 1999;16(10):903–13.
23. Singh IN, Sullivan PG, Deng Y, Mbye LH, Hall ED. Time course of post-traumatic mitochondrial oxidative damage and dysfunction in a mouse model of focal traumatic brain injury: implications for neuroprotective therapy. J Cereb Blood Flow Metab. 2006;26:1407–18.
24. Di Pietro V, Amorini A, Tavazzi B, Hovda D, Signoretti S, Giza C, et al. Potentially neuroprotective gene modulation in an in vitro model of mild traumatic brain injury. Mol Cell Biochem. 2013;375:185–98.
25. Peskind E, Petrie E, Cross D, Pagulayan K, McCraw K, et al. Cerebrocerebellar hypometabolism associated with repetitive blast exposure mild traumatic brain injury in 12 Iraq war veterans with persistent post-concussive symptoms. NeuroImage. 2011;54 Supplement 1:S76–82.
26. Lifshitz J, Sullivan P, Hovda D. Mitochondrial damage and dysfunction in traumatic brain injury. Mitochondrion. 2004;4(5–6):705–13.
27. Povlishock J, Pettus E. Traumatically induced axonal damage: evidence for enduring changes in axolemmal permeability with associated cytoskeletal change. Acta Neurochir Suppl. 1996;66:81–6.
28. Dawson VL, Dawson TM, London ED, Bredt DS, Snyder SH. Nitric oxide mediates glutamate neurotoxicity in primary cortical cultures. Proc Natl Acad Sci U S A. 1991;88:6368–71.
29. Tamura Y, Sato Y, Akaike A, Shiomi H. Mechanisms of cholecystokinin-induced protection of cultured cortical neurons against N-methyl-D-aspartate receptor-mediated glutamate cytotoxicity. Brain Res. 1992;592:317–25.

30. Vagnozzi R, Signoretti S, Cristofori L, Alessandrini F, Floris R, et al. Assessment of metabolic brain damage and recovery following mild traumatic brain injury: a multicentre, proton magnetic resonance spectroscopic study in concussed patients. Brain. 2010;133:3232–42.
31. Staal JA, Dickson TC, Gasperini R, Liu Y, Foa L, Vickers JC. Initial calcium release from intracellular stores followed by calcium dysregulation is linked to secondary axotomy following transient axonal stretch injury. J Neurochem. 2010;112(5):1147–55.
32. Chung RS, Staal JA, McCormack GH, Dickson TC, Cozens MA, Chuckowree JA, et al. Mild axonal stretch injury in vitro induces a progressive series of neurofilament alterations ultimately leading to delayed axotomy. J Neurotrauma. 2005;22(10):1081–91.
33. Okonkwo DO, Pettus EH, Moroi J, Povlishock JT. Alteration of the neurofilament sidearm and its relation to neurofilament compaction occurring with traumatic axonal injury. Brain Res. 1998;784(1–2):1–6.
34. Holmin S, Soderlund J, Biberfeld P, Mathiesen T. Intracerebral inflammation after human brain contusion. Neurosurgery. 1998;42:291–9.
35. Rathbone AT, Tharmaradinam S, Jiang S, Rathbone MP, Kumbhare DA. A review of the neuro- and systemic inflammatory responses in post-concussion symptoms: introduction of the "post-inflammatory brain syndrome" PIBS. Brain Behav Immun. 2015;46:1–16.
36. Schmidt O, Heyde C, Ertel W, Stahel P. Closed head injury—an inflammatory disease? Brain Res Brain Res Rev. 2005;48:388–99.
37. Hurwitz A, Lyman W, Guida M, Calderon T, Berman J. Tumor necrosis factor alpha induces adhesion molecule expression on human fetal astrocytes. J Exp Med. 1992;176:1631–6.
38. Otto V, Heinzel-Pleines U, Gloor S, Trentz O, Kossmann T, Morganti-Kossmann M. sICAM-1 and TNF-alpha induce MIP-2 with distinct kinetics in astrocytes and brain microvascular endothelial cells. J Neurosci Res. 2000;60:733–42.
39. Stoll G, Jander S, Schroeter M. Detrimental and beneficial effects of injury-induced inflammation and cytokine expression in the nervous system. Adv Exp Med Biol. 2002;513:87–113.
40. Barksby HE, Lea SR, Preshaw PM, Taylor JJ. The expanding family of interleukin-1 cytokines and their role in destructive inflammatory disorders. Clin Exp Immunol. 2007;149(2):217–25.
41. Helmy A, Carpenter K, Menon D, Pickard J, Hutchinson P. The cytokine response to human traumatic brain injury: temporal profiles and evidence for cerebral parenchymal production. J Cereb Blood Flow Metab. 2010:1–13.
42. Casarsa C, De Luigi A, Pausa M, De Simoni M, Tedesco F. Intracerebroventricular injection of terminal complement complex causes inflammatory reaction in the rat brain. Eur J Immunol. 2003;33:1260–70.
43. Shultz SR, Bao F, Omana V, Chiu C, Brown A, Cain DP. Repeated mild lateral fluid percussion brain injury in the rat causes cumulative long-term behavioral impairments, neuroinflammation, and cortical loss in an animal model of repeated concussion. J Neurotrauma. 2012;29(2):281–94.
44. DeWitt DS, Prough DS. Traumatic cerebral vascular injury: the effects of concussive brain injury on the cerebral vasculature. J Neurotrauma. 2003;20(9):795–825.
45. Len TK, Neary JP. Cerebrovascular pathophysiology following mild traumatic brain injury. Clin Physiol Funct Imaging. 2011;31(2):85–93.
46. Ellis MJ, Ryner LN, Sobczyk O, Fierstra J, Mikulis DJ, Fisher JA, Duffin J, Mutch WA. Neuroimaging assessment of cerebrovascular reactivity in concussion: current concepts, methodological considerations, and review of the literature. Front Neurol. 2016;7:61.
47. Bonne O, Gilboa A, Louzounb Y, Kempf-Sherfc O, Katza M, et al. Cerebral blood flow in chronic symptomatic mild traumatic brain Injury. Psychiatry Res. 2003;124:141–52.
48. Buckley EM, Miller BF, Golinski JM, Sadeghian H, McAllister LM, Vangel M, Ayata C, Meehan WP 3rd, Franceschini MA, Whalen MJ. Decreased microvascular cerebral blood flow assessed by diffuse correlation spectroscopy after repetitive concussions in mice. J Cereb Blood Flow Metab. 2015;35(12):1995–2000.

49. Bartnik-Olson BL, Holshouser B, Wang H, Grube M, Tong K, Wong V, Ashwal S. Impaired neurovascular unit function contributes to persistent symptoms after concussion: a pilot study. J Neurotrauma. 2014;31(17):1497–506.
50. Doshi H, Wiseman N, Liu J, Wang W, Welch RD, O'Neil BJ, et al. Cerebral hemodynamic changes of mild traumatic brain Injury at the acute stage. PLoS One. 2015;10(2):e0118061.
51. Mcicr TB, Bellgowan PS, Singh R, Kuplicki R, Polanski DW, Mayer AR. Recovery of cerebral blood flow following sports-related concussion. JAMA Neurol. 2015;72(5):530–8.
52. da Costa L, van Niftrik CB, Crane D, Fierstra J, Bethune A. Temporal profile of cerebrovascular reactivity impairment, gray matter volumes, and persistent symptoms after mild traumatic head injury. Front Neurol. 2016;7:70.
53. Lewelt W, Jenkins LW, Miller JD. Autoregulation of cerebral blood flow after experimental fluid percussion injury of the brain. J Neurosurg. 1980;53:500–11.
54. La Fountaine MF, Gossett JD, De Meersman RE, Bauman WA. Increased QT interval variability in 3 recently concussed athletes: an exploratory observation. J Athl Train. 2011;46(3):230–3.
55. Philip S, Udomphorn Y, Kirkham FJ, Vavilala MS. Cerebrovascular pathophysiology in pediatric traumatic brain injury. J Trauma. 2009;67(2 Suppl):S128–34.
56. Sankar SB, Pybus AF, Liew A, et al. Low cerebral blood flow is a non-invasive biomarker of neuroinflammation after repetitive mild traumatic brain injury. Neurobiol Dis. 2019;124:544–54.
57. Amen DG, Wu JC, Taylor D, Willeumier K. Reversing brain damage in former NFL players: implications for traumatic brain injury and substance abuse rehabilitation. J Psychoactive Drugs. 2011;43(1):1–5.
58. Leddy JJ, Cox JL, Baker JG, Wack DS, Pendergast DR, Zivadinov R, Willer B. Exercise treatment for postconcussion syndrome: a pilot study of changes in functional magnetic resonance imaging activation, physiology, and symptoms. J Head Trauma Rehabil. 2013;28(4):241–9.
59. Fann JR, Ribe AR, Pedersen HS, Fenger-Grøn M, Christensen J, Benros ME, et al. Long-term risk of dementia among people with traumatic brain injury in Denmark: a population-based observational cohort study. Lancet Psychiatry. 2018;5:424–31.
60. Martland HS. Punch drunk. JAMA. 1928;91:1103–7.
61. Geddes JF, Vowles GH, Nicoll JA, et al. Neuronal cytoskeletal changes are an early consequence of repetitive head injury. Acta Neuropathol. 1999;98:171–8.
62. Omalu BI, DeKosky ST, Minster RL, Kamboh MI, Hamilton RL, Wecht CH. Chronic traumatic encephalopathy in a National Football League player. Neurosurgery. 2005;57(1):128–34; discussion 128–34.
63. McKee AC, Stein TD, Kiernan PT, Alvarez VE. The neuropathology of chronic traumatic encephalopathy. Brain Pathol. 2015;25(3):350–64.
64. Cantu RC, Bernick C. History of chronic traumatic encephalopathy. Semin Neurol. 2020;40(4):353–8. https://doi.org/10.1055/s-0040-1713622.
65. Kamins J, Bigler E, Covassin T, et al. What is the physiological time to recovery after concussion? A systematic review. Br J Sports Med. 2017;51(12):935–40.
66. Aubry M, Cantu R, Dvorak J, Graf-Baumann T, Johnston K, Kelly J, Lovell M, McCrory P, Meeuwisse W, Schamasch P. Summary and agreement statement of the first international conference on concussion in sport, Vienna 2001. Phys Sportsmed. 2002;30(2):57–63.
67. McCrory P, Johnston K, Meeuwisse W, Aubry M, Cantu R, Dvorak J, Graf-Baumann T, Kelly J, Lovell M, Schamasch P, International Symposium on Concussion in Sport. Summary and agreement statement of the 2nd International Conference on Concussion in Sport, Prague 2004. Clin J Sport Med. 2005;15(2):48–55.
68. McCrory P, Meeuwisse W, Johnston K, Dvorak J, Aubry M, Molloy M, Cantu R. Consensus statement on Concussion in Sport–the 3rd International Conference on Concussion in Sport held in Zurich, November 2008. J Sci Med Sport. 2009;12(3):340–51.
69. McCrory P, Meeuwisse W, Aubry M, Cantu B, Dvorak J, Echemendia RJ, Engebretsen L, Johnston K, Kutcher JS, Raftery M, Sills A, Kathryn Schneider PT, Tator CH, Benson

BW, Davis GA, Ellenbogen RG, Guskiewicz KM, Herring SA, Iverson G, Jordan BD, Kissick J, et al. Consensus statement on concussion in sport–the 4th International Conference on Concussion in Sport held in Zurich, November 2012. Clin J Sport Med. 2013;23(2):89–117.
70. McCrory P, Meeuwisse W, Dvořák J, Aubry M, Bailes J, Broglio S, Cantu RC, Cassidy D, Echemendia RJ, Castellani RJ, Davis GA, Ellenbogen R, Emery C, Engebretsen L, Feddermann-Demont N, Giza CC, Guskiewicz KM, Herring S, Iverson GL, Johnston KM, et al. Consensus statement on concussion in sport-the 5th international conference on concussion in sport held in Berlin, October 2016. Br J Sports Med. 2017;51(11):838–47.
71. Moser RS, Schatz P, Glenn M, Kollias KE, Iverson GL. Examining prescribed rest as treatment for adolescents who are slow to recover from concussion. Brain Inj. 2015;29(1):58–63.
72. Yang J, Yeates K, Sullivan L, Singichetti B, Newton A, Xun P, Taylor HG, MacDonald J, Pommering T, Tiso M, Cohen D, Huang Y, Patterson J, Lu ZL. Rest Evaluation for Active Concussion Treatment (ReAct) Protocol: a prospective cohort study of levels of physical and cognitive rest after youth sports-related concussion. BMJ Open. 2019;9(4):e028386.
73. Alarie C, Gagnon IJ, Quilico E, Swaine B. Characteristics and outcomes of physical activity interventions for individuals with mild traumatic brain injury: a scoping review protocol. BMJ Open. 2019;9(6):e027240.
74. Register-Mihalik JK, Guskiewicz KM, Marshall SW, McCulloch KL, Mihalik JP, Mrazik M, Murphy I, Naidu D, Ranapurwala SI, Schneider K, Gildner P, McCrea M, Active Rehab Study Consortium Investigators. Methodology and implementation of a randomized controlled trial (RCT) for early post-concussion rehabilitation: the active rehab study. Front Neurol. 2019;10:1176.
75. Andreassen J, Bach-Nielsen P, Heckscher H, Lindeneg O. Reassurance and short period of bed rest in the treatment of concussion; follow-up and comparison with results in other series treated by prolonged bed rest. Acta Med Scand. 1957;158(3–4):239–48.
76. Griesbach GS, Hovda DA, Molteni R, Wu A, Gomez-Pinilla F. Voluntary exercise following traumatic brain injury: brain-derived neurotrophic factor upregulation and recovery of function. Neuroscience. 2004;125(1):129–39.
77. Griesbach GS, Gomez-Pinilla F, Hovda DA. The upregulation of plasticity-related proteins following TBI is disrupted with acute voluntary exercise. Brain Res. 2004;1016(2):154–62.
78. Moser RS, Glatts C, Schatz P. Efficacy of immediate and delayed cognitive and physical rest for treatment of sports-related concussion. J Pediatr. 2012;161(5):922–6.
79. Moser RS, Schatz P. A case for mental and physical rest in youth sports concussion: It's never too late. Front Neurol. 2012;3:171.
80. Goia GA, Vaughan CG, Reesman J. Characterizing post-concussion exertional effects in the child and adolescent. J Int Neuropsychol Soc. 2010;16:178.
81. Brown NJ, Mannix RC, O'Brien MJ, Gostine D, Collins MW, Meehan WP 3rd. Effect of cognitive activity level on duration of post-concussion symptoms. Pediatrics. 2014;133(2):e299–304.
82. Gibson S, Nigrovic LE, O'Brien M, Meehan WP 3rd. The effect of recommending cognitive rest on recovery from sport-related concussion. Brain Inj. 2013;27(7–8):839–42.
83. Purcell L. What are the most appropriate return-to-play guidelines for concussed child athletes? Br J Sports Med. 2009;43 Suppl 1:i51–5.
84. Grady MF. Concussion in the adolescent athlete. Curr Probl Pediatr Adolesc Health Care. 2010;40(7):154–69.
85. McGrath N. Supporting the student-athlete's return to the classroom after a sport-related concussion. J Athl Train. 2010;45(5):492–8.
86. Master CL, Gioia GA, Leddy JJ, Grady MF. Importance of 'return-to-learn' in pediatric and adolescent concussion. Pediatr Ann. 2012;41(9):1–6.
87. Schneider KH. Cognitive rest: an integrated literature review. J School Nurs. 2016;32(4):234–40.
88. Relander M, Troupp H, Af BG. Controlled trial of treatment for cerebral concussion. Br Med J. 1972;4(5843):777–9.

89. Stubbs B, Vancampfort D, Hallgren M, Firth J, Veronese N, Solmi M, Brand S, Cordes J, Malchow B, Gerber M, Schmitt A, Correll CU, De Hert M, Gaughran F, Schneider F, Kinnafick F, Falkai P, Möller HJ, Kahl KG. EPA guidance on physical activity as a treatment for severe mental illness: a meta-review of the evidence and Position Statement from the European Psychiatric Association (EPA), supported by the International Organization of Physical Therapists in Mental Health (IOPTMH). Eur Psychiatr. 2018;54:124–44.
90. Jahangiri Z, Gholamnezhad Z, Hosseini M. Neuroprotective effects of exercise in rodent models of memory deficit and Alzheimer's. Metab Brain Dis. 2019;34(1):21–37.
91. De la Rosa A, Olaso-Gonzalez G, Arc-Chagnaud C, Millan F, Salvador-Pascual A, García-Lucerga C, Blasco-Lafarga C, Garcia-Dominguez E, Carretero A, Correas AG, Viña J, Gomez-Cabrera MC. Physical exercise in the prevention and treatment of Alzheimer's disease. J Sport Health Sci. 2020;9(5):394–404.
92. Pereira AC, Huddleston DE, Brickman AM, Sosunov AA, Hen R, McKhann GM, Sloan R, Gage FH, Brown TR, Small SA. An in vivo correlate of exercise-induced neurogenesis in the adult dentate gyrus. Proc Natl Acad Sci U S A. 2007;104(13):5638–43.
93. Sharma B, Allison D, Tucker P, Mabbott D, Timmons BW. Cognitive and neural effects of exercise following traumatic brain injury: a systematic review of randomized and controlled clinical trials. Brain Inj. 2020;34(2):149–59.
94. Vivar C, van Praag H. Running changes the brain: the long and the short of it. Physiology (Bethesda, MD.). 2017;32(6):410–24.
95. Baranowski BJ, Marko DM, Fenech RK, Yang A, MacPherson R. Healthy brain, healthy life: a review of diet and exercise interventions to promote brain health and reduce Alzheimer's disease risk. Appl Physiol Nutr Metabol. 2020;45(10):1055–65.
96. Mahalakshmi B, Maurya N, Lee SD, Bharath Kumar V. Possible neuroprotective mechanisms of physical exercise in neurodegeneration. Int J Mol Sci. 2020;21(16):5895.
97. De Kruijk JR, Leffers P, Meerhoff S, Rutten J, Twijnstra A. Effectiveness of bed rest after mild traumatic brain injury: a randomised trial of no versus six days of bed rest. J Neurol Neurosurg Psychiatry. 2002;73(2):167–72. https://doi.org/10.1136/jnnp.73.2.167. PMID: 12122176; PMCID: PMC1737969.
98. McCrea M, Guskiewicz K, Randolph C, Barr WB, Hammeke TA, Marshall SW, Kelly JP. Effects of a symptom-free waiting period on clinical outcome and risk of reinjury after sport-related concussion. Neurosurgery. 2009;65(5):876–83.
99. DiFazio M, Silverberg ND, Kirkwood MW, Bernier R, Iverson GL. Prolonged activity restriction after concussion: are we worsening outcomes? Clin Pediatr. 2016;55(5):443–51.
100. Shen X, Gao B, Wang Z, et al. Therapeutic effect of aerobic exercise for adolescents after MTBI and SRC: a meta-analysis from randomized controlled trials [published online ahead of print, 2020 Sep 30]. World Neurosurg. 2020;S1878–8750(20):32162–8.
101. Thomas DG, Apps JN, Hoffmann RG, McCrea M, Hammeke T. Benefits of strict rest after acute concussion: a randomized controlled trial. Pediatrics. 2015;135(2):213–23.
102. Howell DR, Brilliant AN, Oldham JR, Berkstresser B, Wang F, Meehan WP 3rd. Exercise in the first week following concussion among collegiate athletes: preliminary findings. J Sci Med Sport. 2020;23(2):112–7.
103. Wilson JC, Kirkwood MW, Potter MN, Wilson PE, Provance AJ, Howell DR. Early physical activity and clinical outcomes following pediatric sport-related concussion. J Clin Transl Res. 2020;5(4):161–8.
104. Mychasiuk R, Hehar H, Ma I, Candy S, Esser MJ. Reducing the time interval between concussion and voluntary exercise restores motor impairment, short-term memory, and alterations to gene expression. Eur J Neurosci. 2016;44(7):2407–17.
105. Nishijima T, Torres-Aleman I, Soya H. Exercise and cerebrovascular plasticity. Prog Brain Res. 2016;225:243–68.
106. Ding Y-H, Li J, Zhou Y, Rafols JA, Clark JC, Ding Y. Cerebral angiogenesis and expression of angiogenic factors in aging rats after exercise. Curr Neurovasc Res. 2006;3(1):15–23.

107. Barnes JN, Taylor JL, Kluck BN, Johnson CP, Joyner MJ. Cerebrovascular reactivity is associated with maximal aerobic capacity in healthy older adults. J Appl Physiol (Bethesda, MD: 1985). 2013;114(10):1383–7.
108. Moraine JJ, Lamotte M, Berre J, Niset G, Leduc A, Naeije R. Relationship of middle cerebral artery blood flow velocity to intensity during dynamic exercise in normal subjects. Eur J Appl Physiol Occup Physiol. 1993;67:35–8.
109. Larsen TS, Rasmussen P, Overgaard M, Secher NH, Nielsen HB. Non-selective beta-adrenergic blockade prevents reduction of the cerebral metabolic ratio during exhaustive exercise in humans. J Physiol. 2008;586(11):2807–15.
110. Maugans TA, Farley C, Altaye M, Leach J, Cecil KM. Pediatric sports-related concussion produces cerebral blood flow alterations. Pediatrics. 2012;129(1):28–37.
111. Clausen M, Pendergast DR, Willer B, Leddy J. Cerebral blood flow during treadmill exercise is a marker of physiological postconcussion syndrome in female athletes. J Head Trauma Rehabil. 2016;31(3):215–24.
112. Cotman CW, Berchtold NC. Exercise: a behavioral intervention to enhance brain health and plasticity. Trends Neurosci. 2002;25(6):295–301.
113. Pereira AC, Huddleston DE, Brickman AM, et al. An in vivo correlate of exercise-induced neurogenesis in the adult dentate gyrus. Proc Natl Acad Sci U S A. 2007;104(13):5638–43.
114. Guiney H, Machado L. Benefits of regular aerobic exercise for executive functioning in healthy populations. Psychon Bull Rev. 2013;20(1):73–86.
115. Cassilhas RC, Tufik S, de Mello MT. Physical exercise, neuroplasticity, spatial learning and memory. Cell Mol Life Sci. 2016;73(5):975–83.
116. Tari AR, Norevik CS, Scrimgeour NR, et al. Are the neuroprotective effects of exercise training systemically mediated? Prog Cardiovasc Dis. 2019;62(2):94–101.
117. Cotman CW, Berchtold NC, Christie LA. Exercise builds brain health: key roles of growth factor cascades and inflammation [published correction appears in Trends Neurosci. 2007 Oct;30(10):489]. Trends Neurosci. 2007;30(9):464–72.
118. Markham A, Bains R, Franklin P, Spedding M. Changes in mitochondrial function are pivotal in neurodegenerative and psychiatric disorders: how important is BDNF? Br J Pharmacol. 2014;171(8):2206–29.
119. Puglielli L. Aging of the brain, neurotrophin signaling, and Alzheimer's disease: is IGF1-R the common culprit? Neurobiol Aging. 2008;29(6):795–811.
120. Carro E, Trejo JL, Busiguina S, Torres-Aleman I. Circulating insulin-like growth factor I mediates the protective effects of physical exercise against brain insults of different etiology and anatomy. J Neurosci. 2001;21(15):5678–84.
121. Morland C, Andersson KA, Haugen ØP, et al. Exercise induces cerebral VEGF and angiogenesis via the lactate receptor HCAR1. Nat Commun. 2017;8:15557. Published 2017 May 23. https://doi.org/10.1038/ncomms15557.
122. Quistorff B, Secher NH, Van Lieshout JJ. Lactate fuels the human brain during exercise. FASEB J. 2008;22(10):3443–9. https://doi.org/10.1096/fj.08-10610.
123. Chen T, Qian YZ, Di X, Rice A, Zhu JP, Bullock R. Lactate/glucose dynamics after rat fluid percussion brain injury. J Neurotrauma. 2000;17(2):135–42.
124. Davis JE. Exercises in the medical rehabilitation on mental patients. Occup Ther Rehabil. 1947;26(4):225–30.
125. Siegel EV. Movement therapy as a psychotherapeutic tool. J Am Psychoanal Assoc. 1973;21(2):333–43.
126. Diesfeldt HF, Diesfeldt-Groenendijk H. Improving cognitive performance in psychogeriatric patients: the influence of physical exercise. Age Ageing. 1977;6(1):58–64.
127. Lion LS. Psychological effects of jogging: a preliminary study. Percept Mot Skills. 1978;47(3 Pt 2):1215–8.
128. Blue FR. Aerobic running as a treatment for moderate depression. Percept Mot Skills. 1979;48(1):228.
129. Greist JH, Klein MH, Eischens RR, Faris J, Gurman AS, Morgan WP. Running as treatment for depression. Compr Psychiatry. 1979;20(1):41–54.

130. Brown RS. Exercise and mental health in the pediatric population. Clin Sports Med. 1982;1(3):515–27.
131. Finocchiaro MS, Schmitz CL. Exercise: a holistic approach for the treatment of the adolescent psychiatric patient. Issues Ment Health Nurs. 1984;6(3–4):237–43.
132. Leng M, Liang B, Zhou H, Zhang P, Hu M, Li G, Li F, Chen L. Effects of physical exercise on depressive symptoms in patients with cognitive impairment: a systematic review and meta-analysis. J Nerv Ment Dis. 2018;206(10):809–23.
133. Stubbs B, Vancampfort D, Smith L, Rosenbaum S, Schuch F, Firth J. Physical activity and mental health. Lancet Psychiatry. 2018;5(11):873.
134. Ströhle A. Sports psychiatry: mental health and mental disorders in athletes and exercise treatment of mental disorders. Eur Arch Psychiatry Clin Neurosci. 2019;269(5):485–98.
135. Venkatesh A, Edirappuli SD, Zaman HP, Zaman R. The effect of exercise on mental health: a focus on inflammatory mechanisms. Psychiatr Danub. 2020;32(Suppl 1):105–13.
136. Finkbeiner NW, Max JE, Longman S, Debert C. Knowing what we don't know: long-term psychiatric outcomes following adult concussion in sports. Can J Psychiatry. Revue canadienne de psychiatrie. 2016;61(5):270–6.
137. Manley G, Gardner AJ, Schneider KJ, Guskiewicz KM, Bailes J, Cantu RC, Castellani RJ, Turner M, Jordan BD, Randolph C, Dvořák J, Hayden KA, Tator CH, McCrory P, Iverson GL. A systematic review of potential long-term effects of sport-related concussion. Br J Sports Med. 2017;51(12):969–77.
138. Hutchison MG, Di Battista AP, McCoskey J, Watling SE. Systematic review of mental health measures associated with concussive and subconcussive head trauma in former athletes. Int J Psychophysiol. 2018;132(Pt A):55–61.
139. Rice SM, Parker AG, Rosenbaum S, Bailey A, Mawren D, Purcell R. Sport-related concussion and mental health outcomes in elite athletes: a systematic review. Sports Med (Auckland, NZ). 2018;48(2):447–65.
140. Topolovec-Vranic J, Zhang S, Wong H, Lam E, Jing R, Russell K, Cusimano MD, Canadian Brain Injury and Violence Research Team. Recognizing the symptoms of mental illness following concussions in the sports community: a need for improvement. PLoS One. 2015;10(11):e0141699.
141. Chrisman SP, Richardson LP. Prevalence of diagnosed depression in adolescents with history of concussion. J Adolesc Health. 2014;54(5):582–6.
142. Mac Donald CL, Barber J, Wright J, Coppel D, De Lacy N, Ottinger S, Peck S, Panks C, Sun S, Zalewski K, Temkin N. Longitudinal clinical and neuroimaging evaluation of symptomatic concussion in 10- to 14-year-old youth athletes. J Neurotrauma. 2019;36(2):264–74.
143. Yang MN, Clements-Nolle K, Parrish B, Yang W. Adolescent concussion and mental health outcomes: a population-based study. Am J Health Behav. 2019;43(2):258–65.
144. Wangnoo T, Zavorsky GS, Owen-Smith A. Association between concussions and suicidal behaviors in adolescents. J Neurotrauma. 2020;37(12):1401–7.
145. Kerr ZY, Evenson KR, Rosamond WD, Mihalik JP, Guskiewicz KM, Marshall SW. Association between concussion and mental health in former collegiate athletes. Inj Epidemiol. 2014;1(1):28.
146. Gouttebarge V, Aoki H, Lambert M, Stewart W, Kerkhoffs G. A history of concussions is associated with symptoms of common mental disorders in former male professional athletes across a range of sports. Phys Sportsmed. 2017;45(4):443–9.
147. Kerr ZY, Thomas LC, Simon JE, McCrea M, Guskiewicz KM. Association between history of multiple concussions and health outcomes among former college football players: 15-year follow-up from the NCAA concussion study (1999–2001). Am J Sports Med. 2018;46(7):1733–41.
148. Nybo L, Moller K, Volianitis S, Nielsen B, Secher NH. Effects of hyperthermia on cerebral blood flow and metabolism during prolonged exercise in humans. J Appl Physiol. 2002;93:58–64.
149. Sato K, Oue A, Yoneya M, Sadamoto T, Ogoh S, et al. J Appl Physiol. 2016. First published February 4, 2016;;120:766–73. https://doi.org/10.1152/japplphysiol.00353.2015.

150. Sakurai A, Atkins CM, Alonso OF, Bramlett HM, Dietrich WD. Mild hyperthermia worsens the neuropathological damage associated with mild traumatic brain injury in rats. J Neurotrauma. 2012;29:313–21.
151. Hermstad E, Adams B. Traumatic brain injury complicated by environmental hyperthermia. J Emerg Trauma Shock. 2010;3:66–9.
152. Satoh T, Rezaie T, Seki M, Sunico CR, Tabuchi T, Kitagawa T, Yanagitai M, Senzaki M, Kosegawa C, Taira H, McKercher SR, Hoffman JK, Roth GP, Lipton SA. Dual neuroprotective pathways of a pro-electrophilic compound via HSF-1-activated heat-shock proteins and Nrf2-activated phase 2 antioxidant response enzymes. J Neurochem. 2011;119(3):569–78.
153. Liu AY, Mathur R, Mei N, Langhammer CG, Babiarz B, Firestein BL. Neuroprotective drug riluzole amplifies the heat shock factor 1 (HSF1)- and glutamate transporter 1 (GLT1)-dependent cytoprotective mechanisms for neuronal survival. J Biol Chem. 2011;286(4):2785–94.
154. Yata K, Oikawa S, Sasaki R, Shindo A, Yang R, Murata M, Kanamaru K, Tomimoto H. Astrocytic neuroprotection through induction of cytoprotective molecules; a proteomic analysis of mutant P301S tau-transgenic mouse. Brain Res. 2011;1410:12–23.
155. Hoshino T, Murao N, Namba T, Takehara M, Adachi H, Katsuno M, Sobue G, Matsushima T, Suzuki T, Mizushima T. Suppression of Alzheimer's disease-related phenotypes by expression of heat shock protein 70 in mice. J Neurosci. 2011;31(14):5225–34.
156. Jaber AF, Hartwell J, Radel JD. Interventions to address the needs of adults with Postconcussion syndrome: a systematic review. Am J Occup Therapy. 2019;73(1):7301205020p1–7301205020p12.
157. Chen CL, Lin MY, Huda MH, Tsai PS. Effects of cognitive behavioral therapy for adults with post-concussion syndrome: a systematic review and meta-analysis of randomized controlled trials. J Psychosom Res. 2020;136:110190.
158. Snell DL, Surgenor LJ, Hay-Smith EJ, Siegert RJ. A systematic review of psychological treatments for mild traumatic brain injury: an update on the evidence. J Clin Exp Neuropsychol. 2009;31(1):20–38.
159. Miller LJ, Mittenberg W. Brief cognitive behavioral intervention in mild traumatic brain injury. Appl Neuropsychol. 1998;5(4):172–83.
160. Wade DT, Crawford S, Wenden FJ, King NS, Moss NE. Does routine follow up after head injury help? A randomized controlled trial. J Neurol Neurosurg Psychiatry. 1997;62(5):478–84.
161. Ponsford J, Willmott C, Rothwell A, Cameron P, Kelly AM, et al. Impact of early intervention on outcome following mild head injury in adults. J Neurol Neurosurg Psychiatry. 2002;73:330–2.
162. King NS. Post-concussion syndrome: clarity amid the controversy? Br J Psychiatry. 2003;183:276–8.
163. Potter S, Brown RG. Cognitive behavioural therapy and persistent post-concussional symptoms: integrating conceptual issues and practical aspects in treatment. Neuropsychol Rehabil. 2012;22(1):1–25.
164. Whittaker R, Kemp S, House A. Illness perceptions and outcome in mild head injury: a longitudinal study. J Neurol Neurosurg Psychiatry. 2007;78(6):644–6.
165. McCarty CA, Zatzick D, Stein E, Wang J, Hilt R, Rivara FP, Seattle Sports Concussion Research Collaborative. Collaborative care for adolescents with persistent Postconcussive symptoms: a randomized trial. Pediatrics. 2016;138(4):e20160459.
166. Brent DA, Max J. Psychiatric sequelae of concussions. Curr Psychiatry Rep. 2017;19(12):108.
167. McNally KA, Patrick KE, LaFleur JE, Dykstra JB, Monahan K, Hoskinson KR. Brief cognitive behavioral intervention for children and adolescents with persistent post-concussive symptoms: a pilot study. Child Neuropsychol. 2018;24(3):396–412.
168. Tomfohr-Madsen L, Madsen JW, Bonneville D, Virani S, Plourde V, Barlow KM, Yeates KO, Brooks BL. A pilot randomized controlled trial of cognitive-behavioral therapy for insomnia in adolescents with persistent postconcussion symptoms. J Head Trauma Rehabil. 2020;35(2):E103–12.

169. Gothe NP, Khan I, Hayes J, Erlenbach E, Damoiseaux JS. Yoga effects on brain health: a systematic review of the current literature. Brain Plasticity (Amsterdam, Netherlands). 2019;5(1):105–22.
170. McMillan T, Robertson I, Brock D, Chorlton L. Brief mindfulness training for attentional problems after traumatic brain injury: a randomized control treatment trial. Neuropsychol Rehabil. 2002;12(2):117–25.
171. Bédard M, Felteau M, Mazmanian D, Fedyk K, Klein R, Richardson J, Parkinson W, Minthorn-Biggs MB. Pilot evaluation of a mindfulness-based intervention to improve quality of life among individuals who sustained traumatic brain injuries. Disabil Rehabil. 2003;25(13):722–31.
172. Bédard M, Felteau M, Marshall S, Dubois S, Gibbons C, et al. Mindfulness-based cognitive therapy: benefits in reducing depression following a traumatic brain injury. Adv Mind Body Med. 2012;26(1):14–20.
173. Cole MA, Muir JJ, Gans JJ, Shin LM, D'Esposito M, Harel BT, Schembri A. Simultaneous treatment of neurocognitive and psychiatric symptoms in veterans with post-traumatic stress disorder and history of mild traumatic brain Injury: a pilot study of mindfulness-based stress reduction. Mil Med. 2015;180(9):956–63.
174. Azulay J, Smart CM, Mott T, Cicerone KD. A pilot study examining the effect of mindfulness-based stress reduction on symptoms of chronic mild traumatic brain injury/postconcussive syndrome. J Head Trauma Rehabil. 2013;28(4):323–31.
175. Bay E, Chan RR. Mindfulness-based versus health promotion group therapy after traumatic brain Injury. J Psychosoc Nurs Ment Health Serv. 2019;57(1):26–33.
176. Polich G, Gray S, Tran D, Morales-Quezada L, Glenn M. Comparing focused attention meditation to meditation with mobile neurofeedback for persistent symptoms after mild-moderate traumatic brain injury: a pilot study. Brain Inj. 2020;34(10):1408–15.
177. Paniccia M, Knafo R, Thomas S, Taha T, Ladha A, Thompson L, Reed N. Mindfulness-based yoga for youth with persistent concussion: a pilot study. Am J Occup Therapy. 2019;73(1):7301205040p1–7301205040p11. https://doi.org/10.5014/ajot.2019.027672.

Narrowing the Knowledge Gap Between Basic Neuroscience Research and Management of Concussive Injury

21

Jeffrey Wisinski, James R. Wilkes, and Peter H. Seidenberg

Current Clinical Practice

Diagnosis/Evaluation Procedures

At all levels of collision sports, a concussion evaluation is initiated when an athlete has a direct or indirect forceful impact to the head that is associated with visible signs, athlete reported symptoms, or suspicion of head injury by medical staff (athletic trainer or team physician). Officials from the sport may also report possible concussion to team clinicians, and some sports have implemented education programs aimed at training officials to recognize a possible concussion. If adequately trained medical staff is not present at an event, any suspicion by a coach, official, or observer should result in removal of the athlete from play. There should be no return to sport until an appropriate medical evaluation has taken place by qualified medical staff and the athlete is medically cleared for participation. Concussion may be diagnosed immediately but excluding a diagnosis of concussion may take up to 48 hours following the head contact due to delayed presentation. During this period, serial evaluations should continue with medical staff [1].

The diagnosis of concussion involves assessing the nature of the injury, clinical symptoms, physical signs, behavior, balance, and cognition. This evaluation can take place on the sideline or in the clinic. The initial sideline evaluation involves

---

J. Wisinski
Penn State Health Orthopaedics and Sports Medicine, Penn State Health Family and Community Medicine, University Park, PA, USA

J. R. Wilkes (✉)
Department of Kinesiology, Penn State University, University Park, PA, USA
e-mail: jrw5336@psu.edu

P. H. Seidenberg
Department of Family Medicine, Louisiana State University Health School of Medicine, Shreveport, LA, USA

observing the ABC's (airway, breathing, and circulation) and taking cervical spine precautions. Any athlete with midline cervical spinous process tenderness or neurological symptoms (upper or lower extremity numbness/tingling or weakness) should be considered to have a cervical spine injury until proven otherwise and be appropriately immobilized. During a sideline evaluation, the athlete should be observed for their motion and GCS (Glasgow Coma Scale) score, which is comprised of eye response, motor response, and verbal response. The appearance of the athlete should also be taken into consideration, particularly their balance (i.e., gait, motor coordination, labored movements), response to questions (confusion, disorientation), and overall affect (vacant or blank look). For athletes at the age of 13 or older, Maddock's questions should be asked to assess the athlete's memory including their recollection of the injury and specific questions pertaining to the game or participation. For athletes younger than 13, Maddock's questions should not be asked due to questionable reliability and usefulness in young children [2]. The athlete should be assessed for red flag symptoms, including neck pain, double vision, slurred speech, severe or increasing headache, loss of consciousness, seizure or convulsion, focal neurologic deficit, repeated vomiting, deteriorating conscious state, and agitation. The presence of these red flag symptoms warrants emergent neuroimaging.

Based on this initial assessment, if there is concern for concussion, the athlete should be immediately removed from competition and undergo thorough examination in a private area that is distraction free. The 5th edition of the Standardized Concussion Assessment Tool (SCAT-5) has been utilized to evaluate athletes for possible concussion. It is a consensus-based instrument validated for use on the sidelines in athletes of ages 13 and over [3]. The Child SCAT-5 is used for evaluating children of ages 12 and younger, and its format is consistent with the format of the SCAT-5 [2].

Links to the SCAT-5 and Child SCAT-5 are as follows:

- SCAT-5: https://bjsm.bmj.com/content/bjsports/early/2017/04/26/bjsports-2017-097506SCAT5.full.pdf
- Child SCAT-5: https://d2cx26qpfwuhvu.cloudfront.net/wru/wp-content/uploads/2019/03/05114400/SCAT5_Child.pdf

The SCAT-5 lists 22 separate symptoms that each athlete is asked to rate on a scale of 0 (nothing) to 6 (severe). This provides a total number of symptoms (out of 22) as well as symptom severity score (addition of all the scaled numbers throughout the 22 separate symptoms). The athlete is then asked about prior history of concussion(s) including date and the recovery course for the concussion(s). They are also asked about prior history of attention deficit disorder (ADD)/attention deficit hyperactivity disorder (ADHD), learning disability/dyslexia, headache disorder or migraine, depression, anxiety, and other psychiatric disorders. The athlete is then screened for cognitive function via the Standardized Assessment of Concussion (SAC) with tests for orientation, immediate memory, and concentration. To assess concentration in the SCAT-5, each athlete is asked to read the months in reverse order as well as a list of digits backward. There are four different lists of digits that the athlete is asked to repeat. Delayed memory is measured after the physical examination takes place, as the athlete is asked to repeat a list of words that was provided to them as part of the test for immediate memory. The SCAT-5 offers additional 10-word lists for immediate and delayed memory as well as longer digital backward sequencing. This minimizes the ceiling effect that was a previous limitation of the SCAT-3; however, no studies have shown increased sensitivity or specificity for diagnosis of sport-related concussion (SRC) with the SCAT-5 over prior versions [4].

The Child SCAT-5 contains a symptom evaluation section that includes a child report and parent report. It is recommended to be completed with the athlete in a resting state. For the child report, a list of 21 separate symptoms is included and the athlete is asked to rate each symptom on a scale of 0 (nothing) to 3 (severe). This provides a total number of symptoms (out of 21) and symptom severity score (addition of all the scaled numbers throughout the 21 separate symptoms). At the end of the child report, the athlete is then asked to rate how they feel on a scale of 0 (very bad) to 10 (very good). For the parent report, the parent is asked to rate the same symptoms of the athlete on a scale of 0 to 3. The same total number of symptoms and symptom severity score are reported, based on the parent's response. The parent is then asked to rate their child on a scale of 0 to 100%. The child is then screened for cognitive function via Standardized Assessment of Concussion – Child Version (SAC-C) with tests for immediate memory and concentration. Orientation is not included due to its doubtful usefulness in young children. To assess concentration in the Child SCAT-5, each athlete is asked to read the days of the week in reverse order and a list of digits backward. There are five different lists of digits that the athlete is asked to repeat. Delayed memory is measured after the physical examination, as the child is asked to repeat a list of words that was provided to them in the test for immediate memory. Five minutes must pass between the assessments of immediate memory and delayed memory [2].

The physical examination component starts with a neck examination, which consists of inspection of the neck and scalp. This is done to ensure there are no red flag signs that would be concerning for a skull fracture, which would prompt further imaging. At this point, the athlete should have already received palpation of the cervical spine to rule out midline spinous process tenderness and step off deformities, but a more thorough palpation examination can take place to find areas of tenderness within the cervical paraspinal musculature. Active ranges of motion with cervical rotation, side-bending, and flexion/extension are then assessed. Identifying areas of tenderness and monitoring range of motion can help with the rehabilitation and treatment process as an athlete recovers from concussion. Special tests are performed, which include the Hoffman test (tapping the nail of the third or fourth finger and observing for involuntary flexing of the thumb and index finger) to rule out an upper motor neuron lesion, and the Spurling compression test (passively extending the athlete's head and turning to the affected side while providing downward pressure and observing for recreation of radiating upper extremity pain or numbness/tingling) to rule out cervical radiculopathy.

The neurological examination then takes place to rule out signs of focal neurologic deficits. First is assessment of the cranial nerves (two through 12) followed by cerebellum testing, which consists of pronator drift, finger to nose testing, and tandem gait. Next, strength, sensation, and reflexes of the upper extremities are evaluated. The biceps reflex, brachioradialis reflex, and triceps reflex are assessed, followed by strength with shoulder abduction, elbow flexion/extension, wrist flexion/extension, supination/pronation, thumb extension, thumb abduction, pincer grasp, and finger abduction. Sensation is assessed over the cervical spine and thoracic spine nerve root distributions. This is followed by the assessment of strength, sensation, and reflexes of the lower extremities. Hip flexion/extension, hip adduction/adduction, hip internal/external rotation, knee flexion/extension, plantarflexion/dorsiflexion, ankle internal/external rotation, and ankle inversion/eversion strength are measured, followed by assessment of the dermatomal distribution of L1 to S1. The patellar and Achilles reflexes are also checked, in addition to Babinski reflex (stroking the lateral aspect of the sole of the athlete's foot with thumbnail or another sharp object and observing for the great toe dorsiflexing and the other toes fanning out), which is evaluated to rule out an upper motor neuron lesion.

Up to 30% of concussed athletes report visual impairments during the first week after initial injury. Dizziness may represent an underlying impairment of the oculomotor and/or vestibular systems. It is reported in approximately 50% of concussed athletes during their recovery timeline and is associated with a 6.4 times greater risk of predicting recovery beyond 21 days [5]. Thus, vestibular/oculomotor screening (VOMS) is clinically assessed with a careful monitoring of symptoms and eye movement abnormalities. Provoking two or more total symptoms after any VOMS item has a high rate (96%) of identifying concussion [5]. VOMS has also demonstrated internal consistency (Cronbach's alpha = 0.92) in identifying patients with concussion [5]. Furthermore, components of the VOMS may also serve as a prognostic indicator of recovery time in SRC [6].

Initially, VOMS begins with the assessment of vertical and horizontal eye smooth pursuits. The athlete is asked to follow a slowly moving target horizontally to the left and right of the athlete's midline and vertically above and below the midline. While doing this, the examiner is observing the athlete's eye movement for any signs of saccadic eye movement (quick simultaneous movement of both eyes between two or more phases of fixation) or nystagmus (uncontrolled repetitive movements of the eyes, otherwise known as "dancing eyes") (Fig. 21.1). The examiner also asks if this test reproduces dizziness, headache, nausea, or fogginess, and if so, to rate it on a scale of 0–6. This is compared to the athlete's baseline symptom severity score that was reported earlier in the SCAT-5 [5].

Horizontal and vertical saccades are then assessed to test the ability of the eyes to move quickly between targets. Horizontal saccades' assessment involves the examiner holding their fingertips approximately 1.5 feet to the right and left of the athlete's midline. Vertical saccades' assessment involves the examiner holding their fingertips approximately 1.5 feet above and below the athlete's midline. The athlete is instructed to move their eyes as quickly as possible from point to point (first horizontally and then vertically) without moving their head. Again, the examiner is

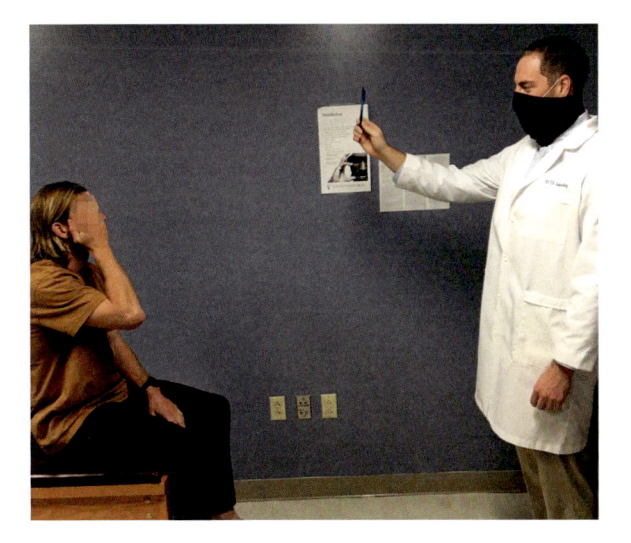

Fig. 21.1 Clinical eye examination as a part of VOMS

observing the athlete's eye movement for saccadic eye movement or nystagmus while monitoring for dizziness, headache, nausea, or fogginess [5].

Vestibular-ocular reflex (VOR) testing is then performed as a means of assessing the ability to stabilize vision as the head moves. The athlete is asked to fully extend their elbow and flex their shoulder to 90 degrees, with their thumb extended in a superior position (thumbs up). The shoulder is adducted, so that the thumb fingertip is midline and at eye level. The horizontal VOR is assessed by asking the athlete to maintain focus on their thumb fingertip while rotating their cervical spine approximately 20 degrees to each side. Ten repetitions are performed, with one repetition consisting of the head moving back and forth to the starting position. The vertical VOR is assessed by holding the thumb fingertip in the same position and asking the athlete to flex and extend the cervical spine 20 degrees while maintaining focus on their thumb. Ten repetitions are again performed, with one repetition consisting of the head moving up and down to the starting position. With both the vertical and horizontal VOR, the examiner is again observing the athlete's eye movement for saccades or nystagmus, while monitoring for dizziness, headache, nausea, or fogginess [5].

Visual motion sensitivity (VMS) testing is performed to assess visual motion sensitivity itself and the ability to inhibit vestibular-induced eye movements using vision. The athlete is asked to stand shoulder width apart, with the examiner standing next to and behind the athlete. The athlete places their thumbs together in front of their eyes with each thumb in the same position done in the VOR testing. While maintaining focus on their thumbs, the athlete rotates their eyes, trunk, and thumbs approximately 80 degrees to the left and right. Five repetitions are performed with one repetition consisting of the trunk moving back and forth to the starting position [5].

Convergence assesses the ability of the athlete to view a near target without double vision. The athlete is seated and wearing corrective lenses only if needed.

The athlete focuses on the examiner's finger, which begins at an arm's length away from the patient. The examiner's finger is then brought toward the tip of the athlete's nose and, throughout this movement, the athlete maintains focus on the examiner's finger. The athlete is advised to inform the examiner when they begin having double vision or seeing two of the examiner's fingers. The examiner also observes for outward deviation of either eye. When this point is reached, the location of this point is measured to the tip of the athlete's nose. This can be repeated three separate times, so that an average length can be recorded [5]. Normal near point convergence (NPC) is considered less than or equal to 5 cm [7]. Although the sensitivity and specificity of NPC as a single measure is unclear, the NPC measurement of greater than 5 cm has a high rate (84%) of identifying concussions [1].

In a study involving youth and adolescent athletes, symptom provocation and eye movement abnormalities in horizontal/vertical smooth pursuits, horizontal/vertical saccades, and VOR testing were associated with delayed recovery from SRC. The reproduction of symptoms and eye movement abnormalities during NPC testing was not associated with delayed recovery in this study [6]. However, a separate systematic review revealed that concussed athletes display impaired NPC acutely, and there is moderate-level evidence that athletes can display impaired NPC for several months postconcussion [8].

The last portion of the physical examination involves the assessment of balance. The Modified Balance Error Scoring System (mBESS) has been validated as part of the assessment of SRC, and it relies on the clinical judgment and observation of the examiner. There are three separate stances (double leg, single leg, and tandem stance) that the athletes maintain for 20 seconds each while standing on a firm surface with eyes closed and hands on their hips. Throughout the 20 seconds, the examiner observes for negative events, which include foot lifting, stepping, falling, removing hands from hips, eye opening, and failing to return to test position for less than 5 seconds. Each occurrence of a negative event is defined as an error and each error is marked as one point that is subtracted from the final score. For the SCAT-5, each stance has a maximum of 10 points, which makes the total maximum mBESS score 30 [4]. For the Child SCAT-5, athletes of ages 10–12 are graded using the same scoring system, but athletes of ages 5–9 are graded with a maximum score of 20. Only the double leg and tandem stances are assessed for the ages of 5–9 [2]. Clinical judgment serves as the gold standard for diagnosing concussion [9], as definitive data are lacking regarding absolute mBESS scores that reliably rule out or rule in concussion [10]. mBESS can also vary throughout a season independent of the concussion status, as it can be affected by environment, fatigue, and lower extremity injuries [5, 7, 10].

Based on the athlete's response to the SCAT-5/Child SCAT-5 and their physical examination findings, the final determination of SRC is made. If an official diagnosis of concussion is not made but there is ongoing clinical concern, the athlete should be held out of participation and undergo serial evaluations for up to 48 hours, due to the possibility of a delayed symptom onset. If an official diagnosis is made, the athlete should not be left alone after the injury and serial monitoring for deterioration should continue over the initial few hours. Monitoring should continue at regular intervals, until the athlete has reached full return to participation (RTP).

An initial evaluation that takes place in the office or subacute setting involves obtaining a comprehensive history, including the mechanism of injury, symptom trajectory, and sleep/wake disturbance. A detailed neurological examination should involve the assessment of gait, balance, neurocognitive function, and a complete cervical spine evaluation. Vestibular and ocular function should also be assessed by using the VOMS tool, VMS, and NPC. Symptom checklists should be used to track symptom trajectory, as the utility of sideline balance and neurocognitive assessments to identify concussion decreases within 3 days after the injury [11]. If computerized neurocognitive testing was performed after the injury, it should be repeated. Making the diagnosis of SRC involves the presence of a clear mechanism of injury along with signs, symptoms, and time course of concussion. In an athlete who has ongoing symptoms during the first clinical evaluation, there should be a focus on excluding other pathologies such as headache/migraine disorder, mood disorder, cervicogenic pain, and peripheral vestibular conditions. There should also be a screening for psychosocial or mental health disorders. These pathologies may be causing the athletes' current symptoms or indicate previous pathology that has been worsened by the presence of concussion [4]. If an athlete is diagnosed with SRC, anticipatory guidance should be provided. It is not atypical for signs, symptoms, and testing to normalize by the time that an office visit takes place [12]. In this case, the visit should focus on establishing a plan for safe return to school and sport.

Return to Participation (RTP) Protocols

The process of return to participation (RTP) is completed with a stepwise progression. After a brief period of initial rest following the injury (approximately 24–48 hours), athletes can be encouraged to become gradually more active while staying below a symptom-reproducing threshold. Preliminary data suggest that early subthreshold aerobic exercise prescribed to symptomatic adolescent males within 1 week of SRC has the potential to prevent delayed recovery and may also accelerate the overall recovery [13]. There are approximately six stages of the RTP protocol:

- *Stage 1*: goal is for the athlete to undergo symptom limited activity, which includes a gradual reintroduction of school and work-related activities.
- *Stage 2*: light aerobic exercise that is done at submaximal exertion with the goal of increasing heart rate. No resistance exercises should be incorporated at this time. Examples of light aerobic activity include walking or stationary bike for no more than 10 minutes at an intensity of 70–80 revolutions per minute (RPM).
- *Stage 3*: may not begin until the athlete is asymptomatic. Sport-specific activity such as skating in ice hockey and running in soccer or football with the goal of adding movement. There is no head impact activity or resistance training permitted.

- *Stage 4*: athlete is permitted to do progressive resistance training. The athlete may also participate in noncontact training drills such as passing drills in ice hockey or football. The goal of this stage is to promote exercise while increasing coordination and thinking.
- *Stage 5*: athlete is permitted to do supervised full contact training, with the goal of restoring confidence and providing a means for coaching staff to assess functional skills. During this full contact training, the athlete is permitted to do all normal training activities.
- *Stage 6*: Return to full participation and normal game play.

For each stage of the protocol, there should be at least 24 hours between the steps in progression. If at any stage the symptoms worsen during the physical activity, the athlete should return to the previous stage. The athlete may then attempt to progress only if symptom free for a 24-hour period at the lower stage. Using this protocol, it takes an athlete a minimum of 1 week to return to full participation once asymptomatic at rest. Athletes who continue to suffer persistent symptoms and inactivity may take longer than 24 hours with each stage due to limitations in physical conditioning [14].

Return to Learn Protocols

Return to learn (RTL) is an important portion of concussion management and there is no standardized protocol of school accommodations that can be provided to teachers, professors, and school administrators. The 2017 Berlin Concussion in Sport Group Consensus Statement recommends that athletes "should not return to sport until they have successfully returned to school" [14]. Currently, students are provided with a list of school accommodations from their physician that can be given to school administrators and disseminated to all teachers and professors. Part of facilitating communication and transition back to school involves obtaining consent between medical and school teams. Accommodations are given with instructions to incorporate as necessary. These depend on the athlete's course of symptoms, academic demands, and preexisting medical conditions (learning disability, mood disorder, or ADHD). The accommodations include the following:

- Extended time on exams/quizzes
- Permission to record lectures/note-taking assistance
- Exams/quizzes in a quiet location
- Absence from class due to scheduled rest periods
- Limit to one exam per day
- Limit the use of electronic screen or adjust screen settings
- Allow the use of headphones or ear plugs to reduce noise sensitivity
- Allow sunglasses or hats to reduce light sensitivity
- Frequent breaks from class, if symptomatic
- Due dates/assignment extensions

- Late arrival or need to leave, prior to the end of class (to avoid crowded hallways)
- Avoid busy, loud, or crowded environments (hallways, lunchroom, assemblies, music room)
- Use of a reader for exams/quizzes
- Defer exams/quizzes

Many athletes recover quickly enough to return to the classroom with no or brief adjustment of academic activities. Schools should be prepared to provide additional support in case recovery takes longer. Athletes who suffer from persistent symptoms should be given an individualized RTL plan that allows for symptom limited activity.

Referral and Management

Multiple symptoms can result from SRC, particularly related to the cervical spine and vestibular system. Most athletes who suffer SRC recover within 10–14 days. However, persistent symptoms are defined as greater than 4 weeks in children and greater than 10–14 days in adults [14]. Prolonged symptoms may result from a primary persistent change in brain function or represent confounding processes, including headache syndromes, depression, and/or oculomotor or vestibular dysfunctions that do not necessarily reflect an ongoing physiological injury to the brain. Psychiatric comorbidities particularly indicate the risk of persistent concussion symptoms and may increase the magnitude of symptoms reported.

Athletes who experience symptoms that are considered persistent or have impairments on physical examination related to the injury may benefit from specific rehabilitation programs. For athletes who have persistent symptoms associated with physical deconditioning or autonomic instability, an individualized symptom limited aerobic exercise program should be instituted. The Buffalo Concussion Treadmill Test (BCTT) is a standardized graded aerobic exercise test that can reliably detect physiological dysfunction in athletes with persistent postconcussive symptoms and quantify exercise capacity to guide treatment [15].

Tilt table testing can also be used to identify autonomic dysfunction in athletes with persistent lightheadedness or vertigo [16]. However, its utilization in the clinical setting is unclear, as there are other simple measures such as orthostatic intolerance or heart rate variability that can be used [17].

There has been evidence of demonstrated benefit with targeted multifaceted physical therapy programs, particularly in patients with cervical spine and/or vestibular causes of symptoms [18]. Athletes with persistent mood or behavioral symptoms should be referred for cognitive behavioral therapy (CBT). A mixed SRC and non-SRC adolescent cohort provided preliminary support for the role of CBT in the management of persistent postconcussive symptoms [17].

Despite widespread use, there is currently no compelling evidence to support the use of pharmacotherapy such as amantadine or peripheral nerve blocks in the treatment of persistent postconcussion symptoms. However, a retrospective study demonstrated that amitriptyline was an effective treatment and was tolerated well in patients with posttraumatic headaches. In this study, female patients were more likely to report posttraumatic headaches, and amitriptyline was found to reduce headache symptoms in 82% of patients [19].

There is evidence that some nutraceuticals may protect or reduce recovery time from concussion in animal models. Vitamin D, omega 3 fatty acids, certain B vitamins, progesterone, and N-methyl-D-aspartate (NMDA) have been investigated. However, there has been no human evidence to show reduced recovery time or protective effect with these agents [4]. Enzogenol®, an antioxidant extracted from the bark of *Pinus radiata* trees, has shown promise as a nutraceutical in the treatment of postconcussion symptoms. Specifically, those individuals who underwent a 6-week Enzogenol supplementation reported reduced mental and physical fatigue and these reports were supported by reduced mental fatigue measures on electroencephalograph (EEG) [20]. If pharmacotherapy or nutraceuticals are begun during the management of SRC, a decision should be made regarding return to play while an athlete is still taking the medication by the treating physician. This is particularly important because the medication may be masking or modifying certain SRC symptoms [17, 18].

Screening neuropsychological testing is often used in the acute setting, and a formal neuropsychological assessment is used when an athlete suffers from persistent symptoms. Paper-and-pencil neuropsychological testing has been used with a variety of test batteries that measure multiple aspects of memory (new learning), cognitive processing speed, working memory, attention, and executive functions. Although the validity of the tests has been well documented, most studies have not demonstrated that paper-and-pencil neuropsychological tests can detect concussion once players are asymptomatic [21]. The tests are extensive and thorough but have increased the cost of administration and interpretation. They are also not ideal for serial use, as a great amount of time is required by the athlete and neuropsychologist. Computerized neuropsychological testing is efficient in the sports medicine setting and useful for serial testing. There are five computerized neuropsychological tests that are available for evaluation of sport-related concussions: Immediate Post-Concussion Assessment and Cognitive Testing (ImPACT), Automated Neuropsychological Assessment Metrics (ANAM), CogSport/Axon Sports Computerized Cognitive Assessment (CCAT), and Headminder Concussion Resolution Index (CRI).

ImPACT is a computerized neuropsychological test that was developed to assess symptoms in addition to cognitive domains such as attention span, working memory, response variability, nonverbal problem-solving, reaction time, and sustained and selective attention. Composite scores are calculated for visual memory, verbal memory, reaction time, impulse control, and processing speed. While it is widely used for baseline testing and in the assessment and management phases of concussion, there are limitations. There is varying test-retest reliability, which can be influenced by the athlete's testing environment and level of academic achievement [22]. Other factors that also influence the testing include gender, level of alertness, effort, and prior testing [23]. In general, testing should not be repeated multiple times in a short time span.

ANAM was developed for serial testing and precise management of cognitive function in the US military. However, a sports medicine battery evolved and includes the assessment of concentration (code substitution and continuous performance test), attention (continuous performance test), mental processing (code substitution-delayed), mental processing speed and efficiency (mathematical processing), reaction time (simple reaction time), and visual memory (match to sample). Several studies have shown that ANAM has consistent correlations with traditional neuropsychological tests, which suggest adequate concurrent validity [21, 24, 25].

The CogSport Axon Sports CCAT is designed to keep the athlete motivated by being brief. It focuses on the speed and accuracy to detect changes in cognitive measures. The four included tests are processing speed task, learning task, working memory task, and attention task. The test developer recommends baseline testing be performed once a year or before each contact sport season. The developer also recommends using this test more often if an athlete sustains a concussion or is going through a period of maturation. This test has been shown to have clinical utility and sensitivity, as 70.8% of concussed patients in a cohort study showed a decline from baseline in one or more tests while symptomatic [17, 26].

The Headminder CRI is composed of six subtests to measure visual recognition, speed of information processing, and reaction time. The subtests include the reaction time subtest, cued reaction time subtest, animal decoding subtest, visual recognition 1, visual recognition 2, and symbol scanning. This has been shown to have a sensitivity of 78.6% for detecting concussion at 24 hours, compared to 68% for self-reported symptoms and 43% for paper-and-pencil tests [27].

Computerized neuropsychological test results should be interpreted by the treating clinician and serve as a single component of concussion management in addition to the athlete's entire clinical presentation [11]. Formal neuropsychological testing can identify persistent brain function deficits in athletes following SRC and can impact the determination of limitations and cognitive capacity with schoolwork. However, there are limited data on the utility of formal testing with athletes who suffer from persistent symptoms and further studies are needed [4]. Overall, athletes with persistent symptoms should be managed in a multidisciplinary setting by healthcare providers (primary care sports medicine neurology, neuropsychology, psychiatry, rehabilitation medicine) with experience in SRC [17, 26].

Other measures have evolved as potentially useful tools; however, they are largely still used in research settings. Virtual reality (VR) has also recently gained attention as a possible neurological assessment tool to detect deficits in balance, spatial memory, immediate memory, delayed recall, and reaction time (Fig. 21.2). The conceptual origins of neurological behavior testing arose in response to behavioral and neurocognitive dysfunction seen in war veterans by Luria, and has since been developed with advances in technology as a way to score and monitor deficits [28]. While this modality proves to have potential in diagnosing concussion and identifying specific deficits, it has only been used in research and has not yet been standardized for clinical use.

Fig. 21.2 Example of a virtual reality setup

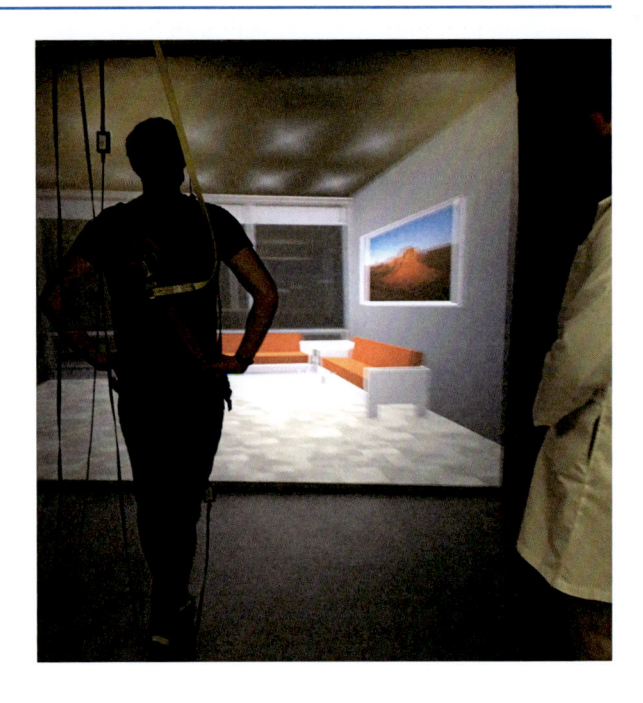

The role of biomarkers (saliva, cerebrospinal fluid, blood) in the diagnosis of concussion is under active investigation, given their potential for predicting the pathophysiology and neurobiological recovery. The overall evidence of using fluid biomarkers for diagnosis of SRC is low, as more research is needed to determine their clinical utility. There is also currently no evidence to support genetic testing as a tool for the evaluation and management of athletes with SRC [29].

Structural imaging techniques, such as magnetic resonance imaging (MRI) or computed tomography (CT), have limited value in athletes with persistent postconcussive symptoms. However, advanced imaging techniques, such as quantitative EEG, magnetic resonance spectroscopy (MRS), diffusion tensor imaging (DTI), and functional MRI (fMRI), have shown changes in brain activation patterns in athletes with persistent symptoms. These findings are shown, even after the athlete has returned to sport and recovered clinically. However, the clinical significance of these findings is yet to be determined. Thus, the use of advanced neuroimaging in the research setting should continue to be encouraged to provide further understanding about the etiology of persistent symptoms [17, 26].

Long-Term Follow-Up/Assessment

Studies pertaining to the long-term consequences of exposure to recurrent head trauma are inconsistent. There is much to learn about the possible cause and effect relationship between repetitive head trauma and concussions. Subconcussive head impacts, which are defined as transfers of mechanical energy to the brain causing axonal or neuronal damage in the absence of clinical signs or symptoms, have been associated with neurologic disorders including chronic traumatic encephalopathy (CTE). CTE is a distinct tauopathy with an unknown incidence in athletic populations. There has been no concrete relationship demonstrated between CTE and SRC or exposure to contact sports. More research is needed to understand the prevalence, incidence, risk factors, protective factors, and clinical diagnostic criteria as well as the extent of neuropathological progression [14].

The short- and long-term effects of repetitive head impacts cannot be characterized using current technology. Future research will focus on developing technologies that can assess any brain changes after repetitive asymptomatic head trauma [4]. Although current impact sensors indirectly monitor linear and angular acceleration forces to the head, they may not consistently record forces transmitted to the brain. Current impact measures are a poor predictor of SRC, as some athletes experience no symptoms with high forces and others suffer a concussion with lower impact forces [30]. Thus, impact monitors are currently only a research tool and require additional study.

A prior history of SRC, participation in collision sport, and being female are considered risk factors for SRC. History of multiple SRCs is associated with more emotional, cognitive, and physical symptoms, prior to participation in a season. Currently, the most consistent predictors of slower recovery from SRC are the initial severity and number of symptoms within the first few days of the injury. Having a low level of symptoms on the first day after the injury is a positive prognostic indicator [14]. For most injured athletes, symptoms improve rapidly during the first 2 weeks after injury. Recent studies have reported longer recovery times, but this may have been influenced by ascertainment bias as well as increased adoption of graduated RTP protocols [14].

According to the 2017 Concussion in Sport Group (CISG) consensus statement, it is reasonable to say that clinical recovery takes place within the first month of injury for most athletes. Children, adolescents, and young adults with a pre-injury history of migraine headaches or mental health disorders are at risk of suffering from symptoms for more than 1 month, while those with history of ADHD or learning disability are not. However, athletes with history of ADHD may need different planning and intervention strategies when returning to school. One concern is the fact that neurobiological recovery may extend beyond 1 month in some athletes [14]. Recent studies have suggested that physiological recovery could exceed the time of clinical recovery, which could lead to an athlete returning to play while still having ongoing brain dysfunction. This highlights a significant challenge to the clinician, who needs to be mindful of the potential risks of returning athletes to sport too early. It also brings and highlights some limitations with current clinical practice.

Issues and Drawbacks from Current Practice

Rule changes have taken place in the sports of ice hockey and American football with efforts to reduce SRC. The Ice Hockey Summit III recently provided updates regarding SRC in ice hockey and discussion on rule changes. In June 2011, USA Hockey approved a rule that banned body checking in youth hockey until the bantam level (ages 13–14). Subsequently in September 2013, Hockey Canada also announced a body checking ban in the peewee youth hockey (ages 11–12). Implementing these bans in the USA and Canada has reduced the incidence of SRC in peewee hockey by 67% [31]. The American Academy of Pediatrics (AAP) has also recommended restricting body checking in boys' youth ice hockey to the highest competition levels (Tier 1, Tier 2, AA, AAA), starting no earlier than 15 years of age. Furthermore, the AAP has recommended reinforcement of boys' youth ice hockey rules to prevent body contact from behind (especially into or near the boards), strict enforcement of zero-tolerance rules against any contact to the head, and a continued emphasis on coaching education to prevent body contact from behind [32].

In American football, kickoff rule changes at the collegiate and professional level have taken place recently. At the collegiate level before the 2012 season, kickoffs were moved from the 30-yard line to the 35. The starting position of the team receiving a touchback was also moved from the 20-yard line to the 25. In 2016, the Ivy League passed a conference-specific rule change that moved the kickoff line from the 35-yard line to the 40. With this rule, the team who received a touchback would start from the 20-yard line, instead of the 25. The intent of this rule was to have more kickoffs land in the end zone and reduce the likelihood of the receiving player in advancing the ball. However, there was a possibility that the movement of the touchback line would lead receivers to try and advance the ball, even when kicked into the end zone. A before-after study took place that examined the annual concussion rates before and after this rule, change was implemented. The mean annual concussion rate per 1000 kickoff plays was 10.93, prior to the rule change and 2.04 after. Although results of this study may not be generalized beyond the Ivy League, it does provide insight for further consideration of kickoff rule changes in all collegiate conferences [33].

The National Football League (NFL) also moved the kickoff line from the 30-yard line to the 35 in 2011. In 2018, further kickoff rule changes included multiple changes for blocking and line-up locations for the kicking and receiving teams (Fig. 21.3). These current rule changes are still in effect and include the following:

- The kickoff team must have five players on each side of the ball and cannot line up more than one yard from where the ball is kicked.
- On each side of the ball, at least two of the players must be lined up outside the yard line number and at least two players between the yard line number and inbound lines.
- For the receiving team, eight players must be lined up in the 15-yard setup zone (15 yards away from where the ball is kicked) and three players are permitted outside this setup zone.
- Double team blocking can only be performed by members of the receiving team located in the setup zone at the time of kick.
- Wedge blocks (two or more players intentionally aligning shoulder-to-shoulder within two yards of each other, and who move forward together with the purpose of blocking for the runner) are not allowed.

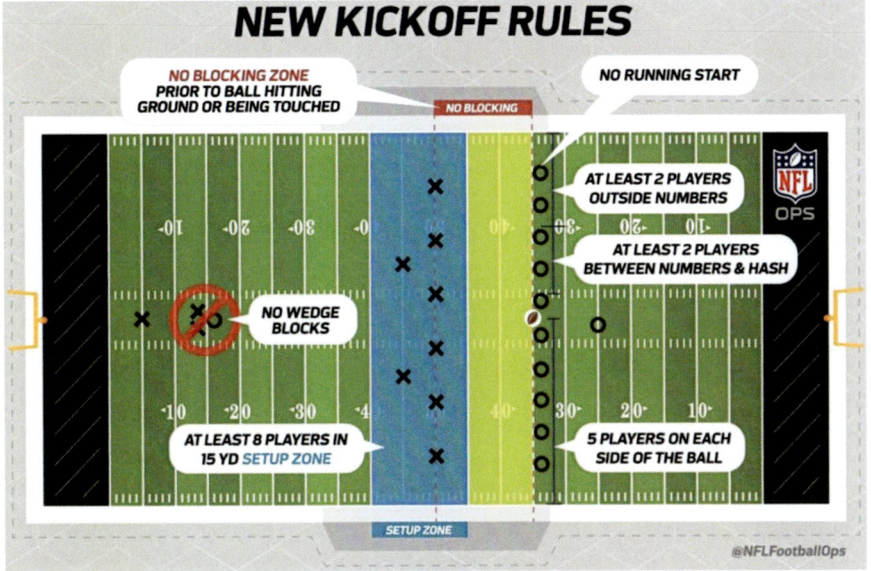

Fig. 21.3 Diagram of NFL kickoff rules

- No player from the kicking or receiving team can block within the 15-yard area from the kicking team's restraining line, until the ball is touched or hits the ground.
- A touchback is called if the ball is not touched by the receiving team but touches the ground in the end zone.

A major limitation with current clinical practice includes inconsistencies with symptom reporting in athletes who suffer SRC. At the high school level, access to athletic trainers can vary, and athletes without access to athletic trainers tend to have lower knowledge of SRC symptoms. Furthermore, these athletes may report their symptoms to a head coach, which is different to reporting to a medical professional. It has also been found that increased knowledge does not necessarily lead to increased reporting behaviors. Many athletes fear that coaches will remove them from a starting position if they report symptoms. Other reasons for not reporting symptoms include not wanting to lose playing time, fear of letting their team down, and feeling that an injury is not serious enough to require medical attention [34].

At the collegiate level, many athletes have a basic understanding of SRC but still fail to identify all the signs and symptoms. Many athletes also continue participating in practices and games after sustaining a possible injury, which suggests a potential lack of understanding of the consequences of SRC. Both female and male athletes have had decreased reporting of symptoms due to not knowing if an injury was a SRC or not believing SRC to be serious [35]. Male athletes have been shown to report less symptoms in comparison to female athletes. Reasons for this discrepancy include not wanting to let their team down in addition to male athlete identity, stigmas, and perceived perceptions of coaches and teammates [35].

Previous experience with concussion (i.e., a greater number of previous concussions) has been shown to negatively impact athlete disclosure of and attitude toward concussion. This may stem from prior experience of being removed from play or from the way that previous concussions were managed. Attitudes may also be driven from perceptions of social, school, or team environment norms. Thus, addressing negative attitudes to concussion may help in improving disclosure in young athletes [36].

Policy changes that have taken place to reduce the health impact of SRC include prevention, education, and rule change programs. The Centers for Disease Control and Prevention (CDC) Heads Up (HU) program was introduced as an educational outreach program, with the goal of improving player safety for youth and high school players (Fig. 21.4) [37]. As part of this program, coaches are trained and certified on safety fundamentals, including proper tackling techniques, ensuring appropriate equipment fitting, and teaching others involved in football (other coaches, players, and parents) on how to recognize and respond to injuries. Additionally, parents, officials, and other athletes have access to the CDC's HU program to protect athletes from concussion or serious brain injury by learning how to spot a concussion and knowing what to do if a concussion takes place. In May 2009, the state of Washington passed the "Zackery Lystedt Law" to address concussion management in athletes, and this was the first state law to require a "removal and clearance to return to play" among youth athletes. According to the Centers for Disease Control and Prevention (CDC), all 50 states now have a return to play law.

A prospective cohort study that took place during the 2015–2016 high school football season evaluated the impact of the HU program on SRC incidence. The SRC incidence of 14 high school teams with one coach who underwent training in the HU program (HU programs) was compared to 10 control teams who did not have training in the HU program (non-HU programs). The HU programs demonstrated a 33% lower concussion rate and 27% faster return to participation in comparison to the non-HU programs. However, limitations of this study were the nonrandomized assignment to each group and the fact that team sizes in the non-HU programs were smaller than the HU programs. Exact game exposures were also not available and specific SRC game incidence rates could not be created [38]. Larger studies with equal sample sizes over longer periods of time are needed to provide more data on the impact of HU programs with SRC incidence.

Despite access to the CDC's HU program, not all collegiate coaches receive basic training regarding SRC. In a cross-sectional online survey, two-thirds of US collegiate coaches reported receiving instructional material about concussion from their respective institutions. The material typically contained information about symptoms and proper management of concussion. This survey also contained a test that assessed the overall general knowledge regarding SRC of the coaches. Female coaches of noncontact or collision teams more frequently answered correctly in comparison to male coaches of male contact or collision teams [39]. This is concerning but not surprising as qualitative evidence has shown that in Division I football programs (all of which are coached by men), competitive pressures can lead to a conflict of interest in the care of concussed athletes [40].

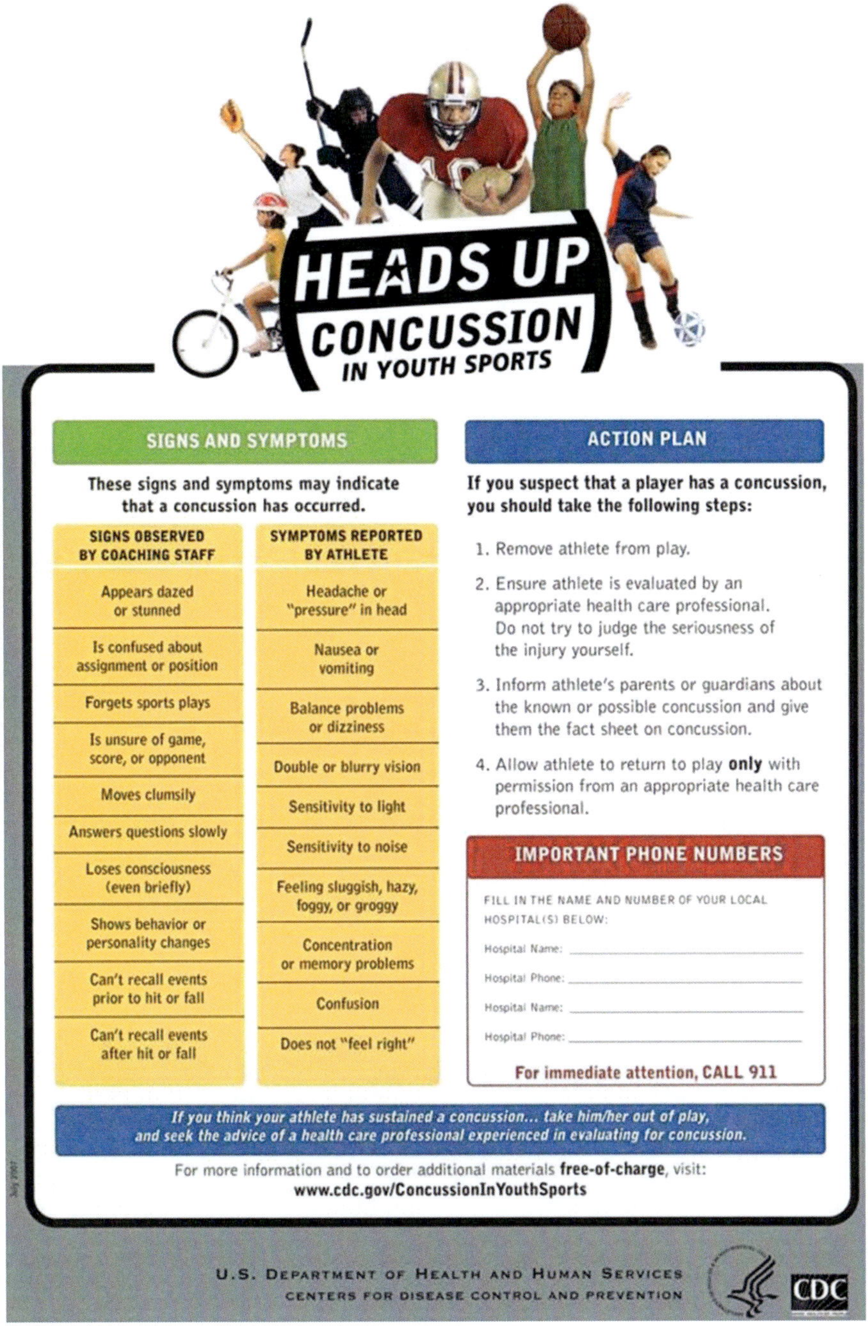

Fig. 21.4 CDC's Heads Up concussion initiative

Clinical testing for concussion also has its limitations, including reliance on the subjective nature of athlete reported symptoms, variability of presentation, and varying sensitivity and specificity of sideline assessment tools. It is also difficult for healthcare providers to establish a timeline of recovery after SRC. Suboptimal neuropsychological testing, as well as the lack of a gold standard diagnostic tool, limits the clinician's ability to make this determination. As mentioned previously, physiological recovery may continue after clinical recovery has taken place. Modalities that provide insight into physiological recovery include fMRI, MRS, DTI, cerebral blood flow (CBF), electrophysiology, fluid biomarkers, heart rate, measures of exercise performance, and transcranial magnetic stimulation (TMS). However, at this time, these modalities are not used clinically but are available for use in the research setting. Going forward, it is recommended that studies are designed longitudinally and follow both clinical and physiological recovery. This may help with correlating neurobiological modalities with clinical measures and allow clinicians to better treat athletes suffering from SRC.

References

1. Rahn C, Munkasy BA, Barry Joyner A, Buckley TA. Sideline performance of the balance error scoring system during a live sporting event. Clin J Sport Med. 2015;25(3):248–53.
2. Davis GA, Purcell L, Schneider KJ. The child sport concussion assessment tool 5th Edition (Child SCAT5): background and rationale. Br J Sports Med. 2017;51:859–61.
3. Yue JK, Phelps R, Ankush C. Sideline concussion assessment: the current state of the art | Neurosurgery | Oxford Academic. Neurosurgery. 2020;87(3):466–75.
4. Harmon KG, Clugston JR, Dec K, Hainline B, Herring SA, Kane S, et al. American Medical Society for Sports Medicine Position Statement on Concussion in Sport. Clin J Sport Med. 2019;29(2):87–100.
5. Mucha A, Collins MW, Elbin RJ, Furman JM, Troutman-Enseki C, DeWolf RM, et al. A brief vestibular/ocular motor screening (VOMS) assessment to evaluate concussions. Am J Sports Med. 2014;42(10):2479–86.
6. Anzalone A, Blueitt D, Case T. A positive vestibular/ocular motor screening (VOMS) is associated with increased recovery time after sports-related concussion in youth and adolescent athletes. AJSM. 2016;45(2):474–9.
7. Santo A, Race M, Teel EF. Near point of convergence deficits and treatment following concussion: a systematic review. J Sport Rehabil. 2003:1–5.
8. Scheiman M, Gallaway M, Frantz K. Nearpoint of convergence: test procedure, target selection, and normative data: optometry and vision science. J Am Acad Optomet. 2003;80(3):214–25.
9. Furman GR, Lin C-C, Bellanca JL, Marchetti GF, Collins MW, Whitney SL. Comparison of the balance accelerometer measure and balance error scoring system in adolescent concussions in sports. Am J Sports Med. 2013;41(6):1404–10.
10. Docherty CL, Valovich McLeod TC, Schultz S. Postural control deficits in participants with functional ankle instability as measured by the balance error scoring system. Clin J Sport Med. 2006;16(3):203–8.
11. Echemendia RJ, Meeuwisse W, McCrory P, Davis GA, Putukian M, Leddy J, et al. The sport concussion assessment tool 5th edition (SCAT5): background and rationale. Br J Sports Med. 2017;51(11):848–50.
12. Kamins J, Bigler E, Covassin T. What is the physiological time to recovery after concussion? A systematic review. Br J Sports Med. 2017;51:935–40.

13. Leddy JJ, Baker JG, Merchant A, Picano J, Gaile D, Matuszak J, et al. Brain or strain? symptoms alone do not distinguish physiologic concussion from cervical/vestibular injury. Clin J Sport Med. 2015;25(3):237–42.
14. McCrory P, Meeuwisse W, Dvorak J, Aubry M, Bailes J, Broglio S, et al. Consensus statement on concussion in sport—the 5th international conference on concussion in sport held in Berlin, October 2016. Br J Sports Med. 2017;51(11):838–47.
15. Leddy JJ, Haider MN, Hinds AL, Darling S, Willer BS. A preliminary study of the effect of early aerobic exercise treatment for sport-related concussion in males. Clin J Sport Med. 2019;29(5):353–60.
16. Heyer GL, Fischer A, Wilson J, MacDonald J, Cribbs S, Ravindran R, et al. Orthostatic intolerance and autonomic dysfunction in youth with persistent postconcussion symptoms: a head-upright tilt table study. Clin J Sport Med. 2016;26(1):40–5.
17. Makdissi M, Schneider KJ, Feddermann-Demont N, Guskiewicz KM, Hinds S, Leddy JJ, et al. Approach to investigation and treatment of persistent symptoms following sport-related concussion: a systematic review. Br J Sports Med. 2017;51(12):958–68.
18. Schneider KJ, Meeuwisse WH, Nettel-Aguirre A. Cervicovestibular rehabilitation in sport-related concussion: a randomised controlled trial. Br J Sports Med. 2014;48:1294–8.
19. Bramley H, Heverley S, Lewis MM, Kong L, Rivera R, Silvis M. Demographics and treatment of adolescent posttraumatic headache in a regional concussion clinic. Pediatr Neurol. 2015;52(5):493–8.
20. Walter A, Finelli K, Bai X, Arnett P, Bream T, Seidenberg P, et al. Effect of Enzogenol(R) supplementation on cognitive, executive, and vestibular/balance functioning in chronic phase of concussion. Dev Neuropsychol. 2017;42(2):93–103.
21. Randolph C, McCrea M, Barr WB. Is neuropsychological testing useful in the management of sport-related concussion? J Athl Train. 2005;40(3):139–52.
22. Resch J, Driscoll A, McCaffrey N, Brown C, Ferrara MS, Macciocchi S, et al. ImPact test-retest reliability: reliably unreliable? J Athl Train. 2013;48(4):506–11.
23. Brown CN, Guskiewicz KM, Bleiberg J. Athlete characteristics and outcome scores for computerized neuropsychological assessment: a preliminary analysis. J Athle Train (Natl Athl Train Assoc). 2007;42(4):515–23.
24. Segalowitz SJ, Mahaney P, Santesso DL, MacGregor L, Dywan J, Willer B. Retest reliability in adolescents of a computerized neuropsychological battery used to assess recovery from concussion. NeuroRehabilitation. 2007;22(3):243–51.
25. Cernich A, Reeves D, Sun W, Bleiberg J. Automated Neuropsychological Assessment Metrics sports medicine battery. Arch Clin Neuropsychol. 2007;22(Suppl_1):S101–14.
26. Makdissi M, Darby D, Maruff P, Ugoni A, Brukner P, McCrory P. Natural history of concussion in sport: markers of severity and implications for management. Clin J Sport Med. 2019;18
27. Broglio SP, Macciocchi SN, Ferrara MS. Sensitivity of the concussion assessment battery. Neurosurgery. 2007;60(6):1050–8.
28. Luria AR. Neuropsychology in the local diagnosis of brain damage. Cortex. 1964;1(1):3–18.
29. McCrea M, Meier T, Huber D, Ptito A, Bigler E, Debert CT, et al. Role of advanced neuroimaging, fluid biomarkers and genetic testing in the assessment of sport-related concussion: a systematic review. Br J Sports Med. 2017;51(12):919–29.
30. Broglio SP, Lapointe A, O'Connor KL, McCrea M. Head impact density: a model to explain the elusive concussion threshold. J Neurotrauma. 2017;34(19):2675–83.
31. Smith A, Alford P, Aubry M, Benson B, Black A, Brooks A, et al. Proceedings from the ice hockey summit III: action on concussion. Curr Sports Med Rep. 2019;18(1):23–34.
32. Council on Sports Medicine and Fitness. Reducing injury risk from body checking in boys' youth ice hockey. 2014;133(6):1151–7.
33. Wiebe DJ, D'Alonzo BA, Harris R, Putukian M, Campbell-McGovern C. Association between the experimental kickoff rule and concussion rates in ivy league football. JAMA. 2018;320(19):2035–6.

34. Wallace J, Covassin T, Nogle S, Gould D, Kovan J. Knowledge of concussion and reporting behaviors in high school athletes with or without access to an athletic trainer. J Athl Train. 2017;52(3):228–35.
35. Wallace J, Covassin T, Beidler E. Sex differences in high school athletes' knowledge of sport-related concussion symptoms and reporting behaviors. J Athl Train. 2017;52(7):682–8.
36. Register-Mihalik JK, Guskiewicz KM, McLeod TCV, Linnan LA, Mueller FO, Marshall SW. Knowledge, attitude, and concussion-reporting behaviors among high school athletes: a preliminary study. J Athl Train. 2013;48(5):645–53.
37. Heads Up | HEADS UP | CDC Injury Center [Internet]. 2020 [cited 2020 Oct 5]. Available from: https://www.cdc.gov/headsup/index.html
38. Shanley, E, Thigpen C, Kissenberth M, Gilliland R, Thorpe J, Nance D, et al. Heads up football training decreases concussion rates in high school football players. 2019 [cited 2020 Oct 5]; Ahead of Print. Available from: https://journals-lww-com.ezaccess.libraries.psu.edu/cjs-portsmed/Abstract/9000/Heads_Up_Football_Training_Decreases_Concussion.99063.aspx
39. Kroshus E, Baugh CM, Daneshvar DH. Content, delivery, and effectiveness of concussion education. Clin J Sport Med. 2016;26(5):391–7.
40. Kroshus E, Baugh CM, Daneshvar DH, Stamm JM, Laursen RM, Austin SB. Pressure on sports medicine clinicians to prematurely return collegiate athletes to play after concussion. J Athl Train. 2015;50(9):944–51.

Index

A
Acceleration/deceleration forces, 56
Achilles reflexes, 418
Active rehabilitation, 366
Advanced Artificial Athlete (AAA), 126
Affective Word List (AWL), 29
Alpha blocking, 60
Alzheimer's disease (AD), 11, 401
American Academy of Pediatrics (AAP), 428
Amino group containing compounds (AGCC), 199
Amyotrophic lateral sclerosis, 11
Anticipatory postural adjustment (APA), 103, 104
Apolipoprotein E (*APOE*), 287, 288
Apolipoprotein E (*APOE*) gene, 339
Apoptosis, 394
Apparent diffusion coefficient (ADC), 179, 180
Asperger's disorder, 325
Asymptomatic injury, 339
    biological and environmental factors, 342
    competition/skill level, 342
    exposure monitoring, 343, 344
    genetics, 339, 340
    physical activity/sport, 341
    protection, 346–348
    sex, 340, 341
    structural health monitoring, 342, 343
    training and rules changes, 345, 346
Athletic exposures (AE), 119
Australian Football League (AFL), 86, 87

B
Behavioral regulation, 325
Biomarkers, 426
    blood test, 271, 272
    proteomic biomarkers
        GFAP and UCH-L1, 272–275
        neurofilaments, 277
        S100β, 276
        Tau protein, 276, 277
    transcriptomic biomarkers, 277, 278
Biomechanics, 195–197
Bottleneck theory, 97
Brain Derived Neurotrophic Factor (BDNF), 288
Brain donation, 10
Buffalo Concussion Treadmill Test (BCTT), 423

C
Calcium voltage-gated channel subunit alpha1 (*CACNA1A*), 290
Capacity theory, 97
Caspase 8 (*CASP8*), 291
Catechol-O-methyl Transferase (COMT), 289
Cellular adhesion molecules (CAM), 395
Center of mass (COM), 96, 97, 103, 104
Center of pressure (COP), 43, 103, 104
Cerebrovascular response, 395
Cholines (Cho), 323
Chronic traumatic encephalopathy (CTE), 396
    Boston University School of Medicine, 9–11
    brain trauma, 12
    historical perspective, 9
    slurred speech, 12
    subconcussive blows, 11
    suicide, 12
    support network building, 12
Chronic traumatic encephalopathy (CTE), 427
Coefficient matrices, 132
Cognitive behavioral therapy (CBT), 403, 404

Collegiate athletics
　concussion education and baseline
　　assessment
　　　AMSSM, 361
　　　NATA, 360
　　　NCAA, 360
　　　sport group, 360
　documentation and legal aspects, 372, 373
　injury management
　　　AMSSM, 365, 366
　　　NATA, 364, 365
　　　NCAA, 364
　　　sport group, 365
　prevalence, 359
　RTL
　　　AMSSM, 368, 369
　　　NATA, 368
　　　NCAA, 367
　　　sport group, 368
　RTP
　　　AMSSM, 371
　　　NATA, 370, 371
　　　NCAA, 370
　　　sport group, 370, 371
　sideline assessment
　　　AMSSM, 362, 363
　　　NATA, 361, 362
　　　NCAA, 361
　　　sport group, 362
　student-athlete's, 359
Complicated mild traumatic brain injury, 37
Concussion in Sport Group (CISG), 390, 391
Concussion Legacy Foundation, 7
Concussion management
　long-term risks (see Chronic traumatic
　　encephalopathy (CTE))
　myths about concussion, 13, 14
　　　blast victims, 12
　　　CTE risk, 14, 15
　　　helmets, 13
　　　loss of consciousness, 12
　　　mild concussions, 13
　　　mouth guards, 13
　　　signs and symptoms, 14
　short-term risks
　　　acceleration, 5, 6
　　　baseline cognitive assessments, 5
　　　coaching preventive strategies, 7, 8
　　　epidural hematomas, 5
　　　focal blow, 5
　　　laboratory and clinical studies, 4, 5
　　　linear and rotational accelerations, 4
　　　linear forces, 6
　　　overview, 3, 4
　　　post-concussion patients, 4
　　　reports vs. pure evaluation, 7
　　　rotational forces, 6
　　　SIS, 8, 9
　　　structural *vs.* functional brain
　　　　disorder, 6
Continuous wavelet transform (CWT), 44
Controlled Oral Word Association Test
　(COWAT), 29

D

Decision rules, 308, 309
Default-mode network (DMN), 229
Diffusion Kurtosis Imaging (DKI), 204
Disability-Stress-Coping Model, 300
Dizziness, 418
Dopamine receptors (DRD), 288, 289
Duffy antigen receptor of chemokines
　(DARC), 291

E

Effective acceleration, 124, 125
Electroencephalogram (EEG)
　absolute amplitude, 64
　asymptomatic concussed athletes, 66
　benefits, 66
　brain lateralization, 72, 73
　clinical diagnosis/management, 57, 58
　in clinical settings, 61, 62
　cognitive symptoms, 63
　coherence analysis, 62
　coherence values, 64, 66
　compensatory mechanism, 69, 70
　correlation coefficient, 64
　cortical potentials, 67
　detecting electrical signals, 59
　EEG-wavelet entropy, 67, 68
　electrophysiological deficits, 62, 63
　Enzogenol, 68, 69
　evaluation, 67
　evidence, 63, 64
　findings, 67
　frequency band, 60, 61, 66
　healthy controls, 61
　immediate post-injury period, 61
　International 10-20 system, 58, 59
　neuronal network, residual disturbance, 68
　on field concussion assessment, 67
　overview, 58
　patterns and cognitive domains, 66
　power, 64
　psychological disorders, 72, 73

quantitative methods, 62
reproducibility level, 66
return to play, 70–72
rs-EEG, 67
SPCN amplitude, 64
Energy metabolism
　AGCC, 199
　biochemical/metabolic/molecular targets, 201, 202
　biomechanics, 195–197
　bio-molecular vulnerability, 201
　chronic mitochondrial malfunctioning, 201
　degree of reversibility, 201
　FAA, 199
　fusion, fission, and mitophagy, 200, 201
　glucose consumption, 198
　^{1}H-MRS, 199, 200
　mitochondrial dysfunction, 198
　MQC, 200
　NAA homeostasis, 199
　patient history, 206–210
　PDH, 198, 199
　return-to-play, 202–204
　structural neuroimaging techniques, 210–213
Enzogenol®, 424
Evoked activation, 224, 227, 228
Excitatory amino acids (EAA), 393

F

Finite element (FE) modeling, 348
Focal encephalomalacia, 166
Fourier Amplitude Sensitivity Test (FAST), 136
Fractional anisotropy (FA), 156, 157, 179, 180
Free amino acids (FAA), 199
Functional cognitive testing, 57
Functional magnetic resonance imaging (fMRI)
　abnormal brain activation, 227
　analytic methods, 225, 227
　BOLD, 222
　clinical manifestation and prognosis, 221
　definition, 221
　DMN, 229
　dynamic connectivity analyses, 231
　hypoactivation, 227, 228
　multimodal imaging, 231–233
　overarching issues, 233–235
　physiology and putative effects, 222–224
　static connectivity analyses, 229
　symptom intensity, 228
Functional recovery, 57

G

Gadd Severity Index (GSI), 124, 125
Gait termination (GT), 105, 106
Gait velocity, 101
Genetics
　APOE, 287, 288
　asymptomatic injury, 339, 340
　BDNF, 288
　biology of, 286, 287
　CACNA1A, 290
　CASP8, 291
　COMT, 289
　DARC, 291
　DRD, 288, 289
　GRIN2A, 291
　implications, 292, 293
　interleukins, 289
　KIAA0319, 290
　NEFH, 291
　NGB, 291
　PARP1, 291
　role of, 285, 286
　SLC17A7, 290
　Tau protein, 290
　TPH2, 291
Glial Fibrillary Acidic Protein (GFAP)
　concussion and subconcussive brain injury, 274, 275
　traumatic brain injury, 272–274
Global sensitivity analysis (GSA), 136
Ground reaction force (GRF), 133

H

Head Impact Telemetry System (HITS™), 259
Head impact threshold
　motivation, 119
　playing surface
　　dynamic models, 128
　　GSI, 124, 125
　　head injury severity, 120, 122
　　Hertz contact theory, 132–134
　　HIC, 125, 126
　　input parameters, 134, 135
　　issues, 127
　　Monte Carlo sensitivity analysis, 134
　　one link model, 128–130
　　results, 136–139
　　sensitivity analysis, 136
　　severity outcomes, 134
　　single particle model, 128, 129
　　testing standards, 126, 127
　　two link model, 128, 131, 132
　　WSTC, 122, 123

Head injuries, *see* Repetitive head acceleration events (rHAE)
Head Injury Criteria (HIC), 125, 126
Headminder Concussion Resolution Index, 425
Heat Shock Protein-27 (HSP-27), 401
Heat shock protein-70 (HSP-70), 401, 402
Heat shock proteins, 402
Heat shock transcription factor-1 (HSF-1), 401
Helmet protection
   age specific tolerance, 92
   angular acceleration, 92
   Australian Football, 86, 87
   characteristics, 84
   combat sports, 87–89
   correlations, 91
   in cricket and baseball, 89
   cycling, 89, 90
   epidemiological studies, 82, 83
   in football/soccer, 90, 91
   laboratory studies, 92
   performance requirements, 84, 85
   research findings, 92
   sub-concussive impacts, 92
   World Rugby's performance regulations, 86
Hemodynamic response function (HRF), 223, 225
Hopkins Verbal Learning Test-Recall (HVLT-R), 156
Hypercapnia, 227
Hyperphosphorylated tau protein, 9, 10

I
Immediate Post-Concussion Assessment and Cognitive Testing (ImPACT), 424
Impact severity indices, 127
Injury risk indices, 127
Insulin-like growth factor 1 (IGF-1), 399
Interleukin 6 (*IL6*), 289
International Classification of Disease (ICD) coding, 203
Intraclass correlation coefficients (ICCs), 66

K
KIAA0319 genotype, 340
King-Devick (KD) test, 363

L
Lactate, 400
Learning disability (LD), 380, 383, 384
Long-term injures, 55, 56

Loss of consciousness (LOC), 153–155

M
Mental illness, 400
Metabolic dysregulation, 393
MicroRNAs (miRNA), transcriptomic biomarkers, 277, 278
Microtubule-associated protein tau (MAPT), 290
Mild traumatic brain injury (mTBI), 194
   axon segments, 166, 167
   balance symptom, 43
   blood vessels, 167
   clinical management, 38
   clinical practitioners, 38
   clinical research studies, 195
   clinical trials, 194
   cognitive and neuroimaging findings, 156–158
   computed tomography, 158, 159
   deformation, 156
   deformation biomechanics, 167–169
   external force, 166
   GCS, 153
   graph theory, 149, 150
   heterogeneity, 151–153
   LOC, 153–155
   neural cells, 166, 167
   neuroimaging (*see* Neuroimaging)
   neuron integrity, 155
   pathology detection, 148, 149
   pathophysiology, 155
   PCS (*see* Post-concussive symptoms (PCS))
   post-resuscitation Glasgow Coma Scale, 148
   postural stability, 38
   practice effect, 38
   quantitative MR abnormalities, 162, 164, 165
   residual lesion, 166
   Rich Club network, 150, 151
   structural and functional pathologies, 156, 157
   structural neuroimaging, 155, 156
   symptom onset, 154
   symptoms, 194
   testing modalities, 38
   visible abnormalities, 147–149
   visible macroscopic abnormalities, 159–162
   visual, vestibular, and somatosensory systems, 38

Index 439

volumetry findings, 169, 170
WM hyperinsensitivies, 153
Mindfulness-based stress reduction (MSBR), 404, 405
Mitochondrial quality control (MQC), 200
Modified balance error scoring system (mBESS), 98, 420
Motor vehicle crash (MVC), 173
Musculoskeletal (MSK) injury, 102, 103

N

N-acetyl aspartate (NAA), 199, 323
National Academy of Neuropsychology (NAN), 19
National Football League (NFL), 7, 428
Near point convergence (NPC), 420
Neurofibrillary tangles (NFTs), 396
Neurofilament heavy (*NEFH*), 291
Neurofilaments, 277
Neuroglobin (NGM), 291
Neuroimaging
  acute stage, 180, 181
  advantages, 174
  chronic stage, 181, 182
  connectomic assessment, 184–186
  DTI-derived WM injury topography, 182–184
  hemorrhagic lesions, 175, 176
  impact to medicine, 186, 187
  incidence, 180
  insurance reimbursement, 180
  longitudinal studies, 182
  neuropsychological deficits, 182–184
  QSM, 176–179
  subacute stage, 181
  TAI, 179, 180
  traumatic vascular injury, 174, 175
Neuroinflammation, 394, 395
Neuropsychological (NP) tests, 39
Neuropsychology, 33
  acute concussion phase, 27, 28
  algorithm, 22
  baseline testing, 20, 21
  Best-Practice guidelines, 22
  computerized tests, 24
  decision rules
    base rates for males and females, 25, 26
    PCSS, 26, 27
    test battery, 24, 25
  evidence-based model, 19, 20
  fact-to-face administration, 23
  limitations, 28
  neurocognitive tests, 19
  Not Recovered group, 32
  outcomes, 29

paper-and-pencil tests, 24
participants, 28, 29
post-concussion testing, 21
post-hoc analyses, 31, 32
preliminary analyses, 29, 31
primary hypothesis, 28, 31
Recovered group, 32
self-report, 24
value added of, 21, 22
Neuroscience research and management
  clinical practice, 429
  clinical testing, 432
  collegiate level, 429
  diagnosis/evaluation procedures
    dizziness, 418
    education programs, 415
    examiner's finger, 420
    horizontal and vertical saccades, 418, 419
    mBESS, 420
    neurological examination, 418, 421
    NPC testing, 420
    patellar and Achilles reflexes, 418
    physical examination component, 417
    SCAT-5, 416, 417, 420
    sensation, 418
    sideline evaluation, 415, 416
    symptom checklists, 421
    VMS, 419
    VOMS, 418
    VOR, 419
  HU program, 430
  long term follow up/assessment, 426, 427
  policy changes, 430
  referral
    ANAM, 425
    biomarkers, 426
    CogSport Axon Sports CCAT, 425
    computerized neuropsychological test, 425
    Headminder CRI, 425
    ImPACT, 424
    neuropsychological testing, 424
    nutraceuticals, 424
    persistent symptoms, 423
    physical therapy, 423
    post-concussion symptoms, 424
    structural imaging techniques, 426
    tilt table testing, 423
    virtual reality, 425
  RTL, 422, 423
  RTP, 421, 422
  rule changes, 427–429
N-methyl-D-aspartate receptor 2A sub-unit (GRIN2A), 291

O
Oxidative damage, 394

P
Patellar reflexes, 418
PCSS, *see* Post-Concussion Symptom Scale (PCSS)
Peak angular acceleration (PAA), 341
Peak translational acceleration (PTA), 136–139, 341
Pediatric mild traumatic brain injury (mTBI)
  behavioral deficits, 318
  cognitive impairment, 320–323
  developmental processes, 319, 320
  educational and social activities, 319
  head injury symptoms, 319
  long-term functional deficits, 318
  metabolic abnormalities, 322, 323
  neuronal myelination and frontal lobe maturation, 320
  neuropathological changes, 317
  post-concussion recovery and assessment challenges
    attentional control and literacy mature, 324
    executive system, 324
    long-term effects, 323
    long-term symptoms, 324
    neuropsychological assessments, 326, 327
    neuropsychological evaluation, 326, 327
    plasticity and functional reorganization, 323
    post-TBI deficits, 325, 326
    professional guidance, 327
    psychotherapy, 327
    school work, 325
  rates of, 317
  regulatory functions and efficiency skills, 319
  short-term *vs.* long-term post-concussion symptoms, 318
  skill development, 320
  social and academic demands, 318
  structural abnormalities, 320–322
Poly(ADP-ribose) polymerase 1 (PARP1), 291
Post-concussion postural control
  adverse effects, 97
  in Australian rules football, 100
  as biomarker, 95, 96
  clinical assessment, 97, 98
  COM, 96, 97
  diffuse axonal injury, 97
  dual-task gait, 102, 103
  gait initiation, 103–105
  gait termination, 105, 106
  motor control strategies, 97
  neurological pathologies, 100
  single-task gait, 101
Post-Concussion Symptom Scale (PCSS), 24, 26, 27
Post-concussive symptoms (PCS), 153, 391
  clinical management, 299
  clinical presentation, 299
  future research, 310, 311
  model for, 300, 301
  occurrence, 299
  prediction, 301
    injury factors, 301–304
    non-injury factors, 302–304
  prognostic models and decision rules, 308, 309
  research issues
    individual outcomes, 307, 308
    mild TBI, 304
    outcome measurement, 305
    prediction vs. moderation, 306
    response validity, pain, and symptom exaggeration, 306
    risk factors, 305, 306
    timing of outcome assessment, 306, 307
Potassium (K^+), 393
Practice effect, 38
Preparticipation exam (PPE), 361
Prognostic models, 308, 309
Proton magnetic resonance spectroscopy (^{1}H-MRS), 199, 200
Psychoeducation, 402, 403
Punch drunk syndrome, 396
Pyruvate Dehydrogenase (PDH), 198, 199

Q
Quantitative electroencephalogram (QEEG)
  activation/arousal measures, 378
  classification matrices, 381, 382
  discriminant analysis, 380, 381
  gender and sex effects, 382, 383
  head injury discriminant approaches, 378, 379
  learning disability, 383, 384
  methods, 380
  placebo effects, 387

Index 441

rehabilitation, 385, 386
TBI population, 382
theorical considerations, 385
Quantitative susceptibility mapping (QSM), 176–179

R

Rapid eye movement (REM) sleep, 61
Reaction time (RT), 45, 46
Regional homogeneity (ReHo), 229
Regulation attributes, 122
Rehabilitation, 364
Reliable change indices (RCIs), 20
Repetitive head acceleration events (rHAE)
   asymptomatic injury, 339
      biological and environmental factors, 342
      competition/skill level, 342
      exposure monitoring, 343, 344
      genetics, 339, 340
      physical activity/sport, 341
      protection, 346–348
      sex, 340, 341
      structural health monitoring, 342, 343
      training and rules changes, 345, 346
   brain structure and function, 334
   diagnosis, 334
   fMRI, 334, 335
   genetic and lifestyle factors, 335
   neuroimaging, 333
   pathophysiology and symptomatology, 334, 336–339
   prevention and intervention, 348, 349
   subconcussive and asymptomatic events, 334
Repetitive head impacts (RHI), 9
Resting state electroencephalography (rs-EEG), 67
Return to learn (RTL), 422, 423
   AMSSM, 368, 369
   NATA, 368
   NCAA, 367
   sport group, 368
Return to participation (RTP), 421, 422
Return to play (RTP) decisions, 21, 22
Return to sport participation (RTP)
   AMSSM, 371
   NATA, 370, 371
   NCAA, 370
   sport group, 370, 371
Rivermead Behavioral Memory Test (RBMT), 29

S

Second-impact syndrome (SIS), 8, 9, 203
Sensory Organization Test (SOT), 97
Short Fourier transform (STFT), 44
Single particle model, 128, 129
Sports-related (SR) traumatic brain injury, 194
Structural health monitoring, 342, 343
Subconcussive head trauma
   animal models, 250, 251
   biomechanical studies, 251–253
   clinical practice, 250
   cognitive assessment
      acute and chronic effects, 254
      encephalopathy, 256
      eye tracking research, 255
      headache, dizziness, and feeling lethargic, 255
      history, 253
      ImPACT, 254, 257
      impaired brain function, 254
      motor speed and reaction time, 254
      neurocognitive dysfunction, 256
      neuro-psychological testing, 253–255
      oculomotor deficits, 255
      preliminary study, 253
      quality-of-life, 256
      repetitive head impacts, 255
      rugby players and athletes, 256
      SAC, 257
      signs/symptoms, 253
      symptoms, 255
   incidence, 250
   neuroimaging
      computed tomography, 257, 258
      CTBI, 263
      DTI, 259, 261, 262
      fMRI, 257, 259, 260
      magnetic resonance imaging, 257, 258
      magnetic resonance spectroscopy, 262, 263
   postmortem studies, 250
   signs and symptoms, 250
   traumatic brain injury, 249
   widespread media coverage, 249
Susceptibility weighted imaging and mapping (SWIM), 176–179
Sustained posterior contralateral negativity (SPCN) amplitude, 64

T

Tau protein, 276, 277, 290
Thatcher discriminant function, 378

Transactional Stress and Coping Model, 300
Traumatic axonal injury (TAI), 161, 179, 180
Traumatic encephalopathy syndrome (TES), 9
Traumatic vascular injury, 174, 175
Treatment
  cerebrovascular response, 395
  chronic traumatic encephalopathies, 396
  clinical manifestation, 389, 390
  concussion
    biomechanics of, 392, 393
    CBT, 403, 404
    definition, 390, 391
    early activity/exercise, 398
    MSBR, 404, 405
    psychoeducation, 402, 403
    rest for, 397
  heat acclimation and neuroprotection, 400–402
  inflammation, 394, 395
  intervention strategies, 396
  metabolic dysregulation, 393
  neurophysiologic adaptation to exercise
    in concussion, 399
    mental illness, 400
    neuroplasticity and neurogenesis, 399, 400
  neurophysiologic cascade of injury, 393
  oxidative damage and apoptosis, 394
  PCS, 391
Tryptophan hydroxylase 2 (TPH2), 291

U

Ubiquitin C-Terminal Hydrolase (UCH-L1)
  concussion and subconcussive brain injury, 274, 275
  traumatic brain injury, 272–274
Unaffiliated neurotrauma consultant (UNC), 7
Uncomplicated mild traumatic brain injury, 38

V

Vascular endothelial growth-factor (VEGF), 399

Vestibular/oculomotor screening (VOMS), 418
Vestibular-ocular reflex (VOR) testing, 419
Vestibulo-ocular motor screening (VOMS), 363
Virtual corridor, 40
Virtual elevator (VE), 42, 43
Virtual reality (VR), 425
  attention module, 50
  balance, 43, 49
  clinical practitioners, 50
  comprehensive score, 50
  cost reductions, 39
  data transferability, 39
  ecological validity, 39
  fatigue assessment, 47–49
  fatigue effect, 51
  postural stability assessment, 43–46
  practice effect, 51
  reaction time, 50
  recognition A test, 40, 41
  recognition B test, 41
  sense of presence, 46
  sensitivity and specificity, 51
  spatial memory test, 40
  spatial navigation module, 50
  sustained attention, 41–43
  3D virtual environment, 50, 51
  2D environment, 39
Visual motion sensitivity (VMS) testing, 419

W

Wayne State Tolerance Curve (WSTC), 122, 123
White matter (WM), 151, 152
World Health Organization (WHO) task force, 70
World Rugby (WR), 120

Z

Zackery Lystedt Law, 430

Printed by Books on Demand, Germany